Diseases of the Oral Mucosa
A Color Atlas

Second Edition

Manfred Strassburg, Dr. med. dent.

Professor of Dental, Oral and Maxillary Diseases
Director, Clinic for Dental, Oral and Maxillary Diseases
– Westdeutsche Kieferklinik –
University of Düsseldorf
Germany

Gerdt Knolle, Dr. med., Dr. med. dent.

Associate Professor
Clinic for Dental, Oral and Maxillary Diseases
– Westdeutsche Kieferklinik –
University of Düsseldorf
Germany

Translated by
Hannelore Taschini Loevy, CD, MS, PhD
Professor of Clinical Pediatric Dentistry
University of Illinois at Chicago
Chicago, Illinois

quintessence
books

Quintessence Publishing Co, Inc

Chicago, Berlin, London, Tokyo, Moscow, Prague, Sofia, and Warsaw

Notice

Because governmental regulations differ throughout the world and because they may change, readers need to verify the use of equipment, supplies, drugs, and drug dosages before using the information presented in this book. Although the authors and the publisher have made every attempt to ensure that the information presented is current and correct, the reader should confirm particulars and heed all manufacturers' instructions and warnings.

Library of Congress Cataloging-in-Publication Data

Strassburg, Manfred.
[Farbatlas und Lehrbuch der Mundschleimhauterkrankungen. English]
Diseases of the oral mucosa : a color atlas / Manfred Strassburg and Gerdt Knolle : translated by Hannelore Taschini Loevy. — 2nd ed.
    p. cm.
  Translation of the third German ed.
  Includes bibliographical references and index.
  ISBN 0-86715-210-9
  1. Oral mucosa—Diseases—Atlases. I. Knolle, Gerdt. II. Title.
    [DNLM: 1. Mouth Mucosa—atlases. 2. Mouth Diseases—diagnosis
    —atlases. 3. Oral Manifestations—atlases. WU 17 S897f 1994a]
  RC815.S77313 1994
  616.3'1—dc20
  DNLM/DLC   93-31256
  for Library of Congress   CIP

First English-language edition, 1972

This book was originally published in German as **Farbatlas und Lehrbuch der Mundschleimhaut-erkrankungen,** 1991, by Quintessenz Verlags-GmbH, Berlin.

© 1994 by Quintessence Publishing Co, Inc, Carol Stream, Illinois.
All rights reserved.

Composition and printing: Kösel GmbH & Co., Kempten/Allgäu
Binding: Lüderitz & Bauer, Berlin
Printed in Germany

Preface to the Second Edition

With the first appearance of *Diseases of the Oral Mucosa: A Color Atlas* in 1968 (in English in 1972), we tried to present oral pathology from a dental viewpoint. The first edition, which was translated into several languages, was quickly exhausted, taking the concepts of the book and the recognition of the field far beyond the frontiers of German-speaking regions.

This long-awaited new edition has been delayed because of the authors' many obligations. In this edition, the authors' many years of clinical experience in regard to interdisciplinary work in oral mucosal diseases is incorporated. The great increase of knowledge required a complete revision and sometimes rearrangement and major enlargement of the content. Instead of the short accompanying text of earlier editions, we have included newly considered basics and have placed them according to their practical importance. Relevant dental aspects (such as "conclusions for the dentist") are presented without losing sight of the medical viewpoint. At the same time, the gap between dentistry and adjacent fields of medicine is bridged to establish a broader base. With the illustrative material, the proven concept of showing the classic appearance of a disease and its frequent and often misinterpreted variations as well as course of duration has been retained. To present as many differential diagnostic examples as possible, the concept of "oral mucosal diseases" in the strict sense was exceeded. We have considered diseases of the lip and perioral region as well as disease processes within the oral cavity that affect the oral mucosa only secondarily or indirectly. The color images number over one thousand—more than twice of that in the previous edition.

The organization of the material, although far from complete, follows different introductory principles in part for readability and in part for practical considerations. In some cases, we considered it worthwhile to remove frequently occurring diseases from their classification group and to consider them in a separate chapter so that we could better describe the course of development of the special clinical and therapeutic problems.

To do justice to the significance of early signs of prognostically serious diseases and to emphasize the responsibility of the dentist as the first examiner, great emphasis is given to malignant tumors of the oral cavity together with their precursors and systemic diseases with their early and accompanying oral symptoms. More space is given to viral diseases and dermatoses, with their possible oral mucosal participation; internal diseases and autoimmune diseases with associated oral findings; and undesirable drug side effects.

The text takes into consideration the position of amplified differential diagnosis questions, indications of interdisciplinary action, indications, and therapeutic recommendations.

For each disease we provide the Anglo-American nomenclature as well as the code number according to the second edition (1978) of the World Health Organization (WHO) *Application of the International Classification of Diseases to Dentistry and Stomatology* (ICD-DA) or, in a few cases, according to the 1977 edition of the WHO *International Classification of Diseases* (ICD). In this manner, literature searching is simplified. We abandoned literature citations in the text as well as a detailed bibliography; the reader interested in further information will find a list of standard publications and basic contributions according to the different specialty groups at the end of the book. From the publisher's point of view and the endeavors of the authors, this new edition is an attempt to satisfy the demands and probably high expectations of the readers. We hope we are successful.

Our efforts were supported by a balanced group of colleagues in different fields and in different areas. Our very special thanks go to Professor Dr. Günter Goerz, Dermatology Clinic of the Heinrich-Heine University of Düsseldorf, for his many valuable suggestions and critical comments on the text of the manuscript. We also received advice and assistance from (in alphabetic order): Professor Dr. Theodor Brüster, director of the Institute for Blood Coagulation and Transfusion Medicine; Privatdozent Dr. Peter Kind, Dermatology Clinic; Professor Dr. Dr. Peter Pfitzer, director of the Institute of Cytopathology of the Pathologic Institute; Professor Dr. Hans Reinauer, director of the Division of Clinical Biochemistry of the Diabetic Research Institute; Professor Dr. Karlheinz A. Rosenbauer, director of the Institute of Histology and Embryology; Professor Dr. Wolfgang Schneider, director of the Clinic of Hematology, Oncology and Clinical Immunology; as well as Professor Dr. Georg Strohmeyer, director of the Clinic of Gastroenterology (all of the Heinrich-Heine University, Düsseldorf). We are thankful to them. We also thank our colleagues at our institution: Professor Dr. Armin Herforth, Professor Dr. Franz Schübel, and Professor Dr. Walter Weise, for supplementary assistance and the willing loan of slides; Professor Dr. Dr. Jürgen Lentrodt for making his patient charts available; Dr. Michael Trüpel for his circumspect suggestions for correction. Our thanks also go to the physicians of Professor Knolle's practice, and to Mrs. Rosemarie Tho Al Ghina and Mrs. Christa Lausberg for careful manuscript preparation.

A color atlas and textbook of this magnitude demands much of the publisher. It is a special pleasure for us to thank our publisher, Mr. H. W. Haase, for his excellent cooperation. Our requests could be accomplished only because he, in spite of many delays in the completion of the manuscript, showed patient understanding. Considering the demand for a new edition, this position was not an easy one. We would like to also thank the staff of the publisher, particularly Mr. Gerhard Kirsten, who took care of the printing and setting of the book in a model manner. Finally, we thank Dr. Hannelore T. Loevy, Professor of Clinical Pediatric Dentistry at the University of Illinois at Chicago, who translated the book into English, and to Dr. Henry O. Trowbridge, Professor of Pathology, School of Dental Medicine, University of Pennsylvania, who provided editorial consultation.

From the Introduction to the First Edition

Our experience makes us believe that no irrelevant difficulties exist in dental practice concerning the differential diagnosis of oral mucosal diseases. Additionally, discussions after continuing education presentations speak to the need for help that is close to the clinical situation and suggest that a color atlas could close this gap. To fulfill this demand for information, we endeavored to put together a diagnostic guide directed to dental concerns particularly.

Contents

Introduction

Dentists frequently are the first medical professionals to examine patients who have oral mucosal changes. They are thus responsible for recognizing the signs of disease, transforming them into a diagnosis, and planning the therapy.

Dentistry is one of several areas of medicine concerned with oral mucosal diseases. In a complete clinical examination, the intraoral findings establish the differential diagnostic position. Together with the dermatologist, internist, otolaryngologist, pediatrician, and neurologist—to name only some specialists—the dentist must address several questions about major symptoms appearing in the oral cavity of a serious disease so that a diagnosis or suspected diagnosis may be made.

Our aim is not to establish the limits of a specialty and to discuss the areas of overlap, but rather to emphasize the connections. Only in close, interdisciplinary work can complex disease pictures be perceived and the danger of an isolated point of view be avoided.

The dentist in his or her office starts the real examination by obtaining the patient's history and evaluating the oral mucosal disease based on the results of palpation and examination. Obtaining the findings based on dental tissues and using dental equipment does not end the procedure. The recording of disease findings in the oral mucosa and perioral region is the duty of the dentist. Even if the therapy of the diagnosed disease is in the area of the medical specialist, she or he must be thoroughly prepared for the duty of recording disease findings. Hence the recognition and determination of visible changes is probably more difficult than it seems. To use the diagnosis some knowledge in basic medicine is assumed. Here, there must be referral to textbooks and the corresponding specialists.

While maxillofacial surgery has a firm and specific place within the surgical discipline, there is a recognizable demand for the nonsurgical subjects of dentistry in the area of oral medicine. In this area there should be cooperation and the possibility of further cooperation with other medical fields. This book has as one aim the acquainting of the medical reader with the dental aspects of diagnosis and therapy of oral mucosal diseases.

Chapter 1

Basic Principles for Diagnosis of Diseases of the Oral Mucosa

History taking

Examination process

Normal oral mucosa

Efflorescences

From findings to diagnosis

Careful history taking combined with systematic, consistent, detailed, and thorough examination continues to be the cornerstone of the development of a diagnosis. The relationship of these points is reviewed. A short discussion of the structural and physiologic peculiarities of the oral cavity is presented to facilitate understanding of the disease processes of the oral mucosal tissues. Indispensable for the interpretation of diseases of the oral mucosa is the systematic observation of efflorescences of the oral mucosa, shown here with selected examples. In interpreting morphologic changes it is important to consider that symptoms are not always caused by major organic diseases but can be caused by psychological problems as well.

History taking

Knowledge of the patient's history (family history, patient history, and other special data) facilitates the task of obtaining clinical findings and making a diagnosis. A printed history form (particularly for a patient being examined for the first time) speeds the process, because it forces the patient to organize his or her thoughts while showing the range of possibilities of the problem area. Even with the written presentation, the experienced and psychologically educated dentist allows the patient to talk and owes him or her the patience to pay careful attention *(consultation does not mean treatment time only!)*. If, for example, because of lack of time, the dentist is reluctant to listen to a patient who is willing to talk, a door may be closed, even during the first visit, which may not be reopened in future visits.

Information must be sorted out, evaluated, and in some instances completed, by directed questioning. Vagueness of data presented by the patient can be clarified by carefully posed questions. The more complex the problem presented by the patient, the more complete must be the history obtained. The dentist should not be unduly impressed by the patient's fears but should also not dismiss the patient's worries as unimportant and without foundation. Two examples, of many, are:

1. References to a patient's "sensitivity" or "excessive sensitivity" should not be considered synonymous with allergy (documented with an allergy test), but should also not be discounted without further consideration.
2. The discovery during an interview that the patient has cancerphobia does not mean that a malignancy may not be present.

In each of these instances, as in others, the cause of the complaint must be carefully evaluated. Each preconceived idea of the examiner results in superficiality and can harm objectivity. Only those who ask receive answers. Directed evaluation contributes to the reduction of complications that may be expected based on known disease history. History of therapy and medication must be obtained in detail, including the use of home medications. In some cases, details must be obtained of professional activities, after-hours activities, and social environment.

In regard to infectious diseases, patients' information is not always dependable and therefore must be carefully considered. Care must also be given to evaluation of reference to time. Experience shows that changes said to have been present for many months can be reduced to a few weeks, or vice versa, upon questioning the patient. In doubtful cases, during the course of the examination, one must repeat the questions of the first appearance and duration of a change.

Obtaining the patient's history is the beginning of all the other steps.

Examination process

During clinical instruction, each dentist learns the systematic examination of the oral cavity and perioral areas. He or she may remember the various instructions. The experienced dentist may allow shortcuts as long as important facts are not disregarded.

Evaluation of the patient usually starts by making an approximate determination of the general condition of the patient based on external appearance. The actual examination is done from the outside to the inside. Initially, one looks at the face, and the perioral area in particular, for conspicuous color changes, pathologic changes in the skin and skin appendages, as well as other deviations from the norm. This is routinely followed by palpation for examination of the regional lymph nodes. This requires sufficient experience to be able to draw conclusions in borderline situations. After evaluation of the lip vermilion and the angle of the mouth, as well as control of mouth opening, the intraoral examination is performed.

In the same manner, all tooth surfaces are carefully examined and probed, followed by several areas of the oral mucosa, tongue, and floor of the mouth. Maintaining a certain order avoids an incomplete examination and is therefore indicated for oral evaluation.

First, the vestibular region is evaluated. Lips and cheeks must be separated so that the whole vestibular area, including the vestibular gingiva, can be visualized. Then the oral mucosa of the oral cavity is inspected, first in the upper region, then in the lower region. Examination of the hard and soft palate is not difficult. For evaluation of the palatal arch, the tonsils, and the posterior wall of the fauces, the dorsum of the tongue must be pressed caudally with the examination instrument. Examination of the dorsum of the tongue does not offer any problem and ends with a transition to the base of the tongue with the help of a mirror. The anterior part of the floor of the mouth is easily accessible if the patient touches the tip of the tongue to the front teeth with the mouth open. The sides and posterior part of the oral cavity are visible by displacement of the body of the tongue with a mirror or spatula. To observe the tongue margins, the tongue undersurface, and the transition area of the tongue base in the floor of the mouth, it is advisable to hold the tongue with gauze or a tongue depressor and to place the tongue in the desired position. If the inspection demonstrates a mucosal change, palpation must be done to determine consistency, mobility, distention, pain on compression, and fluctuation, among other conditions.

Other methods of examination and diagnostic procedures will be discussed in later chapters.

Normal oral mucosa

A detailed discussion of the histology, cytology, physiology (sense physiology), and immunology of the oral mucosa is beyond the scope of this book. We limit ourselves to a few fundamental remarks and direct readers who are interested in further details to the literature, in particular the detailed description of the oral structural biology by H. E. Schroeder, which is essentially being followed in this book.

Knowledge of the oral mucosa depends in part on knowledge of the structure of the skin. The skin is composed of:

- Epidermis (skin surface)
- Dermis (corium)
- Subcutis (subcorium)

The epidermis as the epithelial component of the skin is composed of several layers that represent sequential steps of its biologic proliferation as follows:

- Basal layer (basal cell layer)
- Stratum spinosum (spinal cell layer)
- Stratum granulosum (granular cell layer)
- Stratum lucidum (glassy layer, not found in the mucosa but only in the external skin)
- Stratum corneum (horny layer)

The basal cells are placed in a single palisadelike layer and are responsible for the mitotic activity and continuous substitution of the cells of the upper layers of the skin (average turnover rate is 20 to 28 days). Between the fully vital highly prismatic basal cells and the scaly, lifeless, flat, horny scale is the spinal cell layer. It is of four- to eight-cell thickness and is where the cells acquire a polyhedric form. The spinal cells are in contact by means of interdigitating microvilli (once erroneously considered as intercellular bridges) and desmosomes. Above the thick spinal cell layer is the stratum granulosum. It is made up of two to five cell layers in which the keratocytes begin to be visible and demonstrate initial stages of keratinization. The almost homogeneous stratum lucidum is present only in heavily keratinized skin regions such as the inner surface of the hands and feet. The most superficial layer of the skin is the stratum corneum, composed of superimposed keratinized lamellae, without cell nuclei and granules. These so-called cornified cells scale off continuously (desquamatio insensibilis).

The epidermis consists of keratinocytes in addition to other cells important for the maintenance of the normal functions of the skin. The "nonkeratinocytes" make up about 10% of the cell population of the epidermis. They are the melanocytes, Merkel's cells, Langerhans' cells, and migrated lymphocytes, which are also present in the epithelium of the oral mucosa.

In the area of the cheek skin, for example, there are $1,300/mm^2$ melanocytes in white individuals. Because of the intensity of the pigmentation in dark-skinned people, the number of melanocytes is less important than is the size and degree of melanization of the melanosomes in the cells. The intraepidermal melanocytes located next to the basal layer regularly supply the synthesized melanin to the neighboring keratin cells. The melanocyte forms a functional unit through its dendritic extensions with about 36 surrounding keratocytes. Normal oral mucosa also contains melanocytes, which as a rule do not form melanin.

Merkel's cells, like melanocytes, are derived from the neural tube and are located between the basal cells, particularly in the area of the epithelial ledge. They are not fully understood but seem to act as mechanoreceptors for tactile and pressure reception, and are known to be particularly numerous in the lips and tongue.

In the lower layers of the epidermis there are also Langerhans' cells, which are considered to be part of the monocyte-macrophage system. Langerhans' cells are numerous in the oral epithelium. In the gingiva there are $40/mm^2$ to $200/mm^2$ Langerhans' cells. In the cheek and lip mucosa, there are about $380/mm^2$ to $520/mm^2$ cells. These Langerhans' cells, in association with the lymphocytes present in the epidermis (to be discussed later), have an important role in the immune defense of the mucosa. The lymphocytes, which have a self-recognition controlling function, reach the epidermis after leaving the blood vessels.

A basal membrane—separating complex connects the epidermis and dermis. The papillary bodies (stratum papillare) in the upper portion of the corium that nurture the epidermis with its blood vessels have a wavelike appearance. In this manner the border region is increased and assumes a peg-shaped configuration. In the deep and middle corium (stratum reticulare) there are the skin-appendage structures (sebaceous glands, eccrine sweat glands, and hair) as well as blood vessels, lymph vessels, nerves, and muscles.

As a cushion between muscle fibers and cutis, there is the sub-cutis, which is made up of a system of connective tissue in septal form and contains a large number of fat cells and blood vessels, lymph vessels, nerve endings going to their end organs, and vibra-tion receptors.

In the mouth region, the lip vermilion functions as a transition zone between skin and mucosa. This tissue separation is noticeable through the thin corneous layer and through the connective tissue papillae because of their richness in capillaries, which give the typical red color to the lips. In addition, the lip border region often shows mucous glands and small seromucous salivary glands. In contrast to the lip skin, the appendages of the skin are absent, with the exception of occasionally occurring sebaceous glands and melanin pigmenta-tion. Other information on the morphology of the lip and the oral aspects of the corner of the mouth due to its epidermal origin and the tendency to keratinization of the retroangular mucosa will be discus-sed in chapter 34.

Conceptually, the epithelium of the oral mucosa corresponds to the epidermis (mucoepidermis), the lamina propria of the dermis, and the submucosa of the subcutis. The mucosa of the gastrointestinal tract contains an additional layer, the tunica muscularis mucosae (smooth muscle), which separates the lamina propria from the connective tissue below the submucosa and which is present only in a limited form in the area of the palate.

Structurally, the mucosa and skin have regional differences, i. e., thickness, degree of keratinization of the covering epithelium, disposi-tion of the fibers of connective tissue, and organization of the lamina propria and submucosa. It is customary today to divide the oral mucosa according to the classification of Orban and Sicher into *covering, masticatory*, and *specialized mucosa* (see schematic rep-resentation).

The covering mucosa (Fig. 1-9) is the basic form of oral mucosa. Its thickness is variable, with several layers of noncornified flat epithelium over a thin lamina propria. This epithelium shows the epidermis with a single basal cell layer and a relatively thick spinal cell layer while the stratum granulosum and stratum corneum are not present. Instead, there is a thickened zone on the surface from which nucleated cells desquamate.

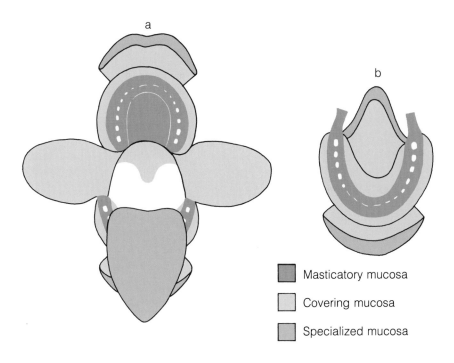

Schematic representation of the distribution of the covering, masticatory, and specialized oral mucosae.
(a) Upper lip, gingiva, hard and soft palate, cheek, and dorsum of the tongue
(b) Lower surface of the tongue, floor of the mouth, gingiva, and lower lip
(Modified from *Squier CA, Johnson NW, Hackemann M. Structure and function of normal human oral mucosa.* In: Dolby AE (ed). *Oral Mucosa in Health and Disease.* Oxford: Blackwell, 1975:15.)

The thickness of the epithelium over the papillae varies: the mucosa of the floor of the mouth and undersurface of the tongue is about 190 μm thick whereas the mucosa of the alveolar area is about 270 μm, the mucosa of the lips about 550 μm, and the mucosa of the cheeks about 580 μm. Number (in mm^2) and height (in μm) of the connective tissue papillae follow the same sequence. The average values are 16/mm^2 and 30 μm for the mucosa of the floor of the mouth, 46/mm^2 and 165 μm for the alveolar mucosa, 76/mm^2 and 245 μm for the lip mucosa, and 73/mm^2 and 340 μm for the cheek mucosa.

In the floor of the mouth, in the area of the vestibule, and in the region of the soft palate, the covering mucosa is movable and deformable. This can be explained by the high number of elastic nets in the lamina propria and by the loose submucosa. Such limited independent movement is not present in the lip and cheek mucosa regions because the fiber systems are closely connected to the fibers of the mimic muscles. Therefore, these areas of mucosa follow the movements of the mouth without folds because they are anchored in the deeper layers.

Like the mucosa of the cheeks, the alveolar mucosa also contains cytoplasmic-stored glycogen, while the noninflamed gingiva is glycogen free. With the aid of Schiller-iodine solution, the alveolar mucosa can be colored and the mucogingival margins precisely established (Figs. 1-2 and 1-3).

The zones of the masticatory mucosa, which are raised due to function (free and attached gingiva, mucosa of the hard palate), contain a stratum corneum as a demonstration of continuing keratinization. This masticatory mucosa is in contact with the periosteum either through a cell-rich and collagen-rich lamina propria—as in some areas of the palate—or is fixed to a submucosa with collagen bundles (periosteal fixed mucosa).

The thickness of the epithelium at the level of the hard palate is about 310 µm, and at the level of the gingiva about 300 µm. The stratum corneum is 10 µm to 15 µm high, which corresponds to eight to ten layers of scaly cells. The increased thickness of the horny layer of the epithelium accounts for the lighter color of the gingiva and the mucosa of the hard palate.

In about two-thirds of the population, a *parakeratinization* (flat horny scales with dissolving of the corresponding nuclei and remnants of cytoplasmic organelles) is seen in healthy gingiva; in the other third, *orthokeratinization* (very flat horny scales that no longer have cell nuclei) is present in the mucosa of the hard palate.

Complete renewal of the epithelial cells occurs in the gingiva considerably sooner than is the case for keratinized cells of the epidermis. The turnover time of these gingival cells from basal to surface layer is about 6 to 12 days, which correlates with the epithelial regeneration in wound repair.

The ability to load the masticatory mucosa is dependent on the remarkably stable ledges and peglike interdigitation of the epithelium and the connective tissue. In comparison with the lip and cheek mucosa the number the of connective tissue papillae in the mucosa of the hard palate (about 114/mm^2) and the gingiva (about 119/mm^2) is one-third larger. Relative to this, the connective tissue papillae are considerably shorter (hard palate about 190 μm, gingiva about 170 μm). The difference is further noticeable when the percentage of passages of connective tissue into the epithelial basic layer is evaluated. It is about 8% at the level of the alveolar mucosa, about 15% at the lip level, about 23% at the hard palate, and about 35% at the gingiva.

As opposed to the gingiva, whose special structural characteristics are considered in detail in Figs. 1-1 to 1-7, the submucosa of the hard palate (Fig. 1-8) presents laterally contained fat tissue and pure mucosal glands.

A specialized mucosa is present at the dorsum of the tongue. The thick, multilayered epithelium of the mucosa of the dorsum of the tongue is located on top of the tongue muscle above a thin (but firm and rich in blood vessels and nerves) lamina propria that cannot be moved. The four types of tongue papillae (papillae filiformes, papillae fungiformes, papillae foliatae, and papillae vallatae) are described more closely according to their morphologic characteristics, distribution, and function in Figs. 1-10 to 1-12. Discussion on the lingual tonsils, found on the lateral side of the tongue behind the vallate papillae, and made up of lymphepithelial tissue, can be found in chapter 2 as well as in the legend to Fig. 19-42.

The lip border region (vermilion of the lip) is interpreted differently and considered either as modified skin or as specialized mucosa because this area does not follow the criteria of covering nor of masticatory mucosa.

The oral cavity is not only the beginning of the digestive tract with a special highly sensitive tactile component, it is also a region of the reduction and mixing and storage of nutrients. The transport of nutrients (mastication and swallowing) takes place in the oral cavity at the beginning of movement with transmission to the pharynx, which is coordinated with breathing. The oral cavity is also used for speech.

The detection of taste is not associated only with the specialized mucosa of the dorsum of the tongue but is a combined action of the sense organs of the oral cavity and the nose. Also, in the epithelia of the soft palate and the pharynx, single taste buds are found that are constantly being renewed. The mechanoreceptors and thermoreceptors are compressed at the tip of the tongue.

In addition to its duty as a sense organ, the mucosa of the oral cavity also has the function of a secretory organ (small and large salivary glands). Composition and quantity of the saliva (according to general data, about 0.7 to 1.5 L/d) is controlled by the autonomic nerve system. The protective function of saliva, mucus, and secreted IgA and complement combine with the hormonal and cellular excretions in the protection of the immunologic integrity of the body.

The covering mucosa of the oral cavity and the cheeks has resorption functions in which the absorbed materials are transmitted via the venous system through the superior vena cava into the heart and from there to the periphery of the body. This mechanism of transport of emergency medication is of clinical importance (e.g., sublingual administration).

Some important perculiarities of the morphology and physiology of the oral mucosa are summarized once more in the following overview:

Peculiarities of the Morphology and Physiology of the Oral Mucosa

- There are genetically determined differences in the structure and function of the masticatory mucosa, specialized mucosa, and covering mucosa.
- The gingivodental connection is at the area of least resistance.
- There is a gingivoperiodontal vessel supply in cases of thrombotic occlusion.
- The mucous-covered environment has an individual-specific and location-dependent composition of oral cavity flora (permanent and transitory flora).
- Saliva has a protective influence via the mucin layer and immunoglobulin (especially IgA) as well as a diluting and rinsing effect.
- There is special cellular and humoral cleansing mechanims of damaged areas of the oral mucosa and in particular of previously damaged epithelial attachments.
- There are unavoidable physical and chemical microtraumas.

Efflorescences

The clinical classification of the diseases of the oral mucosa as in dermatosis is mostly based on morphologic criteria. The basic element of the morphologic changes of skin and oral mucosa is called an *efflorescence* ("blossom"). Efflorescences can vary in color, form, size, surface, and consistency. The close observation of efflorescences results in a "sign language" that must be learned. Because it is like an alphabet, this visual language is not built only on the basis of the clinical morphologic diagnosis but is also useful in interdisciplinary understanding.

While there are *primary efflorescences* and *secondary efflorescences,* they cannot always be distinguished. First, the overall findings must be used to locate the primary efflorescence and to rate its dynamics. One must take into consideration the fact that oral mucosal reactions are less expressive than those of the skin and that the changes are usually more monotonous. Without knowledge of the pathophysiologic reactions of the skin and mucosa, interpretation of the disease findings is impossible.

Primary efflorescences are changes of the skin or mucosa that develop in healthy tissue (e.g., spots, wheals, nodules, and vesicles). They may heal immediately or after transformation into secondary efflorescences with or without noticeable consequences. In addition to the basic morphologic elements, the number, distribution, and arrangement of the efflorescences are also important. Another important clinical point is whether the lesion is monomorphic or polymorphic.

Spots (maculae)

A spot (macula) is level with the surface of the skin (i.e., mucosa) and can be differentiated only from the surrounding tissue as a color change. The color difference is usually less evident in the mucosa than on the skin. In melanin-dependent pigmentation, for example, the color tone is influenced by the location of the pigment (e.g., basal or subbasal). The causes that may determine the color change include body pigments, foreign colored material, vascular changes (such as erythema), and extravascular blood collection. Erythemas and telangiectasias lose color under the compression of a glass spatula (i.e. diascopy) but extravascular accumulation of blood does not.

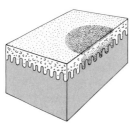 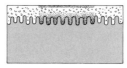

Spot due to melanin deposit in the basal layer

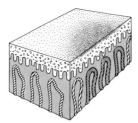 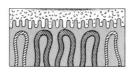

Spot due to erythema (hyperemia)

Wheals (urticaria)

A raised lesion, often associated with a color change (wheal) is the expression of a circumscribed edema caused by a change of capillary permeability. The serum loss can take place in the cutis, that is, in the lamina propria or subcutis or submucosa. An efflorescence occurs rapidly and disappears quickly. On the surface of the lips and eyelids as well as on the mucosa covering the oral cavity, pharynx, and larynx, wheals can become large though relatively flat. Involvement of the larynx can be life-threatening.

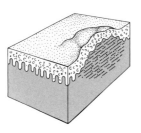 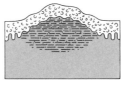

Submucosal papule

Nodules (papules)

A nodule is located above the surface of the skin. It is an efflorescence that can be palpated from 1 mm to a maximum of 1 cm in diameter. The usually sharply limited papule can be flat, pointy, or barrel shaped or have the form of a disk. It can be oval, round-to-oval, or even polygonal in shape. It can appear on the skin as epidermal papules, epidermocutaneous (mixed) papules, or as cutaneous papules.

The *epidermal papule* results from a circumscribed thickening of the epidermis, as in the common wart. If there are also cell infiltrates in the cutis, there is an *epidermocutaneous papule* as is the case in lichen ruber planus. If the nodule consists exclusively of a cellular infiltrate in the cutis, it is a *cutaneous papule*, as can be found in the case of the secondary stage of syphilis.

Efflorescences of the oral mucosa correspond to those of the skin. They are, however, easier to palpate than they are to see with the naked eye. The visible forms of nodules on the oral mucosa vary from a discrete epithelial dimness to unequivocal leukoplakial changes.

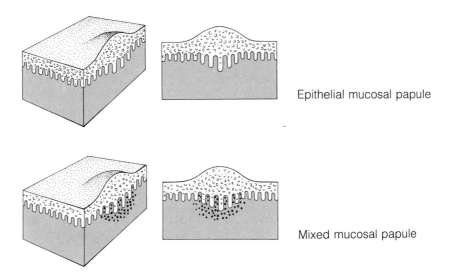

Epithelial mucosal papule

Mixed mucosal papule

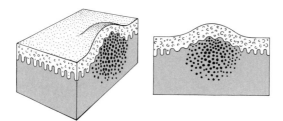

Submucosal papule

Blisters (vesicula or bulla)

Blebs and blisters are raised above the skin and mucosal level as liquid-filled efflorescences. One or several formations with a diameter up to 5 mm (about the size of a pea) are considered blisters. Blebs are larger and are single-chambered. The content of the blister generally is serum, seldom blood. The location can vary. Subcorneal efflorescences are extramucosal only. Of special importance to the skin and oral mucosa are the *intraepidermal blebs* (e.g., in pemphigus vulgaris) and the *subepidermal blebs* (e.g., in the pemphigoid group). Persistence and duration of the vesicles depends on the thickness of the vesicle roof and possible maceration. In the oral cavity there are vesicles and blebs of short duration. Secondary efflorescences (erosions, ulcerations) with remnants of blister roof are usually found there.

The break in continuity of the epithelium is caused by intercellular edema and cell death (e.g., herpes vesicles), because of the separation of the keratinocytes and the prickly cells (e.g., spongiosa in eczema) or because of the absence of desmosome cell contact in the case of acanthoses (e.g., pemphigus vulgaris).

Subepithelial blisters with separation of the epithelium from the papillary body develop because of basal cell degeneration (e.g., bullous lichen planus), because of poor adhesion of the dermoepithelial junction (e.g., junctional blister in diseases of the pemphigoid group), or because of loss of continuity under the basement membrane (e.g., blister due to mechanical conditions is a friction blister).

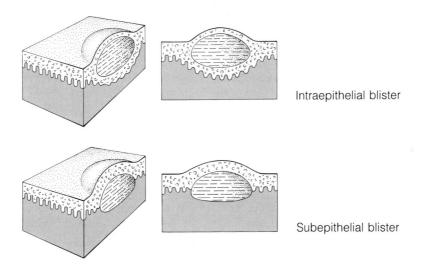

Intraepithelial blister

Subepithelial blister

Pustules

If there is secondary colonization with germs and the previously clear blister becomes cloudy or purulent, a pustule develops. These findings are, for example, found in impetigo contagiosa. The localization of pustules on the skin corresponds to a vesicle or bulla. In the case of psoriasis pustulosa pustules, the lesion is a pustule from the start even if the efflorescences, which are not common in the oral cavity, are not infected.

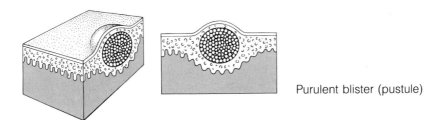

Purulent blister (pustule)

Secondary efflorescences appear by transformation or regression of the primary efflorescences (i.e., erosions, ulcerations, crusts, scales, scars, atrophies, among others).

Erosions

An erosion is defined as the loss of superficial cells of the epidermis or of the mucosa. The light-red, wet, glistening, and often painful epithelial defect can reach as deep as the basement membrane. Erosions develop from secondary efflorescences from intraepidermal, that is, intraepithelial blisters or blebs that have lost their blister cover as well as from trauma (i.e., abrasion). The extravasated intracellular fluid in the area of the damaged epithelium can cause dampness of the skin and a covered area of erosion on the mucosa. Erosions repair without scar formation. The *excoriation* is a deeper epithelial loss, which is tangential to the papillary body and has a punctiform bleeding area derived from some of the capillary loops. Between excoriations, which can be observed in scratch and scrape wounds and traumatic erosions, there are many transition forms.

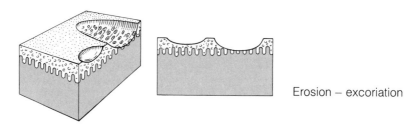

Erosion – excoriation

Ulcers

The ulcer shows a tissue defect that has penetrated the epithelial-connective tissue border and the mucosa and occurs deep in the submucosa or in the muscle and can reach the periosteum. Important for the clinical evaluation are the number (single or multiple), depth, and shape of the lesions, especially the appearance of the base of the lesion and its borders. Inspection, evaluation, and palpation must complement each other. The base of the ulcer can be necrotic, granular, purulent, or covered with mucus. With palpation it is possible to determine the consistency of the base of the ulcer (soft, firm, or hard) and its mobility over underlying structures.

   With the borders of the ulcer, one must carefully observe whether the edge appears flat, rugged with loose epithelial fragments, undermined, or infiltrated. To this are added the aspects of touch (soft, firm, hard, painful, loose, bleeds easily). It is then important to determine if the surrounding mucosa is reaction-free, altered by inflammation, or is infiltrated in other ways. If oral ulcerations develop following sub-epithelial blisters, wall remnants of the blister cover can usually be demonstrated. The remnant scar after healing of the ulcer is much less noticeable on covering mucosa than on skin. Ulcerations can heal without leaving traces in the area of the masticatory mucosa.

The carcinomatous ulcer is schematically represented in chapter 19.

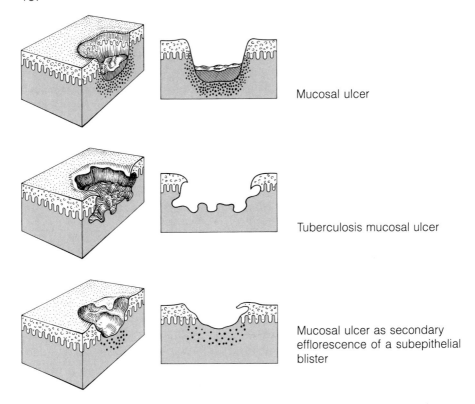

Mucosal ulcer

Tuberculosis mucosal ulcer

Mucosal ulcer as secondary efflorescence of a subepithelial blister

Tears (rhagades)

Rhagades are splitlike tears in the skin that take advantage of body openings or occur in areas of the skin by stretching. A decrease in elasticity of the soft tissues together with brittle skin facilitates the formation of rhagades, which can penetrate the dermis and develop into a painful disabling lesion. Dentists often find rhagades at the corners of the mouth.

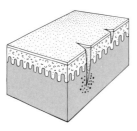 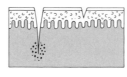

Rhagades of different depths

Crusts

Crusts develop on epithelial defects of the skin by deposit of hardened secretions, blood, or pus. They can be differentiated depending on the color of the dominating part of the deposit. Common examples in the perioral area are crusts following herpes manifestations and hemorrhagic crusts of the lips in erythema exudativum multiforme. There can be exuded yellow-white fibrin deposits on the oral mucosa that are of short duration.

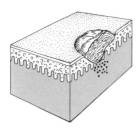 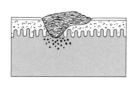

Skin crusts

Scales (squamae)

Pathologic scale formation is caused by a qualitative and/or quantitative disturbance of keratinization. As a consequence of this disturbance, cell masses of the keratin layer become loose, which in form, size, and color can be remarkable in certain diseases. Orthokeratotic and parakeratotic scale formation are distinguishable. Parakeratotic scales appear, for example, in psoriasis where they develop at the same time as the papules, but there are no scales in the oral mucosa.

Scars

A circumscribed scar on the skin is more than a color signal that the normal architecture of the skin was not completely reconstructed after healing of a tissue defect. The epidermis is thinner, the papillary layer has been altered, and the pigmentation has been changed. In the region of the scar, there is also absence of the skin appendages. Continued loss of elastic fiber network causes reduced functional load capacity. Scars in the oral mucosa represent only a partial tissue substitution. The specialized mucosa of the dorsum of the tongue is not repairable.

Keloids are an overdevelopment of connective tissue of scars and are often found on the skin but are unknown on the mucosa.

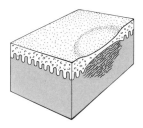 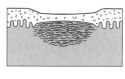

Scar in the area of the covering mucosa

Atrophy

Atrophy of the skin is an involutive process that affects all parts of the integument, including the skin appendages. The regressive changes are an expression of physiologic aging or—if they appear early—a consequence of pathologic changes. A tight atrophic and a nontight atrophic form can be distinguished. The atrophic skin has a thin, creased surface similar to cigarette paper that can be lifted in many folds and is practically devoid of turgor. The tight atrophic skin, while very thin, is hard and stretched due to the collagen fiber bundles; it acts as if glued to the base. This type of atrophy facilitates the development of precancerous lesions. A functional characteristic of the lightly stressed atrophic skin is the development of adjacent hyperpigmented and nonpigmented areas (*poikilodermia*: colorful patching of the skin). The atrophy of the oral mucosa also leads to thinning of the tissue with decreased secretion of the mucous and minor salivary glands.

Specific mucosal efflorescences

In the realm of the theory of efflorescences, only two types of efflorescences characteristic of the mucosa are shown for which a special
chapter is dedicated: *(1) aphthae*, which appear in the mouth and in
the genital mucosa, are special forms of ulcer with characteristic sets
of findings and courses of illness (chapter 12) and *(2) leukoplakias*
(chapter 17).

Cataloging and distribution of efflorescences

The single efflorescence can, in the sense of a division line between
healthy and sick, be sharply or ill defined, as regular and irregular
borders demonstrate. Several single efflorescences can coalesce and
form a common polycyclic focus. Foci in the form of rings can be
formed by centralized healing and simultaneous centrifugal progress
of the border region change.

Efflorescences can appear—depending on skin type or mucosa
type—in smaller or larger numbers or in groups (involving the entire
integument), in flat extensions, as symmetric or asymmetric, as regular
or irregular. In the case of exanthema, there is usually a disseminated
appearance that may be monomorphous or, in the case of multiple
crops of different ages of the same basic efflorescence, polymorphous. The essentially discrete equivalent of the exanthemas in the
oral mucosa as well as in other mucosae is called *enanthemas*. Skin
diseases often have a preferred manifestation, site, for example, in the
stretch or bending areas of the extremities.

The dentist should limit the examination to the oral cavity, the
face, and other sun-exposed areas of skin. Therefore, in some skin
diseases that have oral manifestations, he or she can make only a
limited statement on the disposition and distribution of the efflorescences.

From findings to diagnosis

After an examination has been completed and all findings evaluated, diagnosis begins. While each patient's illness shows its own peculiarities, similar symptoms and similar courses must be unified in a concept (terminology) by grouping together similar clinical courses that have similar pathogenetic and etiologic origins.

We differentiate between *symptoms* and *signs* in differential diagnosis and between subjective and objective findings. The ability to differentiate symptoms and signs, to evaluate them, to be able to translate findings (through visual examination, touch, smell, and sound) into a realization (diagnosis), as well as to make pointed decisions from precise examinations, defines the good diagnostician.

Subjective symptoms usually develop from an organic feeling that the patient often has difficulty in describing ("I notice that there is a difference"; "it is not as before"; "there is no pain but it bothers and disturbs me"). This variable feeling of different duration and intensity is specific for the patient in context and can be primarily *organic, functional,* or *psychic.*

Such physical impressions can be found in the prodromic stages of herpes labialis and the chronic, recurring aphthae, as well as the early phases of blister-forming diseases and allergic reactions of the oral mucosa. In these stages, there are as yet no objective findings on oral inspection. Only later with the appearance of clinical changes is it possible to make a retrospective differentiation.

The classical example of a functional organic feeling of change is the "empty feeling" of the stomach in hunger (caveat: also a symptom of duodenal ulcer). Failing and dysfunctions of the stomatognathic system are sometimes described in the area of the mouth. These functional symptoms are often associated with findings that can be observed on examination.

In the third group of symptoms are complaints of intense pain that do not show any verifiable organic or functional change. At best, one can sometimes find within the physiologic variations a harmless finding that for the average person is unimportant. Up to 50%

of patients seek treatment not because of organic problems or findings that can be documented but because of psychosomatic complaints.

The incidence of psychosomatic illnesses has increased considerably in highly industrialized nations. Also, some skin and mucosal diseases have, in the opinion of the patient, a much greater importance. In the past, disease changes of the skin were associated with lack of cleanliness or bacterial or other infections. Today people with psychological problems or diseases may have an "allergic reaction" that is an expression of an unresolved problem (somatized symptom).

A common psychosomatic complaint in the area of oral cavity is stinging of the mucosa (burning tongue sensation). The patient complains of a feeling of a wound of the mucosa, with a strong burning sensation on (in order of decreasing frequency) the tongue tip, tongue borders, palate, or cheeks. Without other clinical changes, these are subjective findings that cannot be substantiated. They are similar to itching of the skin, which scratching usually exacerbates.

In the oral mucosa it is not possible to obtain improvement with local medication. Extremely frequent self-examination only intensifies pain findings, and the well-informed professional should recognize this untoward effect. The pain can intensify so much from the organic neurosis that a psychosomatic condition or an organopsychic one must be considered a body-fixation symptom or a psychiatric disease. In most of these patients, there is a masked depression. If there is a major discrepancy between objective and subjective findings, the patient's complaints and worries cannot be simply dismissed as unimportant and unfounded ("simulation"). It is necessary—after careful consideration of other possible causes—to demonstrate the existence of a psychosomatic disease. Precipitous embarkation on a course of treatment (e.g., a "take that immediately" approach) in these patients ends in failure and can only result in a repeated change of doctors.

Emotional problems have been discussed in detail because somatic aspects of disease cannot be neglected; they are important in diagnosis and therapy. In summary, dentists in the process of making a diagnosis must consider subjective symptoms in oral mucosal diseases and must conscientiously distinguish them from objective symptoms.

If once again we consider the clinical findings of the diseases in the oral mucosa, the basic morphologic elements are already present in the efflorescence theory. These oral lesions, however, must be considered in relation to the systemic diseases with which they may be associated. They can be classified as:

- Early symptom
- Leading symptom
- Accompanying symptom
- Secondary finding

As an example, consider the uncharacteristic cathartic prodromal findings in acute infectious diseases that are typical findings in the oral cavity or perioral region, for which *early symptoms* are helpful in the final diagnosis.

If oral mucosal changes are regularly found in the early phases of a systemic disease (as in acute leukemias and agranulocytosis) they are considered *leading symptoms*. If they are found together with the systemic disease findings only after the clinical initiation of the systemic disease, they are considered *accompanying symptoms*. Knowledge of the accompanying symptoms is important for the dentist because they remind him or her of the need to include facts usually already known from the history with ideas about dental therapeutic measures and prognosis.

On occasion *secondary findings* are considered those changes of the oral mucosa that do not have a causal relation to the major disease found in the oral cavity.

It should be remembered that *oral manifestations of superimposed disturbances and systemic illnesses* can be decisively influenced by *pre-existing oral changes*. In general, there are already unrelated changes before the onset of the disease in the form of chronic inflammation of the gingiva and periodontium. They are usually the consequence of poor oral hygiene. Previous damage can also be due to other local irritations (e.g., interrupted dental treatment, damaging or inadequate restorative measures).

In all regions of the oral mucosa, the marginal gingiva and epithelial margin are the structures easiest to injure; they are reliable indicators of local and systemic disorders of the body. However, in this area there is a mixture of influences of often-complex etiologic origins. Typical appearances of some special diseases are not considered here and will be presented later in more detail. It is only by a conspicuous progressive gingivoperiodontal inflammatory process and its resistance to local treatment that suspicion of the participation of an endogenous factor may arise. Improvement of diagnostic skills depends on self-discipline, which involves obeying basic rules and adhering to a systematic approach. Professional experience acquired over the years enters here. Willingness to revise a probable diagnosis with new findings and willingness to learn from one's own mistakes are also important to a good diagnostician.

Evaluations of general practices demonstrate that on the basis of precise knowledge of the patient's history, a hypothetical diagnosis is possible in 50% of patients. With the help of the clinical examination, correct diagnoses can be made in 90% of all cases. Only in 10% of patients is there a need for further differential diagnostic measures that will ensure the diagnosis. Data from specialists are less conclusive because the differential diagnosis also depends on different referrals from general practices. The experienced dentist knows when auxiliary diagnostic measures should be requested. Generally, working together with a specialist is desirable as soon as the dentist is unable to make a differential diagnosis.

Referral does not exclude one's own evaluation of the disease findings. It is wrong to assume that a diagnosis can be obtained by manifold examination in different directions. The same is true for additional diagnostic measures, the evaluation of which is above one's own level of competence. A therapy in the absence of a diagnosis must be rejected because it is no more than a treatment of the symptoms. The appearance of a disease, however, may force the initiation of therapy before the diagnosis is complete. The dentist should keep in mind the undetermined nature of the diagnosis and obtain certainty as soon as possible.

The referring professional should provide his or her thoughts on the differential diagnosis to the specialist called on for help so that this professional can use his or her special knowledge and experience to clarify the case. Interprofessional communication, either in proximity or through letters and telephone calls, brings experience and knowledge to both sides, contributes to the interlocking of detailed knowledge of different specialities and is beneficial to all patients.

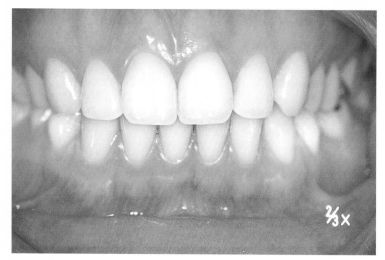

Fig. 1-1 Clinically sound buccal gingival and alveolar mucosa in the area of the anterior teeth of the maxilla and mandible. The clinically normal gingiva is light pink, has a faint, shiny, stippled surface, tight tissue structure, and fills papillary parts completely in the interdental space. Figures 1-1 to 1-6, 1-8, and 1-9 depict the same 23-year-old female patient.

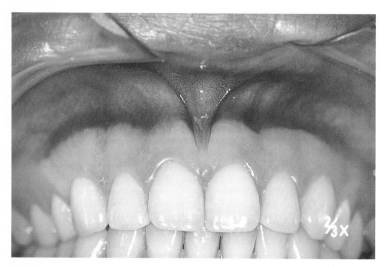

Fig. 1-2 Appearance of the mucogingival borders (transition of the keratinized fixed gingiva to the differently structured noncornified alveolar mucosa) after staining with Schiller-iodine solution. The differential coloring of the tissue demonstrates the alveolar mucosa as opposed to the deposits of glycogen in the healthy gingiva, which can be stained.

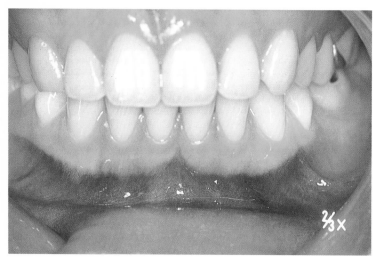

Fig. 1-3 Demonstration of a mucogingival border in the mandible after staining with Schiller-iodine solution. The height of the attached gingiva is individually unique and varies in different areas in the same individual but is bilaterally symmetrical.

Fig. 1-4 Close-up view of the buccal gingiva in the area of teeth 12 (7), 11 (8), and 21 (9) with insertion of the lip frenum. The marginal (free) gingiva forms a 1- to 2-mm rim of smooth tissue, which follows the course of the dento-enamel junction. On the buccal side, the marginal gingiva extends to the attached gingiva while at the tooth level it ends at the marginal epithelium. Marginal epithelium forms the epithelial attachment on the tooth surface that protects the integrity of the epithelial continuity in the mouth.

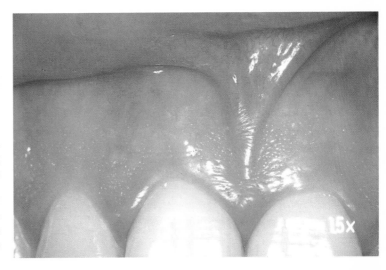

Fig. 1-5 Close-up of the gingiva in the area of teeth 13 (6), 12 (7), and 11 (8). The surface of the clinically healthy alveolar gingiva with its small irregularly distributed depressions is like an orange peel; this effect is also known as stippling. During the mixed dentition stage, the stippling present in the marginal gingiva can disappear in cases of inflammation.

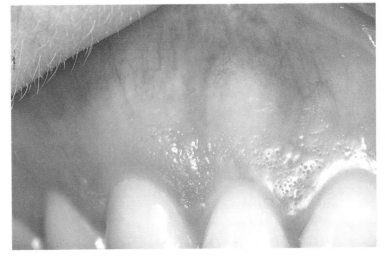

Fig. 1-6 Close-up of the buccal gingiva of the region of the mandibular incisor with frenum insertion. The form of the interdental papillae depends on the position and the closeness of teeth: the closer together, the sharper the papilla. Between buccal and vestibular papilla tips, there is a satellite depression known as a col. In the area of the lateral teeth, the col increases in width and depth. Papillary tips and col are frequent areas of attack.

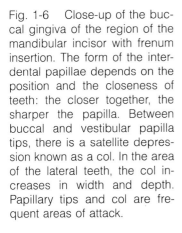

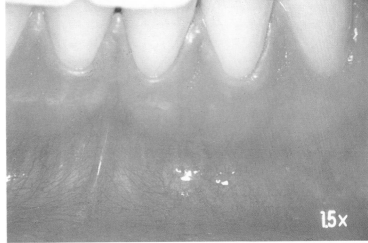

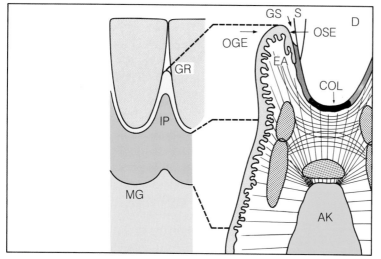

Fig. 1-7   Division of the gingiva and set-up of marginal periodontium in schematic form. AK = alveolar bone; D = dentin; EA = epithelial attachment; GR = gingival margin; GS = gingival sulcus; IP = interdental papilla; MG = mucogingival border; OGE = oral gingival epithelium; OSE = oral sulcus epithelium; S = enamel. (Modified from Schroder HE. *Handbook of Microscopic Anatomy*, vol. 5. Berlin: Springer Verlag, 1988.)

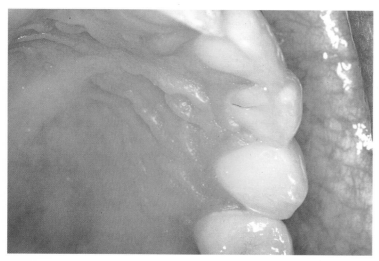

Fig. 1-8   Close-up of palatal mucosa in the region of teeth 21 (9), 22 (10), and 23 (11). The marginal gingiva changes immediately into the periosteal fixed mucosa of the hard palate. Near the palatal raphe and the incisal papilla, the individually different palatal folds (plicae palatinate transversalis) are seen.

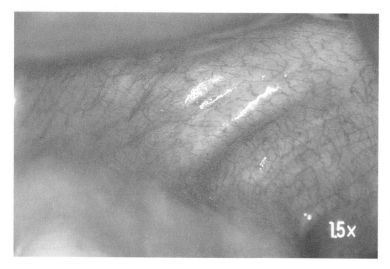

Fig. 1-9   Close-up of the covering mucosa in the area of the maxilla. The deviations of the normal vessel distribution demonstrated here are marked.

Fig. 1-10   Normal papillary relief of a clinically unremarkable tongue. While there are thousands of filiform papillae on the dorsum of the tongue, there are hundreds of macroscopic red points of identifiable fungiform papillae closely scattered together in the region of the tip and sides of the tongue. Also, in the posterior area of both sides of the tongue there are as many as 25 foliate papillae. At the bottom of the papillary borders are the openings of serous salivary glands.

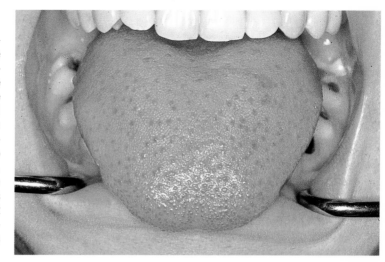

Fig. 1-11   Close-up of the dorsum of the tongue with appearance of the filiform papillae. For each cm^2 there are about 20 basal papillae, which have about 400 to 500 heavily cornified secondary papillae. Filiform papillae are predominantly carriers and transmitters of the sense of taste. The manner of distribution of the bent of the keratinized point that includes the nerve ending allows for an increase of taste value of a factor of 1.6 with stereognostic perception simultaneously.

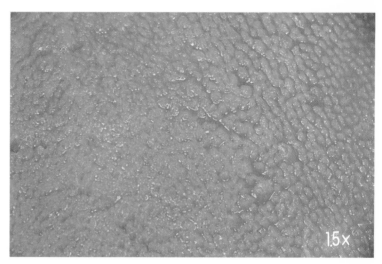

Fig. 1-12   Close-up of the posterior third of the tongue with a direct view of vallate papillae parallel to the terminal sulcus. These eight to 12 knotty, prominent, large tongue papillae (average diameter of 2 mm to 3 mm, height approximately 1 mm) carry many taste buds that transmit bitter taste. On the bottom of the mounds of these papillae, there are the openings of irrigating serous glands (von Ebner's glands). At the dividing line of the terminal sulcus is the foramen cecum (not shown here).

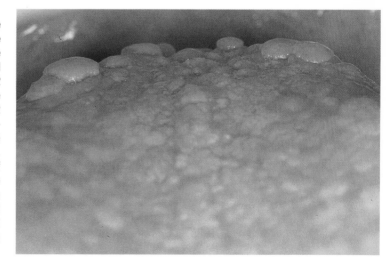

Chapter 2

Clinical Peculiarities of Oral Mucosa Without Real Diseases, but with Borderline Abnormalities

---

Linea alba

Fordyce's spots—Heterotopic sebaceous glands

Epstein's pearls; gingival cysts in newborns

Fissured tongue

Geographic tongue

Crenated tongue

Lateral lingual tonsils; hypertrophy of foliate papillae

Sublingual varices

Median rhomboid glossitis

Coated tongue

Hairy tongue

Oral mucosal and tongue changes are presented here independent of their nosologic and morphologic classifications. A departure from the normal concept, this is useful for diagnoses in dental practice.

Despite their different etiologies, the findings in all the conditions described show minimal disease character. Many findings are borderline between normal and pathologic. Another point in common is that without exception these conditions require more differential diagnosis than therapy. They are by their nature harmless, which nevertheless, does not exclude the fact that they can frequently be zones of least resistance for further disease processes. These harmless conditions have the common feature that patients often believe they have a serious problem and are very disturbed by it. In addition to anatomic variations of normal (e.g., plicated tongue) and physiologic variations (e.g., geographic tongue), a few variations of the soft tissues of the oral cavity have their origin in unique peculiarities of embryology (e.g., linea alba) and defective formation (e.g., median rhomboid glossitis, Epstein's pearls). Also, some findings considered heterotopic conditions that are characterized by the presence of normal tissue in an unusual location (e.g., lateral lingual tonsils, heterotopic sebaceous glands) will be mentioned here. Finally, we will discuss borderline conditions of the tongue (e.g., lateral tongue impression, coated tongue, hairy tongue).

Linea alba (ICD-DA 528.90)

Linea alba is located in the cheek region at the level of occlusion, is a phylogenetic remnant of embryonic development, and indicates the area of fusion between the cheeks and the lips. This area is often a slightly raised white line with some increase in thickness, making it higher than the rest of the cheek mucosa (Fig. 2-1). Color intensity is determined by the amount of keratinization of the epithelium. Originally, linea alba was attributed to the interaction of several factors. Among these was the special biomechanical needs of this tissue, which experiences pressure from the vestibule and the rest of the oral cavity, as well as the possible position of the mandible. It appears that roughness on the buccal surface of the lateral teeth has no effect.

Motor activity, chewing, and mental stresses may cause additional changes, such as impressions of the lateral teeth or proptosis superimposed on the presence of linea alba (see chapter 22). In some cases it can be associated with trauma from cheek-biting (Fig. 2-3). In these cases patients should be directed to stop chewing on the cheek mucosa (see chapter 32).

Fordyce's spots–heterotopic sebaceous glands (ICD-DA 750.25)

Within physiologic variations, single or small groups of sebaceous glands not associated with hair can be found in the oral mucosa. The favored location of these heterotopic sebaceous glands is the cheek mucosa, particularly in the area of a linea alba (Figs. 2-5 and 2-6), the fusion area of the upper lip (Fig. 2-4), and less frequently in the lower lip. In some cases they are also present in the gingiva and tongue. Larger single lesions are sometimes found in the vestibular region of the mandible. Heterotopic sebaceous glands appear clinically as slightly raised, round-to-polygonal, and are usually the size of a pinhead. Color varies from whitish-yellow to yellow to egg yolk. The mucosa in which they are embedded has a somewhat knotty appearance and shows an epithelial surface without interruption. Heterotopic sebaceous glands in children have not been described, but they are often seen in adults. They are usually larger in men than in women.

Epstein's pearls; gingival cysts in newborns (ICD-DA 528.40)

Epstein's pearls demonstrate an embryologic developmental defect, with epithelial nests embedded immediately under the mucosal epithelium (inclusions), which can change into small cysts containing keratin. Because of their superficial position, these formations, usually numerous, are seen as small knots of firm consistency the size of rice kernels and shine through the mucosa as white spots. They do not increase in size. The main locations, with decreasing incidence, are the middle line of the palate, the alveolar process of the maxilla (Fig. 2-7), and the mandible. These harmless findings, seen extensively in newborns and infants, have no clinical importance. They decrease in number in a few months due to resorption (Fig. 2-8) or are eliminated during the normal growth period.

Fissured tongue (ICD-DA 529.5X)

The tongue usually has a regular small-grained velvety surface covered with papillae. The pink fungiform papillae stand out individually because of their richness in capillaries (see Fig. 1-10).

The small deviation from the normal tongue surface consits of a visible long median fissure. There are all types of variations, with the appearance of many fissures originating from this deep median anchorage line. The lateral fissures can also be the starting point of smaller fissures. These branching, varied fold reliefs can give the appearance of lingua plicata when the tongue is extended. The pattern of the tongue surface is like a leaf (Fig. 2-9), brain convolutions, or the treads of automobile tires (Fig. 2-10). When highly convoluted, it is like a contracted scrotum (therefore also described as scrotal tongue). The changes in the tongue musculature are limited to the front two-thirds of the tongue. Forms involving only the lateral aspects of the tongue are frequently seen (Fig. 2-11).

The painless plicated tongue does not require treatment and is a variation of the normal dorsum of the tongue. It should be considered a constitutional marker and be differentiated from all acquired forms of inflammation, particularly from inflammatory fissures. In Melkersson-Rosenthal syndrome (see chapter 30), it is considered one of the symptoms in fewer than half of all cases; here plicated tongue is only considered a pointer to a congenital condition. The fissured tongue whose depressions and elevations are covered with squamous epithelium is considered an area of reduced resistance. In deep fissures (Fig. 2-12), food lodges and bacteria and fungi can cause a local chronic inflammation. The plicated tongue can also function as a point of entry for specific infections.

Fissured tongue is present in 10% to 15% of the general population, including patients with minimal findings. In 20% of cases, geographic tongue is also present.

Geographic tongue (ICD-DA 529.1X)

Geographic tongue represents changes of the tongue dorsum and border of the tongue caused by focal increase of the "desquamation process" of the filiform papillae. With the loss of the cornified tips, a focal massive erythema develops and contrasts with the areas where the fungiform papillae are not participating in the process, giving the impression of a lighter or darker reddish color of the exfoliated areas. The contrast with the normal tongue surface is intensified by a whitish to white-yellow border that appears coagulated or brushed together (epithelial curls) and that surrounds the desquamated areas (Figs. 2-13 to 2-18). The "desquamations" originating from one or several primary areas wander in different directions (e.g., circle, semicircle, or garlands) with varying extensions and spread toward the periphery (hence also the name "wandering plaques"). At the same time, in the center of the lesion the normal surface epithelium regenerates. In this manner, there is the development of a colorful changeable appearance that looks like a map (hence, the name "geographic tongue"). The appearance can change from day to day or even within a day. In some cases changes are limited to some areas of the tongue, and the involved areas contrast with the uninvolved background.

Geographic tongue can appear suddenly at any age. Often it starts at a young age (and in this instance is not noticed) (Fig. 2-13). The duration cannot be predicted. The recurring lesion can remain for months, years, or decades and can disappear for periods of time.

The etiology of geographic tongue is unknown. None of the suggested causes (among them psychologic, neurohumoral, and genetic) provides clear-cut proof of causal relationship. Possibly it is a physiologic variant of the desquamation process of the epithelial surface, which is usually unnoticed. It is remarkable that geographic tongue is often associated with a plicated tongue. There have been some reports of increased appearance of geographic tongue in patients with psoriasis and atopic diseases.

Complaints of burning from eating sour fruits or heavily spiced food are reported by patients in whom the changes were not present since childhood. The appearance of geographic tongue in these individuals is an unpleasant but not severe nuisance. Geographic tongue can be found with superimposed conditions, but the basic condition cannot be treated.

Patients with geographic tongue must be informed of the harmlessness of the condition in order to save them from continuous and useless therapeutic measures. This is also important because in-creased self-observation can result in cancerphobia, which will in-crease the use of unnecessary, useless medications.

Diagnosis must differentiate, among others, mechanically caused scouring of the papillary reliefs (Fig. 2-19) and trophoneurologic changes of surfaces (Fig. 2-20). Also, all variations of leukoplakia of the specialized mucosa of the tongue must be differentiated.

Crenated tongue (ICD-DA 529.80)

Some individuals habitually press the normal tongue against the teeth. Pressure behavior can occur without the patient's conscious know-ledge in cases of functional disturbances as a means of avoiding dental closure in an unstable retrograde contact position (e.g., in empty deglutition). As a consequence of this chronic dysfunction, depressions corresponding to the contours of the teeth can be seen on the border of the tongue (Fig. 2-21). Depending on the intensity of the mechanical irritation (e.g., sharp tooth corners) it is possible to have, in areas of these lateral tongue impressions, an additional irritative change that can create small swelling of the involved area of the tongue. These changes increase the stimulus to continue the tongue pressure, resulting in a vicious circle. It is a trying task to break the patient's habit. It is important to distinguish lateral tongue impressions caused by a discrepancy between the size of the tongue and the oral cavity and therefore formed without active participation of the patient. These are usually cansed by an enlargement of the tongue (macrog-lossia). Macroglossia can be the result of a tumor, an acromegaly, or systemic diseases (see Fig. 26-23).

Lateral lingual tonsils; hypertrophy of foliate papillae (ICD-DA 529.32)

At the base of the tongue one regularly finds abundant lymphoid tissue, which is part of the Waldeyer's ring of the throat. As a harmless, anatomic variation one often sees heterotopic tongue tonsils on the lateral border of the tongue, which are usually bilaterally symmetrical at the level of the anterior palatal arch.

These nodules of lymphoid tissue often have a light-red–colored surface with clefts of a light-red color reminiscent of brain convolutions (Figs. 2-22; see Fig. 19-42).

The lateral tongue tonsil can participate in infections of the throat but can also be affected alone–unilaterally or bilaterally (e.g., angina tonsillae linguae). The size and consistency of these tonsils depends on the degree of inflammation. In some cases there are pea-sized knotty thickenings that can be palpated. The accidental discovery of the lateral tongue tonsil can cause patient concern. Differential diagnosis may be difficult. Lesions caused by prostheses or dental treatment may resemble the early stages of carcinoma of the tongue (see chapter 19). When the dentist is not convinced ot the harmlessness of the change, he or she should refer the patient for a consultation.

Sublingual varices (ICD-DA 456.80)

On the underside of the tongue under normal conditions there is a distinct venous network (Fig. 2-23). In advancing age, with weakening of the walls of the vessels, phlebectasias can be formed even in the absence of venous stasis. These enlargements of the veins form a varicose picture of violet tortuous veins and can be observed in a large percentage of 60-year-old people. It occurs most frequently on the underside of the tongue (Fig. 2-24) but sometimes on the border of the tongue and floor of the mouth (close to the exit of the sublingual salivary gland) as well as on the mucosa of the mouth vestibule. As blood vessel alterations, these lesions can be compressed with a glass spatula. Differential diagnosis must include hereditary hemorrhagic telangiectasia, e.g., Osler's disease (see chapter 25).

Median rhomboid glossitis (ICD-DA 529.2X)

It is generally assumed that median rhomboid glossitis is a developmental abnormality of the tongue because of a persistent tuberculum impar. In this case the tuberculum impar is not completely covered, as normally occurs during ontogenesis by the lateral projections of the tongue anlagen of the first branchial arch. Because of this developmental abnormality, there are then mucosal changes of varying size—rhomboid to oval but sametimes round or long—in the midline on the posterior third of the tongue (Fig. 2-25 and 2-26). Due to the absence of filiform papillae, the surface is usually smooth, salmon to red in color, shiny, and distinct from the surrounding normal papillary area. The area can be located at the level of the mucosa or be elevated (Fig. 2-29), with an extremely varied clinical picture. It is also possible to observe bumpy ridges (Fig. 2-28) and patchy and grapelike (Fig. 2-30) tissue formations. Also, histologic findings vary greatly. Besides sinuslike vascular ectasias, which when severe are reminiscent of hemangiomas, chronic inflammation can almost always be seen (hence the name glossitis).

Median rhomboid glossitis is an area of reduced resistance to exogenous irritants. It is possible for a *Candida albicans* infection to develop on its underside (Figs. 2-31 and 2-32). It was previously thought that median rhomboid glossitis was not a developmental anomaly but a localized *Candida* infection. Different forms of leukoplakias can also be observed (Fig. 2-27). There are some reports of malignant changes of a median rhomboid glossitis with development of a carcinomatous ulcer of the tongue. These instances are rare.

By all rules, median rhomboid glossitis is a harmless, usually asymptomatic, abnormality of the tongue without actual disease. Therapy can be witheld in most cases. The task of the dentist is to explain this to the sometimes worried patient. In cases of proven candidiasis, antifungal therapy should be initiated. In cases of persistent chronic infections, particularly in bumpy tongues with varicose or papillomatous appearance but also in cases that are suspicious at palpation (e.g., with wall-type raised border), surgical intervention is indicated. The patient should be referred for this purpose.

Coated tongue (ICD-DA 529.30)

Coated tongue can be found as an incidental finding in many of the images shown in this book (e.g., Fig. 2-21), hence special photographic documentation is not necessary. More important is the fact that there are several causes for coated tongue. Coated tongue was once considered a symptom of disease of the gastrointestinal tract. Today coated tongue is considered not so much a sign of a gastrointestinal disorder as the result of a deficient or failing function of tongue self-cleaning. Many factors can be important.

Certain inadequate eating habits (rapid swallowing of food) as well as a diet predominantly composed of soft food favor the formation of coated tongue because there is a decrease of normal physiologic scouring on the dorsum of the tongue. Evidence for this can be found in patients with jaw fractures and severely ill patients who are nourished with liquid food. Deficient oral hygiene also favors the development of coated tongue. Another cause is altered mobility of the tongue. Coated tongue occurs frequently in paralyzed, brain-damaged, and unconscious patients. It is also known that with alterations of body heat and fluid intake (e.g., with fevers, desiccation) as well as in marasmic conditions, massive coating of the tongue can occur.

The somewhat altered filiform papillae, food particles, cellular debris, and microorganisms of the oral flora together can cause tongue coating changes within 1 day. It is more intense in adults than in young patients. With increased age there is a decrease in the occurence of coated tongue: during old age, with the age-related atrophy of the tongue papillae, tongue coating is seldom observed. In some illnesses (e.g., Sjögren's syndrome—see chapter 30—and in the now rare Moeller-Hunter glossitis of pernicious anemia) the tongue always remains uncoated.

Hairy tongue (ICD-DA 529.31)

Hairy tongue is a harmless epithelial hyperplasia and hyperkeratosis of the filiform papillae, which here have longer cornified extensions. The preferred location of the change is the middle of the dorsum of the tongue and on the anterior two thirds of the tongue. Extensive areas of the tongue surface, or even the entire surface, are often involved.

The closely packed threadlike cornifications of the filiform papillae, which can attain a length of 2 cm, give the impression of "hairs" or "bushes of wet grass." They appear to be "combed" toward the tip of the tongue. The color of the tongue is usually brown or black (Figs. 2-33 to 2-36) but can also be yellowish-brown (Fig. 2-38), reddish-yellow, blue-green, or in exceptional cases, even white (Fig. 2-37). The name "black hairy tongue" is therefore only correct in some cases. The varying color is caused by the type of pigment of the colonizing chromogenic bacteria, from colored food remnants, and in the case of smokers, depends on the amount of tobacco used.

Hairy tongue has a complex etiology and consists of increased keratinization of the filiform papillae. The causal relationship with antibacterial therapy is certain. In this event there is a change in oral flora with predominance of fungi. Hairy tongue can also occur with systemic use of corticosteroids or after infectious diseases and other serious disease leading to debilitation. Chemical influences (e.g., extensive tobacco consumption or chronic use of aggressive peroxide-containing mouthwashes may also play a role as cofactors). In a remarkable number of cases, however, the determining factor of hairy tongue is completely unknown.

The condition is usually asymptomatic. Sometimes patients complain of an unpleasant feeling when the "hairy" surface of the area of the tongue closer to the pharynx touches the mucosa of the palate. Hairy tongue can persist for several years or can disappear after a short time.

As far as it is possible to find causative factors, they must be eliminated. After termination of antibiotic therapy, hairy tongue disappears completely in a few weeks. In "idiopathic" cases, therapy is unsatisfactory. Suggested treatments are many. The removal of the hairs with wet gauze or a toothbrush, or in massive cases, careful removal by means of superficial curettage, are as effective as symptomatic therapy but the favorable result is short-lived.

The dentist can explain the harmlessness of hairy tongue so that the patient does not suffer unnecessary anxiety or develop psychological problems.

Differential diagnosis must be made between hairy tongue and the coated tongue of hairy leukoplakia. This latter condition may occur in AIDS and AIDS-related complex. In hairy leukoplakia the lesions are white, cannot be removed from the tongue, and appear on the lateral side of the tongue (see chapter 11).

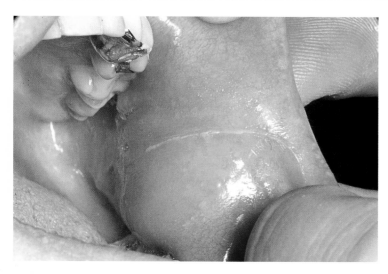

Fig. 2-1   Linea alba in the form of a ledge epithelial thickening.

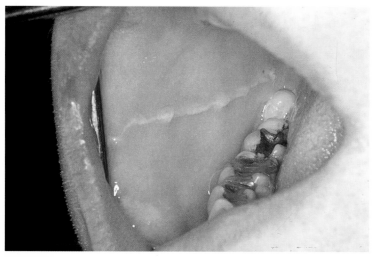

Fig. 2-2   Easily distinguishable linea alba with outlines of dental impressions.

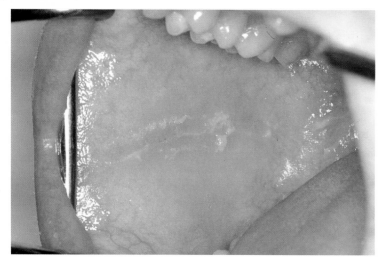

Fig. 2-3   Linea alba with border of bite defect. The epithelial lesion with discrete bleeding in the center can be seen.

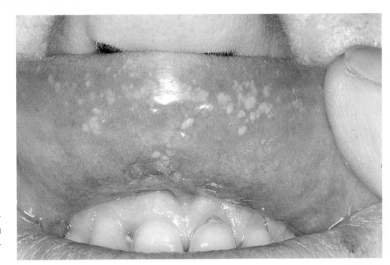

Fig. 2-4 Heterotopic sebaceous glands mainly located in
the mucosa close to the vermilion of the lip.

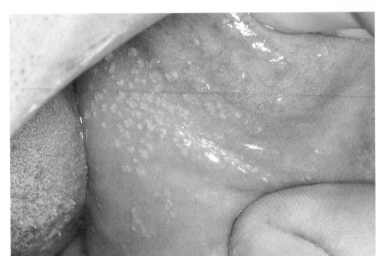

Fig. 2-5 Yolk-yellow heterotopic sebaceous glands in the
area of a linea alba with intact
epithelial surface.

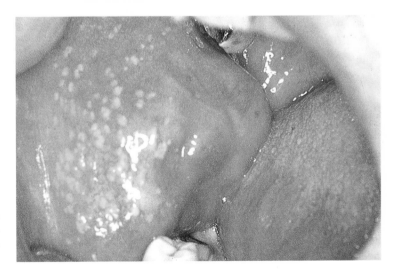

Fig. 2-6 Heterotopic sebaceous glands of the cheek mucosa, above a bulging cavernous hemangioma.

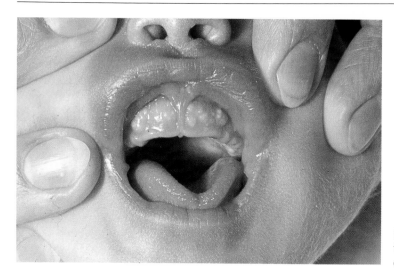

Fig. 2-7   Epstein's pearls on the maxillary alveolar process of a 10-day-old infant.

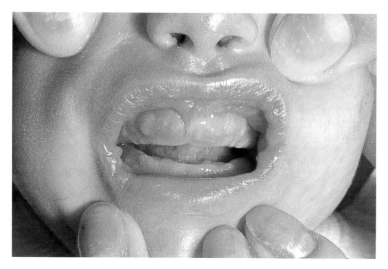

Fig. 2-8   The same infant of Fig. 2-7 8 weeks later; note the distinct spontaneous decrease of keratinized lesions.

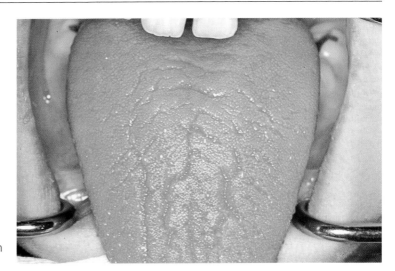

Fig. 2-9   Plicated tongue with leaflike appearance.

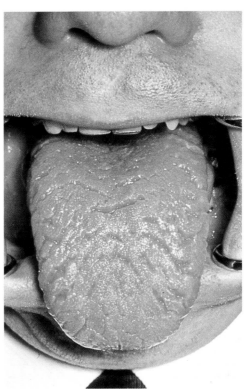

Fig. 2-10   Plicated tongue with the appearance of car-tire treads.

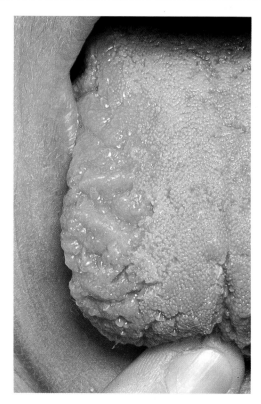

Fig. 2-11 Lateral type of plicated tongue with central anterior fissure.

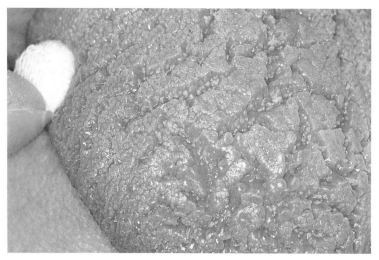

Fig. 2-12 Plicated tongue. With increased magnification, it is possible to see the many differently appearing fissures in which food becomes entrapped as do bacteria and fungi, which can cause and maintain local chronic inflammation (area of decreased resistance).

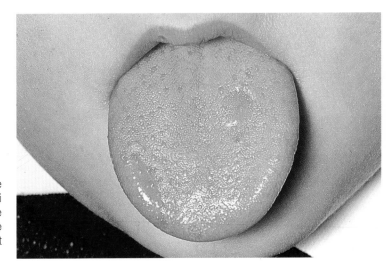

Fig. 2-13 Geographic tongue in a 4-year-old child. Two foci are seen, one at the middle (right side of picture) and one close to the tongue margin (left side of picture).

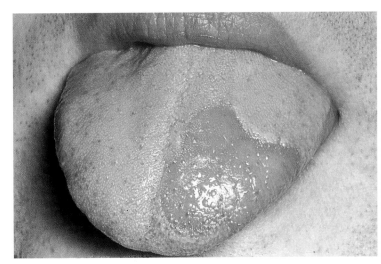

Fig. 2-14 Geographic tongue present since childhood in a 17-year-old boy. In the exfoliated area, the cornified tips of the filiform papillae have been lost so that the fungiform papillae that are not involved are higher on the mucosal level.

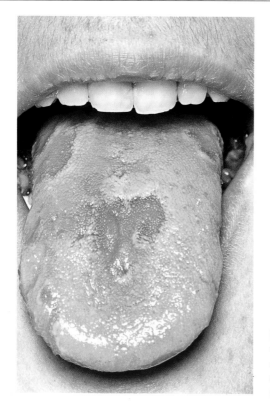

Fig. 2-15 Geographic tongue with a pattern that changes daily. This condition was present for 8 years in the 26-year-old woman.

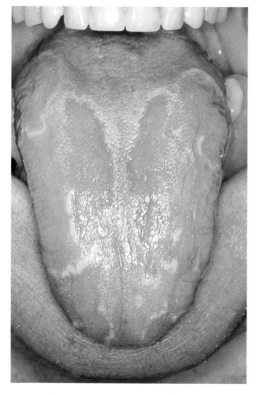

Fig. 2-16 Extensive, almost symmetrical, geographic tongue with foci converging in some areas.

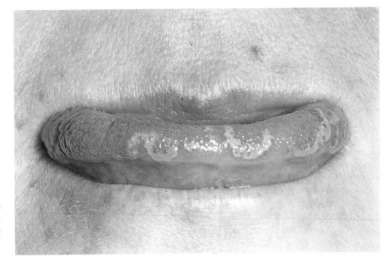

Fig. 2-17   Geographic tongue with garland-shaped manifestations on the anterior margin of the tongue.

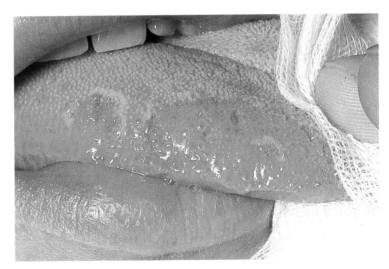

Fig. 2-18   Geographic tongue with focal erosion on the lateral margin of the tongue.

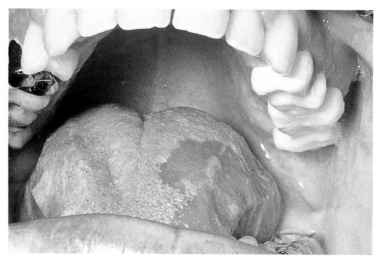

Fig. 2-19   Differential diagnosis of geographic tongue: circumscribed mechanical abrasion of the tongue papillae. After placement of a provisional acrylic resin bridge from teeth 24 to 27 (13 to 20), the 30-year-old man acquired a dysfunctional pressure behavior of the tongue. This mechanical stress caused temporary unilateral abrasion of the normal texture of the tongue papillae. The absence of slightly elevated, whitish margins permits differentiating this condition from that of geographic tongue. Insertion of the final prosthesis allowed regrowth of the tongue papillae, leading to the correct diagnosis.

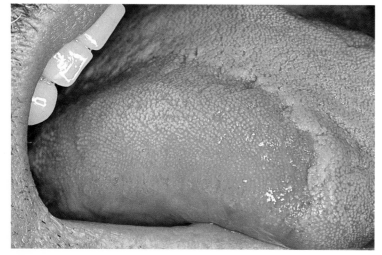

Fig. 2-20   Differential diagnosis of geographic tongue: changes in the relief of tongue papillae, strictly confined unilaterally and regressing relatively quickly. This condition resulted after injury to the lingual nerve in a 60-year-old man. A trophoneurotic disturbance must be assumed to be the cause. Compare these findings with those of a zoster of the third trigeminal branch with involvement of the tongue (chapter 11).

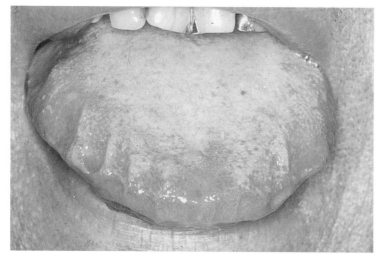

Fig. 2-21   Lateral tongue impressions from constant pressure of the tongue against dental ridges. The depressions on the margin of the tongue correspond to lingual contours of the teeth. Additional findings: major tongue coating caused by rapid eating habits. Macroglossia could be excluded.

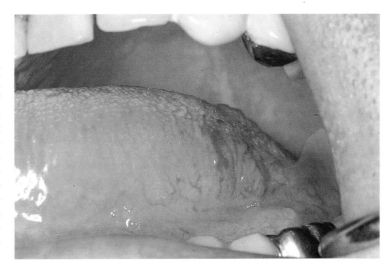

Fig. 2-22   Tongue margin with lateral lingual tonsil. The correct determination of the disease requires extensive knowledge of normal findings and their physiologic variations. The dentist should therefore routinely examine the area of possible lateral lingual tonsils. The heterotopic lymphoid tissue can take part in an inflammatory process. In case of diagnostic doubts (e.g., suspicion of carcinoma), a referral is always required. See also Fig. 19-42.

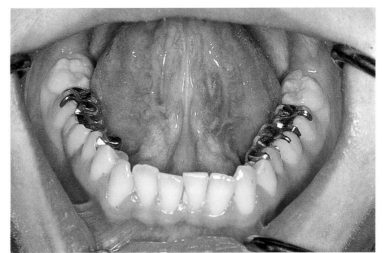

Fig. 2-23   Normal appearance of sublingual venous pattern.

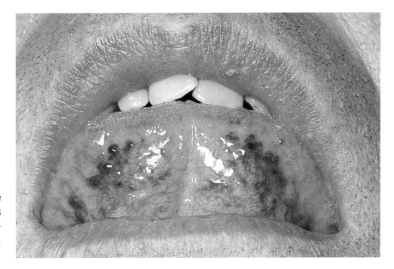

Fig. 2-24   Sublingual varicose veins without obvious venous blockage. Differential diagnosis: Osler's disease (see Figs. 25-13 to 25-17).

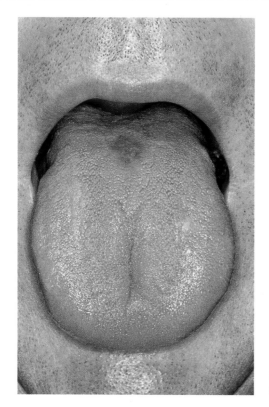

Fig. 2-25   Discrete form of a median rhomboid glossitis.

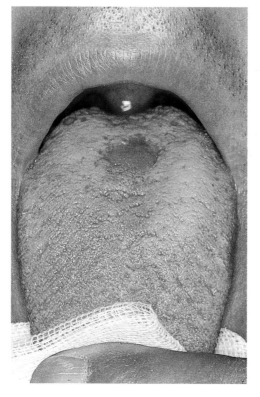

Fig. 2-26   Median rhomboid glossitis with varnishlike surface contrasting sharply with the areas of the normal papillae. In the posterior third of the tongue, some vallate papillae are present.

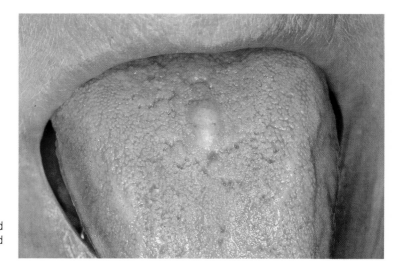

Fig. 2-27   Median rhomboid glossitis with superimposed leukoplakia.

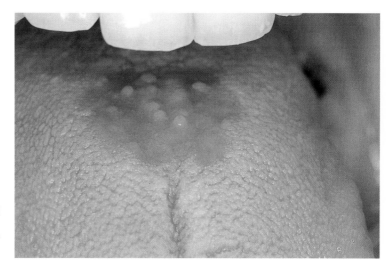

Fig. 2-28   Median rhomboid glossitis with partially smooth, partially bumpy elevations of the mucosal surface.

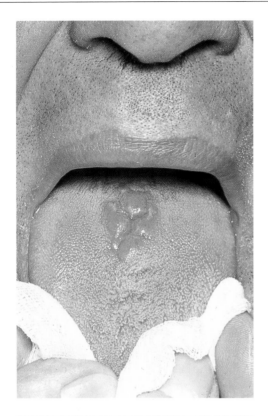

Fig. 2-29 Median rhomboid glossitis with typical localization of bulges and furrows.

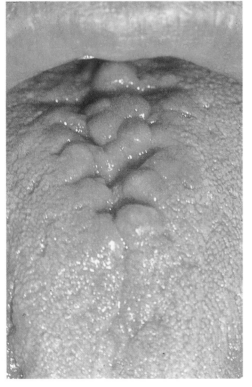

Fig. 2-30 Median rhomboid glossitis with raised grapelike tissue masses.

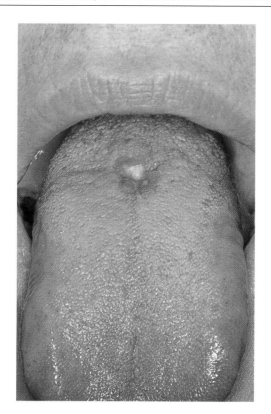

Fig. 2-31   Median rhomboid glossitis with demonstrable localized chronic candidiasis.

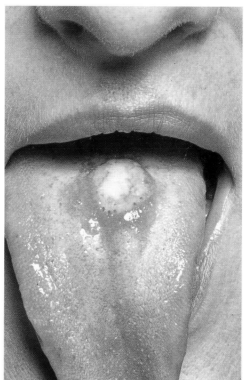

Fig. 2-32   Median rhomboid glossitis with massive chronic mycosis due to *Candida albicans*. Fungal infection produced proliferative changes of tissue; differential diagnosis in each case requires a histopathologic evaluation.

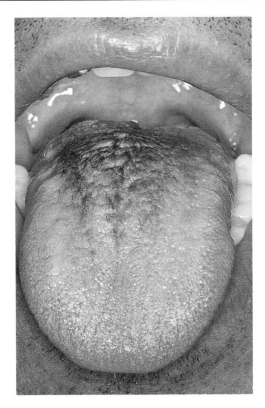

Fig. 2-33 Massive extended hairy tongue of unknown cause.

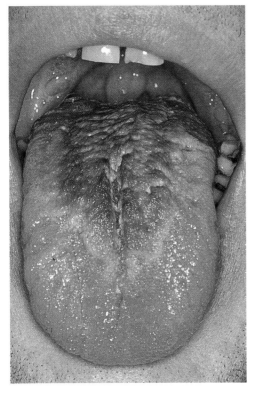

Fig. 2-34 Brownish hairy tongue of unknown cause. The appearance reminds one of a "wet grass patch."

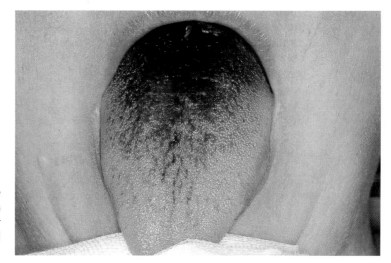

Fig. 2-35   Typical black hairy tongue of unknown cause. The patient was a heavy smoker for years. The condition occurred only recently.

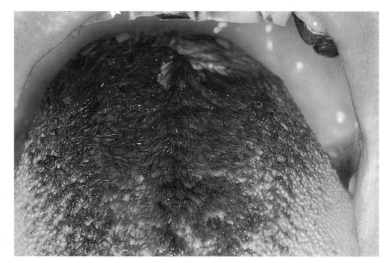

Fig. 2-36   Higher magnification of Fig. 2-35. The greatest changes take place in the median region and decrease in intensity toward the margins and tip of the tongue.

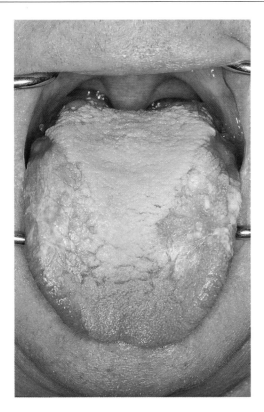

Fig. 2-37 Under a hairy tongue caused by antibacterial therapy are leukoplakial changes of the dorsum of the tongue. The whitish, hairy tongue disappeared within 3 weeks after termination of antibiotic therapy.

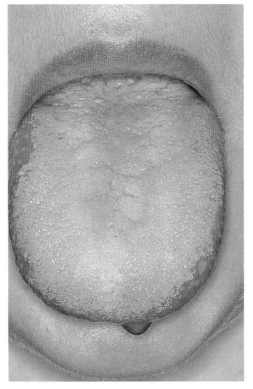

Fig. 2-38 Hairy tongue that has persisted for 1 month in a young patient. Heavy, chronic recurring herpes scales.

Chapter 3

Nevi and Systemic Nevoid Abnormalities of Neurocutaneous Localization (Phakomatoses) in the Maxillofacial Area

Nevi
  Pigmented nevi
  Organoid nevi
    Nevus flammeus

Phakomatoses
  Encephalofacial angiomatosis (Sturge-Weber syndrome)
  Angio-osteohypertrophy syndrome (Klippel-Trenaunay syndrome)
  von Hippel-Lindau disease
  Tuberous sclerosis (Bourneville's disease)
  Neurofibromatosis (von Recklinghausen's disease)
  Multiple endocrine neoplasia
  Basal cell nevus syndrome (Gorlin-Goltz syndrome)

Nevi

Nevi (birth marks) are circumscribed, benign, usually not inherited abnormalities of the skin or mucosa based on an embryonic developmental disturbance. Nevi can appear at birth or later in life. There are two types of nevi. *Pigmented nevi* can be divided into junctional nevi, compound nevi, and interdermal nevi. *Organoid nevi* can be divided depending on the predominant type of tissue: epithelial nevi (e.g., sebaceous glands nevi), connective tissue nevi, and blood vessel nevi. Within the blood vessel nevi, port wine (nevi flammei) are the most common and of major differential diagnostic importance in the maxillofacial region, because they can be combined with other malformations that cannot be observed by the naked eye.

Pigmented nevi

Pigmented nevi that are located on the skin in the areas that the dentist examines or are part of a syndrome that manifests itself in the maxillo-facial region will be discussed briefly.

Lentigo simplex is a small spot, sharply limited, of dark brown hyperpigmentation of the skin caused by increased deposit of pigment with an increase of the melanocytes in the basal cell layer. These pigmented lesions can attain the size of a lentil. They occur singly, in groups, or are diffused over the whole body, and can be found in all age groups. They do not show any preference to skin exposed to the sun and unlike freckles develop independently of ultraviolet radiation. As partial manifestations of a syndrome, there are lentigo-type hyper-pigmentations in characteristic diffusion and location, as in len-tigopolyposis (Peutz-Jeghers syndrome; see chapter 4).

Cafe-au-lait spots can appear singly or in groups (e.g., in neurofib-romatosis) but are not present on the mucosa. They have an even light-brown color and are usually larger than 1.5 cm. They appear in early childhood and become larger with body growth. They are caused by an increased deposit of pigment as well as an increased number of melanocytes in the basal layer. In some cases, the number of melanocytes may be normal. If the cafe-au-lait spot contains nevus cell nevi in a splash pattern of dark pigmented cells, the clinical picture is that of a *nevus spilus.*

Classical examples of dermal melanocytic nevi are those described in chapter 4 as *blue nevus.* Nevi of special forms of this congenital condition are usually resorbed by the time the individual reaches puberty. Mongolian spots (over the sacrum) as well as the nevi that appear in children or young adults are called *nevi of Ito* and *nevi of Ota.* The latter that are in the area supplied by the first two branches of the trigeminal nerve occur with an additional blue-black pigmentation of the conjunctiva and iris and in this way indicate a systemic develop-mental defect (oculodermal melanocytosis). The oral mucosa rarely has a blue-black pigmentation.

Nevus cell nevi are composed of nevus cells (nevocytes) that normally are not components of the skin. The nevus cells also have the ability to form melanin, are located in the upper area of the dermis, and probably develop from epidermal melanocytes. Depending on loca-tion, they can be divided into three types. As a result of intraepidermal proliferation of melanocytes at the dermoepithelial border, there is the *junctional nevus.* According to the so-called trickle theory, the cells arrive at limiting layers of the corium and form new nests there *(compound nevus).* If there are nests only in the corium without connection to the epidermis, the lesion is an *intradermal nevus.* A special form is the *congenital giant pigmented nevus* (Fig. 3-12).

Nevus cell nevi can be congenital or can develop during life and gradually enlarge. With aging there is often regression. From the dermatologic viewpoint it is estimated that each white adult usually has 20 nevus cell nevi that can be formed anywhere on the skin or the mucocutaneous borders. Nevus cell nevi are usually small (less than 5 mm) and flat or only slightly raised. Intensity of pigmentation varies and ranges from dark brown to light-skin color.

A special problem in relation to a possible malignant change can be found in nevi formed during puberty or young adulthood, when first discovered in the oral cavity. *Dysplastic nevus cell nevi* can be distinguished clinically by their unusually large size, indistinct borders, and irregular pigmentation. Histologic findings demonstrate different levels of severity of the dysplasia. Some forms are considered precursors or markers of malignant melanomas. People with a family history of dysplastic nevus syndrome (multiple dysplastic nevi) or a positive history of melanoma are considered in particular danger of having a malignant melanoma.

Organoid nevi

The main organoid nevi are the blood vessel nevi. Isolated lesions as well as the partial manifestations of vascular phakomatoses have, in principle, a similar etiopathogenesis.

Also important to the dentist are the epithelial nevi, for example, the sebaceous nevi as a partial manifestation of tuberous sclerosis.

Nevus flammeus; port-wine nevus (ICD-DA 759.68)

Nevus flammeus is a sharply circumscribed condition that is usually unilateral at the skin surface and of varying size. The color varies from light red to wine-red color. This is due to the many enlarged blood vessels, the level of oxygenation of the blood, and the position of the lesion. The lesion changes color under pressure of a glass spatula. There is no vessel proliferation as seen in a true vascular tumor, but rather vascular ectasia. There are transitional forms between typical nevus flammeus and actual vascular tumors (capillary or cavernous hemangioma).

Median, symmetrically distributed birth marks with a predilection for the back of the head and neck region ("stork bite") or the middle of the forehead or the base of the nose are very rarely associated with visceral or skeletal abnormalities. The congenital lesions usually regress or fade during the first 2 years of life.

The lateral asymmetric forms of nevus flammeus on the face usually show unilateral location along the distribution of the trigeminal nerve, particularly of the second branch (Fig. 3-1) and also involve a part of the mucosa of the mouth (Fig. 3-2). This vascular lesion grows with growth of the body and continues to enlarge even after the individual is fully grown.

In dental extractions when there is an angiomatous lesion of the jaw there is the possibility of serious bleeding complications.

Phakomatoses

Phakomatosis (from the Greek *phakos:* pea) is the collective concept for complex congenital abnormalities with neurocutaneous localizations. *Hamartias* are limited developmental abnormalities caused by a defective combination of normal tissue components; they are the consequence of an abnormal development of embryonic material and do not show autonomous growth. If the defective structure assumes a tumorous growth, it is a *hamartoma.*

This chapter considers the main findings and possible differential diagnoses of many clinical syndromes with manifestations in the maxillofacial region and of their many abortive forms. The first two

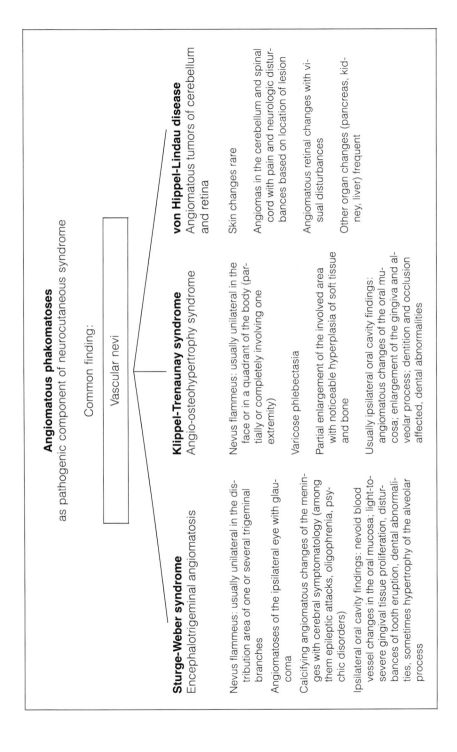

Angiomatous phakomatoses
as pathogenic component of neurocutaneous syndrome

Common finding:

Vascular nevi

Sturge-Weber syndrome
Encephalotrigeminal angiomatosis

Nevus flammeus: usually unilateral in the distribution area of one or several trigeminal branches

Angiomatoses of the ipsilateral eye with glaucoma

Calcifying angiomatous changes of the meninges with cerebral symptomatology (among them epileptic attacks, oligophrenia, psychic disorders)

Ipsilateral oral cavity findings: nevoid blood vessel changes in the oral mucosa; light-to-severe gingival tissue proliferation, disturbances of tooth eruption, dental abnormalities, sometimes hypertrophy of the alveolar process

Klippel-Trenaunay syndrome
Angio-osteohypertrophy syndrome

Nevus flammeus: usually unilateral in the face or in a quadrant of the body (partially or completely involving one extremity)

Varicose phlebectasia

Partial enlargement of the involved area with noticeable hyperplasia of soft tissue and bone

Usually ipsilateral oral cavity findings: angiomatous changes of the oral mucosa; enlargement of the gingiva and alveolar process; dentition and occlusion affected, dental abnormalities

von Hippel-Lindau disease
Angiomatous tumors of cerebellum and retina

Skin changes rare

Angiomas in the cerebellum and spinal cord with pain and neurologic disturbances based on location of lesion

Angiomatous retinal changes with visual disturbances

Other organ changes (pancreas, kidney, liver) frequent

phakomatoses, which are caused by vascular nevi (angiomatoses), are always accompanied by soft tissue and bone hypertrophies, which can also involve the oral cavity. A survey of the symptoms of the angiomatous phakomatoses can be seen in the table on page 79.

Encephalofacial (encephalocutaneous) angiomatosis (Sturge-Weber syndrome) (ICD-DA 759.60)

Encephalofacial angiomatosis is a defective neurocutaneous development that takes place early in embryonic life and is characterized by a combination of vascular malformations on the skin and mucosa in the meninges and in the eye.

The main symptoms are:
- *Nevus flammeus:* usually unilateral, spread over an area supplied by one or more rami of the trigeminal nerve (Figs. 3-3 and 3-5). The angiomatous changes often manifest themselves ipsilaterally on the oral mucosa (Figs. 3-4 and 3-6). The gingiva may show slight-to-marked hyperplasia.
- *Glaucoma of the eye of the affected side* (Figs. 3-3, 3-5, and 3-14): this occurs in a significant number of patients due to angiomatous change of the choroid, often with loss of sight.
- *Headache* and sometimes *atypical neuralgias,* which cannot be explained otherwise.
- *Epileptic attacks:* can start during youth or later in life. They are caused by calcified capillary and venous angiomas in the pia mater of the brain (most commonly in the occipital area).
- *Mental developmental regressions* leading to *oligophrenia* in about one-third of cases.

Depending on the time of onset of the embryologic defect, there are often cases of incomplete syndromes (Fig. 3-7). Abnormalities of dental eruption are frequently noted in the area of the nervus. Discrete enamel hypoplasias are also possible, as are dental dysplasias and aplasias (Fig. 3-8).

In relation to enlargement of the gingiva and the alveolar process, there are transitional changes to the angio-osteohypertrophic syndrome.

Angio-osteohypertrophy syndrome (Klippel-Trenaunay syndrome) (ICD-DA 759.68)

This nonhereditary syndrome is characterized by the following symptoms:

- *Vascular nevi:* color depending on vascularity and duration, usually unilateral in the face or, more frequently, uneven distribution in one quadrant of the body (involving one extremity in part or completely); hence, the name "quadrant syndrome."
- *Venous varicosities:* various findings reminiscent of a hemangioma.
- *Partial enlargement with hyperplasia of soft tissue and bone* in the area affected by the blood vessel defect.

The combination of localized tissue hypertrophy (Fig. 3-11) and blood vessel changes, which may also involve the oral mucosa (Figs. 3-9 and 3-10), may lead to noticeable occlusal dysfunction and a more or less marked asymmetry of the facial bones. Often there is an early pattern of tooth eruption.

Incomplete forms (Fig. 3-10) or syndrome variants (vascular nevi on one side, hypertrophy and varicosities on the other side) can in some instances create diagnostic problems. The peripuberty phase brings about rapid development of the syndrome. After puberty, the changes generally do not progress further.

von Hippel-Lindau disease (ICD-DA 759.68)

This rare phakomatosis, probably inherited in a dominant form, involves multiple blood vessel defects primarily involving the retina, the cerebellum, and the spinal cord. Angiomatous changes may be found in the kidneys, pancreas, and liver. Skin findings are very rare. There are no typical changes in the oral cavity.

Tuberous sclerosis (Bourneville's disease) (ICD-DA 759.5)

A major symptom of this dominantly inherited progressive disease is *sebaceous nevi,* which are angiofibromas with numerous embedded sebaceous glands *(adenoma sebaceum).* They appear on the skin as yellowish to yellow-brown elevations the size of a pinhead to that of millet corn on an inflammation-free background. On the face, the sebaceous adenomas are primarily present in the perioral region:

nasolabial folds, mental sulcus (Figs. 3-15 and 3-19). In 10% to 15% of all cases, there are changes of the oral mucosa and lips in the form of small bumps, pigmentation of the mucous membrane, and angiofibromas of varying size (Fig. 3-16). The affected region of the gingiva has a more or less bumpy appearance (Fig. 3-17). Variant flat lesions are present on the palate, cheeks, and tongue (Fig. 3-19).

Other symptoms, in addition to single cafe-au-lait spots, are leaf-like hypopigmentations, connective tissue nevi of the lumbosacral area, and angiofibromatous nodules in the area surrounding the nail plate of fingers and toes *(periungual fibroma)* (Fig. 3-18).

Numerous organs in addition to the skin can be affected. The prognosis for the fully developed syndrome depends on the neurologic sequence of the tuberous cerebellar sclerosis (glia hamartomas, intracranial calcifications) with epileptic attacks, spastic paralysis, and progressive personality disintegration.

Neurofibromatosis (von Recklinghausen's disease) (ICD-DA 237.7 and ICD-M 9540/1)

In neurofibromatosis there is a phakomatosis with neurocutaneous localization and the following clinical findings:

- *Cafe-au-lait spots:* appear at birth or in the first year as five or more pigmented defects larger than 0.5 cm in size. In adults, six or more 1.5 cm in size can be found. This is a pathognomonic finding of neurofibromatosis.
- *Multiple neurofibromas* of the skin (cutaneous, subcutaneous), mucosa, and bone with possible deformation of the affected tissue.
- *Neurofibromatous changes of the central nervous system* with the following neurologic and psychological disturbances.

In one-third of individuals, the disease is inherited as a dominant asymptomatic neurofibromatosis. Another third requests medical help for reasons of esthetics. One-third of patients have primary neurologic problems with an unfavorable prognosis. The knotty, soft, brownish or light-skin colored neurofibromas of varying number, size, and appearance can be located along the peripheral nerves and be limited to circumscribed regions of the skin (Fig. 3-20) or can be distributed over the whole integument. Poorly defined, flat growth in subcutaneous tissue of the face may cause a patchy elephantiasis (molluscum fibrosum) (Fig. 3-23), which finally deforms the face (Fig. 3-22). A picture of marked hemihypertrophy of the face with participation of the bone is also possible.

Intraorally, enlargement of the gingiva can take place (Figs. 3-24 and 3-25) with lingual localization of the growth and macroglossia. In edentulous areas of the jaw, the neurofibromas must be differentiated from prosthodontic irritative hyperplasias (Fig. 3-21). In general, neurofibromatosis findings in the oral cavity are difficult to evaluate.

When impairment of speech or chewing function occurs, palliative measures include surgical correction.

Multiple endocrine neoplasia

Previously, multiple endocrine neoplasms (MEN) were considered endocrine polyadenomatosis. This genetic dysplastic syndrome consists of synchronous or metachronous appearance of hyperplasias or neoplasias, benign or malignant, in several endocrine organs. The multiple endocrine neoplasias are divided into:

- Type 1 *(Wermer's syndrome)* with benign parathyroid gland tumors, islet cell tumors, and hypophysis adenomas with varied frequency.
- Type 2a *(Sipple's syndrome)* with appearance of a medullary thyroid carcinoma (C-cell carcinoma), a pheochromocytoma (hyperplasia of the adrenal glands), and parathyroid hyperplasia.
- Type 2b *(multiple mucosal neuroma syndrome [MMN])* where in addition to gastrointestinal neuromatosis there is development of plexiform mucous membrane neuromas followed by life-threatening medullary thyroid carcinoma (C-cell carcinoma) and pheochromocytoma.

The multiple mucous membrane neuromas appearing only in type 2b in midface distribution are the first and earliest manifestations and therefore are a key finding of this disease. Early determination is vital to the prognosis. Multiple endocrine neoplasias can be congenital but usually develop in early childhood and are usually found on the lips (Figs. 3-26 and 3-27), tongue (anterior third—Fig. 3-27), mucosa of the cheeks, and eyelids. On the lips the neuromas appear as swellings, which give children and youths a characteristic appearance (Fig. 3-26). Dental findings appear before the eighth year of life. Aside from the regions already mentioned, the nasal and pharyngeal mucous membranes as well as conjunctiva and cornea (Fig. 3-28) can be affected.

The common embryonal derivation of the different affected cell populations of the neural tube points out that multiple endocrine neoplasias and a neuroendocrinal dysplasia syndrome are involved. The inheritance pattern of the hereditary familial disease is not yet sufficiently explained.

Basal cell nevus syndrome (Gorlin-Goltz syndrome) (ICD-DA 759.62)

The basal cell nevus syndrome may fall in the area of surveillance of the dentist. It is sometimes found in the *multiple nevoid basaliomas* of the skin (especially in the face) and *multiple keratocysts* in the jaw region (more often in the mandible than maxilla) and which often recur. Often associated with these major symptoms are degenerative or dysplastic findings such as rib anomalies (split ribs), hypertelorism (abnormally separated eyes), intracranial calcifications, and other changes. The disease is inherited by autosomal-dominant inheritance and first appears in childhood. Besides the fully developed syndrome, many abortive syndrome forms are described. Recognition and therapy require interdisciplinary management.

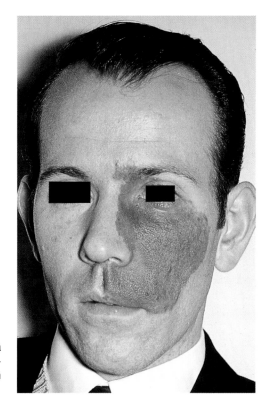

Fig. 3-1   Nevus flammeus in a 30-year-old man, with the distribution area the second division of the left trigeminal nerve.

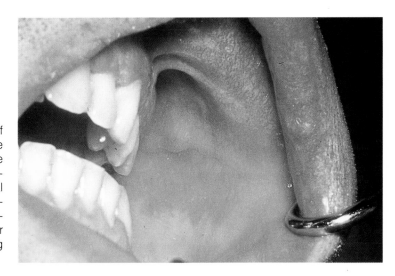

Fig. 3-2   Intraoral findings of the patient in Fig. 3-1 at the same time of examination. The vascular nevus (vascular hyperplasia) is seen on the oral mucosa supplied by the maxillary division of the left trigeminal nerve. However, the color contrast here is less striking than on the skin.

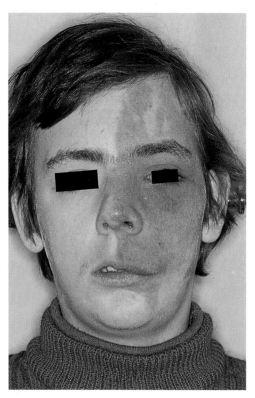

Fig. 3-3   Encephalotrigeminal angiomatosis   (Sturge-Weber syndrome) in a 17-year-old patient. The distribution area of the second division of the trigeminal nerve is completely affected and that of the first and third division incompletely affected. A predominantly midface hyperplasia is noticeable (i.e., upper lip, nose, and orbital area). The left eye is blind; there are no neurologic symptoms.

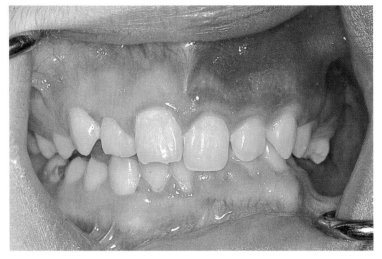

Fig. 3-4   Intraoral findings of the patient in Fig. 3-3 at the same time of examination. There is nevus flammeus with metameric distribution in the left maxilla that is enlarged with occlusal interference. Note the gingival enlargement in the mandible.

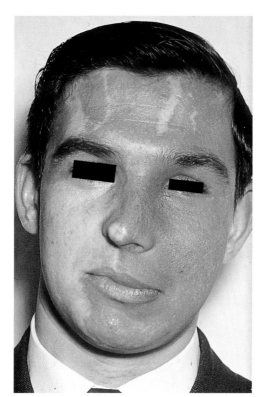

Fig. 3-5   Massive vascular nevus, located chiefly on the left side of the face—a partial manifestation of encephalotrigeminal angiomatosis (Sturge-Weber syndrome). The angiomatous involvement of the left ocular area necessitated enucleation and replacement with an artificial eye. The lesion, also involving the central nervous system, led to convulsive seizures in this 24-year-old man, who had no psychological abnormalities at the time of examination.

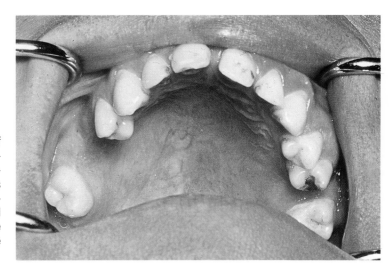

Fig. 3-6   Intraoral findings of the patient in Fig. 3-5. Corresponding to the facial angiomatosis, nevoid vascular changes also appear on the oral mucosa. Malocclusion and facial asymmetry resulted from the associated hypertrophy of the related jaws.

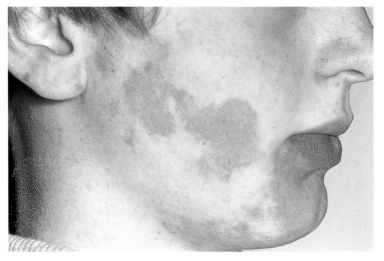

Fig. 3-7 Abortive type of Sturge-Weber syndrome in a 14-year-old girl. There are relatively pale vascular skin nevi in the parts of the region supplied by the mandibular division of the right trigeminal nerve. A moderate angiomatous enlargement of the lower lip is also present.

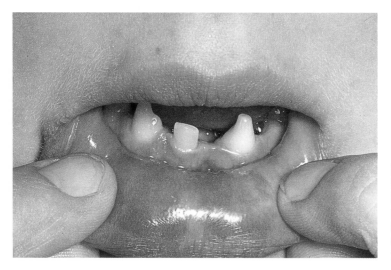

Fig. 3-8 Intraoral findings illustrate the involvement of the lower lip and oral mucosa in the patient in Fig. 3-7. Note the aplasia and dysplasia of individual teeth, a nonobligate symptom in this syndrome.

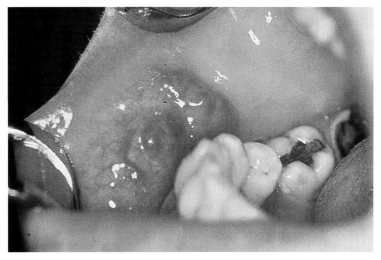

Fig. 3-9   Intraoral findings in a 31-year-old woman with angio-osteohypertrophy syndrome (Klippel-Trenaunay syndrome). Note varicose angiomatosis of the right cheek and marked osteophypertrophy (gigantism) of the right side of the mandible. Segmentally arranged vascular nevi of the skin are found on the same side.

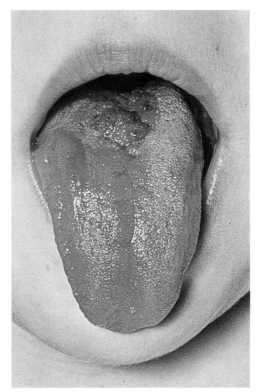

Fig. 3-10   Circumscribed vascular hyperplasia and dysplasia on the right side of tongue. Partial manifestation of angio-osteohypertrophy syndrome in a 6-year-old girl.

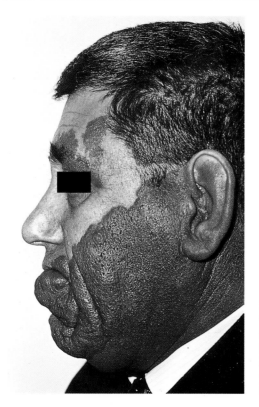

Fig. 3-11 Extensive nevoid varicosities located on the left side of the face, head, and neck with macrocheilia of the lower lip. Partial manifestation of angio-osteohypertrophy syndrome in a 45-year-old man.

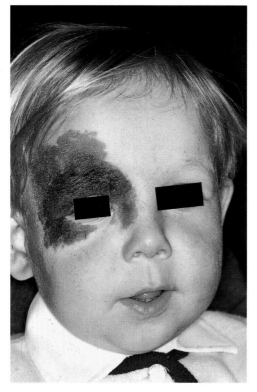

Fig. 3-12 Large congenital nevus cell nevus (congenital giant pigmented nevus) on the forehead and periorbital region. If the surface shows papillomatous or wart-type changes, this congenital deformity is designated a *nevus pigmentosus et papillomatous.* A pigmented nevus containing hair is designated a *giant hairy nevus.* Not only blood vessel nevi but pigmented nevi too can be localized on the face, assuming different shapes and sizes.

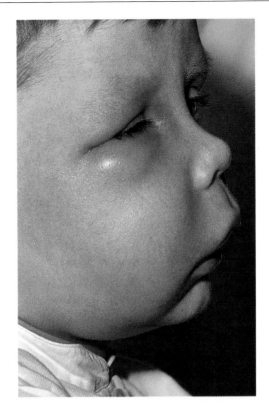

Fig. 3-13   Inflamed soft tissue of an acute osteomyelitis of the right maxilla in a 6-year-old boy. The diagnosis was made more difficult because of the nevus flammeus associated with the area of the second trigeminal brach, which had been treated 2 years previously with radioactive materials. Other differential diagnoses are discussed in chapter 7.

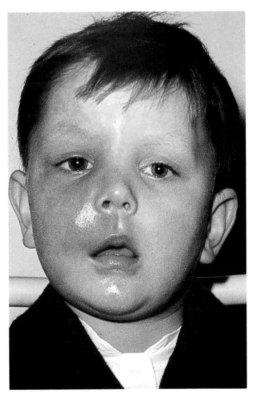

Fig. 3-14   The boy in Fig. 3-13 after 2 weeks. After resolution of the acute inflammatory process there is reappearance of the earlier finding of the irradiated nevus flammeus as a partial manifestation of Sturge-Weber syndrome. The boy has neurologic findings (epileptic seizures); the eye is almost blind.

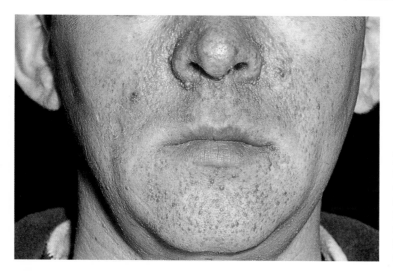

Fig. 3-15   Typical localization of angiofibromas in a 42-year-old man with tuberous sclerosis also involving the brain (Bourneville's disease). The perioral region is affected predominantly in the nasolabial fold and mental sulcus.

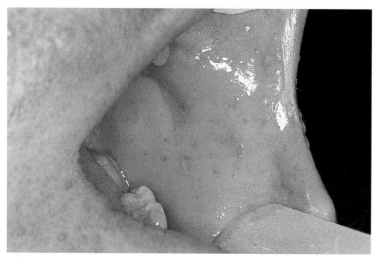

Fig. 3-16   The patient in Fig. 3-15 at the same examination time. The oral mucosa of the cheek has many flat angiofibromas of varying size.

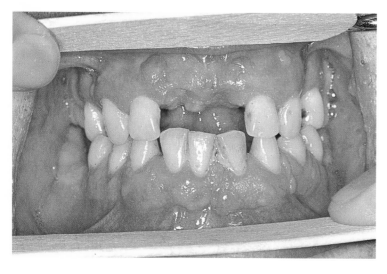

Fig. 3-17   The patient in Figs. 3-15 and 3-16 at the same examination time. The findings are small angiofibromatous nodules in the gingiva.

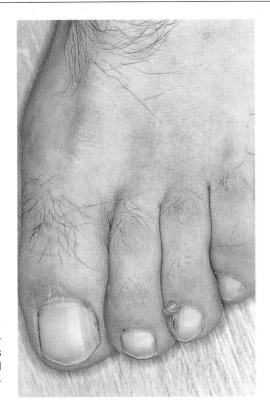

Fig. 3-18　The patient in Figs. 3-15 to 3-17 at the same examination time. Note fibromatous nodules bulging from the nail bed of the toes (Koenen tumors).

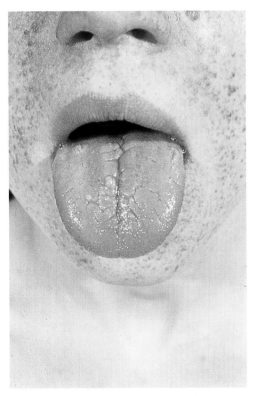

Fig. 3-19　Bourneville's disease in a child with typical localization of the angiofibromas in the facial region. Several small fibromas that are part of the syndrome are on the dorsum of the tongue.

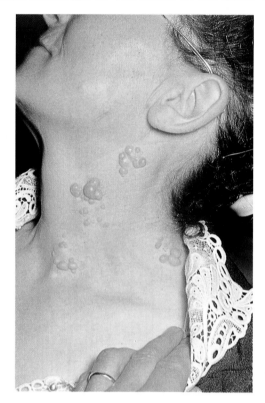

Fig. 3-20   Neurofibromatosis (von Recklinghausen's disease) in a 53-year-old woman. Nodular tumors are arranged in groups, and there are discrete café-au-lait spots. This form with metameric distribution is a variant of neurofibromatosis.

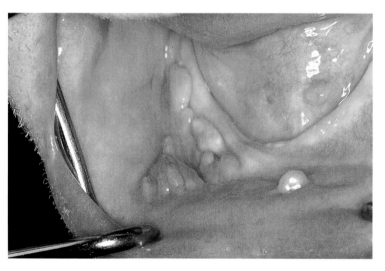

Fig. 3-21   Intraoral findings of neurofibromatosis. The knotty and cylindrical patchy neurofibromas in the mouth vestibule and in the mucosa of the alveolar area of the edentulous mandible must be differentiated from a prosthesis-induced hyperplasia.

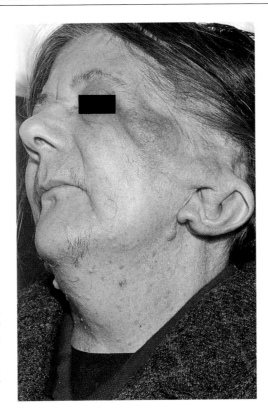

Fig. 3-22   Facial manifestation of neurofibromatosis. Aside from several neurofibromas of the skin of varying sizes, there is focal elephantiasis of so-called molluscum fibrosum, which has caused a deformity of the face and the outer ear.

Note

Phakomatosis must be evaluated, supervised, and sometimes treated by a multidisciplinary team because of the variability of the findings involving different organ systems.

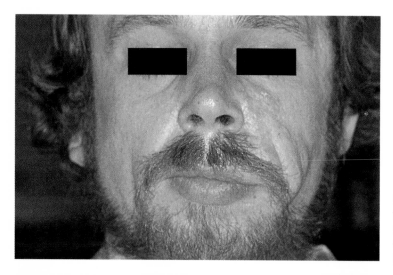

Fig. 3-23   Facial manifestations of a left-sided neurofibromatosis with enlargement and
early elephantiasis of the soft
parts in a 43-year-old man.

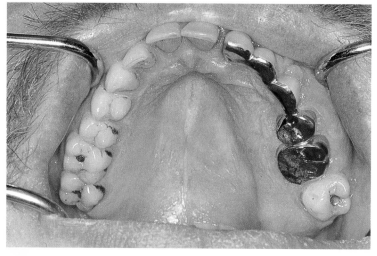

Fig. 3-24   Intraoral findings of
the patient in Fig. 3-23 at the
same time of examination. Hypertrophy of the left maxilla and
enlargement of the bone of the
alveolar process.

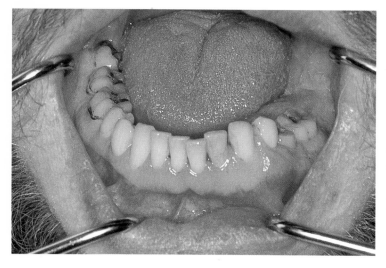

Fig. 3-25   Intraoral findings of
the patient in Figs. 3-23 and
3-24. The lateral dentulous
areas of the left mandible also
clearly show the neurofibromatous changes. The findings
must be differentiated from a fibrous gingival hyperplasia (see
chapter 15).

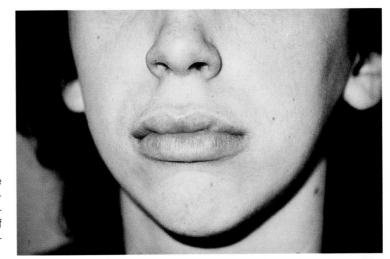

Fig. 3-26   Multiple endocrine neoplasia type 2b in a 16-year-old girl. Note the typical midfacial enlargement, particularly of the upper lip, because of mucous membrane neuromas.

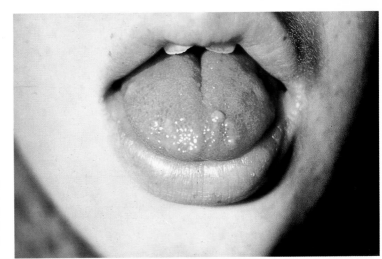

Fig. 3-27   Multiple endocrine neoplasia type 2b in an 8-year-old girl. Mucous membrane neuromas of the maxilla and tongue tip can be seen as bumpy elevations.

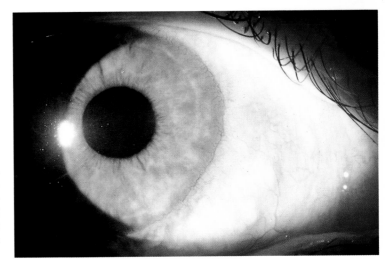

Fig. 3-28   Multiple endocrine neoplasia type 2b. The mucous membrane neuromas can also be found in the eyelids, the cornea, and conjunctiva where they form bulgings. They can easily be diagnosed in the corneal region with the aid of a slit-lamp. Multiple mucous membrane neuromas in midfacial distribution are the first detectable clinical symptoms suggesting multiple endocrine neoplasia type 2b.

Chapter 4

Endogenous and Exogenous Pigmentations of the Oral Mucous Membrane and Perioral Region

Endogenous pigmentations
    Melanin pigmentations within physiologic conditions
    Melanin pigmentations as an accompanying symptom in
        other major changes and systemic diseases
    Circumscribed (hyper-) pigmentations of other origins
    Depigmentation
    Pigmented nevi of the oral mucosa
        Nevus cell nevi
        Blue nevus

Exogenous pigmentations
    Gingival pigmentation resulting from toxic effect of heavy
        metals
    Tattoos
        Amalgam tattoo
        Self-inflicted wounds with colored pencils
        Ritual, deliberate tattooing

The color of the oral mucosa is determined by several factors, including the distention, ramification, and filling of the blood vessels, the chemical and physical composition of the blood, and the thickness and degree of keratinization of the oral mucosal epithelium. Changes in color of the oral mucosa can take place because of deposits of particles of colored foreign material, which have their own color as either a uniform spot or as distinct speckles. They are considered pigmentations, and their origin can be endogenous or exogenous.

Pigmentations of the oral mucosa occur less frequently than pigmentations of the outer skin, and their findings are not as varied. Their significance for the dentist is primarily in differential diagnosis.

Endogenous pigmentations

Endogenous pigments include, among others, products originating from blood, muscle, and bile (e.g., hemoglobin, myoglobin, and bilirubin), but those of major interest are the degradation products of melanin. The following discussion is limited, therefore, to some of the more important melanin pigmentations.

Melanocytes as pigment-forming cells are derived from the neural crest. During early embryonic development, the precursors of melanocytes—melanoblasts—migrate from the neural crest to pre-determined positions of the skin, among others, where during the eighth and tenth weeks of gestation they differentiate into dendritic melanocytes. At this point they can also be demonstrated in the oral mucosa.

The morphologic and biochemical development of melanin production and delivery is well understood. Regulation of the activity of the melanocytes and the biosynthesis of melanin depends—over and above genetic conditions—on the systemic control acting through the hypophysis hormones (adrenocorticotropic hormone and melanocyte-stimulating hormone) as well as on local control. Under the effect of copper-containing oxidase, tyrosinase, insoluble melanin is synthesized from the amino acid tyrosine in several steps with dihydroxyphenylalanine (dopa) as intermediary. The finished melanin is formed through coupling with protein. Via cell extensions (dendrites), the melanocyte delivers the material that has been synthesized and stored in the cytoplasmic organelles (melanosomes) to the neighboring basal epithelial cells (keratinocytes). Depending on the number and depth of the melanin deposits in the tissue, the density of pigmentation in the oral mucous membrane varies from a deep blue-black to a light gray-brown.

The number of melanocytes is not influenced by sex or race. In dark-skinned people, the melanosomes are larger and, because of a high activity level, are completely melanized.

In the skin, there can be many different melanin-determined changes such as hyperpigmentation, hypopigmentation, and depigmentation, but the oral mucosa is different. Here, the clinician must remember that some variability in the degree of melanin pigmentation may represent physiologic variation. Furthermore, increase of melanin pigmentation may represent a symptom caused by another lesion of the mucosa or by systemic disease, but pigmented nevi are seldom seen on the oral mucosa.

Malignant melanomas that develop from melanocytes are highly malignant tumors of the skin and mucosa and are important in differential diagnosis. They are discussed in chapter 21.

Melanin pigmentations within physiologic conditions

In the clinically pigment-free oral mucosa, there are also melanocytes. Under normal conditions, however, they form no melanin.

Morphologic and biochemical determining factors for melanin formation are always present, so that the clinical manifestation of pigmentation on oral mucous membranes is not exceptional and can definitely be within normal physiologic variations. However, physiologic hyperpigmentation may be mistakenly interpreted as caused by an illness.

Experience shows that physiologic pigmentation forms the major portion of the melanin pigmentations found on the oral mucous membrane. Such physiologic oral mucosa pigmentations appear not only in dark-skinned individuals where they are often very distinct; they can also frequently be seen in light-skinned individuals. They are usually discovered by accident by the patients and cause a certain amount of concern even though they are harmless. Their major importance in differential diagnosis is their distinction from pathologic findings. Their intensity, distribution, and classification vary from individual to individual and can also change with time.

When the gingiva is the primary location, these so-called idiotypic pigmentations can appear as a distinct band, be garland-like, or spotty (Figs. 4-1 to 4-8) and light brown (in superficial locations) to blue-black (in deep locations). Even in cases of spotty pigment deposits, the marginal gingiva generally is not involved. This is an important differential diagnostic criterion with a heavy-metal border, for example in lead poisoning, which is still the most frequent incorrect interpretation of these idiotypic pigmentations (Fig. 4-22).

Circumscribed melanin spots, which are also called melanotic spots, can also appear on the mucosa of the cheeks and lips or on the vermilion of the lip (Fig. 4-9) without clinical significance. In spite of atypical localization and arrangement, this is usually a physiologic variation.

Melanin pigmentations as an accompanying symptom in other major changes and systemic diseases

Melanin pigmentations of the mucosa and lips can be caused by systemic diseases and in some cases can even be an early sign of more important symptoms. Their diagnostic value, however, is often limited, so that suspicion of a systemic disease can be justified only when a typical distribution (e.g., in Peutz-Jeghers syndrome) and/or general symptoms are present.

Pigmentations of the mucous membrane in neuroectodermal dysplasias

The common ectodermal origin of melanocytes and nerve cells may explain certain embryonic developmental defects. In the resulting tissues, both differentiating elements can be affected, and their pathologic changes present a characteristic syndrome.

For the autosomal-dominant inherited Peutz-Jeghers syndrome (ICA-DA 759.63) where there is development of small-intestine polyposis, there are extensive melanin pigmentations of the face with preference for the perioral and periorbital regions.

The pigment spots, which are present at birth or appear in early childhood, resemble freckles although are darker, and are often brown-black and sharply delineated. They do not change under the influence of light, and they show an irregular, splashlike distribution (Fig. 4-10). In general, they are located on the oral mucous membrane (particularly on the lip and cheek, seldom on gingiva, palate, and tongue) as a heavy pigmentation in the form of many dark-brown to brown-black melanin spots. These pea-sized pigmentations on the skin and mucosa usually appear before the development of intestinal polyposis as detectable by radiographic and endoscopic examination. Malignant transformation seldom occurs in the multiple intestinal polyps that are hamartomas. Later in the course of the disease, however, these polyps can become threatening complications because of intestinal bleeding or small bowel invaginations. Therefore, the early detection of this syndrome is important.

The cafe-au-lait-colored spots of the skin in *neurofibromatosis* have already been discussed in chapter 3. Additional spotty melanin pigmentation of the cheek mucosa is frequently reported. Because of their inconstant presence, they do not have great diagnostic importance.

In *Albright's syndrome,* a rare combination of polyostotic fibrous dysplasia, hyperpigmentation of the skin, and precocious puberty, the oral mucous membrane can also have spotty melanin pigmentation. As a single symptom, the relatively nonspecific mucosal findings are not sufficient for a diagnosis.

Pigmentations of the oral mucosa in diseases of endocrine or other origin

In *Addison's disease* (ICD-DA 255.4), there is adrenal cortex insufficiency caused by a bilateral destruction or damage of the adrenal glands with loss of glucocorticoid production. The disease is usually chronic, caused by autoimmune problems, tuberculosis, leukemic infiltrates, or tumor metastases. Due to failure of the feedback mechanism between the adrenal cortex and the hypophysis, there is an increased secretion of adrenocorticotropic hormone (ACTH) and melanocyte-stimulating hormone (MSH) from the hypophysis. This leads to stimulation of melanin formation, which can be seen on the hand as lines of brown color changes (Fig. 4-14). The increasing generalized diffuse hyperpigmentations of the skin ("bronzed disease") initially prefers light-exposed and mechanically stressed regions. Even before the appearance of the brown skin there are usually flat melanin pigmentations on the oral mucosa, which are therefore an important early symptom. Their predominant localizations on the cheek mucosa (Figs. 4-11 and 4-12) or on the dorsum of the tongue (Fig. 4-13) are caused by the additional functional-mechanical stimulation. However, the findings are of variable intensity and can be used only in conjunction with generalized symptoms (e.g., increased muscle weakness, loss of weight, hypotonia, anemia) to formulate a tentative diagnosis.

On the other hand, pigmentations of the oral mucosa in hypophysary-determined Cushing's disease, acromegalia, hypothyroidism, and other endocrine diseases have an even more questionable diagnostic position.

In other systemic diseases, the oral mucous membrane can sometimes be facultatively affected together with hyperpigmentation of the skin. Examples of this are the dark skin color (caused by an increased melanin synthesis) in liver cirrhosis, in storage diseases, in chronic kidney insufficiency where there is an additional deposit of urochrome, as well as in cachexia. In all these conditions, the noticeable pigmentation is a secondary phenomenon irrelevant to diagnosis.

Pigmentations of the oral mucosa in hormonal changing phases

In hormonal changes of the female body during pregnancy there is often increased pigmentation (e.g., at the site of warts, linea fusca, genital organs) known as *chloasma* (ICD-DA 709.0). In the area of the face (forehead, temples, cheeks) during pregnancy there can also be an arrangement of selective symmetrical spotty hyperpigmentations of irregular appearance (Fig. 4-15). These will intensify with exposure to the sun and will regress speedily and spontaneously, as a rule, at the end of the pregnancy. Estrogens are responsible for the increased melanin formation. Similar changes may be seen in women who regularly take ovulation-inhibiting, estrogen-containing pills (*pill-chloasma*). In our experience, this type of hyperpigmentation has not involved the oral mucosa during pregnancy or after lengthy use of hormonal contraceptives.

Not all spotty chloasma-like hyperpigmentations of the face, and particularly of the oral cavity, are caused by hormones. Often they are the result of a skin irritation caused by petroleum jelly components or photosensitivity to cosmetic skin creams (so-called *chloasma cosmeticum*).

Circumscribed (hyper-) pigmentation of other origins

Various local factors can, by their activity on tyrosinase, increase melanin formation through increased oxidation. Remarkable is the erythema caused by ultraviolet irradiation and ionized rays that stimulates melanin formation (indirect pigmentation). The slow UVA (320 nm to 400 nm) influences pigmentation, however, without erythema (direct pigmentation).

Among the chemical compounds worth noting are the phototoxic substances, such as furocumarine, bergamot oil, and eugenol and the perfumes, sprays, creams, mouthwashes, and breath fresheners that contain them. They produce a phototoxic reaction with resulting brownish hyperpigmentation *(berloque dermatitis; perfume dermatitis)* when the contact areas are exposed to light.

Also known are *postinflammatory hyperpigmentations* of the skin, which can appear at the end of zoster (Fig. 4-16) and other inflammatory skin conditions and in particular in scarring dermatoses. These inflammatory conditions also stimulate the melanocyte system with increased production of melanin.

In the oral mucosa, corresponding extensive findings are rarely found (see Fig. 16-31). There are also reports that point to a correlation between the frequency of melanin pigmentations of the gingiva and inflammatory alveolar diseases and smoking habits (smoke melanosis). There is the possibility of an inflammatory or chemical stimulation of melanin synthesis of the oral mucosa similar to that observed in the skin.

Depigmentation

Depigmentations result from the lack or loss of the normal melanin pigmentation-producing ability of the skin. The disturbance in pigment content can be congenital or acquired and can be local or generalized.

The most remarkable example is *albinism* (ICD 270.2). In this inherited disease, the melanocytes are present in the same number as in normal individuals, but because of an enzyme defect (genetic blockage of the metabolism through tyrosinase deficiency), their melanin-forming function is disturbed. They remain metabolically inactive. Complete absence of melanin in skin, hair, and eyes is found along with other symptoms in total albinism (Fig. 4-17). There are also partial forms, which show a white piebald of the skin or formation of a white hair curl. The mucous membranes are of normal color, and here, albinism is not noticeable.

An acquired pigment loss is *vitiligo* (ICD-DA 709.0). The insidious onset of this disease of unknown etiology (autoimmune mechanisms are considered) develops with damage to the melanocytes in circumscribed, sharply limited, very irregular white spots. The foci increase in number, join together, and then appear as bizarre patches. In the often-hyperpigmented border zone, the cosmetic disturbance is even more intense and contrasts with the adjacent involved skin. Preferentially affected are the physiologically more highly pigmented skin regions of the face, neck, dorsum of the hand, anus, and genital regions. The depigmentations can appear generalized or limited to certain skin regions (Fig. 4-18). The mucous membrane is always unchanged. Circumscribed depigmentations as signs of a systemic disorder with decrease of the melanin formation can develop after inflammatory dermatoses (e.g., lupus erythematosus, lichen planus, medication exanthemas, zoster). These are usually temporary changes, which—as in postinflammatory hyperpigmentation with which they can associate themselves—can be observed relatively frequently in the mouth and other facial regions. These findings, called *leukodermas,* regress after healing of the dermatoses. On the other hand, there is damage caused by ionizing irradiation as well as atrophies, leading to chronic inflammatory skin diseases with permanent depigmentation.

Pigmented nevi of the oral mucosa

While pigmented nevi of the skin can be demonstrated in everyone, they are much rarer on the oral mucosa. Nevertheless, observations made during the past years demonstrate that their appearance in the oral cavity is somewhat more frequent than previously thought. This is valid for the types described in the literature as intramucosal or intramucous nevus cell nevus and blue nevus.

Because of their usual small size and the absence of pain, they are usually not considered important by the patient and often are not noticed in the dental examination or are simply considered a harmless incidental finding.

Junctional nevus (ICD-M 8740/0); intramucosal nevus (ICD-M 8750/0); compound nevus (ICD-M 8760/0)

Nevus cell nevi are discussed in chapter 3. Depending on the position of the small nests or row arrangement of nevus cells in the tissue, there are three types that can be distinguished in the oral mucosa: the junctional nevus (located on the border between epithelium and connective tissue), the compound nevus (located on the epithelium-connective tissue border with involvement of the lamina propria), and the so-called intramucosal (intramucous) nevus cell nevi (located in deeper connective tissue of the lamina propria without contact with the epithelium).

These oral intramucosal nevus cell nevi are most frequently encountered on the mucosa of the hard palate (Fig. 4-19) and on the cheek mucosa. They are usually slightly raised (but can also be located on the level of the mucosa) and are sharply limited from the adjacent mucosa. Their pigment formation is different. As a rule, it is brown to dirty gray-brown, or sometimes a shiny black color. Pigmentation can be absent.

Compared to intramucosal nevus cell nevi, the compound type on the mucous membrane is rarer, and the junctional type is observed only in a few cases.

For differential diagnosis one must first consider other types of melanotic spots, amalgam tattoos, angiomas (which empty under glass spatula pressure), and an early malignant melanoma (see chapter 21).

Even if according to present knowledge nevus cell nevi only rarely transform into a malignant melanoma on the oral mucosa, prophylactic excision in toto is recommended because mechanical irritation cannot be ignored in the oral cavity. For this reason the patient should be referred to a specialist.

Blue nevus (ICD-M 8780.0)

A blue nevus is a tumorlike formation of pigment-forming melanocytes located deep in the connective tissue of the skin or mucous membrane, which became stuck midway through the embryonic migration from the neural crest to the predetermined skin and mucous membrane region. Three forms can be distinguished on the skin: simple, cell-rich, and a combination blue nevus. The combined form (blue nevus plus nevus cell nevus) frequently appears on the face but only seldom on the oral mucosa. The simple blue nevus is made up of spindle cells—fibroblastlike or with dendrites. It consists of some melanocytes containing much pigment, which is located, together with many melanophages, between collagen fiber bundles. Clinically they are the second most frequently occurring of all oral nevi. They are found as blue nevi that are slightly raised nodules (at the most pea-sized) of firm consistency. Typically they are steel-blue to blue-black in color (Fig. 4-20), hence their name.

Blue nevi, which intraorally occur primarily on the palate, usually appear during childhood or young adulthood. They are seldom congenital and represent benign nevoid abnormalities. Malignant transformation of a blue nevus is rare in the skin. Transformation in a malignant blue nevus on the oral mucosa has thus far not been described, to the best of our knowledge.

Differential diagnosis must include small venous angiomas and an implanted foreign body.

Exogenous pigmentations

Exogenous pigmentation involves the storage of foreign bodies or color-releasing substances in the skin or mucous membrane. Exogenous pigmentation occurs in different ways. The determining substances arrive in the body through the gastrointestinal tract, respiratory tract, or parenterally. They move from the blood-lymph vessel system to the area of manifestation, where they are stored in the tissue. This is the case in intoxication with heavy metals.

Foreign bodies and color-releasing substances can also enter the connective tissue due to wounds or tattooing.

Gingival pigmentation resulting from toxic effect of heavy metals (ICD-DA 984, 985.0, 985.8)

The use of mercury and bismuth medications for the treatment of chronic diseases (e.g., syphilis) has long ago been abandoned. Prolonged application of those substances can cause chronic poisoning with deposition of mercury or bismuth sulfide in the inflamed gingiva. In particular, blue-gray to blue-black color changes (e.g., *mercury margin, bismuth margin;* Fig. 4-21) of the marginal attachment can occur. Thanks to better supervision of hygiene, appropriate protective measures, and more accurate diagnosis, these findings are rare today even among workers who are involved in the mining of, or the industrial application of, these metals.

The lead margin—a sign of a chronic lead poisoning in the past—is today an exceptional finding. It can be found in workers in lead mines and lead mills, but only when industrial hygiene procedures have been grossly disregarded.

Heavy-metal sulfide deposits such as lead sulfide appear only in the oral cavity in patients with totally inadequate oral hygiene. Their location is nearly always associated with the inflammation of altered marginal gingiva (Fig. 4-22). In edentulous jaws, these changes are not present.

The frequency and importance of heavy-metal margins have been grossly exaggerated. Such suspicion is warranted only when, according to the patient's history and accompanying general symptoms, the marginal gingiva demonstrates the absence of care and associated inflammatory changes. Dark calculus shining through the gingival sulcus (Fig. 4-23) or harmless melanin pigmentations located in the perimarginal area can often be mistaken for a heavy-metal border.

Tattoos

Tattooing on the face usually occurs through accident and by embedded particles of street dust, coal dust, powder, tar, or metallic splinters.

In the oral cavity the possibilities are more limited. Possible tattoo causes are amalgam and sometimes self-inflicted wounds with colored pencils. Ritual (decorative) tattoos are rarely found in the gingiva.

Amalgam tattoo (ICD-DA 998.40)

In amalgam tattooing there is a slate-gray or gray-blue to blue-black stain of the mucosa caused by localized deposits of amalgam components (mostly silver, but also tin, copper, and mercury) in the tissue. These amalgam tattoos are relatively frequent in gingival areas around posterior teeth (Figs. 4-24 to 4-26). They are usually caused by small amalgam particles that enter the tissues during the preparation of crowns of teeth containing amalgam restorations.

Amalgam tattoos can also frequently be found in the cheek mucous membrane (Fig. 4-27), a result of wounds caused by rotating dental instruments and contamination by amalgam. Mucous membrane discolorations close to teeth and where amalgam is in immediate contact with the gingiva can also be frequently traced back to inclusion of amalgam particles in the periodontal tissue during restorative dentistry.

In a small number of cases, corrosion can be the causative factor (Fig. 4-28). Corrosion-liberated amalgam components can reach the tissue and embed themselves. Amalgam tattoos found in the area of corroded gold alloys cannot be explained by the presence of gold alloy and are probably unrelated to it (Fig. 4-29).

Amalgam tattooing may also occur when amalgam is accidentally left in the tissue during or after the extraction of amalgam particles lodged in the alveolus (Figs. 4-30 and 4-31). It can also occur when retrograde amalgam filling is improperly placed. The resulting slate-gray to blue-gray discoloration is not necessarily limited to the mucosa (Fig. 4-32). In some cases it can occur in the periosteum and involve the bone (Fig. 4-33).

Radiographs should be used for diagnosis. However, attention must be paid to the fact that amalgam tattoos can sometimes remain for a long time after removal of amalgam remnants from the mucosa and after tooth restoration (Fig. 4-34).

In differential diagnosis an important criterion is that the amalgam tattoo be at the level of the mucosa. In cases in which there is doubt about the clinical importance of the pigment change, the patient should be referred.

Self-inflicted wounds with colored pencils (ICD-E 920.9)

Self-inflicted wounds on the mouth mucous membrane with colored pencils are most frequent in children. Fragments of the tip remain embedded in the tissue. The prognostic evaluation of the tattooing is based on the chemical composition, solubility, and quantity of the coloring material. The graphite present in lead pencils usually remains in place and usually causes only a small foreign body reaction without further major expansion of the tattoo.

Acid and base color materials usually present in colored pencils (e.g., methylblue, methylviolet, and others) are water soluble and used in food manufacture (e.g., ink stamps for meat). They tend, because of their water solubility, to expand rapidly but also resorb and disappear rapidly (Figs. 4-35 and 4-36). The once-used aniline coloring substances left behind an obstinate tattoo (Fig. 4-37).

With felt-tip pens, the pigment is usually dissolved in glycerine or glycol. When these alcohols contact damaged mucosa, they act in a dehydrating manner because of their osmotic diluting action. Hence in addition to possible impregnation, chemical tissue irritation is also possible.

The pigment present in ball-point pens is not water soluble but alcohol soluble. There is therefore almost no color exchange during short-term contact with the wet mucosa (as opposed to what occurs with the skin) because of the small spreading coefficient.

Large pigment quantities as well as broken leads should be removed during wound revision and care in cases of penetrating injury. This is important when the chemical composition of the material is unknown and, therefore, the effect on the tissue of the pigment cannot be determined.

Ritual, deliberate tattooing (ICD-DA 528.98)

Today, as in the past, decorative tattooing with paint, soot, and metallic pigments is in fashion with youths of certain population groups. On the oral mucosa these findings are rare. In young persons of some African groups, there are also certain ritual tattoos of the gingiva. They are considered beauty marks. For this purpose, soot obtained from burned wool soaked in oil is introduced into the oral mucosa using needle bundles. The soot particles introduced in this manner create a lasting darkening of the gingiva (Figs. 4-38 and 4-39), which fades only after many years (Fig. 4-40).

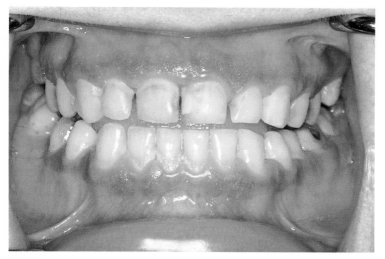

Fig. 4-1 Discrete physiologic melanin pigmentation of the gingiva of a Middle European individual with brown hair.

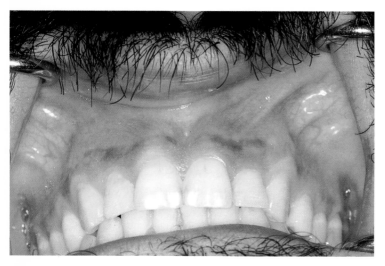

Fig. 4-2 Obvious garland-type melanin pigmentation of the gingiva in a dark-haired Middle European. These findings, within the range of physiologic variation, are also called idiotypic pigmentations.

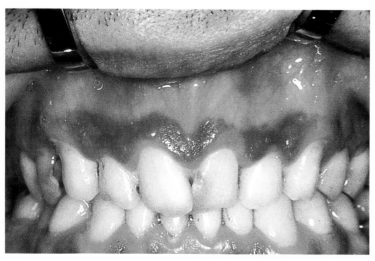

Fig. 4-3 Extended spot-shaped-to-bandlike physiologic melanin pigmentation of the gingiva in a Middle European with blond hair. The marginal gingiva is free in contrast to metallic pigmentation resulting from heavy-metal intoxications (so-called heavy metal border). Compare to Figs. 4-21 and 4-22.

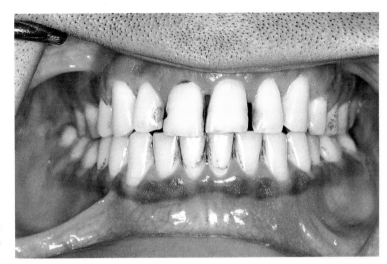

Fig. 4-4   Racially determined band-type melanin pigmentation of the gingiva of an Arab.

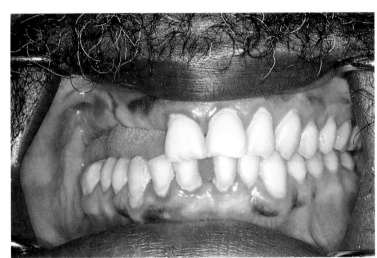

Fig. 4-5   More racially conditioned spot-forming melanin pigment of the gingiva of an African.

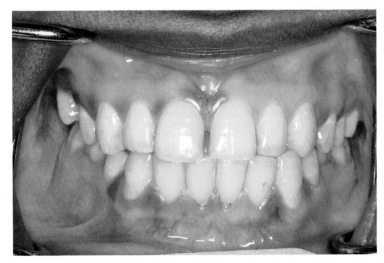

Fig. 4-6   Racially conditioned spots of melanin pigment of the gingiva in an Indian. In cases of marked spot-like pigmentation, the marginal gingiva can be involved.

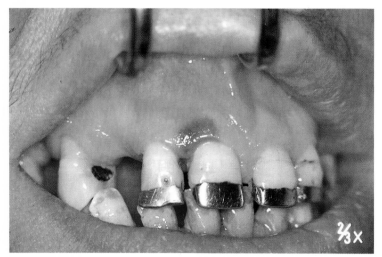

Fig. 4-7 Circumscribed histo-logically determined melanin spot of the gingiva in the area of tooth 11 (8) as a physiologic variant. In the clinical differ-ential diagnosis, the possibility of an amalgam tattoo must be considered.

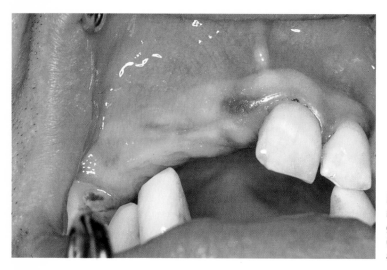

Fig. 4-8 Spotty physiologic melanin pigmentation of the gingiva in the area of tooth 11 (8). These pigmentations are also called melanotic spots.

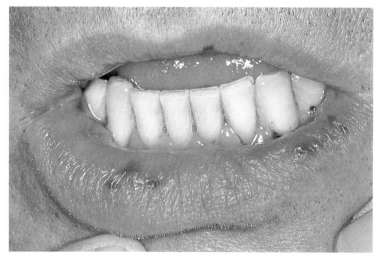

Fig. 4-9 Melanotic lip spots. A relation between these chang-es and a systemic disease can be ruled out.

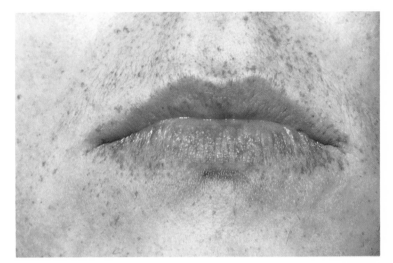

Fig. 4-10   Many small, spray-like dark brown spots of the lip and oral mucosa in a patient with Peutz-Jeghers syndrome. The findings on the face and oral cavity show an early relevant symptom of this syndrome in which multiple intestinal polyps develop later.

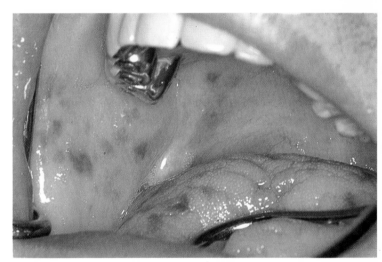

Fig. 4-11   Extensive melanotic spots in the area of the right cheek and the dorsum of the tongue in a Middle European with Addison's disease. The adrenal gland cortex insufficiency in this is caused by adrenal damage from leukemia.

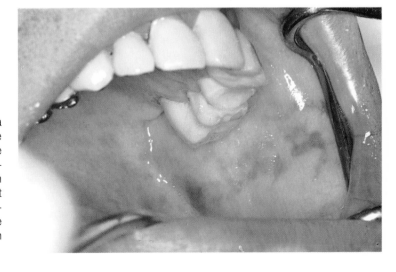

Fig. 4-12   Left cheek mucosa of the patient of Fig. 4-11 at the same time of examination. The spotty-to-large areas of intraoral melanin pigmentation can long precede the development of generalized diffuse hyperpigmentation and therefore may be an important early sign of the disease.

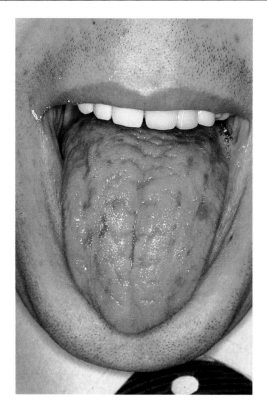

Fig. 4-13 The patient of Figs. 4-11 and 4-12 at the same time of examination. There are many pigment spots on the dorsum of the tongue. Their early appearance on the oral mucous membrane is connected with additional functional-mechanical stimuli.

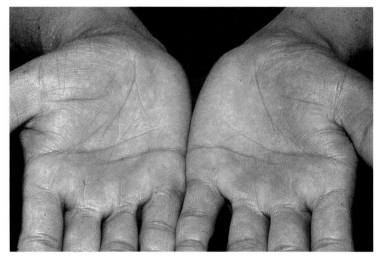

Fig. 4-14 Manifestation of Addison's disease. There is the appearance of diffuse brown color on the skin on areas exposed to the sun and mechanical influences (palms of hands).

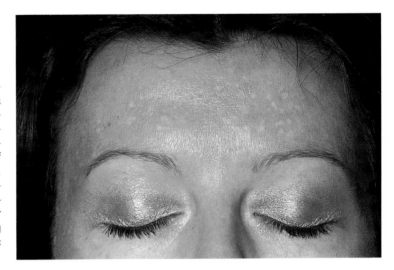

Fig. 4-15   Pregnancy chloasma of the forehead area on a 29-year-old patient. These chloasma yellow-brown hyperpigmentations on the face also appear after long-term use of estrogen ovulation inhibitors. They can also result from infections, a skin reaction to petroleum jelly-type compounds, or from photosensitivity resulting from components in cosmetic creams.

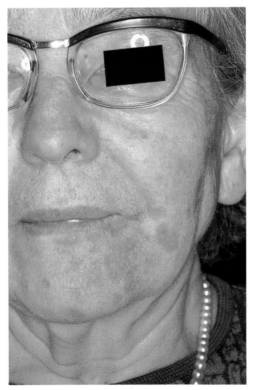

Fig. 4-16   Large spots; postinflammatory hyperpigmentations of the skin with scar formation in association with a zoster of the left second and third trigeminal branch.

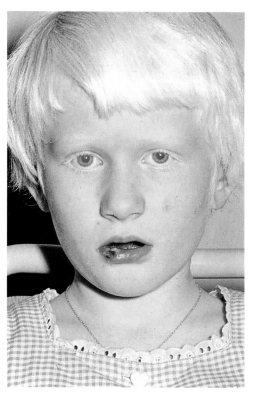

Fig. 4-17   Oculocutaneous albinism in an 8-year-old girl. Note the complete absence of pigment in the skin, hair (of head and eyebrows), and eyes (bright red fundus). As a secondary finding, a circumscribed necrosis is present on the lower lip (bite wound following local anesthesia).

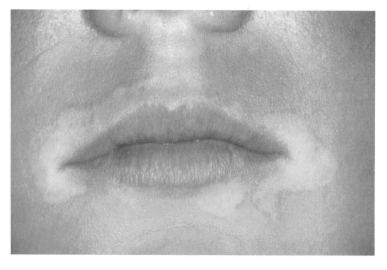

Fig. 4-18   Perioral depigmentation in vitiligo. At the hyperpigmented border, note the disturbing cosmetic defect.

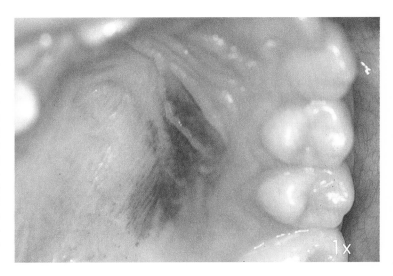

Fig. 4-19   So-called intramucosal nevus cell nevus of the palate of a 10-year-old girl. The 2.1 × 1.5-cm nevus is dirty gray-brown, and in some areas black shines through. The pigment spot was level with the mucosa. Because mechanical irritations can never be excluded in the oral cavity, total removal of these formations is advised at present.

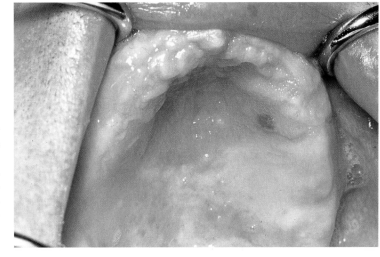

Fig. 4-20   Dark-blue, slightly raised impressive blue nevus on the palate of a 53-year-old patient. In this differential diagnosis, one must consider a malignant melanoma. Radiographs should be taken to exclude the presence of foreign bodies.

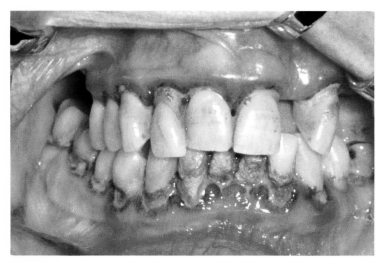

Fig. 4-21   Bismuth border after chronic use of a bismuth-containing medication. This type of metal sulfide deposition is present only with abnormal, inflamed, altered gingiva.

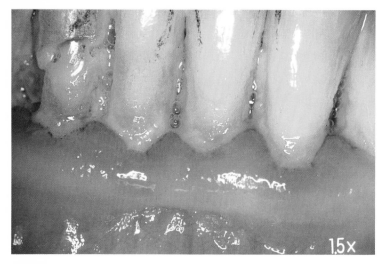

Fig. 4-22   Gingivitis with lead border. This 50-year-old patient works at a lead mill and followed preventive measures (use of a breathing mask). Because metallic lead is milled into small particles in the mill, it enters the body in remarkably large quantities through breathing.

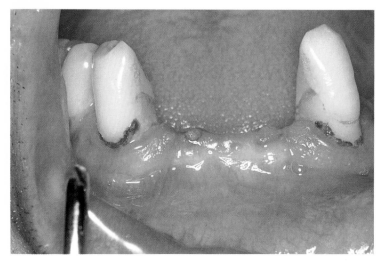

Fig. 4-23   Differential diagnosis of heavy metal borders: subgingival concretions shining through the gingiva can give the impression of a marginal color change. Independent of them is a melanotic spot in the edentulous area.

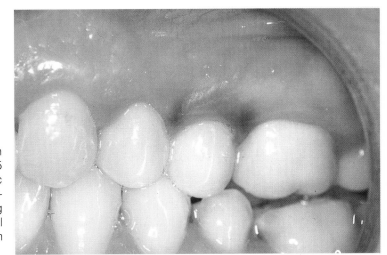

Fig. 4-24   Amalgam tattoo in the gingival region of tooth 25 (11), which has a ceramic crown. Small amalgam particles entered the gingiva during preparation—with slight gingival injury—of the tooth that had an amalgam restoration.

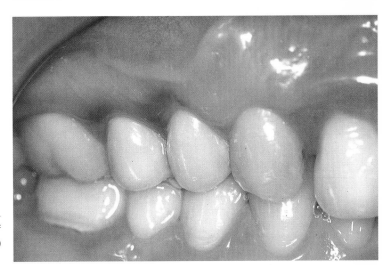

Fig. 4-25   The patient in Fig. 4-24 at the time of examination. There are gingival color changes in the surrounding areas of crowned teeth 14 and 15 (10 and 11).

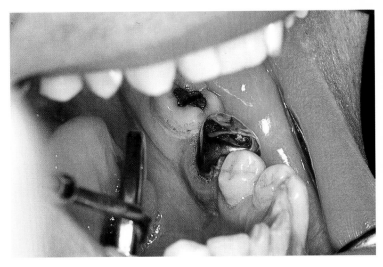

Fig. 4-26   Amalgam tattoo of the gingiva on the left side of crowned tooth 36 (19). Color changes caused by amalgam are always level with the mucosa.

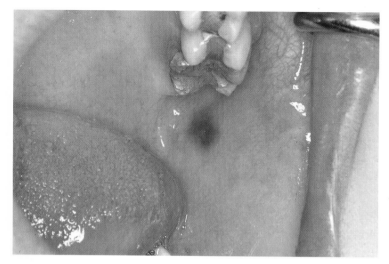

Fig. 4-27 Amalgam tattoo of the cheek mucosa caused by damage from an amalgam-contaminated fissure burr. Differential diagnosis must include melanin spots as well as nevus cell nevus, both of which are usually raised above the surface.

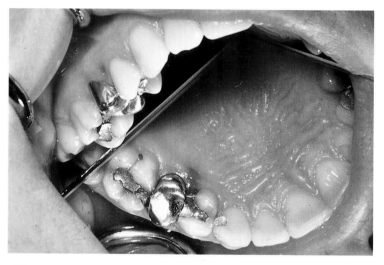

Fig. 4-28 Amalgam tattoo of the gingiva in the vicinity of a silver amalgam restoration that came in contact with a full crown of gold alloy. In this case the deposit of amalgam particles due to corrosion must also be considered.

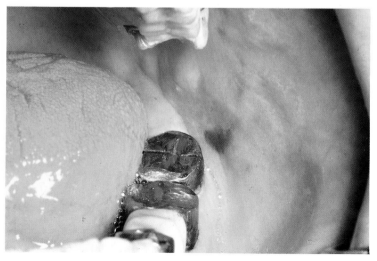

Fig. 4.29 Amalgam tattoo of the mucosa of the cheek in the area of tooth 37 (18). The discolored mucosa was in the area of the corroding precious-metal crown. In addition to the visible gold alloy, there were numerous silver amalgam restorations in the oral cavity.

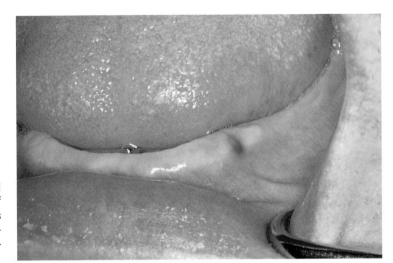

Fig. 4-30 Circumscribed amalgam tattoo in the area of tooth 34 (20) in an edentulous jaw. Amalgam particles had fallen into the alveolus during extraction.

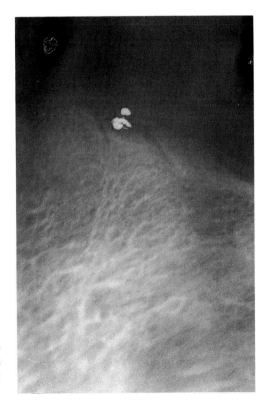

Fig. 4-31 The patient in Fig. 4-30 at the same time of examination. The radiograph shows that the amalgam is embedded in the bone.

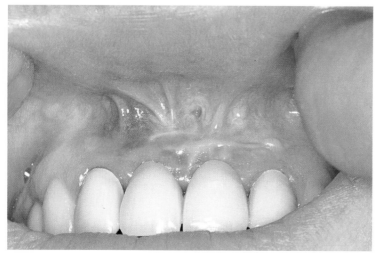

Fig. 4-32 Amalgam tattoo after root tip resection of tooth 11 (8) with defectively applied retrograde amalgam closure. The unfavorable scar formation resulted from poorly approximated wound margins. Retrograde restoration with silver amalgam is no longer recommended.

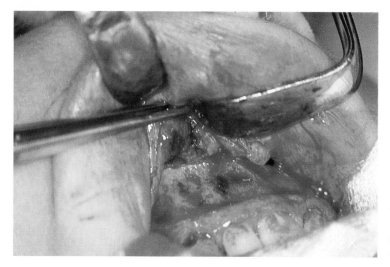

Fig. 4-33 Extensive amalgam tattoo of the alveolar bone, the periosteum, and the gingiva associated with a retrograde amalgam closure.

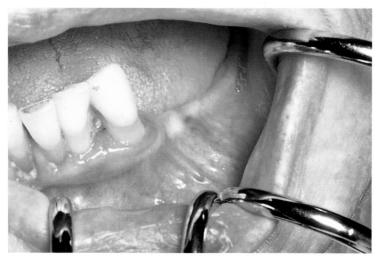

Fig. 4-34 Amalgam tattoo in the edentulous lateral area of the left mandible. The amalgam in tooth 35 (20) had been removed a year before. Radiography revealed no amalgam particles in the bone.

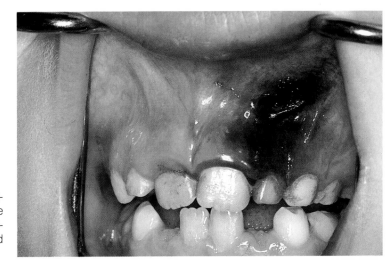

Fig. 4-35 Tattooing after damage to the oral mucosa with the point of a methylene blue pencil. The broken point was found and removed from the tissue.

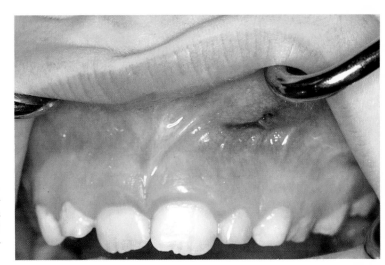

Fig. 4-36   The child of Fig. 4-35 5 days later. The water-soluble coloring material was rapidly eliminated. Some small remnants of the pencil lead remain in the area of injury.

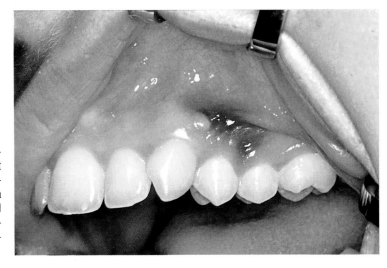

Fig. 4-37   Indelible pencil tattoo of the gingiva and adjacent vestibular fold. In an unintentional self-inflicted injury, a piece of pencil lead penetrated the tissue. In the course of several years, this led to this exogenous discoloration.

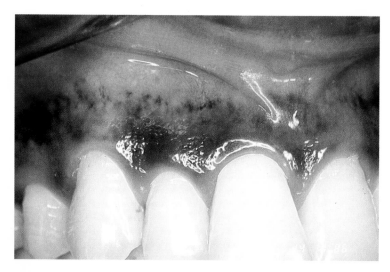

Fig. 4-38   Ritual gingiva tattoo of a 30-year-old Ethiopian woman. The tattoo is considered a beauty mark. At the time of tattooing, the patient was about 15 years old.

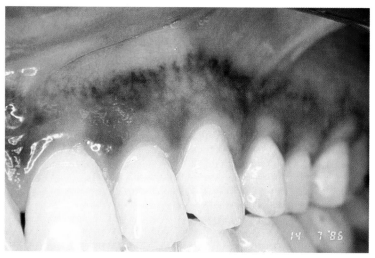

Fig. 4-39 The patient in Fig. 4-38 at the time of examination. The soot particles introduced into the gingiva with needle bundles was made of burned, oil-impregnated wool, which created a slow blackening of the gingiva.

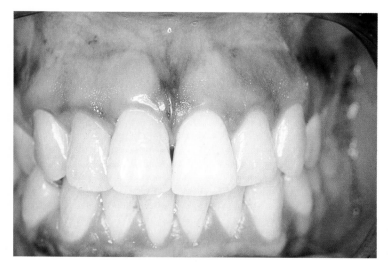

Fig. 4-40   A 40-year-old Ethiopian woman of the same tribe. After about 10 years, the black color of the tattoo has somewhat faded.

Chapter 5

Acute Nonspecific Gingivitis—Periodontitis and Stomatitis

Acute gingivitis

Acute necrotizing ulcerative gingivitis (ANUG)

Acute necrotizing ulcerative gingivostomatitis

Postulcerative periodontitis

Acute gingivitis is the finding with which the dentist is in contact on a daily basis for therapeutic reasons. Development of gingivitis can, in most cases, be traced to local causes. Unsatisfactory oral hygiene with plaque formation is the most important and most frequent factor.

Bacterial deposits are usually the cause of gingivitis, and when they remain for long periods, the acute gingivitis becomes chronic gingivitis and is followed by the development of marginal periodontitis. When the gingivitis has caused attachment loss, it is still considered marginal periodontitis of an inflammatory nature in all parts of the marginal periodontium with increasing loss of supporting tissue.

Opposed to acute gingivitis is acute necrotizing ulcerative gingivitis (ANUG), which is always associated with major or minor involvement of the body. The disease picture shows traits of an acute recurring infection, the spreading and course of which depends on the patient response. In the differential diagnosis, one must keep in mind that severe systemic degenerative diseases can appear first of all as symptoms of an acute nonspecific inflammation of the mouth (e.g., low resistance syndrome); see also chapters 11 and 24.

Untreated or insufficiently treated ANUG can, in a short time, become acute necrotizing ulcerative gingivoperiodontitis (ANUP), which can lead to severe, irreversible periodontal tissue losses with far-reaching consequences for oral health and maintenance of the teeth.

Acute gingivitis (ICD-DA 523.OX)

Many examinations have demonstrated that breakdown in oral hygiene leads within 2 weeks to inflammation, even of healthy gingiva. There is then a correlation between the extent of the gingivitis of the individual and the rate of plaque formation.

The symptoms of gingivitis are: redness, swelling, exudation, increased flow rate of the sulcus fluid, and in some cases, ulcerations (Fig. 5-1). Bleeding can occur on touch or with sulcus probing.

With improvement of oral hygiene and elimination of plaque, these conditions can heal completely in a few days. Extensive observations in young traumatized patients show that after plaque formation and gingival inflammation, resumption of oral hygiene practice led to improvement. In everyday dentistry, however, there is a predominance of chronic gingivitis with subacute or acute exacerbations (Figs. 5-2 and 5-3). The signs of inflammation are variable and, in a chronic course, hyperplastic changes are present. These changes at first are always restricted to the gingiva and do not cause detachment or damage to the bone. Because of insufficient oral hygiene, transition from persistent gingivitis to a marginal periodontitis is in many cases assured (Fig. 5-4). Close to the gingiva there are desmodonts, root cementum, and alveolar bone, which are also affected by the inflammatory reaction. This leads to findings such as pocket formation with loss of attachment and bone damage, and finally increased dental mobility and periodontal abscesses.

There can be different stages of transitions from acute gingivitis to chronic marginal periodontitis in the same patient at the same time. Books on periodontology should be consulted for more extensive information on the subject.

Therapy for gingivitis should ensure clean conditions in the oral cavity. Of primary importance is the mechanical removal of coatings (e.g., materia alba, plaque) and tartar—which can also be removed carefully with ultrasonic instrumentation—as well as instruction and motivation of the patient to effective and controlled home oral hygiene. The use of a 3% H_2O_2 solution is an adjunct measure. Also recommended are chlorhexidine gluconate in a 0.1% to 0.2% solution or gel form for germ-reducing therapy. The duration of chlorhexidine therapy should be limited to 1 week because of reversible side effects (e.g., taste disturbances, tooth discoloration). These procedures and the patient's motivation to cooperate are in accord with present practice. Because of limitations in allowable application time cannot substitute for toothbrushing over the long run, other means of mucosal disinfection are inferior to chlorhexidine in plaque prevention.

Incorrect evaluation of the causative factors is probably the reason that the patient and some dentists consider medication the only possible curative therapy.

The suggestion that phytotherapeutics be used for treatment of gingivitis is not based on controlled studies. Also, the use of plant extracts is associated with the risk of allergic side effects. The alleged curative functions of "cosmetic" mouthwashes as well as periodontal prophylactic additives in toothpaste cannot be demonstrated. In addition, retained plaque that acts as a chronic irritant of the gingiva should be eliminated as far as possible. Modification (removal) of dental restorations that may be a cause of irritation must be considered, as should be the elimination of chronic traumatizing influences due to malocclusion (Figs. 5.5 and 5.6).

Acute necrotizing ulcerative gingivitis (ICD-DA 101.X0)

Acute necrotizing ulcerative gingivitis (ANUG) usually starts in the area of the interdental papillae (Figs. 5-7 and 5-8). Because of the marked destructive character of this disease, the papillae tips recede in few hours (Fig. 5-9). From the fibrin-covered, necrotic, and ulcerated areas, the acute inflammatory process continues, leaving craterlike interdental tissue defects. It also shows a tendency to rapidly invade the other gingival tissues (Figs. 5-8 to 5-11). Transformation to an ulcerative gingivoperiodontitis or necrotizing ulcerative stomatitis is possible.

In accordance with these histopathologic findings are other easily detectable clinical cardinal symptoms in the early stages: bleeding (spontaneous or on very small trauma) and severe pain. Increased saliva flow, bad breath, bad taste, and an acute lymphadenitis of the lymph nodes are typical associated symptoms of this infection, caused by pathogens that are part of the usual flora of the subgingival microbial plaques. A frequently severe feeling of malaise along with fever also suggest acute active infection.

Acute necrotizing ulcerative gingivitis usually develops over a preexisting acute or chronic gingivitis because of a breakdown of the defense mechanism of the organism. It is therefore not infrequently observed as a consequence of febrile diseases of the respiratory tract.

Although this disease has been known for centuries, the pathogenesis is unclear even today. It is certain that ANUG cannot be induced in animals and that it is not contagious in humans. Its sometimes endemic appearance can be explained by similar environmental factors, where many conditions such as inadequate oral hygiene, stress, and exhaustion can contribute as cofactors in the development of the condition.

The differential diagnosis between idiopathic ANUG and ANUG as an accompanying symptom (e.g., to a low-resistance syndrome) in serious systemic diseases such as those of the hematopoietic system has already been discussed.

Dental therapy aims to develop clean conditions of the oral cavity, to stop the progress of necrosis and ulcerations, and to avoid the development of irreversible damage to the dental structures as soon as possible (Figs. 5-13 and 5-14). It starts with a thorough and daily wet cleaning of the oral cavity. Medications derived from oxygen (i.e., 3% H_2O_2 solution) have been very useful because of their foaming effect. Also, careful and tissue-sparing instrumentation to remove hard and soft dental accretions may lead to good results. Also useful is a rinsing solution or gel containing chlorhexidine.

This local treatment can be advantageous only when the patient cooperates with good home oral hygiene, for which she or he must receive instruction and be motivated. Brushing and rinsing with cosmetic mouthwashes is not adequate therapy. In cases of severe ANUG, bed rest is advisable. A vitamin-rich diet of liquid or semiliquid consistency is also advisable.

The prescription of antibiotics should be immediate when there is a high fever and is recommended when there is lack of response after 24 to 48 hours of local therapy. Oral penicillin or a wide-spectrum penicillin in standard preparations and doses is administered over a period of time (at least 5 days). The lack of effect of local treatment can be a determining factor in seeking other underlying causes by the dentist together with a thorough examination by the physician.

Acute necrotizing ulcerative gingivostomatitis (Vincent's stomatitis) (ICD-DA 101.X1)

The extension of the acute necrotizing ulcerative gingivitis to other regions of the oral mucosa can take place by direct extension or by seeding. This is always an unmistakable sign of weakened body defenses.

The initiation point of such a stomatitis is usually the area of half-retained mandibular third molars, which may play a role by causing chronic accumulation of debris and mucosal ulcerations. The lesion spreads from the mucosa covering the molars and grows, often in remarkably short time, to the mucosa of the cheeks, to the gingival region of the teeth bordering the region, and to the retromolar area (Figs. 5-15 and 5-16). If the necrotizing ulceration reaches the palate and Waldeyer's ring, there is development of *Vincent's angina* (ICD-DA 101.X2) (Figs. 5-12 and 5-17). The oropharynx alone can be affected, in which case the lesion must be differentiated from bacterial pharyngitis and tonsillitis.

Any area of the oral cavity, however, can be the initial point of the lesion due to a chronic irritation, for example, in neglected dentitions with deep caries and root remnants. Even now, in immune-suppressed third-world children, nomalike gangrenous lesions that cause extensive areas of necrosis can be found.

Particularly on the lip and cheek mucosa, there is formation of a yellow-white fibrin deposit over the ulceration (hence the old name of stomatitis pseudomembranacea or ulceromembranacea).

The associated regional symptoms are similar to those of acute necrotizing ulcerative gingivitis. Naturally they are more severe and associated with constitutional symptoms.

In differential diagnosis, agranulocytosis and other systemic conditions that lead to a breakdown of cellular and humoral defenses must be considered. Therapy with cytostatic agents and immunosuppressive agents may cause a painful stomatitis with similar findings. Bullous diseases of the oral mucosa may be difficult to differentiate from ulcerative stomatitis. Dental treatment is similar in ulcerative gingivitis and ANUG. For each patient with severe intraoral disease, a complete internal medical examination and therapy of any underlying disease should be provided.

Postulcerative periodontitis

The loss of interdental papillae (negative papillae) and other gingival parts, interdental craters and recesses, as well as a balcony-like padded gingiva with reverse-garland-forming course are typical consequences of acute necrotizing ulcerative gingivitis. Especially heavy irreversible damage of the dental support tissue in the form of a postulcerative marginal periodontitis is to be expected when the treatment is stopped, neglected, or inadequately carried out (Figs. 5-18 to 5-21). Also, the patient must cooperate with home oral hygiene.

Postulcerative periodontal consequences make it harder to carry out oral hygiene, and untreated areas are a classic preferential point for the recurrence of ANUG. They therefore facilitate the progression of periodontal disease and development of cemental or dental caries. Thus it becomes difficult to save the teeth once the gingival and periodontal tissues have been injured or damaged; correction can only be effected through periodontal surgery (gingivoplasty). These postulcerative findings with gingival and periodontal destruction must be differentially diagnosed from ulcerated malignancies that are located on the gingiva (Fig. 5-23). The same is true of manifestations of eosinophilic granulomas in the area of dentulous alveolar processes (see chapter 30).

Fig. 5-1 Acute gingivitis. Reddish, swollen gums are covered focally by exudate. At some points, there are already noticeable ulcerations. Note the massive plaque deposits.

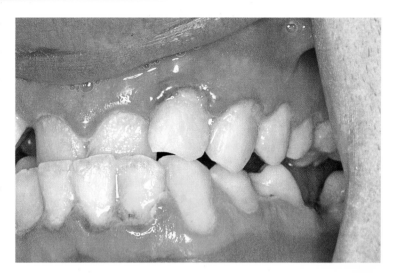

Fig. 5-2 Periodontitis with acute gingival inflammation, located chiefly on the left side of the mandible in a 32-year-old woman. Because of severe toothache (pulpitis of tooth 37 [18] untreated for 7 days), mastication and cleaning were discontinued unilaterally, with intensification of the symptoms. As a consequence of unfavorable marginal conditions from a composite resin crown, gingivitis developed in the area beneath the crowns of teeth 11, 21, and 22 (8, 9, and 10). The right-side posterior teeth show unremarkable gingival conditions. On both mandibular canines are extensive dehiscences.

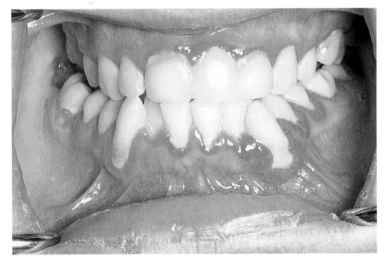

Fig. 5-3 Combination findings of inflamed gingiva and marginal periodontium at various stages of development: acute flare-up of a chronic gingivitis with marginal periodontitis caused by poor oral hygiene. Years of major neglect of oral care created a worsened state of the dentition, permitting microbial plaque activity on the gingiva and periodontium as well as smooth surface caries. The patient made a dental appointment only because of a toothache. Teeth 12, 11, 21, and 22 (7, 8, 9, and 10) were also damaged by caries and were restored with composite resin. Strip crowns satisfy the cosmetic wishes of the patient but do not provide definitive dental care.

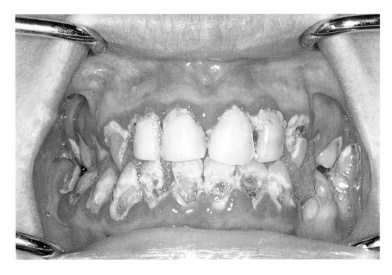

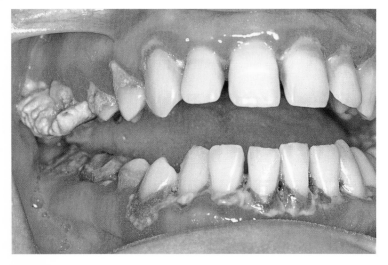

Fig. 5-4   Localized acutely exacerbated chronic gingivo-periodontitis. Disease development was facilitated by extensive plaque and dental calculus deposits, which became massive on the right side.

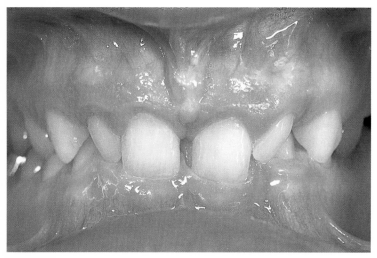

Fig. 5-5   Example of mechanically produced gingivitis. Position of the maxillary incisors in a severe case of vertical overlap of a 15-year-old girl.

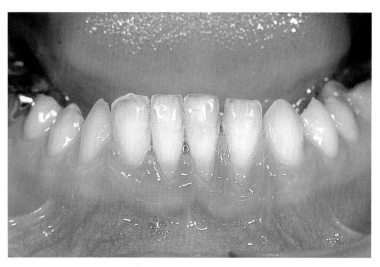

Fig. 5-6   The patient in Fig. 5-5 at the same time of examination. As a result of traumatic occlusion, there are, in the area of the vestibular mucous membrane of the mandibular incisors, recognizable impressions with acute flare-up inflammation and recession of the gingiva. Therapy consists of raising the bite.

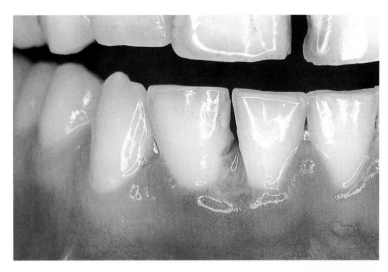

Fig. 5-7   Different stages of an acute necrotizing ulcerative gingivitis (ANUG) in the region of the anterior mandibular teeth: on tooth 31 (24), there is inflammatory infiltration with reddishness, swelling, and exudation; on teeth 42 and 41 (25 and 26), there is total papilla loss with interdental recession. Note the increased vascularity and infiltration in the area around the necrosis.

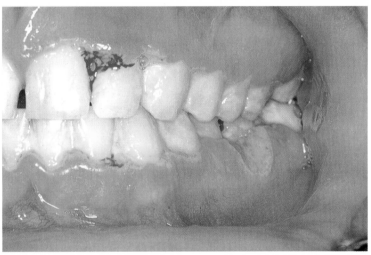

Fig. 5-8   Acute necrotizing ulcerative gingivitis in the background of reduced resistance. The very painful inflammation of the interdental areas began abruptly; later the remaining gingiva was affected by necrosis and ulcerations. Note the already severely damaged gingiva of tooth 36 (30) in the area (deposits of decaying material on interproximal caries).

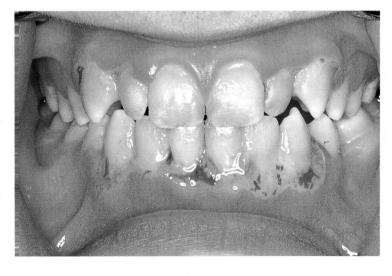

Fig. 5-9   Different stages of an ANUG. Rapidly progressing tissue destruction in the area of the mandibular anterior teeth with extension to the other parts of the gingiva and alveolar mucosa. There are early destructive changes of the gingival architecture around teeth 13, 12, 22, and 23 (6, 7, 10, and 11) with loss of papillae in the maxilla.

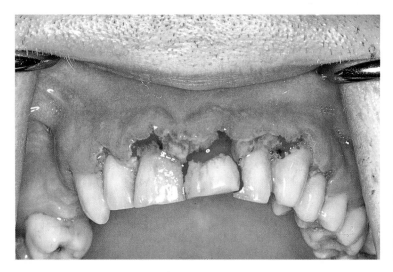

Fig. 5-10   Acute necrotizing ulcerative gingivitis with marked crater formation in the tissues. The disease appeared after an influenza infection.

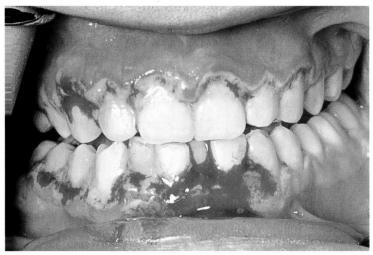

Fig. 5-11   Rapidly progressing ANUG in a patient with moderately compromised general health. Hemorrhage is apparent as a result of slight pressure in newly ulcerated areas. Permanent periodontal tissue losses can be avoided only with prompt and determined dental therapy.

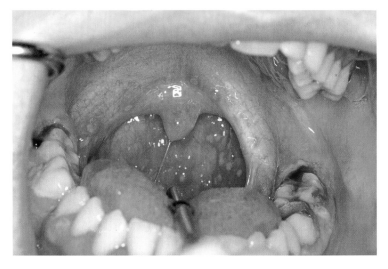

Fig. 5-12 Acute pharyngitis (Vincent's angina) as a partial manifestation of an extensive but already fading necrotizing ulcerative gingivostomatitis. The starting point of the acute inflammation process was chronic ulcerations near the partially retained mandibular third molars.

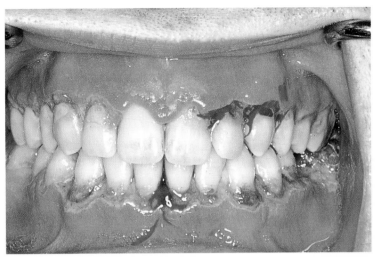

Fig. 5-13 Initial stage of ANUG affecting several teeth. There was a fibrin cover of necrosis and ulcerations as well as spontaneous bleeding. Severe pain, bad breath, bad taste, and painful-to-touch regional lymph nodes were the patient's complaints.

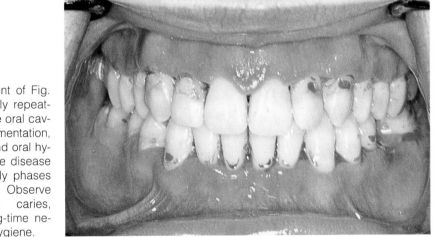

Fig. 5-14 The patient of Fig. 5-13 4 days after daily repeated wet cleaning of the oral cavity, careful instrumentation, dental prophylaxis, and oral hygiene instructions. The disease is stationary, and early phases of healing are seen. Observe the smooth-surface caries, which point to a long-time neglect of proper oral hygiene.

Therapy of ANUG

ANUG—with fever and no considerable damage to general health.

Local therapy:	Several daily wet cleanings of the oral cavity, instrumentation, and dental prophylaxis, with monitoring for the improvement in the findings.
Medication therapy:	H_2O_2, 3%, as solution or spray. Chlorhexidine 0.190–0.2%, solution or gel.
Cooperation of the patient:	Instruction and motivation for effective home oral care.

ANUG—with fever (over 38.5 °C), altered general health and absence of response to local therapy for 24 to 48 hours.

To complement the above-mentioned measures, use systemic antibiotic therapy.

First choice: penicillin G, IM, or oral penicillin, i.e., propicillin 4 × 1,000,000 U/d.

Second choice: wide-spectrum penicillin, i.e., 770 to 1,000 mg of amoxicillin three times per day, when gram-negative bacteria participation is suspected. If the patient is allergic to penicillin, administer erythromycin or clindamycin. *With lack of response to such therapy, the initial diagnosis must be questioned and further examinations (referral) may be necessary.*

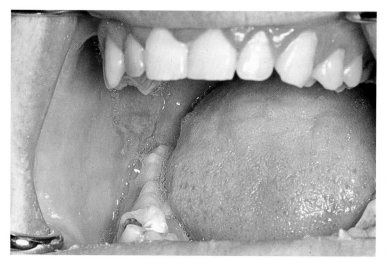

Fig. 5-15 Localized early stage of acute necrotizing ulcerative stomatitits on the cheek mucosa of an 18-year-old woman in the area of a difficult tooth eruption in tooth 48 (32).

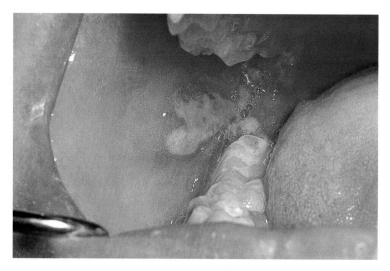

Fig. 5-16 The patient in Fig. 5-15 24 hours later. Tissue necroses have continued to spread to the buccal and retromolar area. Note the extensive increase of plaque. The condition worsened in spite of the use of a hexetidine preparation.

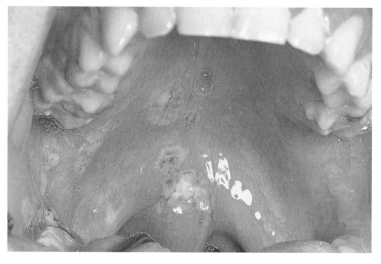

Fig. 5-17 The patient in Figs. 5-15 and 5-16 after a further 24 hours. Acute necrotizing ulcerative lesions have now reached the palatal mucosa and uvula. The rapid course of this disease is characteristic of the extent of the lowered systemic resistance. A medical checkup is indicated.

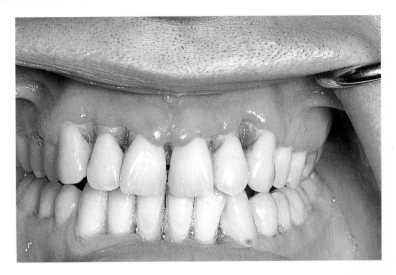

Fig. 5-18   Typical postulcerative findings of untreated ANUG with recesses and craters and an unfavorable gingival contour. In the depths of the recesses and craters are several chronic ulcerations where a recidivating ANUG can develop. The prognosis for maintenance of the anterior teeth is poor. The interdental plaque facilitates the development of root caries.

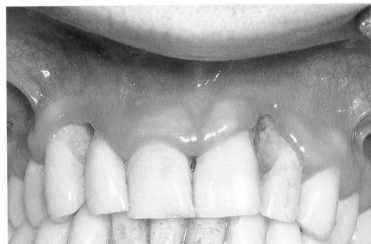

Fig. 5-19   Severe gingivoperiodontal tissue defect with far-reaching interdental craters and recesses after recurrence of ANUG with ulcerated periodontitis.

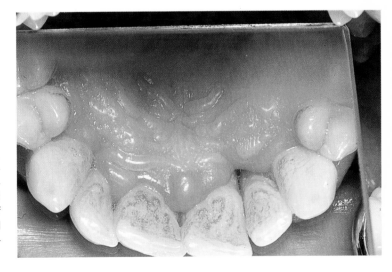

Fig. 5-20 The patient in Fig. 5-19 at the same time of examination. The palate reveals evidence of destruction of dental support tissue. The results of radiographic examination and pocket probing confirm the indication for extraction.

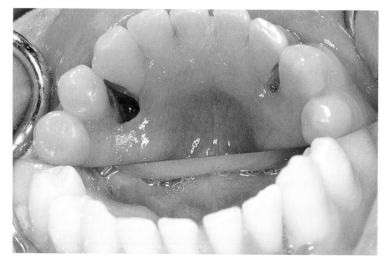

Fig. 5-21   Deep postulcerative interdental craters with extensive periodontal tissue loss in treated ANUG. These findings require differential diagnosis with eosinophilic granuloma (i.e., radiographs). See also Figs. 30-21 and 30-22.

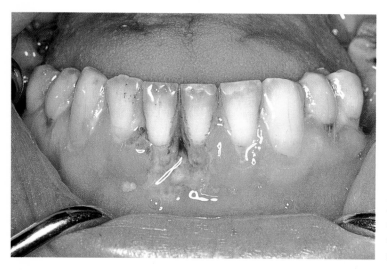

Fig. 5-22   Differential diagnosis of ANUG: appearance after foreign-body impaction between teeth 31 and 41 (24, 25) with subsequent tissue necrosis.

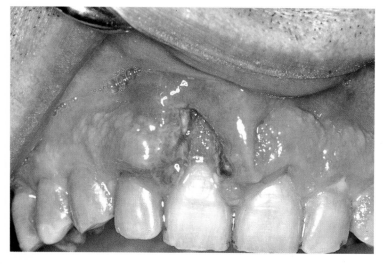

Fig. 5-23 Differential diagnosis of ANUG: keratinized, flat epithelial carcinoma of the gingiva. The deeply infiltrating tumor has destroyed the dental supporting tissue in the area of tooth 11 (8). The central necrosis is surrounded by a thickened margin. Disease duration: 10 months. See also Fig. 19-8.

Chapter 6

Clinical Features of Some Nonspecific Inflammatory Processes in the Oral and Perioral Region

---

Originating in the dentition

Originating outside the dentition

For reasons of differential diagnosis, some special manifestations of nonspecific inflammatory processes in the oral and perioral region that affect the oral mucosa *secondarily* have been included in this chapter.

Originating in the dentition

Inflammatory conditions are frequently observed during pyogenic infections, which as a rule originate in the teeth. The clinical pictures are limited to clinical consequences of chronic apical periodontitis (for nonspecific infections in relation to marginal periodontitis and pericoronitis, see chapter 5).

Chronic apical periodontitis is the reaction of the periapical tissue to the bacterial infection of the root canal of a pulpless tooth. Chronic periapical inflammation (periapical granuloma) can undergo acute exacerbation (seldomly progressing to primary acute apical periodontitis) with the development of a cellular infiltrate and an abscess within the overlying soft tissue. The symptoms associated with acute exacerbation are variable.

Fistulas may be a visible expression of apical periodontitis. Intraoral fistulas (mucosal fistulas) flow into the vestibule (Figs. 6-1 to 6-3), seldom lingually or palatally. Extraoral fistulas can, after spontaneous breakthrough or after incision, remain as subcutaneous abscesses when the affected tooth is not removed or is treated with endodontic-surgical measures.

Odontogenic fistulas of the face develop after a chronic subacute course of periapical inflammation that spreads slowly through cleavage planes in the muscle in the direction of the outer skin. These granulation forms of periodontitis were called chronic-granulating periodontitis by Partsch. Finally, there is the development on the skin of granulation tissue that is rich in collagenous fibers and contains reddish to dark-red nodules that are soft and can give the impression of a fluctuation (Fig. 6-4). If untreated, they usually lead to colliquation followed by spontaneous perforation of the skin. The fistulas that result in this manner are usually in the cheeks, chin, or submandibular region (Figs. 6-6 to 6-8). Usually one can palpate a cordlike connection to the affected tooth in the depth of the vestibular area.

If skin fistulas do not heal after the elimination of the source of dental infection or if a cause cannot be found, differential diagnosis must exclude actinomycosis by examination of fistulous secretion, or in rare cases, fistulas of the thyroglossal duct (medial neck fistulas) or branchiogenic fistulas (lateral neck fistulas).

Of the abscesses secondary to dental lesions, those most frequently observed in dental practice are submucosal abscesses (Fig. 6-9) and palatal abscesses (Fig. 6-10) of the subperiosteal vestibular mucosa of the maxilla and mandible. They have the most favorable clinical course. Their therapy is without problems and seldom has complications.

In abscesses of the canine fossa (Figs. 6-11 and 6-12), care should be taken to diagnose potentially damaging complications (Figs. 6-13 and 6-14), including soft tissue emphysemas (Figs. 6-15 and 6-16).

There is extensive literature on the many possibilities for the spread and manifestations of pyogenic infections in the area around the maxilla and mandible. The same is true for osteomyelitis of the jaw (Figs. 6-17 and 6-18), the incidence of which has noticeably decreased with the development of antibiotic therapy. As a rule, limited osteomyelitic lesions are observed only in circumscribed areas of the mandibular dentition.

Originating outside the dentition

Nonspecific inflammations not caused by the dentition include focal bacterial secondary infections due to injuries of the mucosa, e.g., by piercing with foreign bodies (Fig. 6-19 to 6-21).

There are also examples of oral lesions caused by inflammation of the salivary glands (Figs. 6-22 and 6-23). Salivary stones (Figs. 6-22 and 6-24), which are concretions of the saliva, are most frequently found in the submandibular gland. They are in part the consequence of and in part the cause of sialadenitis.

In the early phases of sialolithiasis in this location, the patient experiences colic-type pain while eating, associated swallowing problems, and a tight swelling of the submandibular area. This symptom decreases after about 2 hours.

With the obstruction of saliva flow by stones in the duct system, there is, as a rule, the development of an ascending infection of the salivary gland. Depending on the early damage to the salivary gland, salivary stones frequently recur after surgical removal. Resection of the gland is indicated in these recurrent cases and when the stone is impacted in the dorsal third of the duct system or inside the body of the gland.

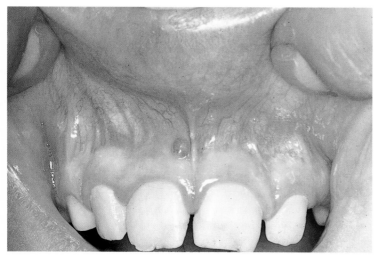

Fig. 6-1   Vestibular mucosal fistula arising from chronic apical periodontitis of tooth 11 (8). Appearance after trauma to the anterior tooth and restoration of the enamel-dentin fracture of teeth 11 and 21 (8 and 9) with composite resin (adhesive technique). Sensitivity tests with carbonic acid snow indicate no reaction for tooth 11 (8). Radiographic findings indicate periapical osteitis for tooth 11 (8). There is incomplete growth of the root compared to vital tooth 21 (9) because of pulp necrosis.

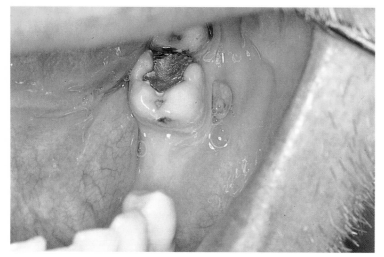

Fig. 6-2 Vestibular mucosal fistula arising from chronic apical periodontitis of tooth 37 (18). Sensitivity testing with carbonic acid snow was negative. Radiographic findings show periapical osteitis. In these cases, there can be an attempt to retain the tooth with endodontic treatment.

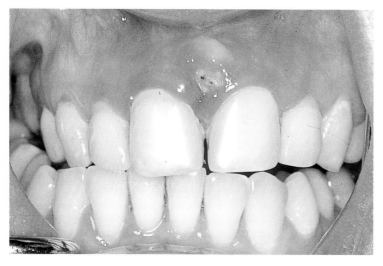

Fig. 6-3   Differential diagnosis for a mucosal fistula: vestibularly erupting mesiodens. Teeth 11 and 21 (8 and 9) were repaired with composite resin after fracture. A radiograph was not taken after the accident nor at the time of crown preparation for one of the teeth.

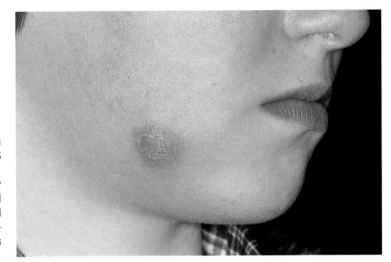

Fig. 6-4   Chronic granulation tissue periodontitis of tooth 46 (30) on the skin of the cheek. The highly vascular, subacutely inflamed granulation tissue led to a soft, circumscribed, and sharply limited reddish swelling. At the incision was no pus discharge.

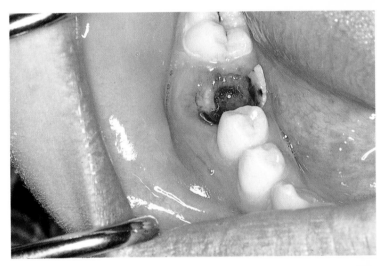

Fig. 6-5   Intraoral appearance of patient in Fig. 6-4 showing the extensively damaged pulpless tooth 46 (30). Between the periapical region of this tooth and the extraoral lesion, it was possible to palpate a cordlike connection in the vestibular region.

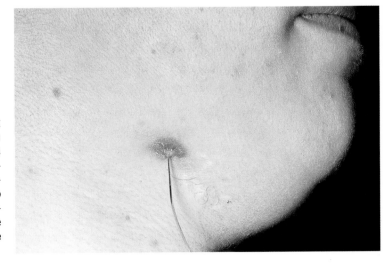

Fig. 6-6   Chronic skin fistula at the base of the mandible (with inserted probe). The cause was chronic granulating apical periodontitis of tooth 46 (30). Patients with this finding often go to a general physician. Treatment for the elimination of the fistula is unsuccessful until the odontologic cause is removed.

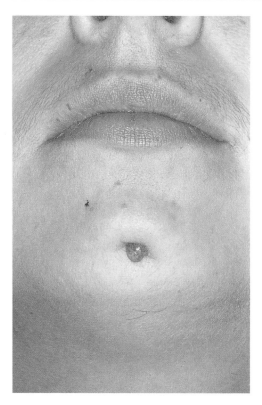

Fig. 6-7   Skin fistula caused by chronic granulating periodontitis. This patient had incomplete luxation of teeth 31 and 41 (24 and 25) due to trauma with consequent necrosis of the pulp. In restabilized teeth without crown damage, clarification of the condition is obtained by radiographs and pulp testing. In cases of persistent leakage of pus and excessive granulation tissue, differential diagnosis includes consideration of actinomycosis (i.e., microbiologic examination of the fistula's secretion using anaerobic culture media).

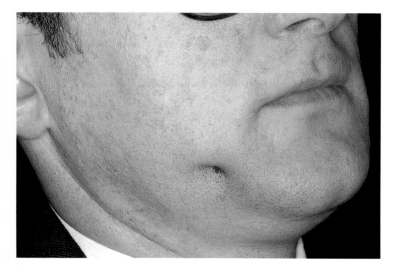

Fig. 6-8   Skin fistula of dental origin with funnel-shaped retracted marginal tissue. The cause was chronic granulating periodontitis from tooth 46 (30), which maintained the extraoral fistula with intermittent secretions for 2 years. Differential diagnosis includes actinomycosis as well as a fistula of a chronic mandibular osteomyelitis. Removal of the affected tooth led to healing of the fistula. Plastic repair of the scar might be indicated.

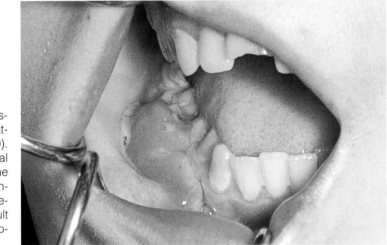

Fig. 6-9   Fully developed vestibular space abscess originating from pulpless tooth 46 (30). The swelling of the mucobuccal fold extends to the area of the right mandibular canine. An incision, which had not previously been done, would result in rapid drainage of the abscess.

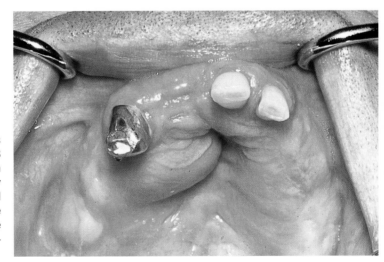

Fig. 6-10   Palatal abscess arising from pulpless tooth 13 (6) before incision. The incision must respect the palatine artery and should be done as an oval excision to avoid rapid collapse of the wound margins on the tight palatal mucosa. The pulpless tooth is to be opened.

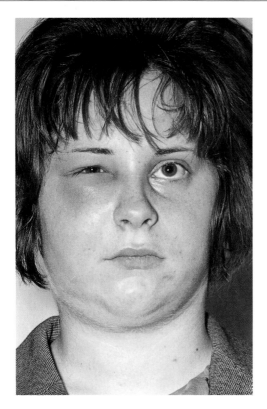

Fig. 6-11 Typical appearance of an abscess of the canine fossa with collateral eyelid edema developing from pulpless tooth 13 (6). The abscess is located above the mucous sulcus. Due to the inflamed, painful-to-pressure swelling of the infraorbital region, the nasolabial fold has disappeared.

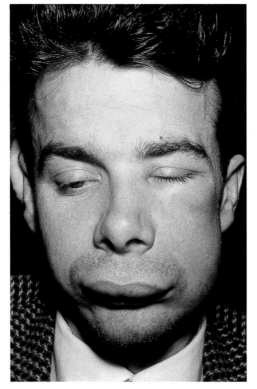

Fig. 6-12 Abscess originating from tooth 22 (7) with distended abscess of the canine fossa and considerable edema of the soft tissue (i.e., under the eyelid). Instead of the required incision, the only measure taken was an incorrect dosage of antibiotics. The abscess spread.

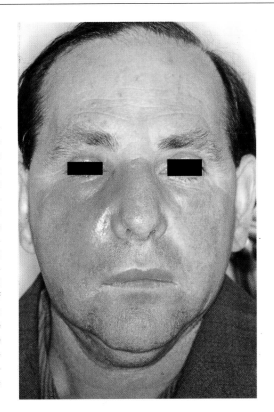

Fig. 6-13   Abscess of the canine fossa with thrombophlebitis of the right angular vein. The cause was acute exacerbation of chronic apical periodontitis of tooth 13 (6). This complication (fortunately extremely rare) warns of the worsening of the general condition (including fever) and an increase of local findings (extreme pain to pressure, palpable blood vessel cords to the internal corner of the eye). With the continuation of the inflammation over the ophthalmic superior vein, there can be a thrombosis of the cavernous sinus. Immediate treatment is required to stop the condition.

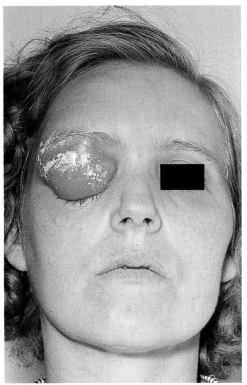

Fig. 6-14   Orbital abscess with protrusion of the bulb and massive eyelid edema (semicircular anterior curvature of the upper lid). The cause was a pyogenic infection of pulpless tooth 17 (2), which progressed from the retromaxillary space over the pterygoid process in the orbit. Proper treatment should be started at the first sign of this condition.

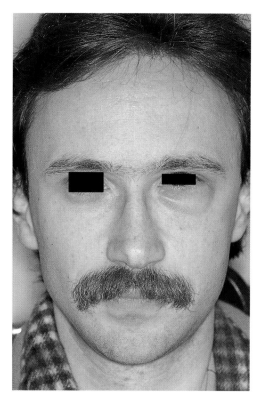

Fig. 6-15   Differential diagnosis of an abscess of the canine fossa: emphysema of the left cheek and lower eyelid region was caused by accidental introduction of forced air during root canal treatment of tooth 22 (10). The air forced under the skin/mucosa collected in the movable soft area of the face and can be palpated as a light movable cushion. On palpation there is characteristic crackling. Massive air accumulations can appear in the maxilla and mandible and provoke temporary eye closure. Because of the danger of bacterial contamination, a prophylactic antibiotic treatment is advisable.

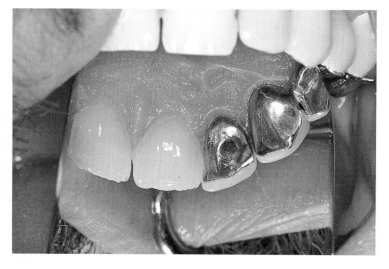

Fig. 6-16   Intraoral situation of the patient in Fig. 6-15 with opened tooth 22 (10). The forcing of air into the root canal by improper handling of the air bubble or uncontrolled use of hydrogen peroxide during endodontic treatment may have occured. Emphysemas can also occur with increased pressure in the nose and paranasal sinuses (particularly maxillary sinuses), for example, with blowing of the nose, or when damaged bone with penetration of soft tissue preexists (after an accident or after a recent plastic closure of a mouth-antrum communication).

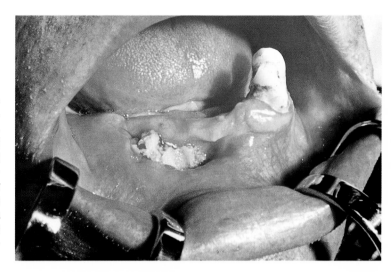

Fig. 6-17 Largely demarcated sequestrum already exposed in the oral area in odontogenic chronic osteomyelitis of the mandible in a 58-year-old patient. Currently, the most-likely chronic, progressing jaw osteomyelitis of adults can be traced, in 90% of cases, to a dental cause. The mandible is six times more likely to be affected than the maxilla.

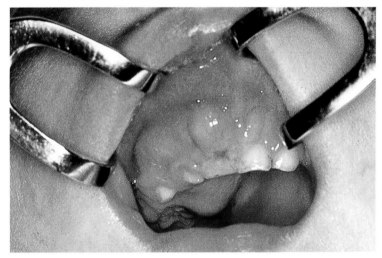

Fig. 6-18 Acute osteomyelitis of the right side of the maxilla with buccal and palatal abscess formation in a 5-year-old boy. This acute infection, following measles, must be considered hematogenous because of the complete absence of caries in the primary teeth. The oral manifestation was speeded by radiation therapy of a nevus flammeus. Maxillary osteomyelitis in newborns and small children develops through hematologic or rhinal routes. Dental microorganisms are only secondarily involved in the disease. The old terminology "dental germ osteomyelitis" is incorrect.

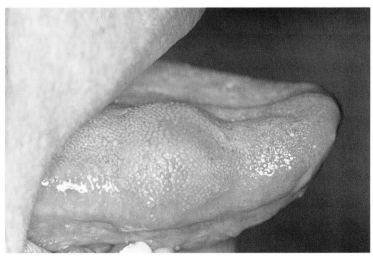

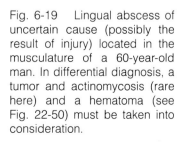

Fig. 6-19 Lingual abscess of uncertain cause (possibly the result of injury) located in the musculature of a 60-year-old man. In differential diagnosis, a tumor and actinomycosis (rare here) and a hematoma (see Fig. 22-50) must be taken into consideration.

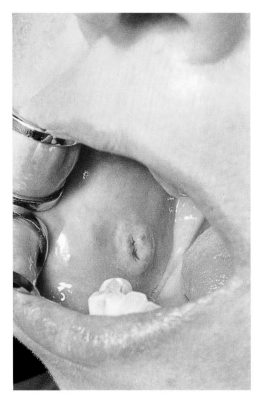

Fig. 6-20   Wound damage by chewing of the right cheek with subsequent damage from a fish bone that pierced the buccal mucosa was followed by deep-seated intraoral tissue necrosis. Extraorally there was a firm inflammatory swelling of the cheek infiltrate extending to the submandibular region that could be thought of as derived from a pyogenic dental lesion.

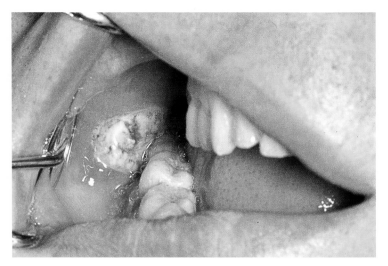

Fig. 6-21   Fibrin-covered ulceration with necrosis after the cheek mucosa was injured by a sharp poultry bone. The spread of the infection was facilitated by considerable plaque retention, mechanical irritation influences, and absence of treatment of tooth 48 (32).

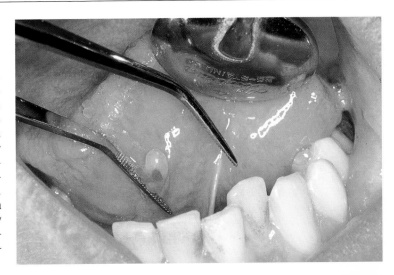

Fig. 6-22   Sialoadenitis of the sublingual gland with small salivary stones shortly before pressing. Sialolithisis of the sublingual salivary gland is rare. Over 80% of the salivary stones are in the submandibular gland with preferential localization in the duct system. Only stones up to the size of a pinhead can be eliminated by provocation of the salivary secretion without resulting in obstruction of the ductal system.

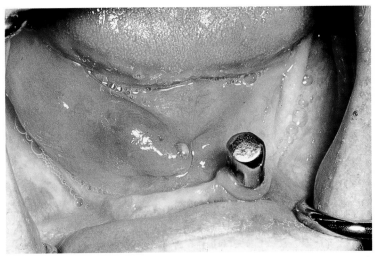

Fig. 6-23   Bulging swelling on the floor of the mouth caused by salivary calculus in the excretory duct of the submandibular gland. As a sign of inflammation of this salivary gland, there is a suppurative secretion that drains from the sublingual papillae. This is an important differential diagnostic symptom from, for example, a sublingual abscess derived from the teeth.

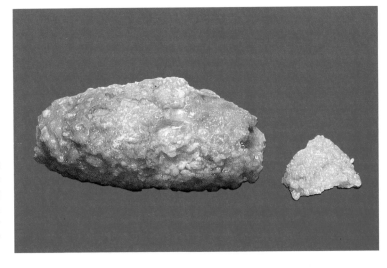

Fig. 6-24   Specimen of the patient from Fig. 6-23. The palpable sialolith, consisting mainly of calcium phosphate, was situated in the anterior portion of the duct and was removed surgically.

Chapter 7

Manifestations of Some Pyodermas of the Skin and Bacterially Caused Erythematous Infections in the Orofacial Region

Pyodermas
   Acute pyodermas
      Impetigo contagiosa
      Lip furuncle
   Chronic pyodermas
      Pyoderma chancriform
      Pyostomatitis vegetans
   Erysipelas

Bacterially caused exanthematic infectious diseases (scarlatina, scarlet fever)

Pyodermas

Pyodermas are infections of the skin and/or the skin appendages caused by pus-forming microorganisms. Some pyodermas occur within the oral mucosa.

To understand the disease process it should be known that several factors may take place separately or in combination. The pathogenic factors are:

- Virulent germs, usually staphylococci and streptococci
- Port of entry through any wound or localized tissue damage of the skin
- Lowered local or general resistance. Weakened local resistance is possible because of altered conditions of the skin, e.g., through maceration. The systemic defenses of the body can be decreased by diseases such as uncontrolled diabetic metabolic disorders, leukemias, and primary and secondary immunodeficiency conditions (which result in increased susceptibility to infection).

For the dentist, it is important to know that he or she can transmit virulent germs and can also be infected.

Certain pyodermas are secondary bacterial infections of preexisting skin changes (e.g., burning, dermatosis). Such conditions are called *impetigo.*

Acute pyodermas

Acute progressing skin infections may or may not be associated with hair-follicle units (i. e., hair follicles, sweat and sebaceous glands). Differential diagnosis generally includes several different diseases of significance for the dental practice that share similar-appearing symptoms.

Impetigo contagiosa (ICD 684)

This acute progressive infection of the epidermis is, in its small blister form, predominantly caused by pyogenic streptococci (group A) and, in its large blister form, is generally caused by coagulase-positive staphylococci. The disease appears generally in childhood; adults are seldom affected. It is highly contagious and can be endemic in schools and pediatric wards, where it is a feared complication.

Impetigo contagiosa of the face begins as small subcorneal blisters and develops into pustules. The blisters soon burst and turn into erosions with thick, honey-yellow to brown crusts. The changes can be associated with lymphadenitis of the regional lymph nodes. Scratching creates new lesions, which not infrequently melt into larger foci (Fig. 7-1). The area around the mouth is often affected. The angle-of-the-mouth rhagades can be starting points of pyodermas (see Figs. 34-9 and 34-10).

Patients with suspected impetigo should be referred to a dermatologist, whose job is to differentiate impetigo from other dermatoses with superimposed inflammations. In severe cases, systemic antibiotic therapy is indicated, always in conjunction with local therapeutic measures and improved hygiene.

Lip furuncle (ICD-DA 680.0X)

A furuncle is a prototype of staphylococcal infection of the hair follicle. The condition often starts with an infected small nodule or a pustule around the hair shaft *(folliculitis).* If the infection spreads into the surrounding tissue and there is a central purulent colliquation, it is called a furuncle. The clinical picture is dominated by an infiltrate under diffusely reddish skin that is rigid and painful. The area can turn into a large edematous swelling. High fever and chills (bacteremial) suggest systemic involvement.

About one-third of all facial furuncles are located in the upper lip (Fig. 7-2) and can then produce swelling. In this location there is (as in the nose furuncle) danger of a thrombosis of the cavernous sinus through the angular vein (see Fig. 6-13), hence referral of the patient should not be delayed. Any improper manipulation is to be avoided (i.e., the bad habit of squeezing pimples not infrequently favors the development of furuncles). Healing with scarring may occur after the removal of the core of necrotic tissue together with the hair follicle.

When neighboring hair follicles are involved with the deep sub-cutaneous abscess, the formation is called a *carbuncle*. The carbuncle is only infrequently found in the perioral region.

A dermatologist must differentiate a furuncle from, for example, a trichophytosis.

In furuncles in the vascular district of the angular vein, it is always appropriate to use a large dose of antibiotics. Because 75% of *Staphylococcus aureus* infections are resistant to penicillin, initial penicillin therapy is contraindicated. Oral cephalosporins should be administered first. Antibiotic sensitivity should be determined and, depending on the results, therapy may be changed.

Chronic pyodermas

There are also pyodermas that tend to have chronic vegetative courses. Their clinical course is explained by the peculiar properties of the pathogen and an unusual reaction of the body. Although the disease is rare, its preferential location is the facial region and sometimes the oral cavity and is thus of interest to those in dentistry.

Pyoderma chancriform (ICD-DA 686.00)

Staphylococcal-infection-associated pyoderma chancriform is found mainly in the external genitalia and in the face, especially the lip region. The oral mucosa is seldom affected. In the oral mucosa, the lesion is usually a single fatty, shiny, hard, infiltrated erosion or ulceration (Fig. 7-3) that has the appearance of a syphilitic primary infiltrate (therefore the denomination "chancriform"). The fact that regional lymph nodes are completely or almost completely painless but swollen also raises the suspicion of syphilis. To differentiate these findings from the hard chancre of syphilis, repeated detailed examinations must be performed.

Pyostomatitis vegetans (ICD-DA 686.00)

This rare form of a chronic, vegetative pyoderma caused by hemolytic streptococci, *Staphylococcus aureus,* and sometimes gram-negative microorganisms manifests itself in the body openings of the face (mouth, nose, eyes) as well as in the bordering mucosa (particularly oral mucosa), leading to striking lesions (Fig. 7-4). Typical of these lesions are small, pustular, granulating moist vegetations with erosions/ulcerations covered by exudate and with a considerable reactive hyperplasia of the epithelium and connective tissue. As a rule there is also associated ulcerative colitis.

These skin and mucosal lesions, for which there is no real therapy, are not very painful and do not greatly affect systemic conditions. They must be diagnostically differentiated from forms of pemphigus vegetans. Depressed defenses against pyogenic agents are thought to be the cause of this condition.

Erysipelas (ICD 035)

This skin infection is caused by a hemolytic *Streptococcus,* group A, and typically involves the lymphatic network of cutaneous and subcutaneous regions, which is why it is considered here.

Injuries of all types, as well as chronic skin diseases that lead to damage of the epithelial covering, are considered the point of entry. An incubation time of a few hours to 3 days, usually accompanied by high fever and severe malaise, leads to painful infection. The skin areas affected by erysipelas appear red and shiny, feel hot and tense, and exhibit a border raised above the healthy tissue (Fig. 7-5). Peripherally, the acute inflammation proceeds in a tonguelike, flamelike manner.

Favorite localizations of erysipelas are the face (facial rose) and the lower leg. The oral mucosa can in rare cases be affected as a primary area or as an extension from the adjacent inflamed skin. Isolated intraoral lesions are difficult to diagnose.

Erysipela responds well to penicillin. It tends to recur because of infection of the lymphatic vessels and leads to late complications (e.g., macrochelia, elephantiasis). In dental practice, erysipela must be differentiated from the dental and jaw abscesses with soft tissue participation (see Fig. 6-13). Further, a beginning zoster (see Fig. 11-32), an allergic contact dermatitis, and Quincke's edema must be considered (Fig. 7-6; see chapter 31). The very rare disease picture of an erysipeloid (fish handler's disease) can be eliminated based on clinical history.

Bacterially caused exanthematic infectious diseases (scarlatina, scarlet fever; ICD-DA 034.1 and 034.10)

Scarlet fever, measles, and rubella are exanthematic infectious diseases. Of these contagious diseases, scarlet fever is the only one caused not by a virus but by a hemolytic streptococcus, group A.

The acute exanthematic infectious disease is caused by a toxin produced by the streptococcus. This toxin is an antigen and leads to the development of protective antitoxins, so that the symptoms of scarlet fever appear only once in humans. Repeated streptococcal infections can result in a "second disease," with complications (including myocarditis, glomerulonephritis, polyarthritis) of great clinical importance.

According to the immune response to scarlet fever streptococci, three reactions of the organism must be distinguished:

1. Lack of type-specific antibacterial immunity and lack of antitoxin immunity.
   Consequence: scarlet fever as acute infectious disease.
2. Lack of type-specific antibacterial immunity with preexisting antitoxin immunity.
   Consequence: streptococcal angina. Pharyngitis, glomerulonephritis, myocarditis. Diseases of the rheumatic group. Focal infection.
3. Type-specific antibacterial immunity with or without antitoxin immunity.
   Consequence: no clinical disease but possibly a clinically healthy disease carrier.

Scarlet fever develops after an incubation period of 2 to 5 days with nonspecific initial symptoms such as fever, headaches, sore throat, and vomiting. With pharyngitis, there is an associated short-term, spotty enanthema on the palate, as well as lymphadenitis of the regional lymph nodes. The tongue develops a thick, furry coating that results in swollen, fire-red fungiform papillae.

These findings are followed by the typical punctate, spotty scarlet fever exanthemas with spreading on the body, from top to bottom. The perioral region of the face is characteristically pale *(perioral paleness, scarlatine face;* Fig. 7-7).

After the second day of exanthems, the tongue loses its gray-white coating. On the now desquamated and clearly red tongue dorsum, there are also red, edematous, fungiform papillae. This is the so-called *scarlet fever tongue (strawberry tongue;* Fig. 7-8). With decrease of the fever, the exanthemas also lose color. Subsequently there is the formation of large scales on the skin, which are particularly distinct on the palms of the hand and soles of the feet.

Typical of scarlet fever, as well as for exanthematic infectious diseases, are the intraoral manifestations that occur before the appearance of the skin changes. The findings in the oral mucosa are therefore important for early clinical diagnosis.

In differential diagnosis, scarlatiform medication exanthemas must be considered in addition to exanthematic infection.

Scarlet fever decreased worldwide with the discovery of penicillin therapy (maximal dose for 10 days). In the era before antibiotics, the disease had a 20% mortality rate; today it is about 0.5%. Death due to scarlet fever must, however, still be reported.

In the above-mentioned diseases, the focal oral manifestations are of importance in dental practice.

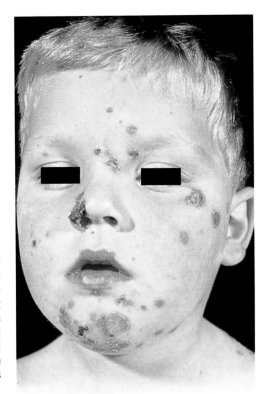

Fig. 7-1 Small blisters of impetigo contagiosa in a child. The infection of the skin started with small red spots followed by blisters that become opaque because of pus and that burst quickly. The clinical picture is dominated by crust-covered erosions. By scratching and smearing, new foci of infection can develop. Healing takes place without scars.

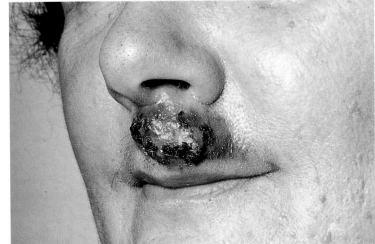
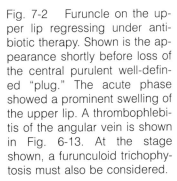

Fig. 7-2 Furuncle on the upper lip regressing under antibiotic therapy. Shown is the appearance shortly before loss of the central purulent well-defined "plug." The acute phase showed a prominent swelling of the upper lip. A thrombophlebitis of the angular vein is shown in Fig. 6-13. At the stage shown, a furunculoid trichophytosis must also be considered.

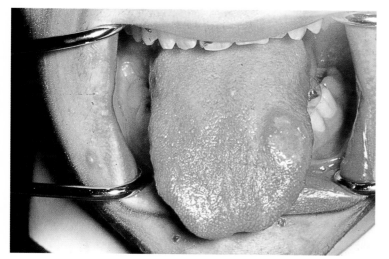

Fig. 7-3 Chancriform pyoderma of the tongue accompanied by painless swelling of the submandibular lymph nodes in a 17-year-old boy. A painless swelling of the submandibular lymph nodes appeared at the same time. Primary syphilis should always be suspected with findings of this type (and the patient should be referred to a dermatologist). For differential diagnosis, see also Figs. 8-1 to 8-3.

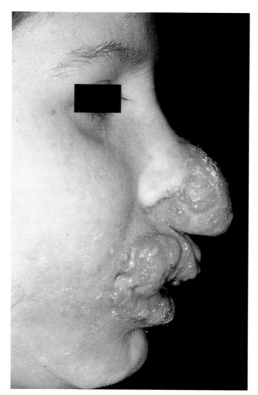

Fig. 7-4 Pyostomatitis vegetans in a 10-year-old boy. Episodes of this chronic pyoderma (practically therapy resistant) over a period of years led to the formation of tumorlike, purulent but almost painless vegetating lesions surrounding the oral and nasal orifices. This patient demonstrates the chronic course of the disease.

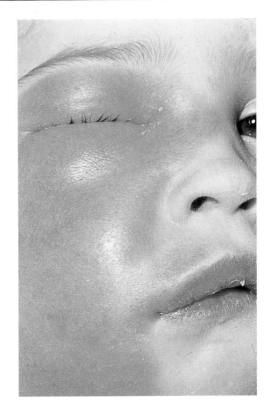

Fig. 7-5 Facial erysipelas in a 6-year-old child. Note the bright red, sharply demarcated skin lesion of this acute streptococcal infection. There are tongue-like extensions of the streptodermia in the area of the nose and the upper lip.

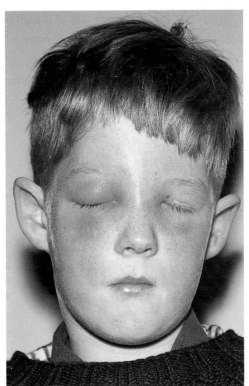

Fig. 7-6 Differential diagnosis of erysipela: allergic reaction with erythema and edema of the eyelid to a sulfonamide-containing intraoral pack.

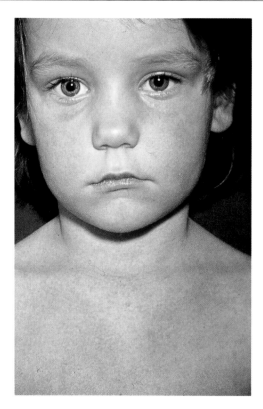

Fig. 7-7   Scarlet fever exanthema on the face (facies scarlatinosa) and trunk of a child. The transmission by droplets of saliva took place in a kindergarden. The exanthema that spares the perioral region (perioral pallor) is typical.

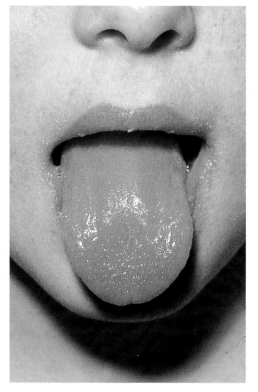

Fig. 7-8   Scarlet fever tongue (strawberry tongue). The reddish dorsum of the tongue is seen after loss of the coating and desquamation of the mucosal epithelium at the beginning of the exanthematous phase of the skin. The edematous enlarged fungiform papillae are easy to distinguish. The skin has a tendency to form scales with progress of the disease.

Chapter 8

Syphilis and Tuberculosis

Syphilis
    Early syphilis
        Primary syphilis; oral chancre
        Perioral lesions and oral mucosal patches in secondary syphilis
    Late syphilis
        Oral and perioral lesions of tertiary syphilis
    Congenital syphilis
        Hutchinson's teeth

Tuberculosis
    Primary tuberculous complex
    Oral tuberculous ulceration
    Tuberculosis cutis colliquativa; scrofuloderma
    Lupus vulgaris
        Carcinomas developing from lupus vulgaris

For rare diseases and diseases that have become rare, there is the danger of lack of clinical experience in recognition and management. For this reason, syphilis and tuberculosis deserve a closer look in the dental practice.

These chronic infectious diseases, which are caused by different pathogens, can be treated with relative success today. They are, however, not strictly limited to fringe groups of the society, as sometimes considered. Additionally, they offer diagnostic as well as therapeutic problems.

Syphilis

Syphilis is caused by *Treponema pallidum* and has a worldwide distribution. Together with gonorrhea, ulcus molle, lymphogranuloma venereum, and granuloma inguinale, syphilis makes up the five historically known sexually transmitted diseases that, according to the law, must be reported to health authorities. Syphilis is predominantly, but not exclusively, transmitted through sexual contact. Untreated, syphilis in the past led to late syphilitic changes of the large vessels (cardiovascular syphilis) and of the central nervous system (neurosyphilis) that can be fatal after a long clinical course.

The prognosis for patients with correctly identified and early treated syphilis is quite good today, aside from rare cases of lues maligna. Because the effectiveness of penicillin is widely recognized among lay people, the danger of transmission of syphilis has become trivialized. The occurrence rate of this infectious disease over the years is practically unchanged in Germany. In New York, there was a sixfold increase between 1985 and 1988 in reported cases of congenital syphilis, and in 1989 there was an elevenfold increase.

After a person has become infected, there is a series of specific cellular and humoral defense reactions, which manifest themselves clinically in a variable, chameleon-like clinical picture. Because the skin and mucous membrane efflorescences of the secondary stage can imitate numerous skin diseases and because of the disease's varied clinical presentation, syphilis was earlier designated as the "ape" among diseases.

The delicate, corkscrew-like *Treponema pallidum,* which is about 5 to 15 µm long, acts as the pathogen of syphilis and is, contrary to other spirochetes, a tissue parasite that uses the circulatory system only as a means of transportation. The port of entry can be any microscopically small lesion of the skin or mouth membrane.

Early syphilis

Early syphilis includes

- The primary stage—lues I—(primary lesion, regional lymphadenopathy)
- The secondary stage—lues II—(eruption generalization stage)
- The early latency stage—lues latens seropositiva— (clinically asymptomatic but with persistent positive serology)

The various clinical pictures of the oral and perioral lesions of lues I and II are shown in the figures.

Primary syphilis; oral chancre (ICD-DA 091.20)

Approximately 10% of patients with primary syphilitic lesions show an extragenital localization, in half of which the lips (frequently) and oral mucous membrane (rarer) are involved.

After a time of incubation averaging 2 or 3 weeks, a well-defined lesion can be found at the pathogen's place of entrance. These lesions are brownish-red bumpy nodules of varying size (seldom larger than a penny), with induration and surface involvement. The change feels, upon palpation with a protected finger, like an embedded piece of hard rubber. It can also initially be covered by epithelium and erodes or ulcerates only later.

Usually a wet erosion (erosive chancre) or a round-to-oval, bowl-shaped, not-painful ulcer, with a lacquerlike surface and a ham-colored, sometimes slimy-covered bottom (Figs. 8.1 to 8.3) exists at the time of examination. On the skin-covered portion of the lips, finely adherent crusty lesions are also possible (Fig. 8-4).

The base and edges of the lesion in typical cases have a firm or cartilaginous-like infiltration (ulcus durum, hard chancre). The classic finding is identified by the texture, painlessness, and, most often, single ulcer. Eroded and ulcerated primary lesions do not bleed upon touch; they ooze a highly contagious serous secretion.

In response to this syphilitic primary lesion, which can occasionally be surrounded by an indurated edema (Fig. 8-2), a clearly visible and palpable painless swelling in the regional lymph nodes (syphilitic primary complex) appears about 8 to 14 days later. Like the skin that covers them, the well-delimited lymph nodes are movable and show, contrary to tuberculosis, no tendency to coalesce and fistulate.

From the point of view of differential diagnosis, in older patients with this type of a hardened ulcer on the lip or the mucous membrane, it is always important to consider an ulcerated carcinoma. Occasionally, corroded giant aphthae can imitate, on inspection but not on palpation, the clinical picture of a primary lesion (see chapter 31, Fig. 31-2).

In primary syphilis, darkfield examination of the secretion obtained from the primary lesion can demonstrate the treponemas. Seroreactions become positive only after 2 to 3 weeks. Serologic tests include the nontreponemal seroreactions of the classic type (among others, Wassermann complement fixation reaction, WaR) and the specific treponemal seroreactions (among others IgM fluorescent treponema-antibody absorption test or IgM-FTA-ABS-test). The serodiagnosis should be performed by an experienced specialist.

During primary syphilis, there is formation of immunizing humoral antibodies of the IgM type. In further course, with the generalization of the disease, there is formation of antibodies of the IgG type, which then results in corresponding specific tissue reactions.

The syphilitic primary lesion is a local spirochetosis. With penetration of the lymph nodes, the disease is transformed into a systemic spirochetosis.

Perioral lesions and oral mucosal patches in secondary syphilis (ICD-DA 091.3 and 091.30)

Secondary lesions occur about 5 to 8 weeks after the appearance of the primary lesion, which if untreated heals with a barely visible scar within a few weeks. After a period of variable length, there is the initiation of the secondary stage with exanthematous clustered skin lesions that may also involve the oral mucosa. These generalized skin and mucous membrane changes of often chameleon-like polymorphism are signs of the early dissemination of the pathogens through lymphatic and hematogenous routes, as well as a result of a changed reaction of the organism, which in most cases includes systemic lymph node swellings (polyscleradenitis).

At this time, a feeling of malaise develops followed by a symmetrically localized, spotty skin eruption *(roseola syphilitica),* which manifests itself on the oral mucous membrane as a spotty, murky-red enanthema. With deep infiltration, round, red-brown, papular efflorescences soon form, most of which are the size of lentils *(papular syphilid)* (Fig. 8-5) whereby macular and papular sources of contagion often exist next to each other *(maculopapulous syphilid).* Pustulous and scaly forms also occur. The skin eruptions, which are all over the body and do not itch, are usually polymorphic and can be confused, in their variable forms, with other clinical pictures (such as infectious dermatitis). Bullous and urticarial exanthemas are missing, however.

Syphilitic papules (Fig. 8-5), which are often observed even in the region of the mouth, undergo changes that are dictated by the environment. In the corner of the mouth, they can lead to wet, vegetating lesions and then to painful, perleche-like fissures (Fig. 8-6) that can most often be differentiated from a trivial infection because of a marked infiltration of the surrounding tissue.

Because of the special conditions of the oral cavity (due to the influence of the saliva), the syphilitic mucous membrane papules show a modified picture (Figs. 8-7 to 8-9). Their surface is macerated and covered by a thin, dull-gray to gray-white veil as a sign of epithelial clouding *(opaline plaques).* On the dorsum of the tongue, due to the flattening of the filiforme papillae, flat papules the size of lentils *(plaques lisses)* appear (Figs. 8-7 and 8-8). Increasing infiltration can cause them to become slightly elevated.

Difficulty in swallowing, without fever, is a demonstration of *angina specifica,* which is an expression of reactive changes of the lymphoid tissue of the throat. The tonsils are reddened and swollen. Their surface shows a veil-like gray-white coating as well, which is delimited from its surroundings by a red margin (Fig. 8-10).

All mucous membrane changes of secondary syphilis are summarized under the term *mucous plaques.* They secrete large quantities of fluid loaded with spirochetes and, therefore, present a dangerous source of infection so that the dentist with unprotected hands (Fig. 8-9) can easily be infected during a patient's care.

Diagnosis is based on clinical findings (syphilis should be considered), proof of the pathogen, and serologic verification, which is always possible in this stage of the disease.

As a result of the immunologic defense of the organism, the relapsing, healing efflorescences decrease in number and finally heal without scar formation after months, but most often after 2 to 3 years into the early latent phase. Lues latens seropositiva stands out by the absence of clinical symptoms with decreasing infectiousness, but seroreactions remain positive and can last indefinitely.

Late syphilis

Thanks to the successful treatment of early syphilis with penicillin, late syphilitic disease in this country is a relic of the past.

The small number of patients observable today with clinically manifested late syphilis is due primarily to persons who, because of unnoticed early symptoms, did not seek a physician and therefore remained untreated.

Not every untreated early case of syphilis necessarily becomes a case of late syphilis. Apparently there are patients who, having had secondary syphilis, remain without symptoms without any therapy (stable latency) and over time have a negative seroreaction, so that spontaneous healing can be assumed. In most patients, the infection progresses because they are asymptomatic and therefore untreated but the seroreaction remains positive. This stage of the seropositive clinical latency can last from 3 to 30 years or more and can then become manifest with the appearance of a tertiary or quaternary syphilis. In contrast to tertiary syphilis, lues IV *(tabes dorsalis, progressive paralysis)*, also called metalues, presents another path of development that can probably be traced to an anergic reaction.

Of the tertiary stage of syphilis (which can cause serious damage to the vascular system and the central nervous system in addition to changes of internal organs), only the findings in the oral cavity are of special importance to the dentist.

Oral and perioral lesions of tertiary syphilis (lues III) (ICD-DA 095)

The late course of syphilis depends on the development of immunity. The interaction between host and pathogen depends on the cellular allergic reaction of the tuberculin type (type IV reaction according to Coombs and Gell; see chapter 31). The organism reacts to the syphilitic antigen with the formation of a typical syphilitic granuloma, which can lie cutaneously or subcutaneously.

In cutaneous localization, brownish-red, hard, obviously raised knots, clustered in groups, develop that can become confluent foci; they are described as *tuberous syphilid (syphiloma)*. They develop slowly and are not painful or contagious. The center heals, leaving scars and atrophic areas, but new knotty infiltrates form at the periphery. As a result of the centrifugal progression, the lesions are arch-shaped, i.e., isolated by serpentine lines *(tuberoserpiginous syphilid)*. If there are ulcerations, they are referred to as *tubero-ulcero-serpinginous syphilis.*

In comparison with lupus vulgaris (see section on tuberculosis), syphilitic granulomas destroy the tissue in relatively shorter time. They can appear anywhere on the skin but definitely prefer the face (Fig. 8-11). Involvement of the bones of the jaws in the form of a nongummy, tertiary syphilitic osteitis is very rare (Fig. 8-16).

Gummas are subcutaneous, sharply delimited, hard and gumlike barely contagious syphilitic granulomas. They tend toward a central coalescence during growth, which leads, over a variable period, to perforation at the outer edge with subsequent ulcer formation. Gummas leave scars and tissue defects on healing.

In the oral cavity, the gummas initiating in the submucosa, periosteum, or bone are observed predominantly on the hard and soft palate as well as on the arch of the palate and on the tongue, where they are first noticeable as hard, relatively sharply delimited, indolent knots. Later they colliquate, resulting in deep ulcers with an often slimy-covered bottom and borders that look stamped out (Figs. 8-12 and 8-15). Gummas of the hard palate can destroy the floor of the nose and can cause perforations into the nasal cavity. It is necessary to differentiate perforations caused by an ulcerated carcinoma (see Fig. 19-28) from those caused by a gangrenous granuloma (see Fig. 30-20) and from those caused by physical trauma due to the wearing of dentures (see Fig. 33-33). Breakthrough of nasal syphilitic gummas into the oral cavity is also possible. A special form of granulomatous tongue infection in tertiary syphilis is *diffuse interstitial glossitis,* which can be superficial or deep. This form leads to a more or less distinctive shrinking or sclerotic hardening of the tongue. In the past, this lesion was considered a dangerous, precancerous stage because findings included disturbance or leveling of the papillae, and leukoplakial changes with irregularities of the tongue contour with fissures and nodular areas (Figs. 8-13 and 8-14). The development of a carcinoma on these atrophic and leukoplakial modified areas, which were damaged by chronic infection, is not unusual, but in light of their frequency were possibly overdiagnosed in the past.

Congenital syphilis

Syphilis can be transferred from an infected, untreated mother through the placenta to the fetus after the fourth month of gestation. Depending on the time of infection of the mother (i.e., stage of syphilis) and the immune status of the mother, the transfer of the infection leads to spontaneous abortion, stillbirth, premature birth, or syphilitic manifestations and complications after birth.

In what is called *precocious congenital syphilis,* the syphilitic disease is detectable in the newborn or develops within the first 2 years of like ("infantile syphilis"). In some cases, the consequences of congenital syphilis are only clinically noticeable in later years. These late stigmata are described as *late congenital syphilis.*

Hutchinson's teeth (ICD-DA 090.51)

Hutchinson's teeth are permanent features of syphilitic infection that occurred during fetal development in the syphilitic mother. The malformations of the crowns of the teeth can be seen on the permanent maxillary central incisors. The crowns are barrel shaped with semicircular indentations of the incisal edge (Fig. 8-7). Other teeth, the first molars and the mandibular central incisors in particular, can show crown abnormalities.

If *keratitis parenchymatosa* (corneal clouding) and difficulty in hearing or inner ear deafness exist in addition to these findings, then the condition is called *Hutchinson's triad*. The complete triad is a certain sign of late congenital syphilis whereas the same certainty of diagnosis is not possible with single symptoms. The changes are often found in late childhood or in young adulthood.

Further classic stigmata of the delayed form of congenital syphilis are—in addition to other skeletal deformities—the saddle-shaped nose, as well as pouchlike perioral radial fissures and scars, which reach the vermilion region of the lips *(parrot wrinkle).*

Syphilis can be associated with gonococcal infection (ICD-DA 098), the most frequently transmitted disease worldwide. Gonococci *(Neisseria gonorrhoea)* are often detected on the mucous membrane of the oropharynx as a result of orogenital contact. The infection course is, however, most often asymptomatic, but on occasion leads to purplish enanthemas or tonsillitis-pharyngitis. It is not certain whether the gonococci can give rise primarily to a specific gingivitis or stomatitis. On one hand, when identified in small numbers, gonococci may be confused with other gram-negative diplococci that may be found in the oral cavity and have similar biochemical reactions. On the other hand, the unequivocal identification of gonoccoci demonstrates, at the most, that they are part of the plurimicrobial bacterial pool of gingivoperiodontitis, i.e., stomatitis, but it is not yet certain that it is the primary cause.

Tuberculosis

Tuberculosis is a chronic and necrotizing bacterial infection caused by *Mycobacterium tuverculosis,* an acid-resistant rod about 2 to 4 μm long. The disease primarily affects the lungs; however, by dissemination it may affect every organ, singly as well as part of generalized disease.

Up to the beginning of this century, tuberculosis was the most frequent fatal chronic infectious disease in Europe. The mortality rate of tuberculosis in the 1920s in Germany was 150 men, 160 women, and a great number of children per 100,000 residents. Fifty years later, tuberculosis affected 13 men (partly because of work-related causes) and four women per 100,000 residents.

After Robert Koch discovered the pathogen in 1882, the disease could be isolated by strict epidemiologic and hygienic measures, which resulted in the development of a separate specialty and branch of the public health service. The impressive reduction of morbidity and mortality associated with tuberculosis was possible with the availability of effective combinations of tuberculostatic medications. Currently in HIV-infected persons, an increase of tuberculosis and mycobacterial infections can occur as opportunistic infections.

The danger of contagion of tuberculosis is comparatively small. Case history details concerning the time of incubation are variable. Vaccination is only partially successful. Today, the contamination occurs aerogenically by droplet infection.

Until a few decades ago, many cases of tuberculosis were triggered by ingestion of milk products infected with the pathogen *Mycobacterium bovis* (food TBC). With the elimination of infected cattle due to supervision by veterinarians, and by pasteurization of milk, which is common today, this path of infection no longer exists in western countries. In people from other regions, the possibility of an oral-enteric primary infection should, however, be considered.

A percutaneous infection by inoculation also occurs, which under some conditions is judged a work-related disease.

Thre stages of tuberculosis can be differentiated:

- Primary stage. Includes the primary complex (parenchymal focus and lymph node focus). With the penetration of the lymph node filter, a lymphogenic-hematogenous dissemination is possible.
- Subprimary stage. As a result of the lymphohematogenous dissemination, multiple disease manifestations occur most often immedi-

ately after the primary stage, whose extent and degree of seriousness depend on the immune condition of the infected person.

- Postprimary stage. Tuberculosis localized to a previously infected organ or a generalized process is known; this is traced back, in most cases, to the endogenous reactivation of an earlier (lung) tuberculosis caused by reduced immunity defenses. In this manner, the renewed increase of tuberculosis as an opportunistic infection with AIDS is understandable. Further, chronic alcoholism plays a frequent and important role in the reactivation of tuberculosis.

Resistance to the tuberculosis infection (no matter in which location the infection enters) is, in the beginning phase, nonspecific with macrophages and, only in the later phase of the disease, is targeted with the help of T- and B-lymphocytes. After 4 to 6 weeks, the cell-mediated immune response *(tuberculin reaction)* can be demonstrated. Necrosis develops under the influence of proteolytic enzymes, which are set free by macrophages. The *tuberculum* is the pathohistologic characteristic of the infection. In this case, a wall is made up of epithelioid cells that are modified macrophages.

The healing phases, which are frequently accompanied by calcifications, allow survival of the tubercular bacteria within the healing *tuberculoma,* which can then become a means of reinfection by reactivation.

The various possible clinical manifestations of tuberculosis are determined not so much by the type of pathogen involved (human or bovine) but by the mode of infection and speed (i. e., aerogenic, hematogenous, lymphogenic, per continuitatem), by the localization, and especially by the immune status of the organism. Diseases by the *Mycobacterium tuberculosis avium* (pathogen of poultry TBC) and other special forms, which are described today as *mycobacterioses,* are not considered here. Leprosy, which proceeds similarly to tuberculosis, is also not described because it is almost never seen in our region.

From the dental point of view, the following are significant:

- The course of the oral primary complex
- Miliary tuberculosis (as expressions of an anergic immune status)
- Tuberculosis cutis colliquativa and lupus vulgaris (as expressions of a predominantly normergic reaction)

Finally, the question of existence of a carcinoma over a chronic skin or mucous membrane tuberculosis is discussed.

Primary tuberculous complex (ICD 010.0)

The primary pulmonary complex results from a parenchyma focus with a lymphangitis and regional lymphadenitis. Among the extrapulmonary manifestations, the skin and mucous membrane are seldom the location of the primary tuberculous infection. The primary focus is favored in the oral cavity as a result of oral-intestinal tuberculosis from contaminated milk, which has become very rare today. It affects the gingiva related to the dentition, as well as the region of the cheeks, lips, and above all the tonsillar ring in children.

A small ulcer a few millimeters in diameter is identified with a soft, flaking, undermined edge and a slimy base that heals after 2 to 3 weeks even without therapy. Because of its limited size, its painlessness, and its brief existence, the ulcer is easily overlooked or is not identified. It is, however, infectious.

In the forefront of the clinical picture, even in oral manifestations, is lymphadenitis, which occurs shortly after the ulcerous disintegration of the mucous membrane tubercle and is accompanied by a high fever. The lymph nodes, which range in size from a pigeon's egg to a hen's egg, are rarely painful at first and adhere to each other and to the skin; they finally colliquate in a cheesy material and can result in fistulation. The lymph nodes (Fig. 8-20) can be of various sizes and progress with no intraoral change or only an unnoticeable scar. In the case of a considerable lymphadenitis lacking a dental cause, the existence of tuberculosis should be considered in every patient, not only in children and foreigners, despite its rarity today.

Differential diagnosis and treatment of all tuberculous forms is the work of the specialist.

In retrospect, the diagnosis of an oral tuberculosis can be reached with proof of sclerosis in the regional lymph nodes (submandibular, cervical), which is seen as a secondary finding in orthopantomoradiographs.

Oral tuberculous ulceration (ICD-DA 017.80)

Ulcerated tuberculosis of the oral mucosa takes place in the anergic terminal phase of a progressive primary, often reactivated, pulmonary tuberculosis when mycobacteria from the lung pass from the bronchi and upper respiratory tract into the mouth, i.e., *bronchogenic tuberculosis* (Figs. 8-18 and 8-19).

By autoinoculation, small nodules (tubercles) initially develop that disintegrate quickly and turn into highly infectious, painful ulcerations. They occur in the larynx, the oropharynx (tonsils, base of the tongue), in the frequently affected oral cavity (tongue, frenum of the tongue, palate at regions of the mucous membrane that border dentures, areas of lesser resistance), as well as in the surrounding areas of the mouth (lips, especially the region of the corner of the mouth) with the appearance of a migrating cheilitis. In older patients, who are preferentially affected, the ulcerous changes are frequently found in relation to removable dentures and poor denture hygiene (Fig. 8-24).

The flat abscess has a soft consistency, an undermined border, and a base with a granular appearance, which is covered with a thin gray-yellow exudate.

Differential diagnosis must particularly distinguish the disease from syphilitic efflorescences.

Tuberculosis cutis colliquativa; scrofuloderma (ICD 017.0)

Tuberculosis cutis colliquativa develops from the chronic tuberculosis infection under normal conditions of immunity in the cutaneous and subcutaneous (or submucous) layers. Its spread is by direct extension or through lymphatics and is preferentially located in the throat. It starts with few painful nodules and progresses through softening and confluence of the tubercular foci and thinning of the epidermis. After the (not unusual) spontaneous perforation, the fistulas discharge a thin liquid pus, which contains tubercular bacteria (Fig. 8-21). The colliquation leads continuously to scar formation with star-shaped, pointed, and bridge-forming scars.

Differentially, one must consider cervicofacial actinomycosis. The colliquative form of tuberculosis can, in rare cases, manifest itself on the tongue (Fig. 8-27), where the findings can be demonstrated by biopsy.

Lupus vulgaris (ICD 017.0 and 017.00)

The term "lupus" points to an extreme chronically developing form of skin tuberculosis of the most destructive character with formation of granulation tissue. Because of the blood flow in the area of the face, the skin of the face (cheeks, nose, forehead, ears) is affected in 90% of cases (Figs. 8-22 and 8-23). Brown-red papillae the size of pinheads develop discretely on the areas of predilection, which correspond to subcutaneously and intracutaneously located tubercles. They progress at the periphery and form larger lesions. The typical yellowish-brownish apple jelly-like color can be seen clearly under pressure of a glass spatula *(glass spatula phenomenon)*. A probe can easily perforate the soft tissue without much pain *(probing phenomenon)*. The untreated disease will penetrate different layers under the skin, such as cartilage and bone, and will be destructive (Fig. 8-28). These lesions are practically noncontagious and can be cured with early therapy.

Lupus vulgaris can advance from the skin into the mucosa. Thus, this lesion, commonly found in the area of the nose, can also be observed in the perioral region (see Fig. 11-19).

Almost every other patient with lupus shows mucous membrane participation, which can be detected by a large ulcerated area. Because of good blood circulation, there is a favorable tendency to spontaneous healing.

In the isolated mucous membrane tuberculosis of the oral cavity (hard and soft palate, cheek, lips, gingiva), there are shiny gray-to-light-red bumps (tubercles) with a reddish base that are usually considered conglomerated tubercles (Figs. 8-25 and 8-26). The granulated-appearing finely bumpy surface shows small embedded white kernels that correspond to blurry epithelial regions. In contrast to hyperplastic gingival changes, palpation reveals a doughy consistency. With colliquation and destruction, there is development of ulcerations, which exhibit the typical picture of tuberculous craters (with irregularly limited, flabby-bordered, purulent-covered bases that bleed easily). New satellite nodules facilitate diagnosis, which must be confirmed histologically. These lesions are practically noncontagious.

Carcinoma developing from lupus vulgaris (ICD-M 8070/3)

On the base of a lesion that has been present for decades, particularly in atrophic and sclerosed skin, a carcinoma can develop (usually a squamous cell carcinoma) from mutilating and scarring lupus vulgaris (Fig. 8-28).

Within the framework of the chronic disease, past treatment must be considered in the development of the carcinoma. This subject is discussed in detail in the description of carcinoma developing over lichen planus (see chapter 16).

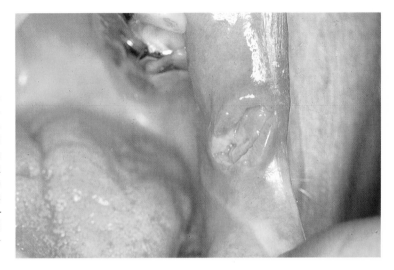

Fig. 8-1 Syphilitic primary lesion in the area of the left corner of the mouth. With extragenital lesions, the patient, and sometimes the physician, does not consider the possibility of a venereal disease. With the help of darkfield microscopy, it is possible to find *Treponema pallidum* in the exudate removed from the lesion and in this manner reach the diagnosis.

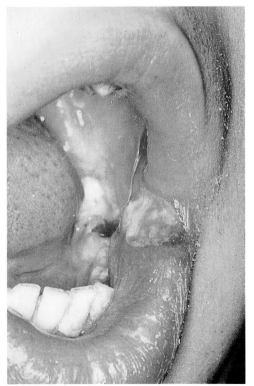

Fig. 8-2 Syphilitic chancre in the left labial angle of the mouth with surrounding indurated edema. In differential diagnosis, it is important to consider an ulcerated carcinoma in older patients.

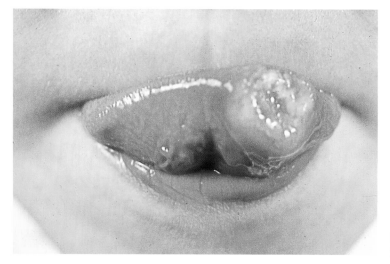

Fig. 8-3 Syphilitic chancre of the tip of the tongue.

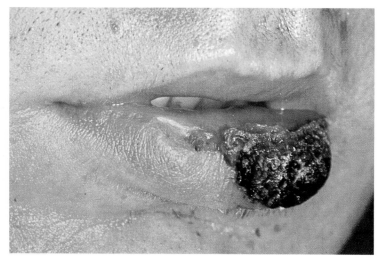

Fig. 8-4 Syphilitic chancre of the lower lip. The chancre is covered by a crusty layer. (From Kruger, E. Lehrbuch der chirurgischen Zahn-, Mund- und Kieferheilkunde, vol. 1. Berlin: Quintessenz, 1988.)

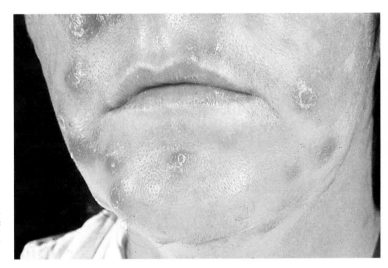

Fig. 8-5 Particularly pronounced papular syphilid of perioral region in secondary syphilis.

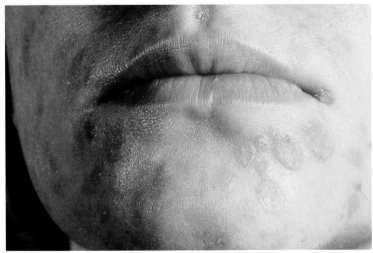

Fig. 8-6 Syphilitic papules of the perioral region in secondary syphilis. Note especially the papule with a central crust, which resembles angular cheilosis, in the left labial angle of the mouth. With this finding, highly infectious secondary syphilis must be suspected. Diagnostic clarification is necessary prior to dental treatment. The patient must be referred to a dermatologist.

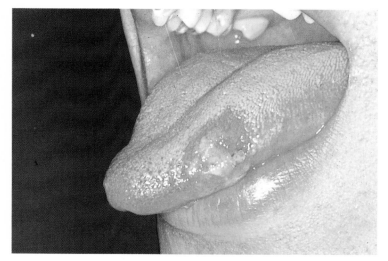

Fig. 8-7 Mucous patch located chiefly on the edge of the tongue in secondary syphilis. The lingual papillae damaged by inflammation are temporarily flattened. Note the typical grayish-white covering as a sign of epithelial opacity (plaques opalines).

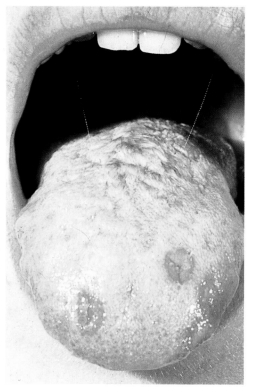

Fig. 8-8 Lesions on the dorsum of the tongue in secondary syphilis. The appearance of the mucous patches is determined by their location: due to flattening of the filiform papillae, they appear on the dorsum of the tongue as sharply delimited smooth red spots. All mucous membrane efflorescences in secondary syphilis are dangerous because of their large pathogen load.

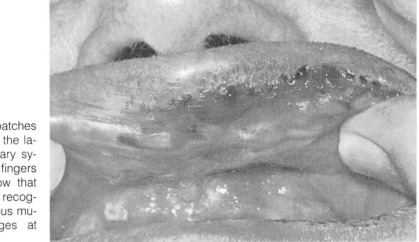

Fig. 8-9 Mucous patches (plaques muqueuses) in the labial vestibule in secondary syphilis. The unprotected fingers seen in the picture show that the examiner failed to recognize these highly infectious mucous membrane changes at first.

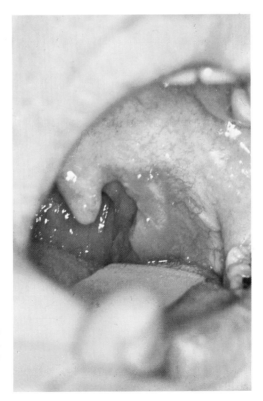

Fig. 8-10 Specific angina in secondary syphilis. (From Kruger, E. Lehrbuch der chirurgischen Zahn-, Mund- und Kieferheilkunde, vol. 1. Berlin: Quintessenz, 1988.)

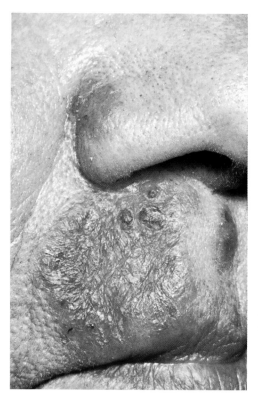

Fig. 8-11   Tuberous, that is, tuberoserpiginosus, syphilid in the upper lip and on the ala of the nose in tertiary syphilis. (From Kruger, E. Lehrbuch der chirurgischen Zahn-, Mund- und Kieferheilkunde, vol. 1. Berlin: Quintessenz, 1988.)

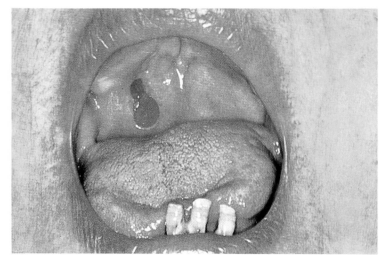

Fig. 8-12   Ulcerated gumma of the soft palate in tertiary syphilis. Note that the border of the lesion has a punched-out appearance.

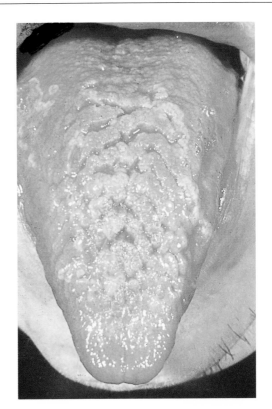

Fig. 8-13 Tertiary syphilitic interstitial glossitis with distinct leukoplakial superficial changes. An asymmetric fissured pattern is seen as result of the sclerosing, inflammatory process.

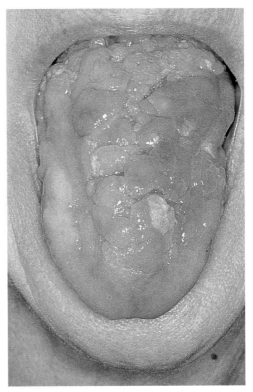

Fig. 8-14 Long-standing profound tertiary interstitial glossitis. As a consequence of the deeply located, chronic, coalescent, granulomatous inflammation, the tongue is deformed and sclerosed (very characteristic). The surface, which became atrophic (i.e., papillae loss), has an irregular, knotty, and pitted appearance.

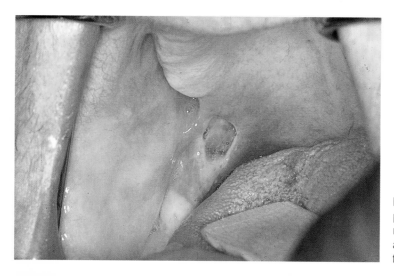

Fig. 8-15 Sharply delimited, partially exudate-covered ulcerated gumma on the anterior aspect of the vestibule in tertiary syphilis.

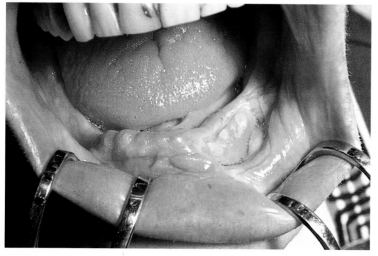

Fig. 8-16 Circumscribed nongummatous osteitis on the edentulous alveolar process of the mandible as the chief organic manifestation of tertiary syphilis. Note the brownish, discolored, superficial osteonecrosis within the mucosal defect with stamped-out appearance.

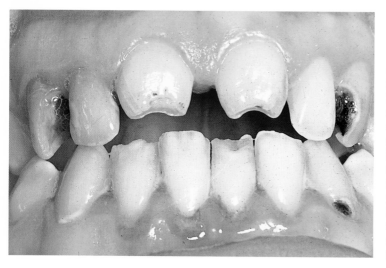

Fig. 8-17 Hutchinson's teeth in congenital syphilis. The maxillary central incisors show the characteristic barrel-shaped crowns with notched incisal edges. In addition, interstitial keratitis and a partial internal ear deafness (Hutchinson's triad) were present in this 18-year-old patient. The first molars can also show coronal dome-shaped abnormalities, with an appearance reminiscent of a mulberry.

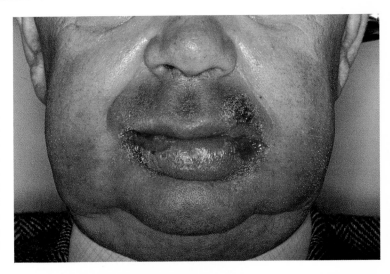

Fig. 8-18 Perioral manifestation of tuberculosis ulcerosa in cavitary fibrocaseous tuberculosis. Autoinoculation by pathogen-containing secretions (sputum: acid fast rods +++) resulted in ulcerative lesions on the lip and perioral area. The endogenous reactivation of a lung tuberculosis often occurs with chronic alcoholism.

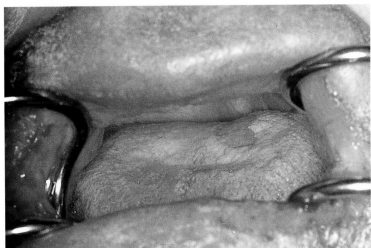

Fig. 8-19 The patient in Fig. 8-18 at the same time of examination. Besides the tubercular mouth angle rhagades, the oral mucosa shows ulcerations with flaccid borders covered with a thin secretion. The painful lesions, which bleed easily on contact, are contagious.

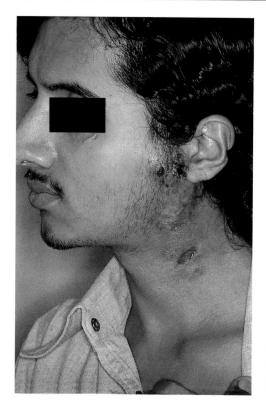

Fig. 8-20 Oral tuberculosis primary complex with cheesy lymphadenitis colli (appearance after incision) in a patient of Asian origin from an area with endemic tuberculosis.

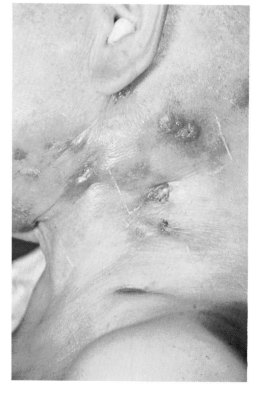

Fig. 8-21 Tuberculosis cutis colliquativa in the area of the soft tissue of the neck. In addition to new well-developed foci (tuberculomas), colliquated and scarred lesions are seen. Frequently, in earlier times, the illness lasted for decades. (From Kruger, E. Lehrbuch der chirurgischen Zahn-, Mund- und Kieferheilkunde, vol. 1. Berlin: Quintessenz, 1988.)

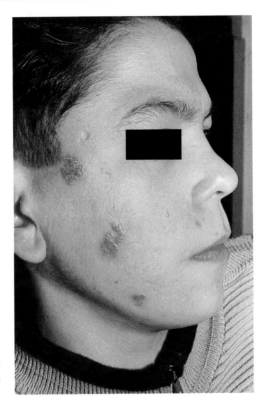

Fig. 8-22   Early tuberculosis of the skin (lupus vulgaris) in a young patient.

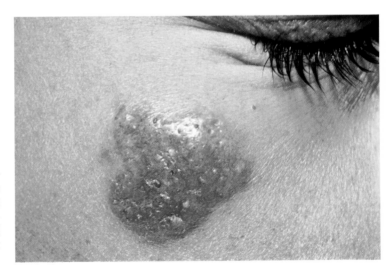

Fig. 8-23   Initial stage of tuberculosis of the skin (lupus vulgaris) on the cheek. (From Kruger, E. Lehrbuch der chirurgischen Zahn-, Mund und Kieferheilkunde, vol. 1. Berlin: Quintessenz, 1988.)

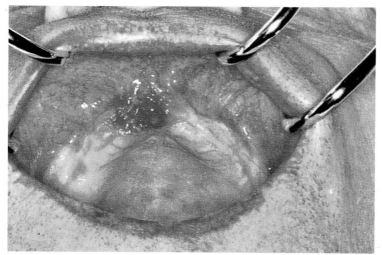

Fig. 8-24 Tuberculous ulcer (tuberculosis miliaris ulcerosa) on an edentulous maxillary alveolar ridge. The shallow ulcer with soft, undermined margins was mistaken for a pressure area (decubitus ulcer) by the dentist and treated unsuccessfully for 3 months. The intraoral lesion was a symptom of active pulmonary tuberculosis, unknown to the patient and his associates. Such tuberculous ulcers of the oral mucosa, most frequently found on the tongue, are the result of coughed-up, swallowed infectious materials.

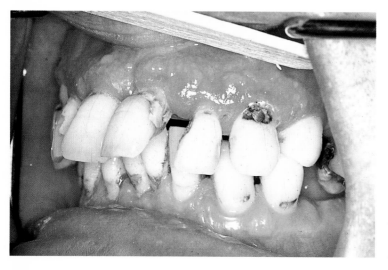

Fig. 8-25 Gingival manifestation of tuberculosis cutis luposa (lupus vulgaris) in the area of the maxillary anterior teeth. Note the numerous conglomerated nodules (tubercles).

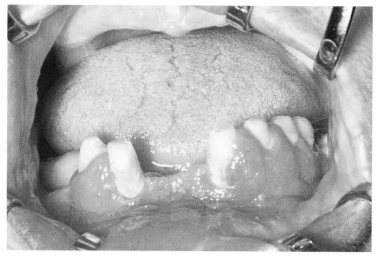

Fig. 8-26 Lupus vulgaris of the gingiva in the vestibular area of a partially edentulous mandible. The tubercular infiltrates cause swelling of the gingiva and have increased the tissue area. They have a doughy consistency. Later they will transform into large ulcerations.

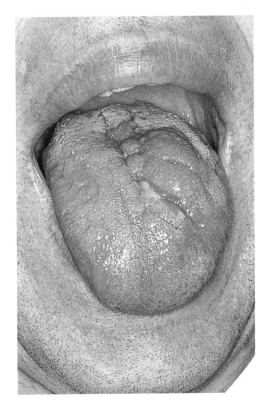

Fig. 8-27 Proliferative tuberculous inflammation (gumma-
tous tuberculosis), not yet in the
stage of liquefaction, on the
tongue. Actinomycosis, syphilitic gumma, and particularly malignant neoplasms should be
considered in the differential
diagnosis.

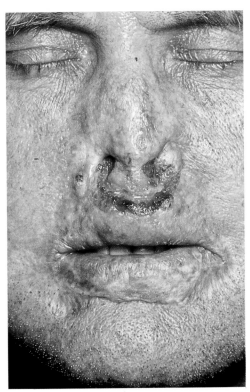

Fig. 8-28 Cornified flat epithelial carcinoma over lupus
vulgaris previously treated with
radiation in a 59-year-old patient.

Chapter 9

Tetanus

Tetanus (ICD-DA 037)

This insidious infectious disease, which is found worldwide, is caused by the exotoxin of the anaerobic spore-forming *Clostridium tetani* (tetanus bacillus). In its spore form, the bacterium has a practically unlimited life duration in all climatic zones. The infection can appear in all types of injuries of the skin or mucosa when the known pathogen (which is present in not only the soil) finds favorable anaerobic life conditions. The size and condition of the injury allow no conclusions concerning the existence of a tetanus infection. Half of all the illnesses are caused by minor injuries. Even today, the illness has a mortality rate of about 25% to 50%. From the prognostic point of view, the disease should be considered to be more serious the shorter the incubation period (a few days, usually 5 to 10, sometimes several weeks).

Because the appearance of inflammation can be absent at the point of entry, noticing the early general symptoms of the onset of a tetanus infection is important. Prodromic symptoms are, among others, fatigue, irritation, agitation, muscle pain, and muscle numbness. The exotoxin (tetanospasmin) initiates a blockage of the nervous system-mediated reflex. Excitability creates a tonic rigidity of the skeletal muscles and clonic reflex spasms ("rigid cramp"). The tonic cramp is first noticeable in the masticatory muscles, leading to cramping of the masseter muscle and then to a locking of the jaw (trismus) (Figs. 9-1 to 9-3). Because of tonic contraction of the mimic muscles, there is a facial rigidity *(facies tetanica)* or an involuntary grinning facial expression *(risus sardonicus)* (Figs. 9-1 and 9-3).

The muscle jamming affects one muscle after another: the neck (causing difficulty in talking and swallowing and rigidity of the neck), the trunk, and the extremities. At the same time, spastic cramps in response to minor stimuli are usually characteristic symptoms. Once the toxin is fixed in the nerve membrane, it cannot be neutralized. Because of the cramps of respiratory musculature, asphyxiation can occur, resulting in death.

The sudden appearance of a jaw spasm can cause a frightened patient to seek the dentist for help. Early recognition of tetanus is essential for preservation of the patient's life. Unmotivated jaw locking should always create suspicion of a cramp due to an injury, particularly when a fixed bilateral hardening of the masseter muscle can be palpated. This finding, even in the absence of tetanic face or rigidity of the neck, among other symptoms, is sufficient to require immediate referral of the patient to a hospital.

Because of the reasons mentioned, active prophylactic immunization against tetanus is important. As a rule, immunization must be renewed after 10 years and also after an injury that may result in infection with tetanus (care of a wound should always be recorded). If the patient is not vaccinated against tetanus, passive immunization with tetanus serum offers, in case of injury only, a questionable transitory protection. It is therefore combined with an active immunization (see table on next page).

The dentist must also remember the importance of these measures when he or she is the first to treat a patient for accidental injury (e.g., trauma to anterior teeth).

Current recommendations for tetanus prophylaxis in case of accident/injury

Previous injection with Tetanol® (last immunization record)	Time elapsed since last injection to the day of injury	On day of injury Tetagam® (Simultaneously on the contralateral side of body)	On day of injury Tetanol®	Interval since other injections with Tetanol® for completion of active protection 2–4 wk	6–12 mo	Every 10 y (renewed inoculation)
0	–	●	○	○	○	○*
1	Up to 2 wks	●		○	○	○*
1	2–8 wks	●	○		○	○*
1	Over 8 wks	●	○	○	○	○*
2	Up to 2 wks	●	○		○	○*
2	2 wks to 6 mos				○	○*
2	6–12 mos		○			○*
2	Over 12 mos	●	○			○*
3	Up to 5 yrs					○*
3	5–10 yrs		○*			○*
3	Over 10 yrs	●	○*			○*

Time interval of the basic immunization: between one and two inoculations, 4 to 8 weeks (minimal interval of 2 weeks). Three inoculations 6 to 12 months later (this equals the complete basic immunization). Routinely renewed inoculation every 10 years.

Explanation of symbols: ● = 250 immunization units of tetanus immunoglobulins from human serum (Tetagam® S) intramuscularly for passive immunization.

○ = 0.5 ml of tetanus-adsorbate inoculation materials (Tetanol®) intramuscularlyfor active immunization.

* = IgG Td-Impfsoll® (tetanus-diphtheria combination inoculation for adults) IM if the last diphtheria inculation was more than 10 years ago.

Source: latest information from Behringwerke AG, August 1989.

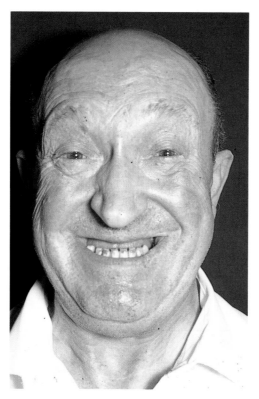

Fig. 9-1   Sardonic smile (mimic stare) of a 66-year-old patient with tetanus 1 week after a small injury of the hand with a wire. The toxin caused a spasm of the facial musculature and resulted in the typical facial expression with a fixed smile and raised eyebrows.

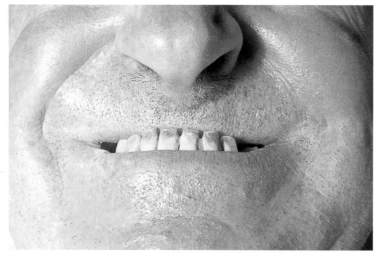

Fig. 9-2   The same patient. Tonic spasm of the masticatory musculature with clamping of the jaw (trismus) is the most frequent early symptom of tetanus. The almost complete jaw lock, which occurred overnight, was misdiagnosed as a disease of the temporomandibular joint by the dentist and physician. The patient died 14 days after this photograph was taken.

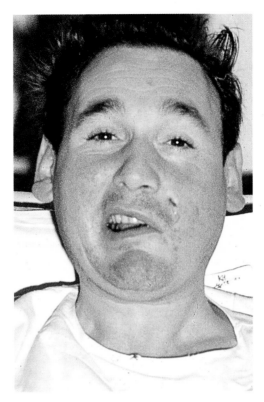

Fig. 9-3 Special clinical course of a tetanus infection: head tetanus (rose disease) with risus sardonicus. Trismus, temporary facial paralyis, and stiffness of the neck is apparent in this 28-year-old patient. Three weeks previously, after tripping over a shrub, the patient injured the left cheek, which subsequently became infected. Hospital treatment for 1 month was followed by recovery.

Note

Even small injuries of the skin and mucosa can produce a tetanus infection. Therefore, tetanus prophylaxis is extremely important. If there is no plausible local explanation, a jaw spasm should always be considered tetanus. When in doubt, immediately hospitalize the patient. Tetanus has a high mortality rate.

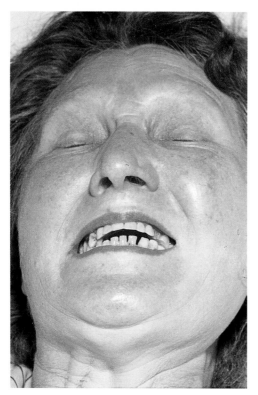

Fig. 9-4 Differential diagnosis of tetanus: demonstration of atypical facial pain and muscular spasm in the facial area of patient with mental problems. Psychogenic appearance of paralysis resembling risus sardonicus and trismus.

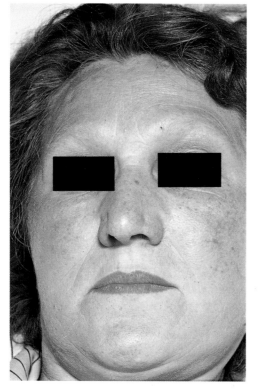

Fig. 9-5 While distracting the same patient during the examination, it was possible to release the facial expression, therefore the spasm was not rigid. The transfer of psychological conflicts and fear into a somatic symptom (by an unconscious process) is called *conversion*.

Chapter 10

Fungal Diseases (Mycosis) in the Oral Cavity and the Region of the Mouth

Candidiasis (thrush)

Trichophytic tinea of the beard

Cervicofacial actinomycosis (as a pseudomycosis)

Yeasts have become increasingly significant as pathogens in all fields of medicine. This is true for fungi that are saprophytes–because of their opportunistic behavior toward altered conditions of health of the host organism–as well as for fungi that are obligatory parasites and appropriately considered true pathogens.

Fungi are a part of the world of plants; approximately 100,000 different types of fungi have predominantly ecologic importance and useful functions (for example, in fermentation and purfication). Only about 50 types of fungi cause disease in humans. These can cause superficial infections (dermatomycosis), deep mycoses, and systemic mycosis. Human pathogens and, with them, medically important types of fungi are differentiated into three groups. However, these groups are not uniformly classified botanically:

- Yeasts (e.g., *Candida* group)
- Dermatophytes (e.g., thread fungi such as trichophytes, microsporum)
- Molds (e.g., aspergillus variants)

According to their botanical origin, the fungi have a different morphology, markedly different requirements for life, and reproductive forms that help in their identification. Even if the clinical pictures of fungal diseases are typical, diagnosis is reached by means of identification of the fungus–initially by a direct microscopic preparation (smear) and, should the need arise, by means of a histologic examination of biopsy material (i.e., PAS staining). Only a culture allows the definitive identification of the fungus type. The differential diagnosis lies in the hands of the dermatologist and an expert laboratory technician.

Fungi, just like bacterial microorganisms, are in many cases harmless companions of the skin, as are inhabitants of the mucous membrane in symbiosis as saprophytes. The transition from existence as a harmless saprophyte to parasite that lives at the expense of the host and attacks living cells does not depend on a change in the fungi's pathogenic ability according to present opinion. More important is the change and decrease in the level of tolerance. As long as the living organism can tolerate the fungi on its surface (i.e., mucous membrane), there is no outbreak of disease. The level of tolerance is decided by the immunologic defense of the host.

Conditions induced by medication, such as antibiotic therapy, immunosuppressive agents, cytostatics, and corticosteroids, and HIV infection (AIDS), have extensively explained this phenomenon of opportunistic infections (see chapter 11). Immune defects, especially in cell-mediated immunity, openly favor the development and progression of fungal diseases. Beside opportunistic *Candida* infections, aspergilli, cryptococci, and histoplasmosis are of significance in HIV infection. In addition to the ubiquitous incidence of the parasitic fungi *(histoplasmosis, blastomycosis, and others),* the occurrence of clinical diseases in the human is influenced by clinical factors (e.g., tropics, subtropics). Mobility of the population (including tourism) leads sometimes to their diagnosis in zones of temperate climate. The dentist should consider the possibilities that are described below:

- Candidiasis; that is, findings in the mucous membrane and skin in the presence of yeast under various conditions of the host defenses (saprophyte, facultative pathogens, opportunistic infection)
- Trichophytosis, parasitic fungal disease of the skin, preferentially the head (common in central Europe)
- Cervicofacial actinomycosis (pseudomycosis), with a typical clinical course in the jaw (but requiring differential diagnostic considerations)

Candidiasis (thrush) (ICD-DA 112.0)

Candida albicans is among the members of the yeasts, with more than 120 types. It is the most frequently found and the most pathogenic aerobic fungus in humans under certain conditions. *Candida albicans* (newly introduced term; *for Syringospora albicans)* is found in every other person—almost certainly in denture wearers—as harmless saprophytes of the oral cavity *(latent thrush).* For this reason, the demonstration of fungi in culture is, by itself, not diagnostic and needs correlation with the clinical condition. A fungal disease (mycosis) will depend mostly on the availability of the fungus and not as much on local factors but on general factors of the host organism. Yeast infections were recognized centuries ago as indicators of an underlying serious illness such as malignant tumors, leukemias (Figs. 10-7 to 10-9), chronic infectious diseases, and diabetes mellitus. Concern about these underlying conditions has increased in the meantime.

An exception to the above rule is found in the development of *Candida* infection in the mouth of a newborn (up to 2 weeks of age); in this instance the *Candida* infection occurred during birth. The fungal spread that develops rapidly ("thrush") covers the bacterial flora that is just developing in scattered areas of the mouth. After a short time, the fungus yields to the normal local bacteria of the oral cavity in the healthy newborn.

During antibacterial chemotherapy, an ecologic gap develops to the advantage of the fungi, because the normal flora is suppressed to the advantage of *Candida* in the oral cavity. These types of clinically manifest colonizations with *Candida* in the oral cavity abate spontaneously with cessation of the bacteriostatic-bactericidal antibiotic chemotherapy. This phenomenon must therefore be considered a side effect of medication (Figs. 10-1 and 10-2) in immunocompetent people.

Even local circumstances such as covering of the mucous membrane with a removable prosthesis (see Fig. 33-36), especially in cases of poor oral hygiene, as well as in the maceration of the skin of the lip commissures (see Figs. 34-20 to 34-22), which require moisture, are pathogenetic factors that favor manifestation of the mycosis. Comparable phenomena are observed around skin folds as a result of sweating, maceration, and chafing, which result in a *Candida intertrigo* (often occurring with diabetes mellitus, obesity, and poor hygienic conditions). These examples make clear that the physical and chemical disturbance of the integrity of the body surface (skin or mucous membrane) can influence the equilibrium of the bacterial flora without a deficiency in the immune system.

The pathogenesis of opportunistic infections is more easily demonstrated with saprophytic fungi than with opportunistic bacterial or viral infections. Congenital or acquired, temporary or permanent immunologic defects of humoral or cellular defenses (for *Candida,* especially in the lymphocyte-macrophage system) sooner or later regularly lead to opportunistic infection, so that the development of candidiasis is considered a clinical indicator of disturbed T-cell function. Candidiasis in the oral cavity begins, especially with HIV infection, with discrete relapsing but later escalating symptoms corresponding to the degree of dysfunction of the immune system (see Figs. 11-49, 11-51, 11-62 to 11-65). As the immune defenses become more compromised, there is also a descending gastrointestinal tract candidiasis, organ mycosis, and finally a *Candida* sepsis as the most generalized form of the opportunistic yeast infection.

The frequency of development of a *Candida* mycosis in the oral cavity as a consequence of therapy for other diseases led to a classification of several types of candidiasis. Today, in oral candidiasis, a *pseudomembranous* form, an *erythematous (atrophic)* form, and a *chronic hyperplastic* form are differentiated.

The clinical picture of the *pseudomembranous* form in the oral cavity consists of white, raised spots and also flat *Candida* membranes over an infected red base (erythema) that can grow to a thickness of several millimeters (Figs. 10-1 to 10-11). They consist of a layer of matted threads of fungi together with desquamated epithelial cells, fibrin, granulocytes, and food residue. The ends of the fungal threads only superficially adhere to the squamous epithelium, so that the brittle, pastelike coating of whitish gray color can be wiped off without much injury and without selective bleeding from the mucous membrane. The thrush can spread to the pharynx and esophagus and cause severe subjective symptoms with the development of erosions and ulcerations (which inhibit nutrient absorption).

Erythematous (atrophic) candidiasis is found particularly on the palate (see Fig. 11-49). Localization on the dorsum of the tongue leads to a loss of papillae. *Candida*-induced *chronic* changes most likely occur at the corner of the mouth (see Fig. 34-20) and can be associated with a papillary variant on the hard palate under ill-fitting removable prostheses, where they are a cofactor of the multifactorial prosthesis stomatitis (see Figs. 33-35 and 33-36). Chronic hyperplastic candidiasis can present hard, plaquelike, sometimes even nodular or wart-forming lesions that resemble a leukoplakia, with which it is also often associated. These forms of *Candida* mycosis are observed in areas of the corner of the mouth (see Figs. 34-21 and 34-22), particularly retroangular areas (Figs. 10-13 and 10-14).

If the fungi penetrate deeper into the subepithelial tissue, depending on the immunologic conditions, it is more difficult to wipe off the fungi, and removal of the coating is associated with punctate bleeding. In this case, the mucosa shows varying degrees of inflammation and often a granulomatous response. The prognosis of these forms is definitely less favorable. With extension of the fungi into the blood vessels, hematogenous dissemination can develop (*Candida* sepsis).

A damp environment with swelling of the stratum corneum, maceration of the skin, disturbance of the physiologic oxygen layer, and with this, the damage of the epithelium are important prerequisites for the development of candidiasis on the skin. Like other dermatophytes, *Candida* fungi require a damp environment for 2 or 3 days in order to germinate and penetrate into the uppermost surface of the skin. If these conditions occur in the skin of the corner of the mouth, this is a region of predilection for a localized *interlabial mycosis* caused by *Candida* infection (see Figs. 34-20 to 34-22). With removal of the local favorable conditions (even a closed occlusion can be considered), the *Candida* loses its pathogenicity (facultative pathogenicity).

In cases of serious immunodeficiencies (among them AIDS), a form of mucocutaneous mycosis can be caused by *Candida albicans* (see chapter 11).

Conclusions for the dentist

If the dentist observes oral candidiasis that cannot be related to a short-term antibacterial chemotherapy, he or she should refer the patient for a more complete consultation. In differential diagnosis, HIV infection is to be considered in young patients. In the location where the sore occurs, disturbance of wound healing is to be expected. Chronic periodontal processes tend toward progression. The reasons for the opportunistic behavior of the saprophytic fungi must be explained in every single instance. Particularly after termination of treatment with *Candida*-specific antimycotic agents (with which there is usually rapid improvement of the clinical findings), recurrences can occur that must raise the suspicion of a thus-far-undetected underlying condition. Identification of a mycosis should therefore act as a signal for the dentist to seek cooperation with the internist.

Trichophytic tinea of the beard (ICD 110.0)

From the group of parasitic fungal diseases of the skin, trichophytosis is mentioned here briefly. At present, all dermatophytic infections of the skin, regardless of type of fungus responsible, are referred to as *tinea* with the addition of their respective localization (tinea capitis, tinea barbae, tinea facies).

Trichophyton mentagrophytes–a thread fungus–is passed on from diseased livestock or house pets (golden hamsters, guinea pigs) but also from person to person and by means of objects on which spores lie. The fungal parasite affects the keratin of the skin, hair, and nails, where it can release many variously shaped fungal elements. The oral mucous membrane always remains free, because the necessary histologic structures (keratin, skin appendages) are missing.

A preferred location is the head/face region. In the beard region is a marked spreading in an especially impressive manner (beard lichen). Clinically, a surface and a deep trichophytosis are distinguished; those afflicting the beard are always deep trichophytoses. Differential diagnosis of the cervicofacial actinomycosis and all other pyogenic skin and hair follicle infections (folliculitis, furuncle, carbuncle) are to be considered.

Tinea barbae (Fig. 10-6) begins with a single, infected, pustulating folliculitis. The pathogens are spread by shaving. The resulting surface infection, which is accompanied by redness and flakes, penetrates deeply into the hair follicle and leads to furuncle-like nodules that occasionally change into confluent or colliquating abscesses. Typically the beard hairs, which look dusty, can be painlessly pulled out of the follicle openings like wicks. The disorder progresses for 4 to 6 weeks, and healing begins under the scars as the immune response develops. As a rule, there is no permanent alopecia and the hair grows back. Serologically, 50% of the population has antibodies against trichophytic fungi, which suggests that trichophytosis is highly contagious.

The differential diagnosis with actinomycosis shows in the latter a firm and deeply rooted infiltrate that as a rule is without relation to the hair follicles. The diagnosis is accomplished by demonstrating the pathogen and, if necessary, by a fungal culture.

Cervicofacial actinomycosis (as a pseudomycosis) (ICD-DA 039.3)

The cause of the human actinomycosis, *Actinomyces israeli,* is a common gram-positive saprophyte of facultative pathogenicity found in the oral cavity of healthy adults. It is classified botanically between fungi and bacteria. Only under anaerobic conditions does it develop parasitic characteristics. Therefore, the prerequisite for the development of an endogenous disease is the transport of the pathogen in tissue layers with an anaerobic environment where an accompanying bacterial flora, also common in the oral cavity, is a *conditio sine qua non (actinomycotic mixed infection)*. Belonging to this group of associated bacteria are *Staphylococcus aureus,* hemolytic streptococci, *Actinobacillus actinomycetemcomitans,* and *Bacteroides melaninogenicus.* The duration of incubation is about 4 weeks. A pyogenic infection serves as a precursor to the development of actinomycosis. These infections may originate in the dental system via the root canal, predominantly from mandibular teeth (Figs. 10-17 and 10-22), as well as via traumatic influences such as tooth extraction (Figs. 10-18 and 10-21). Injuries of the soft tissue and jaw fractures also facilitate entrance of the pathogen.

The cervicofacial actinomycosis manifests itself predominantly in the region of the soft tissue of the jaw with a strong inclination to the submandibular region (Figs. 10-17, 10-19, and 10-20). Actinomycotic disease of the tongue, salivary glands, and bone seldom occurs. Seventy percent of the spreading fungal diseases are observed in the region of the face and soft tissue of the neck; thoracic and intestinal manifestations are comparatively rare.

The actinomycosis of mixed infections may have an acute or subacute onset (Fig. 10-18) under the guise of an initial unspecific pyogenic infection, so that its specific chronic character is revealed only later. In these instances, the clinical suspicion should increase whenever, despite successful extraoral abscess incisions, an unexplained recurrent abscess or a second abscess appears nearby, or the infection, despite adequate drainage, shows induration of the adjacent tissue and persists longer than expected. As a rule, the disease shows a chronic course from the beginnng, with an early deep-seated infiltrate that advances gradually to the outer skin. Later softening results under the thinned, bluish-red skin with the development of one or more subcutaneous abscesses, which can perforate spontaneously. If the process remains untreated, the well-known symptoms appear and there is a tendency to the development of a tough−even hard−surface infiltrate with subcutaneous abscesses, multiple fistulas, scarring, and new peripheral, interconnecting infiltrates. These findings are expressed in the chronic course with continued spreading.

A special diagnostic problem is caused by the unsupervised and often suboptimal use of antibiotics for abscesses, the clinical picture of which can, therefore, be blurred (e.g., cold abscess).

The definitive diagnosis is obtained by microbiologic proof of pathogen by means of *anaerobic culture* (special laboratory). The material to be submitted (e.g., pus, granulation tissue) is preferably obtained by extraoral incision.

Sulfur granules (radially arranged fungi threads, thus the name "ray fungi") cannot be found in one-half of the histologic preparations. The lack of granules therefore does not rule out actinomycosis.

Treatment consists, aside from the necessary surgical intervention, of a directed antibiotic treatment (antibiogram) that in relatively high doses will attack not only the penicillin-sensitive actinomycetes but, above all, the gram-positive and gram-negative accompanying flora that may have a different susceptibility. In addition, supportive measures may be indicated.

The dentist should consider the possibility of actinomycosis in all infiltrates tending to a chronic course and in stubborn recurring abscesses of the deep soft tissue of the jaw as well as of the neck region in order to arrive at a direct diagnosis and determine therapy, which in this age of antibiotics may still create problems.

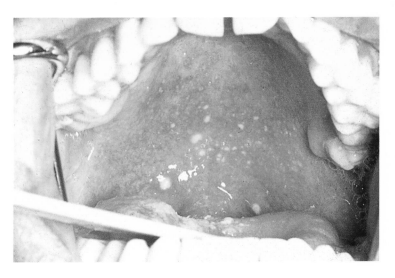

Fig. 10-1   Candidiasis of the palate of a young patient undergoing antibacterial chemotherapy for bacterial tonsillitis. The paint-drop-like deposits, which are removable pseudomembranes, consist of fungi threads (which attach to the epithelium and cause an inflammatory reaction) admixed with fibrin, granulocytes, desquamated epithelium, and food debris. The development of these findings is favored by therapy that eliminates the regular oral flora, which are then replaced by the latent, available fungi (latent *Candida*). Even without a *Candida*-specific therapy, there is regression of these side effects with the discontinuation of the antibiotic therapy (see chapter 31).

Note

In oral *Candida* infections—so far as they are not clearly associated with an antibiotic therapy or cannot be associated with local factors—there must be a search for an underlying disease (opportunistic infection).

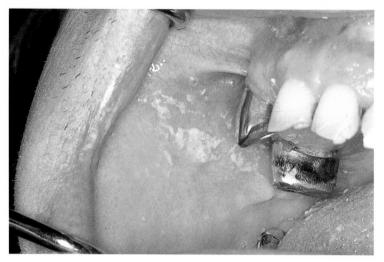

Fig. 10-2 Pseudomembranous candidiasis of the oral cavity of a patient undergoing 10-day antibiotic therapy. Areas of predilection of this form of oral candidiasis are the cheeks, palate, and tongue. Predisposing factors are long-term treatment with antibiotics, corticosteroids, cytostatic and immunosuppressive agents, as well as serious diseases that compromise the immune system. The greater adhesion of the fungal pseudomembrane and the greater the intensity of the mucosal erythema, the more severe the candidiasis. In this case, candidiasis is only the side effect of antibiotic treatment.

Fig. 10-3 Pseudomembranous candidiasis in a typical location on the palate with stippled and plaque-like fungal deposits in a patient undergoing corticosteroid treatment. The whitish cream coating on red

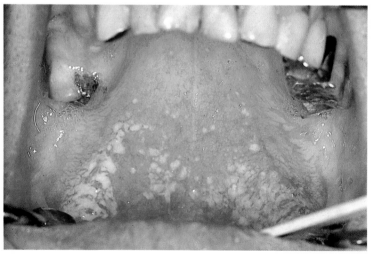

background (erythema) can be scraped off. With changes of the host defenses, the opportunistic behavior of the fungi becomes apparent and an independent disease can develop. The oral cavity, which is easily accessible for examination, allows early and easy detection of the changes of the cellular immune defense system. For this reason, the dentist should constantly seek consultation with the internist upon observation of candidiasis (for explanation of causes, see also chapter 11 under HIV-infection).

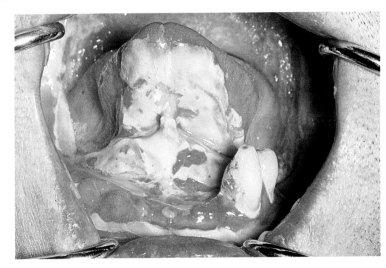

Fig. 10-4   Severe acute pseudomembranous candidiasis in a 57-year-old man after prolonged antibiotic therapy for pulmonary tuberculosis. Extensive, curdlike, whitish patches on the oral mucosa can be scraped off. The mucosal portions, surrounding or lying beneath these patches, are reddish and swollen. Note the cyanotic color of the mucous membrane as an expression of the disturbed function of the lungs.

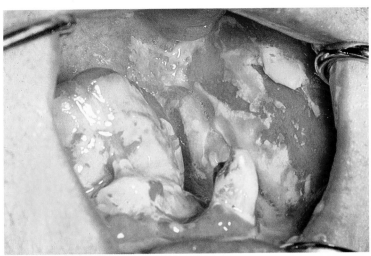

Fig. 10-5   The patient in Fig. 10-4 at the time of examination: the patches of the left buccal mucosa can be scraped off. The greater the adhesion of the mycelium to the mucous membrane, the more unfavorable the prognosis. In this patient, systemic mycosis was not yet present.

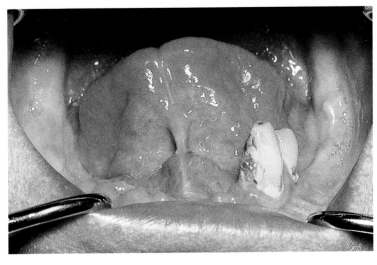

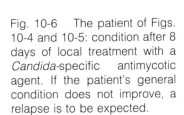

Fig. 10-6   The patient of Figs. 10-4 and 10-5: condition after 8 days of local treatment with a Candida-specific antimycotic agent. If the patient's general condition does not improve, a relapse is to be expected.

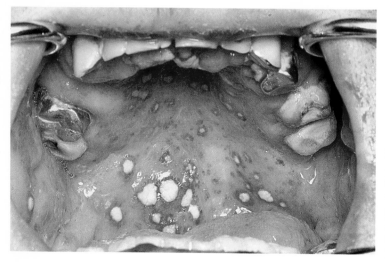

Fig. 10-7   Oral candidiasis in a 64-year-old man: opportunistic infection with a severe underlying systemic disease (acute phase of a chronic leukemia). There is spotty and stipple-like thrush on the dark-red erythema.

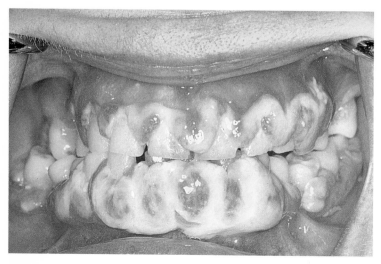

Fig. 10-8   Pseudomembranous candidiasis in the vestibular region of the gingiva of the maxilla and mandible in a 34-year-old woman. The cause is considerable lowering of general resistance due to an acute myelogenous leukemia.

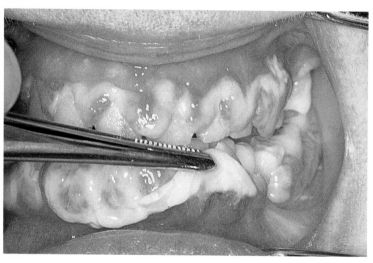

Fig. 10-9   The patient of Fig. 10-8 at the time of examination. After lifting the apron-shaped fungal coating, the reddish adhesive zone is recognizable on the enlarged gingiva, caused by leukemic infiltrate.

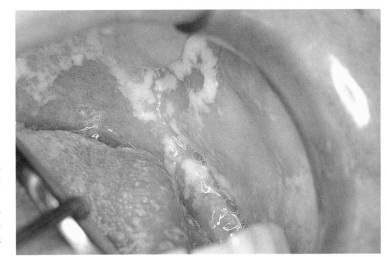

Fig. 10-10 Pseudomembranous candidiasis of the oral mucous membrane (cheeks, palate, and tongue) that has been present for several weeks in a 62-year-old patient with a tumor.

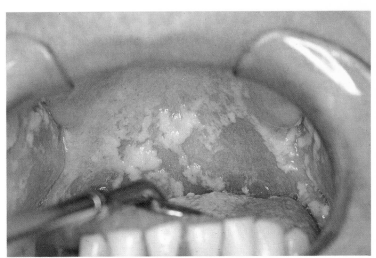

Fig. 10-11 The patient of Fig. 10-10 at the time of examination. The lesions consist of a creamy, removable coating with a small or medium amount of erythema that is slightly painful and hardly noticed or completely ignored by the patient. In contrast, atrophic as well as hyperplastic forms, which often develop rhagades on functionally important regions, cause extensive complications under certain conditions and in some locations (e.g., corner of the mouth, tongue, esophagus).

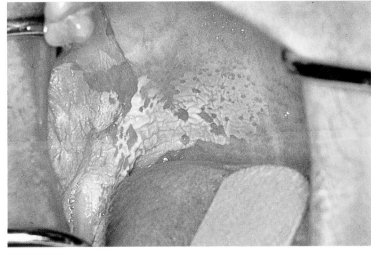

Fig. 10-12 Differential diagnosis of candidiasis. Flat homogeneous leukoplakia. The distinctly palatally located leuko plakia cannot be wiped off. Compare with Figs. 17-19 to 17-29 (flat homogeneous leukoplakia) as well as Figs. 16-2 and 16-3 (basic form of *lichen planus* on the oral mucous membrane).

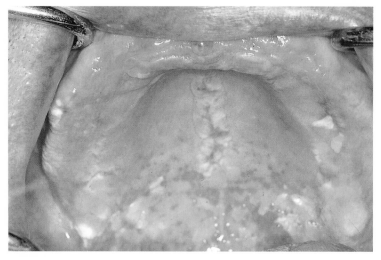

Fig. 10-13 Chronic hyperplastic form of candidiasis of the palate in a wearer of complete dentures. The firm, in some areas wart-forming, plaques have a hard consistency. Note the scattered erosive areas. This form of thrush mycosis, in its clinical picture, resembles leukoplakia, with which it is often confused. (See also chapter 18, "Precancerous leukoplakias.")

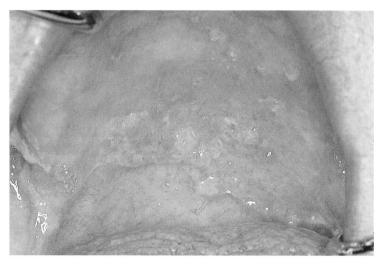

Fig. 10-14 Histologically confirmed chronic hyperplastic form of candidiasis of the palate under a complete denture. Under poorly fitting protheses, there is the development and persistence of local factors for an opportunistic growth of *Candida albicans,* possible even in immunocompetent patients (see Figs. 33-35 to 33-37).

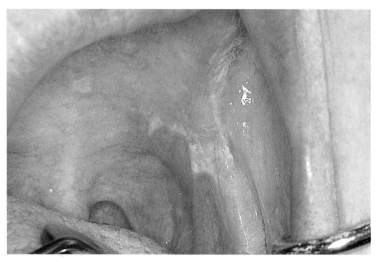

Fig. 10-15 Differential diagnosis of candidiasis: retromolar leukoplakia. Leukoplakias can look like thrush, which is not present in this case, and can be interpreted as risk factors (see chapter 18). Changes such as the ones presented must be clarified by histologic examination.

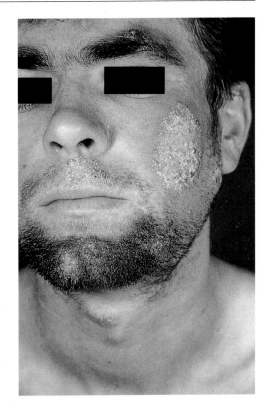

Fig. 10-16   Tinea barbae (trichophyte profunda barbae, spots on the beard area). This fungal disease, which develops in the keratin of the skin and hair, omits the vermilion of the lip and never attacks the oral mucous membrane. Contagion through the obligated parasitic thread fungi takes place from person to person, from diseased animals (in cities, most commonly from fur-bearing house pets) or through objects contaminated by spores. Shown are fresh, fully developed, and spontaneously healing lesions. The hair can be removed like wicks from the infected hair layer. The hair grows back. The degree of endemic distribution of the dermatomycosis is given, according to the reaction of immunity, at about 50%, which translates into a high degree of infectivity.

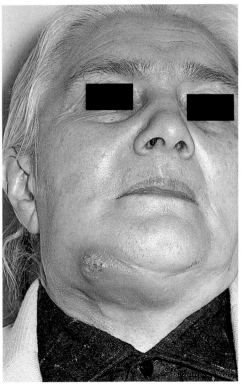

Fig. 10-17   Advanced stage of cervicofacial actinomycosis in a 66-year-old woman. The infiltration developed 6 weeks previously and has since become a marked induration with areas of softening and a central draining sinus. The granulation tissue, removed by extraoral incision, contained colonies of fungi. An antibiogram provided direction for therapy also of the accompanying flora.

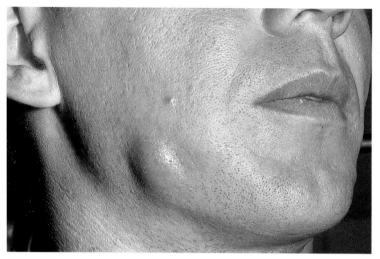

Fig. 10-18 Cervicofacial actinomycosis in the initial stage in
a 27-year-old patient. The hard
infiltrate affects the entire cutis
and allows the identification of
a central softening; the onset
was preceeded by extraction of
tooth 46 (30). Intraoral findings
do not substantially contribute
to the differential diagnosis of
the actinomycosis. A chronic
granulated periodontitis according to Partsch (see Figs.
6-4 and 6-6) is to be ruled out.

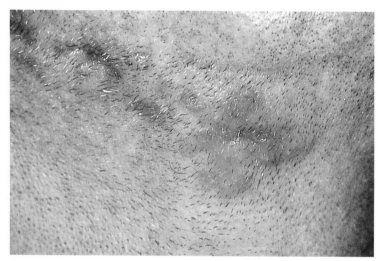

Fig. 10-19 Atypical form of
a cervicofacial actinomycosis
that has been present for 2
years in a 51-year-old patient.
In this clinical picture, the lesion resembles an obstinate folliculitis, which recalls a chronic,
infiltrated, mixed infection with
the presence of the so-called
small actinomycete (identified
by anaerobic culture). This condition, at first resistant to therapy, also spreads to bone.

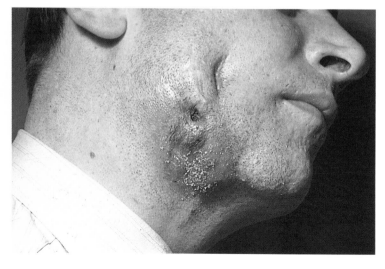

Fig. 10-20 Advanced cervicofacial actinomycosis after repeated surgical intervention,
and recurrent, fresh, hard, and
only slightly painful soft tissue
infiltrates over the mandible.
The bacterial folliculitis is observed as grafted on.

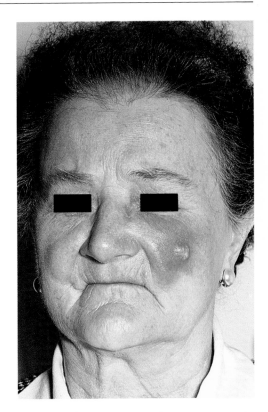

Fig. 10-21   Anaerobic culturally diagnosed cervicofacial actinomycosis of the upper cheek region that occurred after the extraction of tooth 26 (14). This localization is rare. The typical location is the submandibular region on the mandibular angle (in over 90% of cases). The actinomycosis (mostly *Actinomyces israeli*) only becomes a cause of disease as a frequent endogenous saprophyte when, under anaerobic conditions, actinomycosis penetrates deeply into an extraction wound, the periapical bone via a root canal, or a break in the mucosa. Crucial to the manifestation is an accompanying bacterial mixed infection, which provides the proteolytic enzymes that actinomycetes do not have (microbiotic supplementation by means of accompanying bacteria).

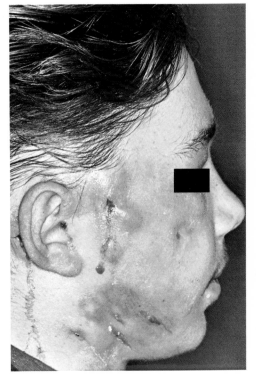

Fig. 10-22   Extensive, draining, cervicofacial actinomycosis of the right side of the face, derived from tooth 46 (30) (condition 6 months after tooth extraction and after multiple incisions). (From Kruger E. Lehrbuch der chirurgischen Zahn-, Mund- und Kieferheilkunde, vol. 1. Berlin: Quintessenz, 1988.)

Chapter 11

Viral Diseases with Oral Manifestations

Smallpox

Diseases caused by herpesvirus
   Herpes simplex virus
      Herpetic gingivostomatitis
      Herpes labialis
      Oral mucosal herpes
   Varicella zoster virus
      Chicken pox
      Herpes zoster
   Epstein-Barr virus
      Infectious mononucleosis
      Hairy leukoplakia
Diseases caused by enteroviruses
   Herpangina
   Hand-foot-and-mouth disease

Diseases caused by human papillomaviruses
   Focal epithelial hyperplasia (Heck's disease)
   Oral verruca vulgaris

Acquired immunodeficiency syndrome (HIV infection, AIDS)

There is no virus known that brings good; as somebody once pointedly noticed, a virus is "protein-wrapped bad news."

From: Medawar P. B., Medawar J. S. From Aristotle to Zoos. Cambridge: Harvard University Press, 1983.

Growth in knowledge has reached a remarkable point not even thought of a few years ago. The new rapidly expanding knowledge in virology, immunology, and molecular biology give justified hope that even little-understood diseases will be deciphered in the future.

Viruses are small pathogens of the order of 20 to 300 nm (1 nm = 10^{-9} m) in size. As obligatory cell parasites, they can only multiply in live cells whose metabolic apparatus they use for reproduction. As opposed to bacteria, which have totally independent synthesis and reproduction systems, viruses have only one set of building instructions, that is, a synthesis program, which they impose on the host cell with loss of their own identify. For the therapist, the difference is significant.

Carriers of genetic information are deoxyribonucleic acid (DNA) or ribonucleic acid (RNA), which are present in single-stranded or double-stranded forms. The surrounding protein cover is termed *capsid*. Many human pathogenic viruses contain an additional configured envelope made up of proteins, glycoproteins, and lipids. Like the capsid, they have antigenic properties important for the immune response of the organism. Particulars of the complicated structures, the multiplication cycles, and the biochemical reactions of the virus in relation to their mode of infection cannot be discussed here. The reader is referred to specialized texts on virology.

Of the many known viral diseases, only a few will be presented here. Those described may represent a local reaction in the course of a systemic viral disease or may be a partial manifestation of a generalized viral disease but as a major finding in the initial phase.

Smallpox (ICD-DA 0.50 and 050.VO)

Smallpox, because it is a large DNA virus, is a contagious exanthematic disease with high lethality. In 1977, the World Health Organization declared the disease eradicated.

The disease is shown in Figs. 11-1 to 11-4 for historical interest, as a reminder of a dangerous disease, and as evidence of the tremendous success of scientific medicine in the past 25 years in Germany. The same could be said of poliomyelitis.

Starting with the work of the English physician Jenner (1796), it was possible, with the development of a vaccination and the consequent development of hygienic measures to conquer an infection feared as a scourge of humankind. It had existed for 3000 years without interruption, and about 400,000 people died from the disease in 18th-century Europe.

Diseases caused by herpesvirus

Currently 40 varieties of herpesvirus are known, of which four are pathogens in the human and are of special importance. These are herpes simplex virus (HSV), varicella zoster virus (VZV), cytomegalovirus (CMV), and Epstein-Barr virus (EBV). These human pathogenic viruses are spheric DNA viruses with a diameter of 100 to 200 nm.

Herpes simplex virus

Worldwide, two serotypes of herpes simplex virus can be distinguished: *oral* type I and *genital* type II.

The primary infection from herpes simplex virus type I usually takes place via the oral cavity (mouth to mouth infection through saliva, smear infection) in early childhood. The greatest incidence is at the primary dentition stage. By the sixth year of age, most children come in contact with this virus. In more than 90% of all cases, the primary infection goes unnoticed, that is, without clinical manifestations. The proof of the "silent" infection can be demonstrated serologically by a rise of the antibodies. In some cases, the primary infection leads to a herpetic gingivostomatitis.

Manifestations in the genital area as a consequence of a first contact with the herpes simplex virus type II are observed usually only after the fifteenth year of life because this type is often transmitted through sexual intercourse (epidemic level of 10% to 20% of the adult population with many recurrences).

It is characteristic of the herpes simplex virus, as well as of all viruses of the herpes group, that after the first infection the virus is not eliminated from the body, despite the demonstrable immune reaction. Rather, an occult infection remains by which the virus remains in a latent state. Some of these viruses remain latent for life, often in neural structures (regional ganglion cells). This fact explains the typical herpes virus recurrence diseases in the sense of a "local recurrence" (exacerbation) as well as the generalization of the viral disease in the presence of immune system depression.

Herpetic gingivostomatitis (ICD-DA 054.2X)

The classical clinical picture as a consequence of primary infection from type I herpes simplex virus is herpetic gingivostomatitis (Figs. 11-5 to 11-11). It appears predominantly in children between the ages of 2 and 4 years but can also be observed in older children and adults.

After the incubation time of 4 to 6 days, there is the development of an acute viral disease with fever, fatigue, vomiting, restlessness, and even cramping, as well as typical changes in the oral cavity ("mouth decay"), which are associated with bad breath, increased saliva flow, and regional lymph node swelling. On the oral mucosa there appear many (about 50 or more) blisters the size of pinheads on a reddish, inflamed background. Because these blisters are short-lived in the oral cavity, they change rapidly into yellowish, fibrin-covered, usually circular but also polycyclic, confluent erosions, which are surrounded by a thin, very red halo and which are very painful. Different stages of development are present in these efflorescences. Most commonly affected areas are the anterior and middle of the oral cavity.

There is always a concurrent, extensive, acute gingivitis (hence gingivostomatitis). The gingiva is very red, inflamed, and often covered with serofibrinous exudate on its marginal parts. In contrast to acute necrotizing ulcerative gingivitis (ANUG; Fig. 11-12), there is no progressive necrosis in the area of the interdental papillae. The lymphatic pharyngeal ring also remains free of necrosis. Concurrent catarrhal inflammations are possible, however. The herpetic gingivostomatitis, with rare exceptions, tends not to recur and has nothing to do with the chronic recurring aphthae (see chapter 12). For this reason, the earlier erroneous terminology "aphthous stomatitis" should not be used. The diagnosis is based on the typical clinical findings and, depending on the case, on virus-specific demonstration methods, including serologic evaluation (i.e., rise in antibodies).

Feared complications such as meningoencephalitis in children, which follow an earlier infectious disease such as measles, whooping cough, or scarlet fever, occur because of weakened defense mechanisms. Children with eczemas usually show severe forms of the herpetic primary infection. A local complication can appear in the form of a herpetic nail bed infection by inoculation of the virus onto the finger by sucking or as a consequence of nail biting. The problem of neonatal infections will not be discussed here. As in infections of early childhood, first infections in adults can lead to complications.

The dramatically developing oral mucosal changes regress within 10 to 14 days, as a rule, under symptomatic treatment (bed rest, medication to lower fever, increase of liquid consumption, careful but thorough oral hygiene). The results of antiviral chemotherapy of the herpetic gingivotomatitis with acyclovir are promising, but chemotherapy should be unnecessary in uncomplicated courses. Antibiotics are useful only when a superimposed bacterial infection can be demonstrated.

In dubious cases, the internist or pediatrician should be called in. Because parents usually first take their children to a physician when there is fever, the sequence of consultation in the practice is often reversed.

Herpes labialis (ICD-DA 054.00)

Herpes labialis is the most common recurring infection from herpes simplex type I in dentistry. Almost every other woman and every third man suffers from a recurring labial herpes infection. The cause is a latent virus that results in "local recurrences." The triggering (provoking) factors are febrile influenza, heavy ultraviolet irradiation, climatic changes, menstruation, microtraumas, and general stress situations. Favorite localizations are the skin-vermilion margin of the lip. Local recurrences, in some cases, for as yet-unexplained reasons, always appear at the same spots.

Prodromal symptoms of herpes labialis can include a feeling of tension, itching, or light pain among others, and an odd "furry" feeling in the area of future manifestation. In a matter of hours, there is the development of blisters the size of pinheads to grains of rice arranged in clusters over a light reddish, edematous background (Figs. 11-14 to 11-16). Larger efflorescences are also sometimes observed (Fig. 11-13). The now-tense blisters filled with a clear material often flow together, become opaque, and burst. Secondarily, there is formation of erosions or flat ulcerations (Fig. 11-17) on which crusts form after several days. Over the rest of the erythema is healing without scar formation. The total time of disease is 8 to 10 days. The regional lymph nodes are usually palpable and painful to pressure. Differential diagnostic problems in herpes labialis are presented in Figs. 11-19 to 11-21.

The not-infrequent complications to be considered seriously from the prognostic point of view include keratoconjunctivitis herpetica as well as postherpetic erythema exudativum multiforme because of possible residual damage (see Figs. 28-7 to 28-9).

It has sometimes been said that herpes labialis lasts a week with therapy and 8 days without treatment. Until now, symptomatic treatment recommendations were as follows: the blister-free initial phase treated with ether or corticosteroid local preparations on cotton swabs to shorten the disease time. In the erosion stage, creams should not be used because they can exacerbate the condition and cause secondary infections. Alcohol solutions and dessicating mixtures are recommended.

With the introduction of antiviral chemotherapeutic agents, there has been the development of other treatments for herpes labialis. Topical application of the virostatic agent acyclovir has decreased viral shedding. In recurrences, however, nothing can decrease the problem, because no vaccination is available. As long as knowledge about the possibilities of prophylaxis and therapy remain incomplete, we will continue to hear of wonder drugs for the treatment of herpes labialis.

Oral mucosal herpes (ICD-AA 054.00)

The less frequent intraoral variation of herpes labialis caused by a recurring HSV infection is herpes of the oral mucosa. On unaltered mucosa, there is the development of short-lived clustered blisters the size of pinheads. At the time of examination, there are already roundish confluences of the individual efflorescences, often also polycystic partially delimited erosions with a fibrin cover (Figs. 11-22 to 11-24), hence "erosive herpes." The masticatory mucosa (hard palate, gingiva, alveolar ridge), where the altered area seldom reaches the size of a quarter, is usually the only area affected. Based on this location, it is possible to exclude chronic recurring aphthae, which prefer the mucosa not fixed to the periosteum.

The patient who is not affected or is only minimally affected experiences local complaints of varying intensity. In 8 to 10 days, the lesions heal without scarring.

If irritation from mechanical causes is present, the offending object(s) should be removed. Because of the relatively rapid spontaneous healing, treatment of herpes of the oral mucosa is superfluous.

In differential diagnosis, one must think first of associated symptoms such as early stages of oral manifestations of zoster of the second and third branches of the trigeminal nerve (Fig. 11-25) as well as a beginning ulcerative stomatitis of the region (Fig. 11-26).

Varicella zoster virus

In the past, chickenpox and shingles were considered two independent illnesses. Today we know that varicella is a consequence of the first infection with the varicella zoster virus in an antibody-free person, while zoster is a recurrence of a latent varicella zoster virus related to imcomplete immunity. The common pathogen is a 150- to 200-nm DNA virus of the herpes group. A patient with zoster can be the source of chickenpox; the opposite infection course is impossible.

Chicken pox (ICD-DA 052 and 052.XO)

Chicken pox is a worldwide viral, infectious disease with an incubation time of 14 days that is transmitted through drops and/or smear infection. Its high level of contagiousness—comparable to other exanthematic infectious diseases such as measles and rubella—is responsible for a large number of cases of chicken pox in children. While the disease in children as a rule has a good prognosis, the infection appearing first in adults has a more guarded prognosis and exhibits a greater degree of complications.

Chicken pox starts with uncharacteristic red spots (maculous exanthema) on the head and trunk in children, usually lacking prodromal symptoms (headache, vomiting, fever). The spots develop to papules and change in a few hours into thin-walled blisters the size of a pinhead or rice grain with light watery content. Contrary to smallpox, this eruption is followed by many primary efflorescences, so that different stages of polymorphic efflorescences (erythemas, papules, blisters, and crusts) usually can be recognized in preferred areas of the face (Fig. 11-27) and trunk; hands and feet remain free.

Examination of the oral cavity (Figs. 11-28 to 11-31) may reveal vesticulated eruptions, which, however, are already fibrin-covered erosions of the palate, gingiva, lips, or cheeks. The findings in the oral mucosa also show a polymorphic form. These findings are equally typical for the diagnostic distribution in chicken pox as well as for Koplik's spots in measles and strawberry tongue in scarlet fever (see Fig. 7-8). With symptomatic treatment (bed rest), patients with chicken pox usually heal well. Because of scratching in response to itching, bacterial superinfections are possible and can cause scar formation.

Herpes zoster (ICD-DA 053 and 053.X0)

Zoster is a secondary manifestation of varicella zoster infection that develops in older patients with incomplete immunization. It manifests itself as a rule on one side ("half shingles") or one skin segment (expansion area of one sensory nerve). The zoster can also take over several skin segments in exceptional cases on both sides. After the thorax and lumbosacral segments, the area of the trigeminal nerve is the second most often affected. The course of the disease is prone to complications. The reason for the different localization is not known.

As a consequence of viremia at the start of the disease, there is always an acute prodromal appearance (fever, weakness, fatigue, poor disposition, stiff neck) as well as neurologic symptoms in the form of severe, sometimes intolerable sharp pain alongside the affected segment, which are brought about by ganglionitis and neuritis.

In this phase of the disease, there is a localization in the affected area of the second and third branches of the trigeminal neve that is often misdiagnosed by the dentist. The intolerable pain is misdiagnosed as being due to dental causes (e.g., pulpitis) and treated accordingly. Usually this occurs in the form of extraction, trephirnation, or root canal therapy, without improvement. A few days later the skin and mucosal eruptions appear, and the patient blames the disease on dental treatment.

In a small number of cases, during the time from the beginning of the general symptoms and neurologic findings, there is the appearance of small areas of dark-red erythema on the skin innervated by the affected nerve (Fig. 11-32). Within this erythema is the development of large groups of clustered papulovesicular efflorescences (Figs. 11-36 and 11-38). The initially water-clear (sometimes hemorrhagic) blisters become cloudy, and limited polycystic erosions or ulcerations remain in the wet crust stage (Fig. 11-39) for a relatively long time (up to 2 weeks).

During the often-long process of healing, erythema of the skin can persist for several weeks and bring about postinflammatory pigmentation. Even in the absence of necrotizing variants, zoster usually leaves scars. Particularly feared is the late sequence of tormenting postzoster neuralgias, which in previous years were associated with therapy-resistant "sacred fire." As local complications in the region of the trigeminal nerve, there can be changes in taste and feeling, and otalgias, paresthesias, and some types of paresis.

The zoster of the second and third branches of the trigeminal nerve as a rule leads to extensive unilaterally localized, extremely painful oral mucosal changes. They usually appear after the eruption on the skin but also represent the initial site. The usually short-lived oral mucosal blisters coalesce and rapidly turn into flat fibrin-covered erosions and ulcerations. While efflorescences in the oral cavity are relatively non-specific in appearance, the developmental stage diagnostic of zoster may be appreciated in fresh lesions of the affected mucous membrane (Figs. 11-33 and 11-40). Necrotizing forms of zoster can often be seen on the oral mucosa (Fig. 11-34), which in severe cases can involve bone (Fig. 11-37). An acute lymphadenitis of regional lymph nodes may be present, secondary to infection of the oral mucosa, and may last 3 to 4 weeks. Scars are more discrete in the oral cavity. While the classic unilateral lesions are easier to diagnose, there are abortive forms—particularly in those with oral symptoms only (Fig. 11-35)—which can complicate the diagnostic process.

Today, antiviral medications (acyclovir) are available, which if used according to instructions, in the early stage and in adequate dosages, can be effective. When in doubt, the dentist should refer to a specialist. Because of possible involvement of the corneal layer, an ophthalmologist should be consulted immediately in cases of localizations in the first branch of the trigeminal nerve *(zoster ophthalmicus)*.

Zoster can be an indicator of depressed immunity in patients receiving immunosuppressive therapy, for example, after a kidney transplant.

The expansion of zoster over several skin segments or its generalization with exanthematic picture *(generalized zoster)* indicates recurrences and is prognostically unfavorable, suggesting severe immunosupression. In these cases, one should search for an underlying debilitating or neoplastic disease. In young patients, the appearance of zoster raises the suspicion of an HIV infection; 10% of AIDS patients have a zoster as a viral opportunistic infection at the beginning of the clinically manifest immunosuppressed stage.

Epstein-Barr virus

The cytomegalovirus is mainly a pathogen of early childhood with intrauterine or perinatal transmission and can also occur by opportunistic infection in severe immunodepression. Oral manifestation of cytomegalovirus infection (for example, thrombocytopenia with bleeding) does not frequently occur. The Epstein-Barr virus is different. This virus, which also belongs to the herpesvirus group, is not only the pathogen of *infectious mononucleosis,* it is considered to be at least an oncogenic cofactor in *Burkitt's lymphoma* (B-type lymphoblastic lymphoma) endemic to Central Africa as well as in *nasopharyngeal carcinoma,* the most frequent form of tumor in some areas of China. In addition, the Epstein-Barr virus probably has an important role in the development of *"hairy" leukoplakias* secondary to acquired immunodeficiency.

Infectious mononucleosis, glandular fever (ICD-DA 075)

Infectious mononucleosis is an acute illness of the lymphatic tissue, usually with associated systemic symptoms, transmitted as a rule through saliva contact or droplet infection.

After an incubation time of 8 to 28 days (about 10 to 14 days in children), the disease starts with generalized fatigue and weakness, slowly rising fever, and a later-occurring sore throat. Main symptoms are the almost regular appearance of angina ("monocyte angina") and pharyngitis of varying severity, as well as the rising fever, or initiation of lymph node swelling (cervical, axillary, and inguinal). A further typical accompanying symptom is a purpura that involves the hard and soft palate and resembles an enanthema of the oral mucosa (petechial bleeding) in addition to exanthematic skin changes. Together with the pharyngitis, there is sometimes gingivitis or stomatitis.

The spleen and liver are often enlarged. Infectious mononucleosis leads to characteristic changes in the peripheral blood picture (i.e., leukocytosis) with marked increase of mononuclear (meaning one nucleus, unsegmented) lymphomonocytic cells.

Different courses are possible; there may be complications (through meningeal, cardial, or hepatic participation) that on an average require 1 or 2 weeks' or possibly several weeks' convalescence, but these are infrequent.

Particularly susceptible are children (often in small epidemics), teenagers, and young adults (sporadic disease cases). The viruses multiply in B cells of the oropharynx and persist in the reticuloendothelial system. By adulthood 80% to 90% all people worldwide are infected with the Epstein-Barr virus. Considering the degree of seropositivity level of the adult population, it must be concluded that most adults' first infection with Epstein-Barr virus was a clinically silent event.

In the presence of depressed immunity, a reactivation of the acute infectious mononucleosis can occur. This disease therefore belongs to the opportunistic infections in acquired immunodeficiency syndrome (AIDS).

Hairy leukoplakia (ICD-DA 279.10)

"Hairy" leukoplakia involves discrete, fairly outlined but not sharply delimited, whitish, nonremovable epithelial changes, which are present particularly on the border of the tongue (Figs. 11-52, 11-54, and 11-55). The changes can also occur on the dorsum (Fig. 11-56) or on the lower side of the tongue.

The irregularly shaped, often rippled or wrinkled surface resembles a hairy surface. In the superficial epithelial layers, several *Candida* hyphae are seen. In older textbooks this lesion was described among the *Candida* infections.

Hairy leukoplakia is an associated symptom of acquired immunodeficiency syndrome and is considered an early, relatively reliable oral indicator of the onset of AIDS (see related part in this chapter).

Using immunofluorescence and hybridization techniques, Epstein-Barr virus particles can be demonstrated almost regularly, hence a viral genesis is assumed. There are also a series of pathohistologic markers suggestive of a virus-induced leukoplakia. The Epstein-Barr virus multiplies apparently in the differentiated epithelial cells of the tongue. The proliferating basal cells, on the other hand, appear to repress multiplication. The significance of the 50-nm particles found in the lesion is unexplained.

Diseases caused by enteroviruses

Enteroviruses are 20- to 30-nm RNA viruses. They are not transmitted only by contact and droplet infection; because enteroviruses are acid stable, an infection–for example after eating contaminated food–is also possible via the digestive system because the viruses can multiply in the intestinal mucosa.

Important enterovirus pathogens such as *polioviruses, coxsackievirus A* (with 24 serotypes), *coxsackievirus B* (with six serotypes), and the echovirus (with more than 30 serotypes) will not be discussed here. The coxsackievirus is named for the city in the United States in which it was first isolated. The name echovirus is a shortening of *enteric cytopathic human orphan* (orphan implies that the virus is known but the diseases for which it is responsible are not). Infections throughout the world that are spread by coxsackieviruses and echoviruses run a nonapparent clinical course. Occasionally, some infections are symptomatic, generally causing minor illnesses, although they are sometimes severe (among others, hepatitis, myocarditis pericarditis, and meningitis). There is seasonal preference for the summer months.

In their clinical symptoms there is a great similarity among coxsackievirus and echovirus diseases. We discuss two caused by coxsackievirus virus A with manifestations in the oral mucosa.

Herpangina (ICD-DA 074.00)

After an incubation of 2 to 6 days, the disease develops suddenly sometimes with sustained fever and often with otherwise nonspecific general symptoms such as lack of appetite, vomiting, fatigue, and headache, stomachache, muscleache, or extremity pain.

Characteristic for herpangina is that after a few hours there is the onset of sore throat with difficulty swallowing. On the anterior palatal arch, often also on the soft palate, the uvula, and the tonsils, there is the formation of pinhead blisters surrounded by a red halo (Fig. 11-41). These blisters, which often have the appearance of pearl necklaces or efflorescences in clusters, usually number six to eight with a maximum of 20. Within 24 hours from onset of the blisters, there is the development of fibrin-coated erosions or ulcerations that have a tendency to heal quickly. About 1 week after the appearance of the disease, patients are well again. Besides the typical forms with acute appearance and mild course, there are also absortive forms. A silent infection is also possible.

The herpangina Zahorsky due to coxsackievirus A type 4 primarily affects infants and small children, among whom epidemics are possible. Sometimes young adults are also affected. The disease leaves behind a life-long immunity against the pathogen. A new infection can, however, take place via other serotypes of the coxsackievirus group A. The diagnosis is usually made on the basis of the typical clinical findings of "herpangina" changes. In the differential diagnosis, one must initially consider that herpetic gingivostomatitis with oropharyngeal localization has a more severe course. The short, mild course as well as the lack of an acute gingivitis is an important point in the differential diagnosis. Also, nonspecific as well as specific pharyngitis tonsillitis must be ruled out. Therapy is limited to symptomatic measures such as a liquid diet, oral hygiene, antipyretic medications, and in some cases bed rest.

Hand-foot-and-mouth disease; vesicular stomatitis with exanthema (ICD-DA 074.3 and 074.30)

This diseases appears sporadically or in small epidemics, especially in children of preschool age, and is transmitted through coxsackievirus group A (as a ruletype 16, seldom types 5 or 10) and sometimes through coxsackievirus group B (types 2 and 5).

After an incubation of a few days, the temperature rises and there is malaise and headache. On the hands, fingers, soles of the feet, and toes (Fig. 11-43), spotty erythemas appear from which there is the development of whitish blisters with clear watery contents. These blisters heal with a crust, as a rule, without complications.

The skin of the buttocks and thighs and the oral mucosa show a papular exanthema and later formation of blisters. They are soon substituted by painful aphtha-like ulcerations (Fig. 11-42). These lesions disappear with time.

The course of hand-foot-and-mouth disease is benign and lasts about 2 weeks. Treatment is symptomatic.

Diseases caused by human papillomaviruses

The human papillomaviruses (HPV) belong to the family of *papovaviruses* that are about 45 to 55 nm in size. They are double-stranded ring forms of DNA and do not have an envelope. The papillomavirus cannot be cultured in tissue culture, infects basal cells of the epithelium, and multiplies only in maturing cells.

The increase in knowledge of HPV in the last few years is remarkable. However, its importance and its consequences for prophylaxis and therapy of associated diseases are not yet fully understood. Thanks to the progress in molecular virology (i.e., use of restrictive enzymes, techniques of blot-hybridization), over 60 viral types can be isolated and characterized. At the same time, it is possible to prove that some of the virus types have oncogenic properties—often acting together with genetic changes in host cells. Such changes can be manifest through different ways. H. zur Hausen and his group determined that various specific papillomaviruses can be associated with benign and malignant neoplasias in the genital area. More research must be done to determine the role that human papillomaviruses play, aside from their definite association with certain carcinomas of the skin and genital organs, and in the origin of other forms of cancer.

Association of human papillomaviruses (HPV) with benign and malignant skin and mucosal diseases*

Disease	Inducing HPV type
Common warts	
Common hand wart	1, 2
Filiform	2
Papillomalike	2, 4, 7
Other forms	2, 4, 7
Plantar warts	1, 2, 4, 60
Juvenile warts	3, 10, 27, 28
Epidermodysplasia verruciformis	3, 5, 8-10, 12, 14, 15, 17, 19-25
Focal epithelial hyperplasia (Heck's disease)	13, 1, 32
Laryngeal papilloma	6, 11
Condylomata acuminata	6, 11, 42
Bowenoid papulosis	16, 18, 31, 33, 35, 45, 51, 52, 56, 58
Cervical changes	6, 11, 16, 18, 31, 33, 35, 45, 51, 52
Squamous cell carcinoma of skin in epidermodysplasia verruciformis	5, 8, 14, 17, 20, 48, 56, 58
Carcinoma of the vulva	6, 11, 16, 18, 33
Cervical carcinoma	16, 18, 31, 33, 39, 45, 51, 52, 56
Penile carcinoma	16, 18, 33
Scrotal skin carcinoma	16

* According to *zur Hausen* (personal communication, 1989) and from *de Villiers*. Reference Center for Human Pathogenic Papilloma Viruses, German Center for Cancer Research, Heidelberg.

Of the large number of benign and malignant skin and mucosal diseases that are currently thought to be caused by HPV, there are two that appear in the oral mucosa: focal epithelial hyperplasia (Heck's disease) and common warts.

Focal epithelial hyperplasia (Heck's disease) (ICD-DA 528.73)

This disease, first described in 1965 as focal epithelial hyperplasia of the oral mucosa, manifests itself on the oral mucosa in the form of multiple papules that are roundish to oval, single or confluent, flat, slightly raised, or bumpy clusters. They have a soft consistency, are broad based on the underlying surface, and are of a maximum size of 1 cm. The surface is finely stippled with a strawberrylike pattern (Fig. 11-46). These slightly keratinized proliferations that are pale, whitish, or of the color of the surrounding mucosa are present on the lip mucosa (excluding the vermilion of the lip and vestibulum), the cheek mucosa, and the dorsum and border of the tongue (Figs. 11-44 and 11-46), and on the gingiva in the area of the incisors (Fig. 11-45). The disease appears predominantly in children but can appear in adults of both sexes.

Focal epithelial hyperplasia that is endemic in Eskimos in Greenland, Canada, and Alaska as well as in Native Americans of North and South America was similarly observed in South Africa and in Turkey. Reports of sporadic cases have appeared in several countries. In Germany, the disease is rare, at least in patients of German origin.

The grouping of focal epithelial hyperplasia within certain populations and the appearance at the same time in different members of the same family (i.e., in the same household or within a group of persons with similar life habits; contact with household animals?) in the past led to the suspicion of a viral disease. Today the viral origin is certain. There is demonstration that the disease is associated with HPV (particularly types 13 and 32, possibly also type 1). The genetic factors involved are still unknown.

These painless mucosal changes that also resemble papillomas histologically can last for years, but can regress spontaneously (which emphasizes the viral origin of the disease). Differential diagnosis must be made between common warts, condylomata acuminata, and other virus-induced papillomas. Because of the possible spontaneous remission, the clinical diagnosis of viral papilloma should be confirmed by a biopsy in order to avoid radical surgery or other unnecessary treatment. Focal epithelial hyperplasia is an opportunistic viral infection when there is acquired immunodeficiency syndrome.

Oral verruca vulgaris (ICD-DA 078.10)

Verruca vulgaris is among the most common skin lesions. These warts, mostly induced by HPV types 1, 2, and 4 appear in children (peaking during school age), young adults, and adults, preferentially on the hands (transmission caused mainly from handshaking) and fingers (not infrequently on the nail bed) but also on the face or anywhere else on the skin. They can be single or multiple. Frequently they are found on the lips (Fig. 11-47) and oral mucosa (tongue, Fig. 22-60; cheeks, Fig. 11-48), where they are probably caused by contact with warts on the hands. As opposed to the findings on the skin, the hyperkeratotic, thick cellular upper layer in oral warts has a more whitish color and often a shaggy structure, so that it is impossible to differentiate them clinically from papillomas (see chapter 22).

Warts can remain for years, but they can regress spontaneously. They are found significantly more often in ill persons with reduced cellular immunity than in healthy persons. *Condylomata acuminata* (pointed condyloma, wet warts) on the oral mucosa have several of the clinical and pathohistologic features of genital warts. They are caused by HPV (types 6, 11, and 42) and probably through orogenital contact.

Acquired immunodeficiency syndrome (HIV infection, AIDS) (ICD-DA 279.10)

The HIV infection and the diseases associated with it have a varied clinical course. It is a chronic disease with an irreversible end stage and is a manifestation of acquired immunodeficiency syndrome (AIDS).

In dental practice, the problem is not the patient in the final phase of infection, for which necessary treatment and emergency measures usually are indicated, but the much greater (at least 10 times higher) number of HIV-positive patients who are asymptomatic or only minimally symptomatic and are, therefore, of great importance for early diagnosis.

HIV (human immunodeficiency virus) belongs to the group of *retroviruses* and within it to the subfamily of *lentiviruses*. Retroviruses (*reverse transcriptase containing oncogen virus*) are roundish 100-nm RNA viruses surrounded by a lipid envelope that has a well-defined structure.

The concept of lentivirus is based on the fact that between infection and the appearance of the disease manifestations, a long time elapses (presently thought to be 10 years or more), which must be considered a time of latency. The incubation time of the HIV infection is 2 to 6 weeks. The following early phase of disease may be completeley asymptomatic; in any case, diagnosis of HIV infection is usually not made at this stage.

HIV as a lymphotropic lentivirus shows an affinity for cells with T4-receptors (B lymphocytes, macrophages, Langerhans' cells of the skin and specific cell groups of the central nervous system). Lentiviruses and HIV in particular have antigenic properties that vary somewhat because of the peculiar structure of the virus surface; this may hinder immunologic recognition of the virus. What hinders diagnosis and therapy is that HIV has a marked "antigen drift": changes/mutations of the surface structure occur that have been known in influenza viruses for decades. This fact complicates serologic proof of infection and the development of appropriate vaccines. While HIV I and HIV II are responsible in humans for the same illnesses, they are not identical from the molecular structure and antigenic point of view. It must be assumed that other mutations will also appear.

Extensive knowledge of the overwhelming number of animal retroviral pathogens has been in existence for a long time. In regard to the appearance of the HIV virus, it is believed that it was first a zoonosis that was able to become endemic in a circumscribed population in Africa and left this endemic area 15 years ago. With increasing sexual activity and mobility of populations, there was rapid dissemination with preference for special groups (risk groups include: homosexuals, drug addicts, heterosexual partners of infected and diseased persons). When the HIV by means of a specific structure of its coat has "docked" on the receptor (T4) cell, it will subsequently be integrated into the cell. There it gives its genetic determining factor of (uncoated) RNA to the "reverse transcriptase" enzyme for transfer into DNA (provirus). As such, it will become part of the host genome and will remain there until the death of the cell. With the help of cellular metabolism, viral components will be reproduced, and other cells infected as HIV is shed from the infected cells. For each virus replicating cell, there are 100 to 1,000 "sleeping cells" with the integrated virus genome.

HIV infection does not lead to a massive viremialike classic viral infection. For example, in the peripheral blood only 1,000 to 1,000,000 lymphocytes are infected. The danger of the infection is that the switch cells of the immunologic system become nonfunctional and are destroyed.

HIV infection takes place by direct entrance of virus-containing body fluids into the blood circulation. HIV has been demonstrated in blood, sperm, vaginal secretions, saliva, liquor, maternal milk, tears, sweat, urine, and other body secretions that contain blood cells, as well as in tissue cells (also in the oral mucosa). The modes of transmission are many.

Of major importance is sexual transmission and mucosal contact by infected blood or other body fluids. Of secondary importance is parenteral transmission through inoculation, transplantation, or the intrauterine or neonatal transmission to the child from an infected mother.

Problems for medical personnel are predominantly needlesticks or cut injuries with possible inoculation of infected material as well as blood contact with previously damaged skin and/or a mucosal contamination.

Retrospective estimates of the danger of physicians and medical personnel contracting HIV during professional activity is based on data of limited reliability. The risk of an HIV infection from a needlestick, for example, is about 1%. For hepatitis B virus (HBV), on the other hand, it is about 25%. Today hepatitis B is avoidable by vaccination (although there is no vaccination against the non-A, non-B hepatitis virus yet).

The use of passive protection measures (protective gloves, mouth protection, protective glasses) is important.

Serologic diagnosis of HIV belongs in the hands of the physician who has special training in this area and who knows the problems of false-positive as well as false-negative findings, the selection of the tests available, and their sensitivity and specificity. This book aims to acquaint the dentist with the clinical and particularly with the oral and perioral findings of HIV-positive patients as well as AIDS patients.

A good medical history offers important clues for diagnosis of a possible HIV infection. It should include history of blood transfusions and blood factor preparations before 1985, history of infectious diseases (zoster in young adults and such suspicious findings as in oral thrush), and systemic symptoms such as fever, fatigue not relieved by rest, night sweats, diarrhea, and weight loss.

The dentist must determine whether he or she needs special information such as drug dependency and sexual tendencies to obtain information that will allow referral for a clarifying serologic HIV diagnosis.

Serologic diagnosis requires the patient's permission; in an unclear disease picture, the proof of HIV status is a necessary clinical measure. HIV infection does not need to be reported in Germany, as does, for example, tuberculosis or a salmonella infection.

According to the classification established in 1986 by the *Centers for Disease Control (CDC)* in Atlanta, Georgia, the disease course can be divided for didactic purposes into four stages and corresponding subgroups (see table on page 240). One must, however, understand that in the early and middle phases of the disease there are no typical clinical courses but a variable clinical picture that in part depends on the medical history of the patient and on therapeutic measures available for opportunistic infections. Only in advanced stages of the infection do certain disease signs and findings dominate, which facilitate the diagnosis. In any phase of the disease after the appearance of seroconversion, the indispensable proof is the result of the serologic examination.

The *acute HIV stage* (group I) may be observed days or weeks after entrance of the virus as a nonobligatory symptomatic expression of the infection. The complaints are nonspecific: malaise, headache, limb pains, fever, nausea, lack of appetite, and weakness, which disappear without treatment. The infected patient then enters the asymptomatic stage of the disease (group II).

In half of the cases when there is a symptomatic early phase, there is a maculoerythematous exanthema, primarily in the trunk, which is reminiscent of other infectious diseases.

The oral cavity findings in acute early HIV infection can resemble those of infectious mononucleosis and can terminate with aphthoid lesions. It is not possible to establish a definite diagnosis. The laboratory diagnosis provides no answer in the first weeks or months prior to seroconversion *(serologic gap)*. The transition from group II (asymptomatic stage) to group III (generalized lymphadenopathy) can, according to present thinking, take years. In 45% of cases, transition to disease manifestation takes from 5 to 8 years. In the asymptomatic phase of HIV infection, the person may be unaware of his or her condition and unknowingly transmit the infection. All groups other than group I include a positive HIV serology, which in 95% of cases should become demonstrable between the sixth week and sixth month after infection *(seroconversion)*.

In group II (asymptomatic stage) there is a change in laboratory parameters, among others, lowering of the ratio between T-helper lymphocytes (T4) and T-suppressor lymphocytes (T8).

The factors that determine the time span between infection and appearance of the disease are presently poorly understood. Also unexplained is how much of a deficit in immunocompetence must be reached for the disease to manifest itself.

With generalized lymphadenopathy (group III), there is the appearance of the first relatively reliable clinical sign. This consists of generalized lymphadenopathy persisting longer than 3 months. Lymph node swelling appears on several parts of the body for which no other cause can be found. The inguinal lymph nodes and submandibular lymph nodes are not useful for diagnosis, because there can be other causes for their enlargement. The dentist should examine the neck and cervical lymph nodes.

Other frequent symptoms in group III HIV-positive patients are nocturnal sweats, fever or subfebrile temperature, diarrhea, and weight loss. In every third patient, there is a noticeable skin change with seborrheic dermatitis in zones rich in sebaceous glands.

Because only 40% of patients in whom AIDS eventually develops show the stage of generalized lymphadenopathy, group III can only be considered a *facultative prodromic stage for AIDS*. All causes of immune suppression (drugs, alcohol, intensive ultraviolet irradiation, deficient diet, chronic infections) can accelerate the disease process. Group IV AIDS is present in HIV-positive patients when there is:

- Opportunistic infection
- And/or otherwise rare malignancies
- Progressive HIV-associated diseases of the central nervous system

The clinical picture of AIDS is the result of the lymphotropic and neurotropic properties of the virus and demonstrates a multiorgan involvement.

Every second patient of group III with lymphadenopathy syndrome progresses in about 3 to 5 years to the final stage of AIDS (group IV). In spite of manifold therapeutic efforts and experiments, a long-term improvement or cure of HIV infection is so far lacking.

The accompanying illustrations deal mainly with oral and perioral findings. There are numerous monographs on the general picture of the disease.

Nearly all HIV-positive patients develop neurologic and psychiatric symptoms in the final phase of the disease. These will be apparent to the dentist who has treated the patient over several years.

The concept of *opportunistic infections* (group IV, class 1) includes infections from protozoans, fungi, bacteria, and viruses, the appearance and/or course of which depends on the severity of immune depression of the host organism. They are caused by facultative pathogens that as a rule do not have any effect or very little effect in an immunocompetent patient. However, here they produce severe or life-threatening diseases. A classic example and most important AIDS marker is *Pneumocystis carinii* pneumonia. Often its appearance indicates the terminal phase of the disease. In dentistry, *oral candidiasis* is an opportunistic infection of great diagnostic importance.

Local treatment is insufficient; after discontinuation of the systemic antimycotic therapy, recurrence soon takes place. The clinical picture of *Candida* infection (seen in Figs. 11-49, 11-51, 11-62 to 11-65) has many different appearances.

Also to be observed are recurring *mucocutaneous herpes simplex infections* in the area of the mouth and perioral areas (Figs. 11-57 to 11-59), which manifest themselves in similar form in the genitoanal region. In spite of a higher degree of penetrance with type 1 herpes simplex virus, type 2 is predominant in serologic testing.

The lesions respond favorably to acyclovir: recurrences, however, take place after medication is discontinued.

Other opportunistic viral infections that appear in the immunodeficiency syndrome are *cytomegalovirus infections* and the already discussed *zoster, hairy leukoplakia* (Figs. 11-50, 11-52, 11-54 to 11-56), and *focal epithelial hyperplasia* (Figs. 11-60 and 11-61).

Other suspicious oral findings are *noticeable worsening of gingivoperiodontal inflammatory conditions* (Fig. 11-53) and *exacerbations of chronic periapical osteitis.*

Of greater importance to public health is the reactivation of *tuberculosis.*

The oncogenic properties of retrovirus are discussed in group IV D. With the incorporation of the provirus in the host genome, there is the associated danger of translocation on a site with "switch-on effect" for the oncogenesis, where the cells and outside stimuli as well as internal inhibitory feedback processes become independent. Thus, the appearance of malignant neoplasias can be explained. Most frequent is dissemination of increasingly aggressive variants of classic *Kaposi's sarcoma;* second most frequent are the *aggressive types of non-Hodgkin's lymphoma.* The preferred location of Kaposi's sarcoma in the oral cavity is the palate (Figs. 11-68, 11-70, and 11-71). The red, violet, dark blue, or black-blue spots of an incipient Kaposi's sarcoma are first without symptoms. Later they enlarge in surface and/or volume and acquire a spongy consistency. Most frequently affected is the skin (95%) (Figs. 11-66, 11-67, 11-72, and 11-73). Second most frequently affected is the oral mucosa (Fig. 11-69 shows the gingival manifestation of an epulis). The gastrointestinal tract and other parenchymal organs can also be affected.

HIV infection in the latency phase without clinically noticeable changes of groups III and IV in general has few reliable signs in dentistry. The key finding in differential diagnosis remains a positive HIV serology. The HIV infection is therefore a challenge for the dental team. The same protective measures are needed as for the hepatitis B virus. The high level of penetrance of dentists with hepatitis B now abating because these protective measures are increasingly being applied with care and consistency. From the widespread increase of the hepatitis B infection in the 1940s until the development of risk-free vaccines, about 40 years have passed. When effective therapeutic and particularly prophylactic measures against HIV infection will be available, we do not yet know.

Complete CDC classification of HIV infection

Group I: Acute infection
2 to 6 weeks after the infection, 3 days' to 3 weeks' duration, "spontaneous healing."

- o Mononucleosislike picture
  with or without acute meningoencephalitis
- o Seroconversion; in 95% of the cases after 4 to 12 weeks, occasionally demonstrable only after many months

Group II: Asymptomatic infection
Duration of the latency phase is months or years.

Positive serology

II A—asymptomatic (however infectious)
II B—plus pathologic laboratory findings (i.e., thrombocytopenia, lymphopenia, reduction of the T4/T8 cell ratio, anergia)

Group III: Generalized lymphadenopathy
Facultative prodromic state to group IV because only 40% of the patients go through this stage. Mild enlargement of inguinal and submandibular lymph nodes of limited significance. In 30% of cases there is a seborrheic dermatitis.

Positive serology

III A—generalized lymphadenopathy
III B—plus pathologic laboratory findings (see II B)

Group IV: Manifest immunodeficiency syndrome
Reversion to a lower stage has not yet been described (principle of the "one-way street").

Positive serology

IV A—general symptoms (at least one of the following):
- o Involuntary weight loss over 10%
- o Fever for longer than a month
- o Diarrhea for longer than a month

IV B—neurologic symptoms

Dementia, encephalopathy, encephalitis, myelopathy, peripheral neuropathy. Over 40% of all HIV-infected persons show neurologic and neuropsychiatric symptoms. In 10% of all cases, these are the first signs of disease. In the final phase, almost all AIDS patients show CNS findings. These findings are:

○ HIV dementia complexes
○ CNS complications of opportunistic infections (i.e., toxoplasmosis) or neoplasms (i.e., B-cell lymphoma)
○ HIV-associated metabolic changes

IV C$_1$—opportunistic infections
Protozoan- and helminth-caused infections
○ *Pneumocystis carinii* pneumonia
○ Toxoplasmosis with pneumonia or CNS involvement
○ Intestinal cryptosporidiosis; diarrhea for longer than 1 month
○ Isosporiasis; diarrhea for longer than 1 month
○ Strongyloidiasis with pneumonia or CNS inolvement or dissemination

Fungal infection
○ Esophageal, bronchial, or pulmonary candidiasis (endoscopic white plaques on erythematous base)
○ Cryptococcosis with lung or CNS involvement or dissemination
○ Aspergillosis with CNS involvement or dissemination
○ Histoplasmosis disseminated (not restricted to lung or lymph nodes)

Of special importance for the dentist
Oral candidiasis with the following patterns of prsentation: pseudomembranous; erythematous; hyperplastic (plaquelike; nodular); angular cheilitis

Bacterial infections
○ Atypical mycobacteriosis, among others, disseminated
Of special importance for the dentist
○ Acute necrotizing ulcerative gingivitis (ANUG)
○ Progressive marginal periodontitis
○ Exacerbation of periapical osteitic process

Viral infections
○ Cytomegalovirus infection with pneumonia and gastrointestinal, rectal, or CNS involvement
○ Herpes simplex with mucocutaneous participation (duration of at least 1 month, ulcerating) or pneumonia, gastrointestinal involvement, or disseminated
○ Zoster (also of the trigeminal branch); sometimes over several dermatomes or generalized

Also of importance for the dentist
○ Hairy leukoplakia (Epstein-Barr virus)
○ Focal epithelial hyperplasia (human papillomavirus)

IV C$_2$−other infections
○ Tuberculosis (extrapulmonary, involvement ot several organs or generalized)
○ Salmonella sepsis

IV D−malignancies
○ Kaposi's sarcoma
For the dentist to observe

One third of all AIDS patients develop Kaposi's sarcoma; preferred site is the skin, secondarily the oral mucosa
○ CNS lymphomas
○ Non-Hodgkin's lymphoma, high grade (diffuse, undifferentiated) of the B-cell line or of undetermined immunologic phenotype
○ Malignancy of lymphatic or reticuloendothelial systems (lymphoreticular malignancy) that appears more than 3 months after onset of HIV-related opportunistic infections

IV E−others
Chronic lymphoid, interstitial pneumonia, and neoplasms that are probably HIV-associated but do not belong in the above groups

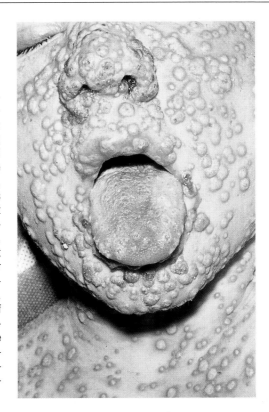

Fig. 11-1   A 19-year-old non-immunized patient with smallpox. Fully developed eruption stage on the third day of skin eruption. The areas close and far from the perioral area are covered with cloudy, pus-filled, centrally depressed blisters (pustules) that are confluent at some points. After an incubation time of about 2 weeks, there is a massive viremia that first appears as a spiking fever and severe malaise with catarrhal changes in the oropharynx. Then there is development of typical skin and mucosal efflorescences that go through the following stages: maculous exanthemas (enanthemas), papules, single-cell blisters, pustules, scabs, and scars.

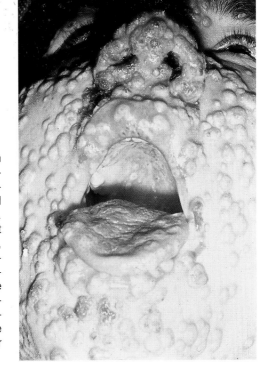

Fig. 11-2   The same patient in Fig. 11-1 also at the time of examination. There are characteristic changes in the oral mucosa (tongue and palate). The umbilicated pustules burst rapidly and result in painful, highly infectious erosion ulcerations. All skin and mucosal efflorescences are at the same stage of development, in contrast with chicken pox where lesions at various stages can be seen. They progress more or less at the same pace.

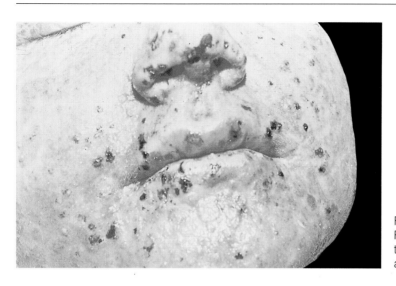

Fig. 11-3   The same patient in Figs. 11-1 and 11-2 six days later. The pustules have burst and scabbed in the meantime.

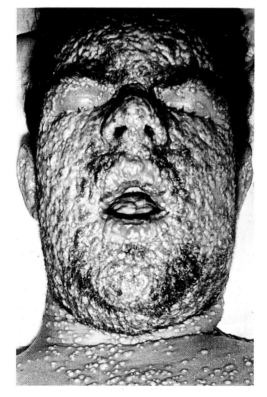

Fig. 11-4   Fully developed pustular stage in another patient during the same epidemic. In the past, the illness had a different degree of severity. It progressed rapidly from mild initial symptoms to a deadly hemorrhagic pox ("black leaves"). Transmission of this smallpox virus, which remains viable for a relatively long period of time, occurred as a result of infected droplets or dust contacting the mucosa of the upper airways.

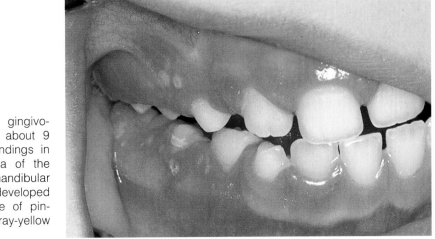

Fig. 11-5 Herpetic gingivo-stomatitis in a child about 9 years of age. The findings in the vestibular gingiva of the right maxillary and mandibular lateral teeth have developed from blisters the size of pin-heads into circular, gray-yellow coated erosions.

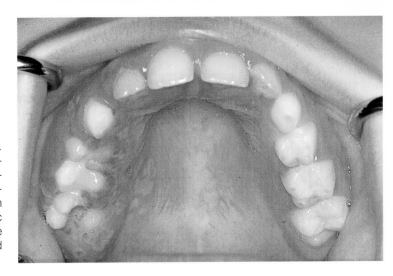

Fig. 11-6 The child in Fig. 11-5 also at the time of exami-nation. There are multiple fibrin-covered erosions on the pala-tine mucosa, which, through confluency, have a polycyclic outline in some areas. Note the acute gingivitis in the affected regions.

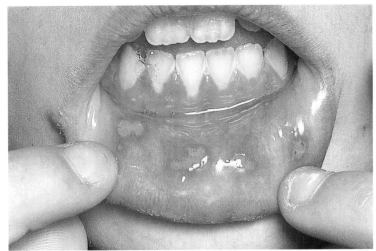

Fig. 11-7 Herpetic stomatitis in a 12-year-old child. Yellow-coated erosions with bright red rims have already superseded the short-lived vesicular stage.

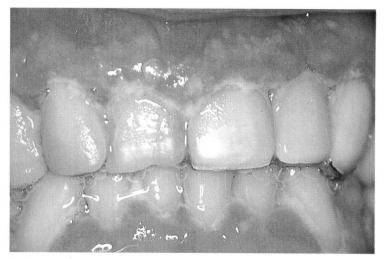

Fig. 11-8 Severe herpetic gingivostomatitis in an adult. The gingiva is covered with many erosions the size of pinheads. The acute inflamed gingiva is very red and swollen. In some cases it must be clarified whether there is a primary infection from herpes simplex virus (i.e., via serology) or an opportunistic infection in an immunodeficiency condition.

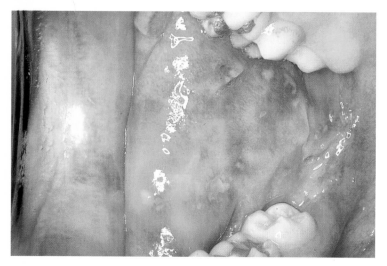

Fig. 11-9 Herpetic gingivostomatitis in a juvenile with severe systemic symptoms including neurologic symptoms (stiff neck and threatening herpetic meningoencephalitis). Shown are findings on the cheek mucosa.

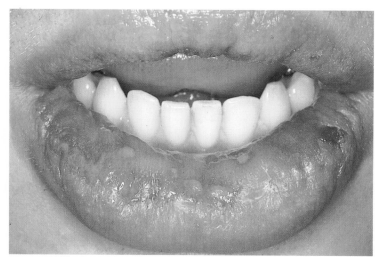

Fig. 11-10 The same patient in Fig. 11-9 also at the time of examination. There are many herpetiform, fibrin-covered erosions with red rims on the mucosa of the lower lip.

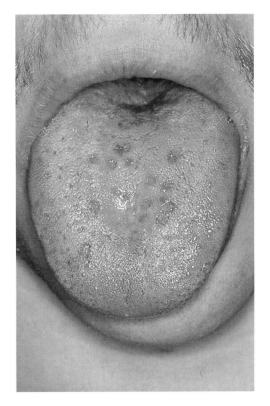

Fig. 11-11 Intraoral partial manifestation of a herpetic gingivostomatitis in a young patient. Multiple, already regressing roundish erosions on the specialized mucosa of the dorsum of the tongue. The differential diagnosis after inspection is with rare herpetiform aphthae (Cooke aphthae) that do not appear in an acute gingivostomatitis and do not have the corresponding associated symptoms (see chapter 12).

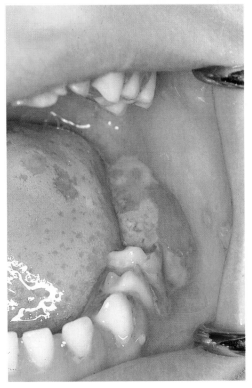

Fig. 11-12 Differential diagnosis of herpetic gingivostomatitis; development of acute necrotizing ulcerative gingivostomatitis (ANUG) following bronchopneumonia. As opposed to the herpetic gingivostomatitis, in this disease there are flat ulcerations with necrosis and later destruction of the gingivoperiodontal tissue (see chapter 5).

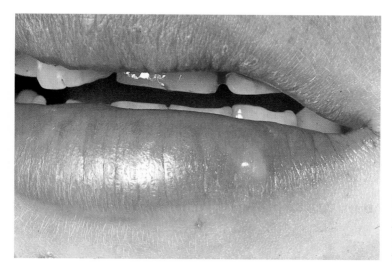

Fig. 11-13   Early stage of herpes simplex (labialis) on the vermilion border of the lower lip. Tense, fluid-filled, single vesicles.

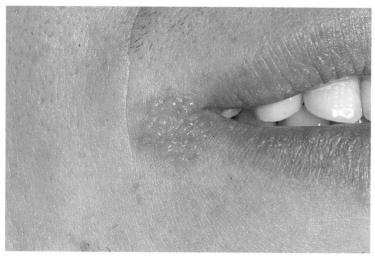

Fig. 11-14   Vesicular stage of herpes simplex (labialis) showing typical grouping at the labial angle.

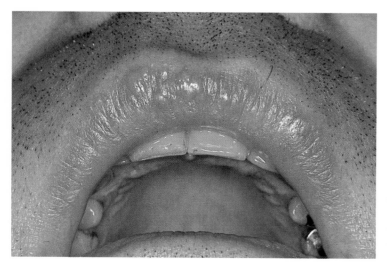

Fig. 11-15   Confluent blisters of labial herpes sometimes cluster at the vermilion border of the upper lip. The patient reported that the herpes labialis always appeared in the same area (herpes recidivans in loco).

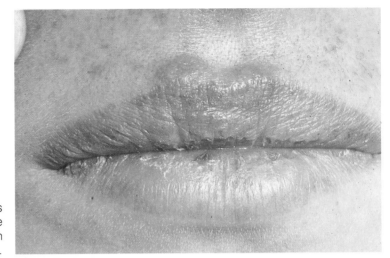

Fig. 11-16   Localized herpes labialis during influenza in the area of the philtrum on the skin of the vermilion of the upper lip.

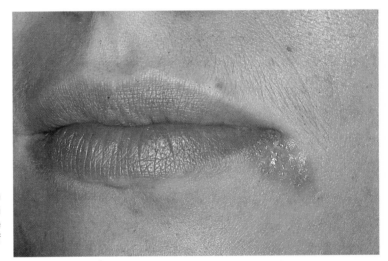

Fig. 11-17   Herpes labialis in the corner of the mouth shown immediately after rupture of the blisters with development of scabs.

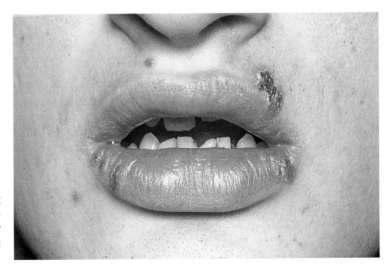

Fig. 11-18   Herpes simplex (labialis) following a febrile infection of the upper respiratory tract. Shown is the healing stage with scabbing.

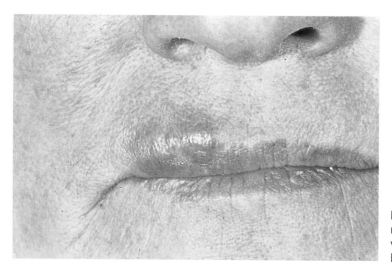

Fig. 11-19 Differential diagnosis of herpes labialis: lupus vulgaris on the vermilion lip border (see chapter 8).

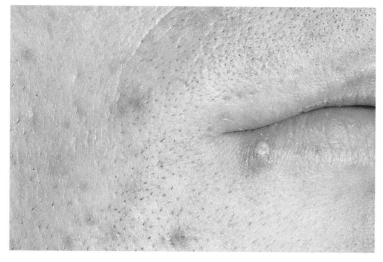

Fig. 11-20 Differential diagnosis of herpes labialis: acne with formation of pustules on the lower vermilion of lip border as a partial manifestation of acne in the perioral region.

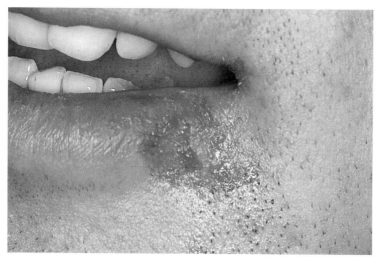

Fig. 11-21 Differential diagnosis of herpes labialis: mechanical tissue damage on the lower lip caused by excessive pull with a blunt wound retractor.

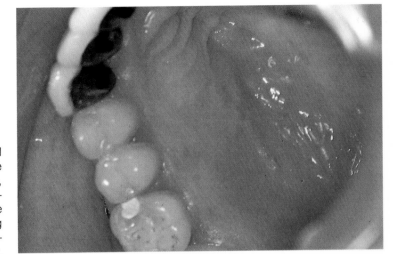

Fig. 11-22 Herpes of the oral mucosa (erosive herpes) on the mucosa of the hard palate, shown 48 hours after the appearance of the blisters. The triggering factor was a feeling of nausea from a dental medication, according to the patient.

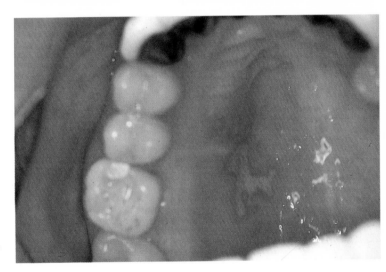

Fig. 11-23 The patient in Fig. 11-22 five days later in the healing stage.

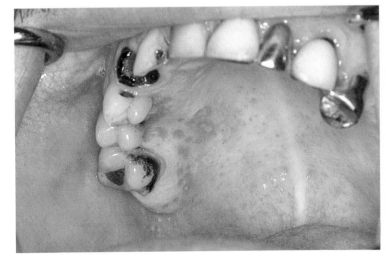

Fig. 11-24 Herpes of the oral mucosa with typical distribution on the mucosa of the hard palate. The short-term blister stage is already superseded by erosions. The affected area is usually no larger than a silver dollar.

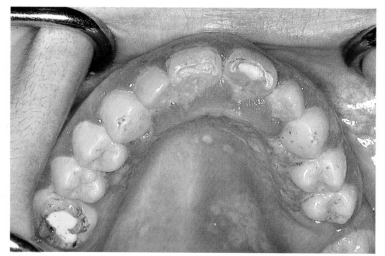

Fig. 11-25   Differential diagnosis of herpes labialis: zoster
of the left second trigeminal
branch. Note the dark-red erythema with advanced herpetiform efflorescences on the
mucosa of the hard palate. The
distribution is limited to one
side of the face. In contrast to
an almost complete absence of
systemic symptoms in herpes
mucosae oris, this patient complained of a severe general
malaise and sharp pain in the
area of the intraorbital nerve.

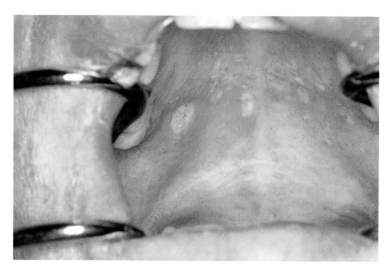

Fig. 11-26   Differential diagnosis of herpes labialis: acute
necrotizing ulcerative stomatitis
of the mucosa of the palate in a
patient with a severe, debilitating systemic disease (Hodgkin's disease).

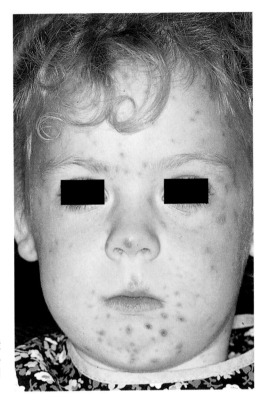

Fig. 11-27   Face of a patient with varicella. Typical polymorphic efflorescences on the third day of exanthema.

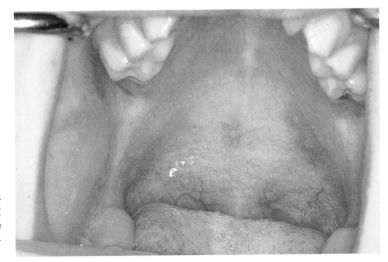

Fig. 11-28   Intraoral findings in the child in Fig. 11-27 also at the time of examination. There are fresh papulovesiculous efflorescences on the palate.

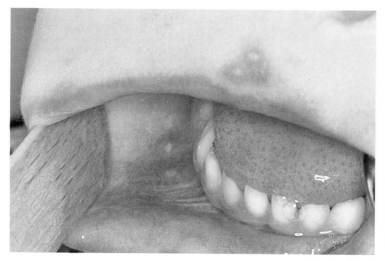

Fig. 11-29   Intraoral findings of the child in Figs. 11-27 and 11-28 at the time of examination. On the oral mucosa as on the skin there are herpetiform efflorescences that are at different stages of development.

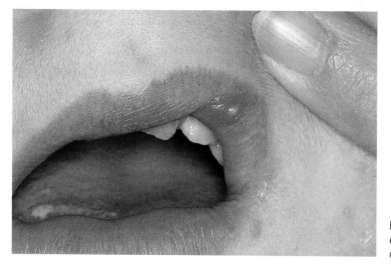

Fig. 11-30   Papulovesicular efflorescences on the upper lip of a child with varicella.

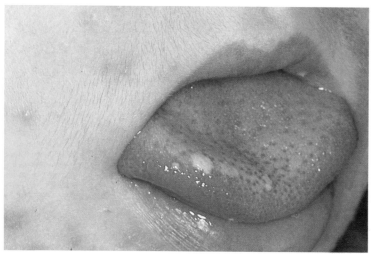

Fig. 11-31   The child in Fig. 11-30 also at the time of examination. There are already erosive, fibrin-covered lesions on the border of the tongue. Note the healing efflorescences in the perioral region.

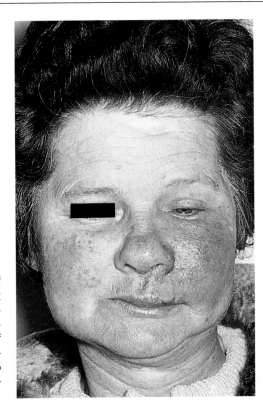

Fig. 11-32   Herpes zoster of the second division of the left trigeminal nerve in a 51-year-old woman. A burning sensation in the innervation area of this nerve was the first symptom of the disease, followed 5 days later by cutaneous eruptions.

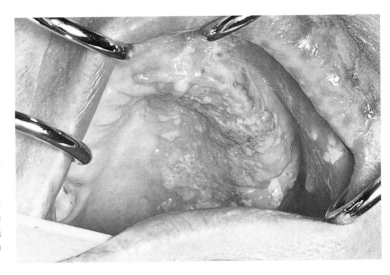

Fig. 11-33   Oral manifestation in the same patient in Fig. 11-32. Note the unilateral arrangement of the lesions, which like the skin efflorescences are strictly confined to the area supplied by the second division of the left trigeminal nerve.

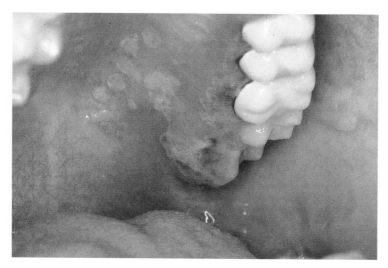

Fig. 11-34　Partial manifestation of zoster of the second trigeminal branch in the palatal mucosa. In addition to groups of typically arranged herpetic-like lesions, note also necrosis and ulcerations in the region close to the gingiva.

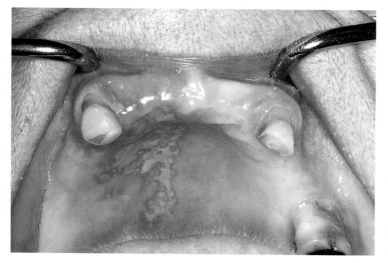

Fig. 11-35　Abortive form of a zoster of the right second trigeminal branch. The impairing general conditions and the severe prodromal pains already present, together with the extensive mucosal changes, allow a definite clinical differentiation from the findings of herpes mucosae oris.

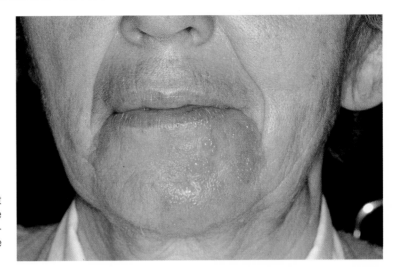

Fig. 11-36   Zoster of the left third trigeminal branch. The skin changes in the area innervated by the mentalis nerve are in the acute eruption phase.

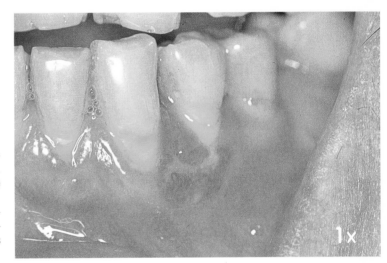

Fig. 11-37   Associated gingival findings in the patient of Fig. 11-36, 4 weeks later. In the areas of teeth 33 and 34 (21 and 22), there was a necrotizing inflammatory process caused by a sequestration of parts of the interdental septum.

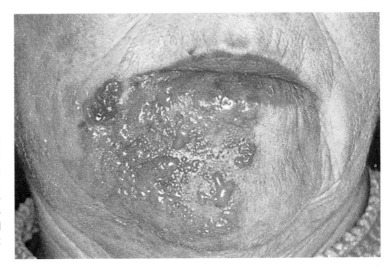

Fig. 11-38   Zoster of the right third trigeminal branch. There is development of dark-red erythema with tense, clustered, coalescing blisters. (From Krüger E. Lehrbuch der chirurgischen Zahn- Mund- und Kieferheilkunde, vol. 2. Berlin: Quintessenz, 1988.)

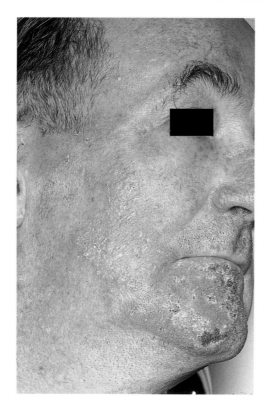

Fig. 11-39   Healing process of zoster of the right third trigeminal branch with ear participation (otic zoster).

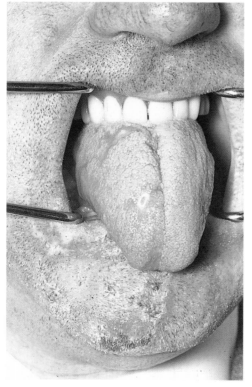

Fig. 11-40   The patient in Fig. 11-39 also at the time of examination. The erosions caused by the herpetic-like blisters involve the dorsum of the posterior part of the tongue. After healing, they leave atrophy of the specialized tongue mucosa (loss of papillae). The patient complained at this time of a persistent loss of taste.

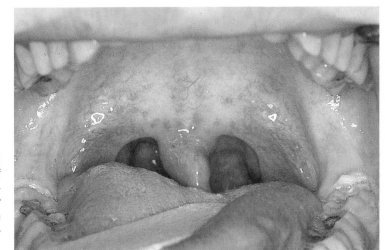

Fig. 11-41 Herpangina. Pearl necklace-like arrangement of efflorescences in typical location, particularly on the anterior border of the palate. Transition from the blister stage to erosions.

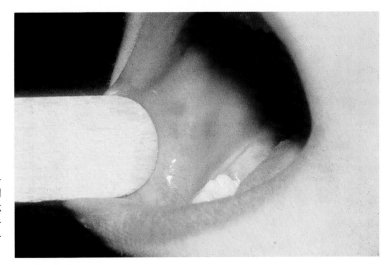

Fig. 11-42 Hand-foot-and-mouth disease in a 4-year-old child. The blisters on the cheek mucosa have advanced to aphthaelike secondary efflorescences.

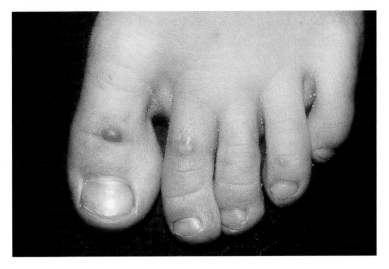

Fig. 11-43 The same child as in Fig. 11-42 also at the time of examination. In addition to the oral mucosal changes, there were painless blisters on the toes. Hand-foot-and-mouth disease was once erroneously called hoof and mouth disease.

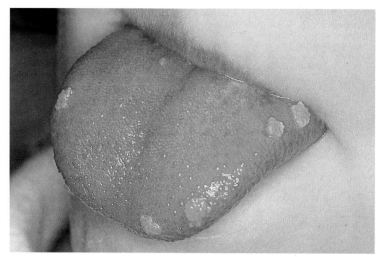

Fig. 11-44   Focal epithelial hyperplasia (Heck's disease) in a 3-year-old girl. On the dorsum of the tongue, particularly on the border of the tongue, are dispersed knotty aggregates resembling white pearls. The German Cancer Center in Heidelberg, section of virology, isolated the human papillomavirus type 13 in a biopsy specimen.

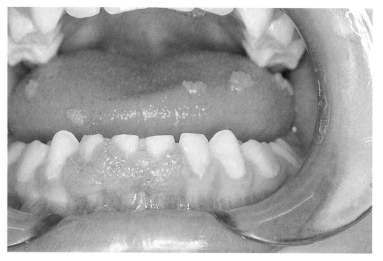

Fig. 11-45 The child in Fig. 11-44 also at the time of examination. Besides the efflorescences visible on the tongue surface, there are grapelike mucosal proliferations that have already covered some of the dental crowns in the area of the vestibular gingiva of the mandibular incisors. Similar changes were found on the palatal mucosa of the maxillary anterior teeth and in the region of the cheek mucosa.

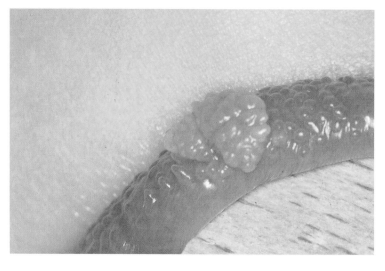

Fig. 11-46   The child in Figs. 11-44 and 11-45 at the time of examination. Clusters of papules the same color as the mucosa are found on the border of the tongue in a magnification of the area. The raspberry pattern of the surface is clearly visible. According to the parents, the mucosal changes regressed under treatment with external homeopathic agents within 4 months. Scientifically, this can be considered spontaneous remission.

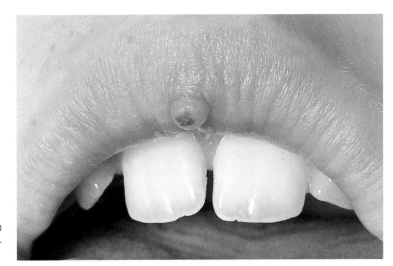

Fig. 11-47 A common wart in the area of the upper lip border.

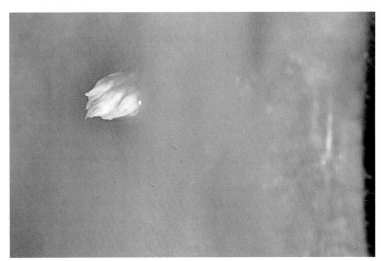

Fig. 11-48 A common wart in the region of the cheek mucosa.

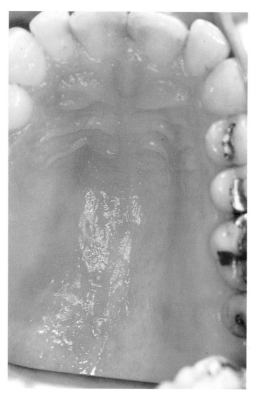

Fig. 11-49 Erythematous (atrophic) candidiasis of the palatal mucosa. Together with hairy leukoplakia, this forms (see Fig. 11-50) the first clinical sign of an HIV infection unknown to the patient. *Candida* infections are an important indicator of disturbed lymphocyte function and are found in almost all AIDS patients.

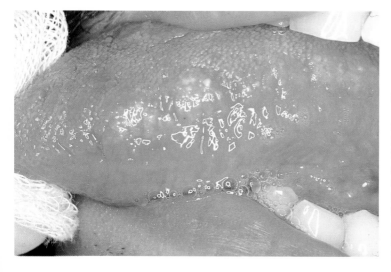

Fig. 11-50 The patient in Fig. 11-49 also at the time of examination. The hairy leukoplakia is found in a typical location on the tongue border. It ranks as an early relatively reliable oral sign of the developing full picture of AIDS. Both findings were grounds to suggest a serologic examination to the patient, who turned out to be HIV positive.

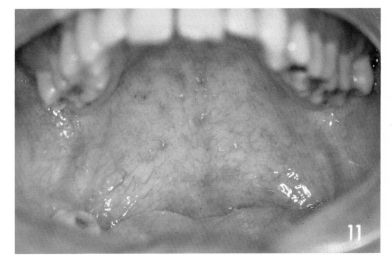

Fig. 11-51 This and the following two figures demonstrate three important AIDS-related changes on the oral mucosa of the same patient. Shown is a stippled pseudomembranous form of an oral *Candida* infection.

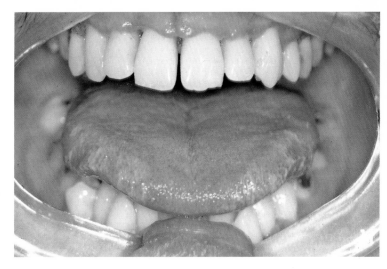

Fig. 11-52 The same patient in Fig. 11-51. Hairy leukoplakia with additional *Candida* colonization predominantly present on the border of the tongue.

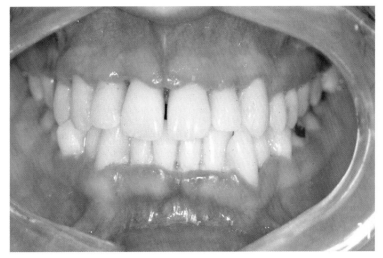

Fig. 11-53 The patient in Figs. 11-51 and 11-52. Shown is gingivoperiodontal tissue destruction caused by acute necrotizing ulcerative gingivitis (ANUG).

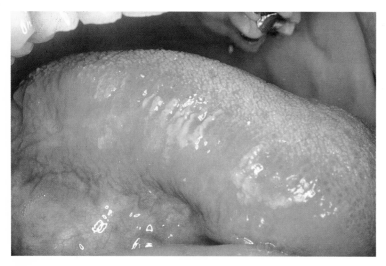

Fig. 11-54 Hairy leukoplakia on the border of the tongue in a patient in the early stages of AIDS. The whitish, nonremovable changes often have a rippled and wrinkled surface. Superimposed *Candida* colonization.

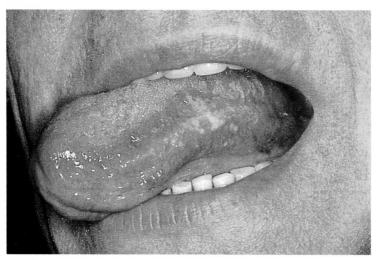

Fig. 11-55 Hairy leukoplakia in a patient with AIDS. The viral genesis of this finding is now considered certain (Epstein-Barr virus). (From Frenkel G. *In:* Knolle G. (ed). HTLV III-infektion. Berlin: Quintessenz, 1986.)

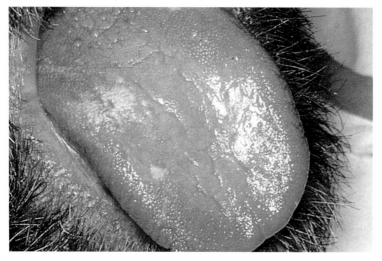

Fig. 11-56 Hairy leukoplakia in an AIDS patient. In addition to the frequent location on the border of the tongue, the dorsum of the tongue and the underside of the tongue can also be affected. (From Frenkel G. *In:* Knolle G. (ed). HTLV III-infektion. Berlin. Quintessenz, 1986.)

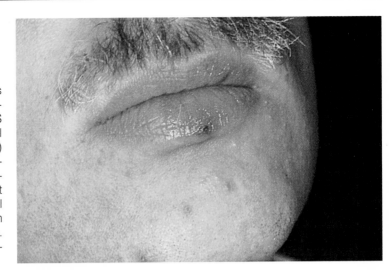

Fig. 11-57 Mucocutaneous herpes simplex as an opportunistic infection in an AIDS patient. Localization in the oral cavity (erosions, ulcerations) results in decreased food intake because of pain (dysphagia). These findings are most often present in the perianal and perigenital region. (From Frenkel G. *In:* Knolle G. (ed). HTLV III-infektion. Berlin: Quintessenz, 1986.)

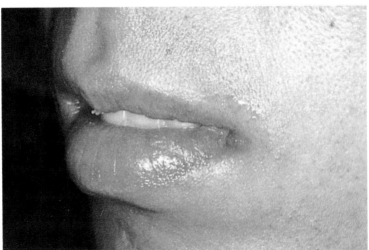

Fig. 11-58 Opportunistic herpes simplex infection in an AIDS patient. Surface ulcerations under a rhagade of the mouth corner. The lesion responds to acyclovir but recurs after cessation of the virostatic agent. (From Frenkel G. *In:* Knolle G. (ed). HTLV III-infektion. Berlin: Quintessenz, 1986.)

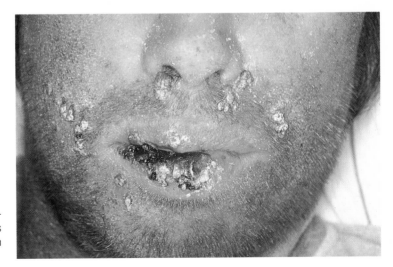

Fig. 11-59 Massive mucocutaneous herpes simplex lesions as an opportunistic infection in preterminal stage of AIDS.

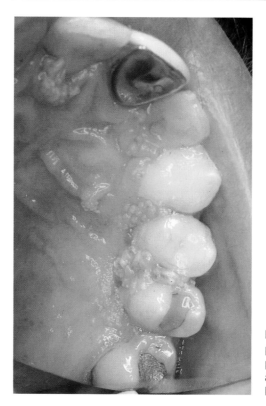

Fig. 11-60 Focal epithelial hyperplasia (Heck's disease) in a patient with AIDS. There are aggregated papules on the palatal gingiva.

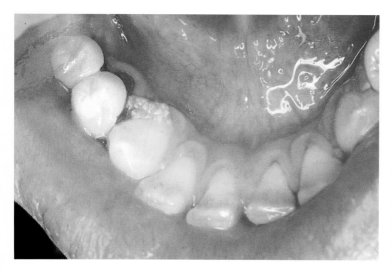

Fig. 11-61   The patient in Fig. 11-60 also at the time of examination. The mucosal proliferation is multilocular and occurs also on the oral gingiva in the area of teeth 43 and 44 (26 and 27).

Fig. 11-62 Stippled-like pseudomembrane caused by oral candidiasis on the palatal mucosa as an opportunistic infection in AIDS. The demonstration of the fungal disease is frequently the first clinical sign of AIDS. In addition to the oral mucosa, the *Candida* infection involves the esophagus and the vagina, but seldom the airways, the intestines, or the skin. Generalization is possible through hematogenous dissemination. (From Frenkel G. *In:* Knolle G. (ed). HTLV III-infektion. Berlin: Quintessenz, 1986.)

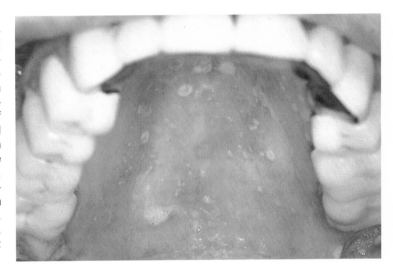

Fig. 11-63 Erythematous (atrophic) form of oral *Candida* infection in an AIDS patient with manifestation on the palatal mucosa under a partial prosthesis. Mycotic opportunistic infections can respond to therapy. They recur, however, after suspension of the systemic antimycotic agent and require continuous treatment. Thrush is caused in 90% of the cases by *Candida albicans* and in 10% by other *Candida* species.

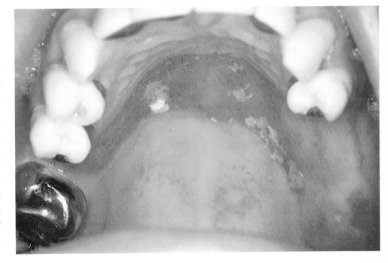

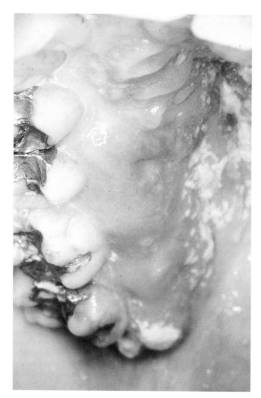

Fig. 11-64 Pseudomembranous form of oral candidiasis in an advanced case of AIDS. Gingivoperiodontal infections and also worsening systemic conditions are evident (rapid deterioration or a marginal periodontitis, sometimes multiple pocket formation; appearance of an acute necrotizing ulcerative gingivitis).

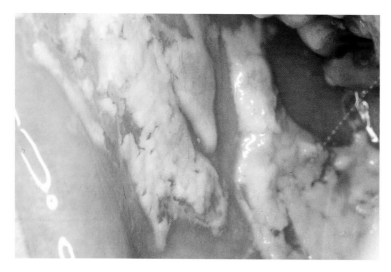

Fig. 11-65 Massive pseudomembranous candidiasis in the final stage of AIDS.

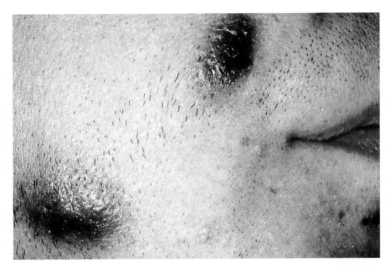

Fig. 11-66 Kaposi's sarcoma of the skin of the right cheek. First described in multicentric form in the immunodeficient or immunodepressed patient by Kaposi in 1872, the malignant vascular tumor involves skin, mucosa, lymph nodes, and/or viscera. It is frequently found today but was rare in the past. About one third of all AIDS patients develop Kaposi's sarcoma in the course of the disease.

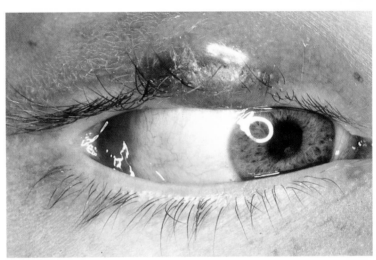

Fig. 11-67 Kaposi's sarcoma on the upper eyelid. The most frequent location is the skin (95% of all cases). The second most frequent is the oral mucosa and after that the mucosa of the gastrointestinal tract. Lymph nodes and internal organs can be affected. It has the appearance of a malignant tumor type IV D and appears most often in patients who have had opportunistic infection.

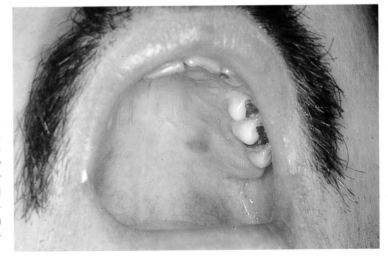

Fig. 11-68 Early Kaposi's sarcoma on the palatal mucosa, which is the most frequent location in the oral cavity. Initially there is a red spot, which later becomes bluish-black and grows in size. The often-multiple tumor nodules can remain flat or grow as exophytic lesions.

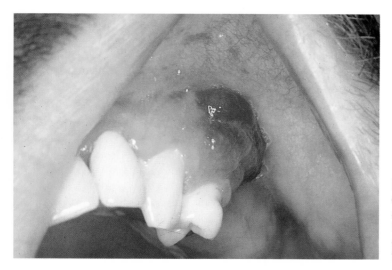

Fig. 11-69   Kaposi's sarcoma on the gingiva with the appearance of an epulis. Among intraoral manifestations, the gingiva is the second most frequent site.

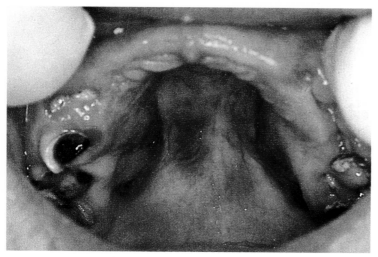

Fig. 11-70   Intraoral partial manifestation of multiple, disseminated Kaposi's sarcomas in typical localization on the palatal mucosa of a female AIDS patient. (From Frenkel G. *In:* Knolle G. (ed). HTLV III-infektion. Berlin: Quintessenz, 1986.)

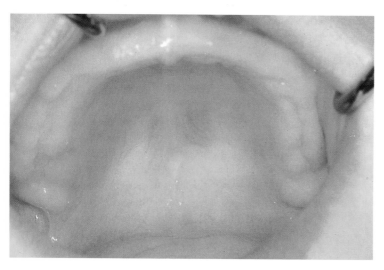

Fig. 11-71   Intraoral findings of the patient in Fig. 11-70 after removal of the root rests and after associated radiation therapy. Condition before prosthetic treatment. The decision for dental treatment—when of palliative nature—should always be done with the treating physician who has an ambulatory AIDS service.

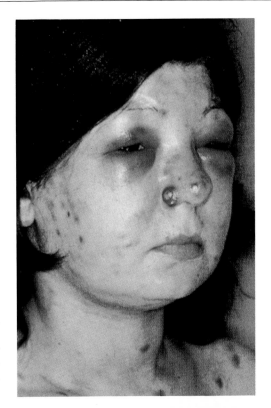

Fig. 11-72 The patient in Figs. 11-70 and 11-71. Note the many disseminated Kaposi's sarcomas of different size and extension in the face. The initial findings were mistakenly diagnosed as eczema of the eyelid. Old and large Kaposi's foci resemble the borders of hematomas because of the color change. (From Frenkel G. *In:* Knolle G. (ed). HTLV III-infektion. Berlin: Quintessenz, 1986.)

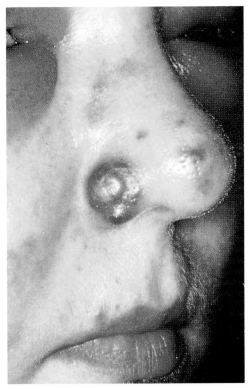

Fig. 11-73 The nose and perioral region of the patient in Fig. 11-72 also at the time of examination. In the area seen by the dentist, there are many nodules of Kaposi's sarcoma at various stages of development. In relation to the etiopathogenesis of Kaposi's sarcoma, there is suspicion of virus-induced oncogenic "switch-on effect" (possibly through cytomegalovirus). (From Frenkel G. *In:* Knolle G. (ed). HTLV III-infektion. Berlin: Quintessenz 1986.)

Nomenclature for HIV infection / Classification	Acute infection Group I	Asymptomatic stage Group II	Generalized lymphadenopathy Group III	Manifest immunosuppression AIDS Group IV (A–E)
Clinical course	Mononucleosislike illness	Appearance of health in spite of infection	Facultative prodromal stage in 40% of cases	Clinical illness with deteriorating condition; lethal prognosis

Cachexia
Progressive failure of immune and organ systems
Unavoidable medical side effects
Neurologic-neuropsychiatric findings
Meningitis-encephalitis, CNS findings
Tuberculosis, salmonellosis
Kaposi's sarcoma and other malignancies
Mucocutaneous manifestations of herpes simplex
Bacterial and pneumocystic pneumonia
Zoster, Candidiasis as beginning of opportunistic infection
Dermatologic findings (erythema, seborrheic dermatitis)
Lymphadenopathy
Headache, conspicuous physical manifestations, neurologic findings
Diarrhea, enteritis, weight loss
Fever, night sweats, fatigue, exhaustion |
Incubation time 2–6 weeks				
Duration of course	3 days–3 weeks	Months or years	Facultative 1–5 years	Undetermined (up to 5 years?), lethal (Stand 1990)
Laboratory findings: HIV serology / Blood workup	– – ± As in other viral infections	+ + + Not observable until T_4/T_8 values begin to fall	+ + + Decrease of lymphocyte regeneration	+ + + + + + + + + + + + + + Includes, among other things, lymphadenopathy, acute decrease or absence of T helper cells, anemia, leukopenia, periodic thrombocytopenia. In late stages and with opportunistic infection there is an increase of cerebro-spinal fluid/serum HIV antibodies.

‖ = Regular finding
╎ ╎ ╎ = Frequent finding (approx. 50%)
⋮ = Infrequent finding (approx. 10%)
⋱ = Recurrent finding

Chapter 12

Aphthae of the Oral Mucosa

Recurrent aphthous ulcerations

Behçet's syndrome

An aphtha is morphologically characterized by a circumscribed erosion or ulceration that is oval, sharply limited, painful, appearing in single or multiple form, with an adhering pseudomembranous fibrin cover and a very red border.

However, not every fibrin-covered ulceration can be considered an aphtha; fibrin-covered changes on the oral mucosa are frequently seen as secondary efflorescences. Many conditions and diseases have a common morphologic expression in such ulcerations. Among the diseases considered aphthous diseases is the so-called *Bedner aphthae,* which are nothing more than lesions caused by an injury, with inflammatory cover, and that appear because of mechanically incorrect oral hygiene in infants.

To differentiate aphthae from similar changes of other cause, it should be known that aphthous lesions commonly chronically recur at various intervals and heal spontaneously. The patient's history and the disease course, in addition to the clinical findings, are therefore decisive criteria for clinical diagnosis of aphthae.

While chronically recurring aphthae are a local illness limited to the oral mucosa, remain harmless, and are painful and often bothersome lesions, Behçet's syndrome is a generalized, severe, systemic disease. Thus in Behçet's syndrome oral aphthae are only partial manifestations of a complex of symptoms involving many organs.

Recurrent aphthous ulcerations (ICD-DA 528.20)

Recurrent aphthous ulcerations occur with the diseases of the oral mucosa most commonly found in dental practice. Because they are probably noninfectious, they should be distinguished from any type of herpes simplex viral infection of the oral mucosa (herpetic gingivostomatis, erosive herpes simplex). Through recurrences they can, in many patients, lead to decades of or lifelong suffering. Primarily young or middle-aged adults are affected, and there is a predominance of females. The first appearance usually occurs in the second decade of life but exceptionally also during childhood.

The onset of the disease occurs with a peculiar feeling of pain in a circumscribed area that soon becomes erythematous. In the center of this area there is formation of a small bump, possibly also an inconspicuous blister, which is usually not observed because it disappears quickly. With increased exudation there is necrosis of the epithelium (Fig. 12-1). The subsequent erosion of shallow-to-deep ulceration is accompanied by an intense burning sensation, which causes the patient to seek help. In this phase, the fully developed aphtha shows a picture of a very red, infiltrated border around an ulceration covered by a dirty-white to more yellow fibrin cover (Fig. 12-2 and 12-3). The mucosal defect usually remains the size of a lentil but can, however, in exceptional cases have the diameter of about 1 cm.

The most frequently appearing *aphthae of the smaller type (Mikulicz's aphthae)* appear alone or in very small numbers (Figs. 12-4 and 12-5). More than five efflorescences is rare.

After 6 to 8 days, the mucosal lesion becomes epithelialized from the border inward (Fig. 12-7). The lesion usually heals in 10 to 14 days, leaving no scar.

Involved are the nonkeratinized areas of the oral mucosa, particularly the lip and cheek mucosa and the area of the vestibular fold, and less frequently the anterior floor of the mouth, the underside of the tongue, and the border of the tongue. The masticatory mucosa (hard palate, gingiva propria) and the dorsum of the tongue usually remain free (exception: Fig. 12-6). Smoking habits appear to negatively influence the appearance of chronic recurring aphthae, which can be explained by the increased keratinization of the mucosa in smokers.

In spite of the chronicity of the disease, the individual efflorescences disappear quickly. The duration of the symptom-free interval can last days, weeks, months, or even years. In short-term attacks, different stages may be observed in the oral cavity of the same patient.

Clinical findings and case history allow, as a rule, the differentiation from other diseases of the oral mucosa. The confusion with herpetic gingivostomatis (caused by the herpes simplex virus) can only be understood in view of the similarity of the terms ("aphthous" stomatitis). This descriptive terminology should be abandoned completely because the classic symptoms of gingivostomatitis as found in the acute viral infection of early childhood (i.e. large number of efflorescences, including masticatory mucosa and fixed in periosteum, progressive spread with associated gingivitis, halitosis, increased salivation, lymphadenitis of the regional lymph nodes, and fever accomanied by malaise, usually not recurring) are absent in chronic recurrent aphthous ulcers.

The differential diagnosis is somewhat difficult when the interval between recurrences is only a few days and therefore many aphthae are present. To be kept in mind, also, is the development of a peculiar, though rare, clinical finding with the formation of multiple foci formed by clusters of aphthae that later partially coalesce. Because of the similarity with the clinical findings of herpes (Fig. 12-8) and particularly with erosive herpes of the oral mucosa (whose main location is, however, the hard palate and the gingiva), the diagnosis of *herpetiform aphthae* (synonym: *Cooke aphthae, herpetiform ulcerations;* ICD-DA 528.21) can only be made when viral cultures and serologic tests for viral infection yield negative results. Another, rare form is *periadenitis mucosa necrotic recurrens* (ICD-DA 528.22). This usually single "giant aphtha" of a diameter up to 3 cm is an extremely painful, deep, craterlike ulceration on the oral mucosa (Figs. 12-9 to 12-12) that usually has a border that is raised, not distinguishable at palpation. Associated findings usually include edema of the adjacent tissues, swelling of the regional lymph nodes, and a slight fever. Not uncommon manifestations of this aphthous form in the oropharyngeal region include complaints of pain on swallowing and a jaw cramp. Because of major tissue necrosis, the course of healing is delayed. It can take up to 8 weeks. Healing leaves scarring or residual tissue defects.

The differential diagnosis of periadenitis mucosa necrotic recurrens includes the blister-forming dermatosis. The blisters in the oral mucosa are rapidly substituted by secondary efflorescences in the form of erosions or ulcerations (see chapter 29). Also included in differential diagnosis are the circumscribed, traumatic ulcerations of acute and chronic type and the erosive changes in syphilis II in the oral mucosa (see chapter 8). Because the ulcerations of major-type aphthae can be very deep with a marked induration and can persist for many weeks, in these special cases, it is always necessary to consider an ulcerated carcinoma.

There is no lack of attempts to find the cause of recurrent aphthous ulcerations. In addition to genetic and constitutional factors (family clustering), psychological (emotional) stress has been considered. Expression of a neurovegetative labile state (vessel neurosis), hormonal influences (menstrual cycle, pregnancy), gastrointestinal dysfunction (among others, dyspepsia), microbial pathogens (reaction to streptococcal antigens), and individual specific hyperergic reactions to minimal tissue traumas have been discussed. Research has suggested the possibility of a lymphocyte-bound autoimmune pathogenic mechanism. It is therefore possible to claim many factors as plausible explanations of the onset of aphthae, but all hypotheses have not changed the fact that the cause of this disease remains unknown.

Generally, the treatment of the recurrent aphthous ulcerations is not very satisfactory. There is so far no way to avoid recurrence. As a rule, symptomatic therapy aims to reduce the pain and decrease the duration of the single episodes. Cauterization, customarily used in the past, should not be done in most cases. It detroys sensitive nerve endings and offers short-term pain reduction, but there is additional tissue damage, a delay of healing, and increased scar formation.

Limited local use of some corticosteroids in the form of sticky ointments and pastes is suitable. Depending on the location of the aphthae, corticosteroid-containing lozenges may be prescribed. But long-term use of corticosteroid preparations may have untoward side effects. Good results are reported with tetracycline powder that can be used on aphthae after removal of the superficial debris. The aphthae so treated are then covered with a corticosteroid-containing ointment.

If the patient finds eating difficult because of pain, local anesthetics may be indicated. These are usually components of preparations that also contain other medications such as antibiotics or phytotherapeutics (plant extracts). The therapeutic value of these combination preparations is debatable. The risk of allergic complications caused by these preparations should be considered.

Behçet's syndrome (ICD-DA 136.1 and 136.10)

Behçet's syndrome is, from the prognostic point of view, a very serious systemic disease that follows a progressive course with periodic relapses. Even though more cases are known in Japan and in eastern Mediterranean nations and are seldom encountered in Germany, Behçet's syndrome is not restricted to foreigners. The disease findings are characterized by the *classic triad* of *aphthae on the oral mucosa, aphthous ulcerative changes in the genital area* (penis, scrotum, vulva, vagina, perineum), and *hypopyoniritis* (pus accumulation on the bottom of the anterior eye chamber with inflammation and pus on the iris).

In addition to this trisymptomatic complex, there are many other possible manifestations *(polyorganotropic disease).* The vascular system (vasculonecrotic inflammatory reaction, thrombophlebitic process), nervous system, skin, gastrointestinal tract, urogenital system, and articulations (among others, polyarthritis) can be affected in different combinations. Particularly feared are the neurologic manifestations (among others, encephalomyelitis with high mortality), ophthalmologic complications (blindness), and conditions leading to "acute abdomen."

Because laboratory findings, while consistent for an inflammatory condition, are not specific for Behçet's syndrome, the diagnosis must be established clinically.

In its fully developed clinical picture, the disease cannot be mistaken. Diagnostic difficulties may arise because there are also monosymptomatic and abortive forms. The constantly recurring oral aphthae are the cardinal sign of early detection (Figs. 12-13 to 12-17). In comparison with the common chronic recurring aphthae, they tend to appear in large numbers (more than five) and to be on the entire oral cavity including the throat ring. The appearance of not a single efflorescence but of many that extend into the depth of the oropharynx is a diagnostic guide. The patient complains of severe malaise (i.e., weakness, loss of weight, sometimes subfebrile temperatures) and other symptoms such as stomatitis (halitosis, excessive salivation, lymphadenitis of regional lymph nodes).

The etiology of Behçet's syndrome is still unclear. For a long time a viral origin was suspected, but to this day there is no positive proof. Present knowledge suggests a chronic inflammatory vascular disease with a possible basis in humoral and cellular autoimmune dysfunction in association with genetic factors. It remains undecided whether the chronic recurring aphthae are a benign form on one hand and Behçet's syndrome the generalized (so to speak) malignant form of the same condition. It is possible that they are extreme variations of the same disease.

Symptomatic therapy should involve high doses of systemic corticosterone, cytostatics, immunosuppressive agents, and anticoagulants. The results are uncertain because the disease course often cannot be controlled.

The dentist must keep in mind that aphthae on the oral mucosa are not always harmless local changes; in some cases, they can be an early cardinal sign as partial manifestation of a serious systemic disease. The dentist should not hesitate to refer the patient to obtain an interdisciplinary opinion.

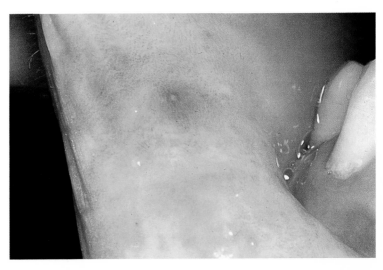

Fig. 12-1 Early stage of an aphtha on the oral mucosa. A dot-sized epithelial necrosis has already started to form in the center of the erythematous macula. This patient experienced a chronic recurrent course over 5 years with asymptomatic intervals of several months' duration.

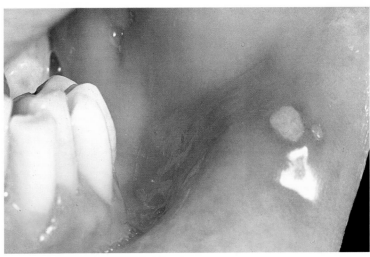

Fig. 12-2 Fully developed, extremely painful aphtha on the lip mucosa with red halo and lentil-sized, fibrin-covered ulceration. On the border of this lesion is another efflorescence, which at the time was undergoing epithelial necrosis and later would lead to a coalescing ulceration.

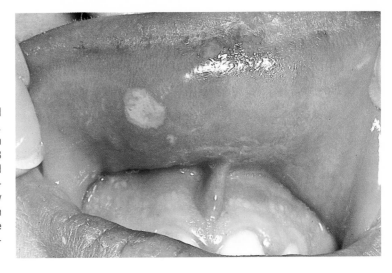

Fig. 12-3 Fully developed large aphtha on the lip mucosa. The chronic recurring lesion appeared at intervals of 1 to 3 months over 10 years and shows at the time of examination a recurrence that is a few days old. On the border zone in the direction of the fold of the vestibule is another small efflorescence.

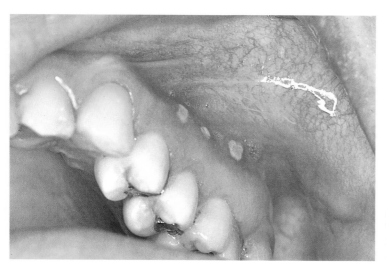

Fig. 12-4 Three fully developed aphthae in the vestibular fold of the cheek mucosa. They have been recurring for several months.

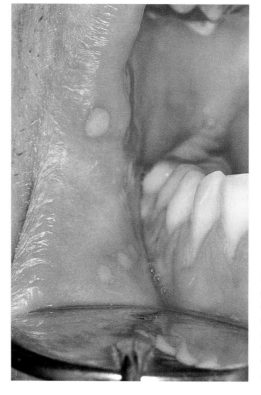

Fig. 12-5 Several chronic recurring aphthae on the lip and cheek mucosa. Characteristic clinical findings include the circular-to-oval, slight, bowl-forming, depressed ulceration with pseudomembranous fibrin coating and red border.

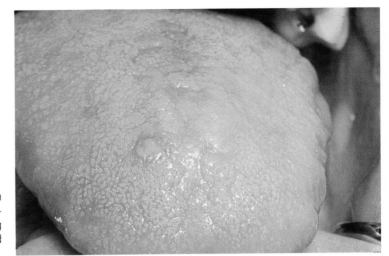

Fig. 12-6   Rare location of an aphtha on the tongue in a patient with frequently occurring aphthae on the nonkeratinized regions of the oral mucosa.

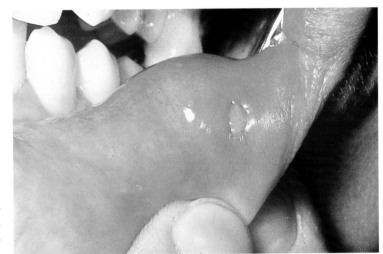

Fig. 12-7   Pain-free repair stage of an aphtha with regrowth of the border epithelium.

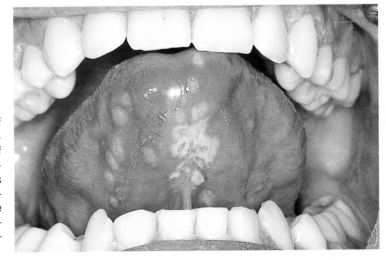

Fig. 12-8   Multiple clusters of partially coalescing, noninfective aphthae on the bottom of the tongue. Because of the similarity with the lesions of herpes simplex, these are called herpetiform aphthae. A viral cause was ruled out because of negative test results for viral infection.

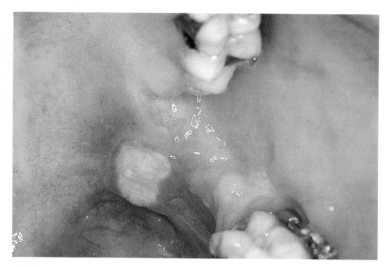

Fig. 12-9 Oropharyngeal manifestation of a major-type recent aphtha. The patient had considerable swallowing problems and swollen regional lymph nodes.

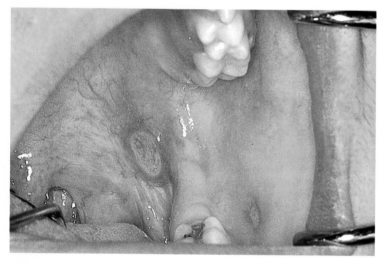

Fig. 12-10 Painful aphthae of the major type on the anterior palatal arch that have been present for 14 days. On the cheek mucosa is the development of other aphthae. Lengthy healing course with scar formation.

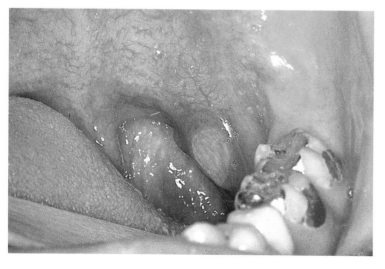

Fig. 12-11 Aphthae of the major type with associated edema. Accompanying symptoms were swallowing problems, jaw cramps, and lymphadenitis of the regional lymph nodes. Note the raised, but not indurated, ulcer border. Because of the protracted healing course of the deep crater-forming ulceration, a carcinoma should be considered in the differential diagnosis if the border of the ulcer has an increased consistency.

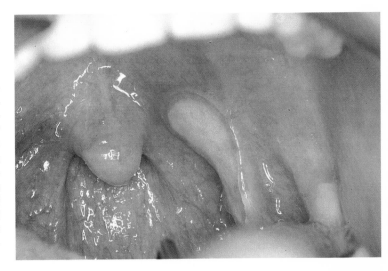

Fig. 12-12 Deep "giant aphtha" at the anterior part of the palatal arch of 4 weeks' duration. The painful lesion is associated with a lymphadenitis of the regional lymph nodes and regresses very slowly. The slightly raised border was unremarkable on palpation. There were no findings suggestive of Behçet's syndrome. Differential diagnosis is with a secondary efflorescence of a blister-forming disease.

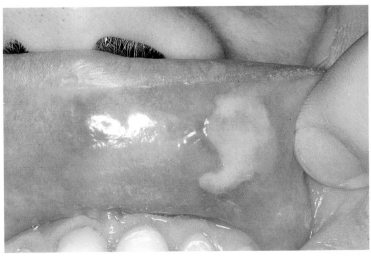

Fig. 12-13 Behçet's syndrome. Large aphthae on the lip mucosa as partial manifestation of several very painful aphthous ulcerations in the oral mucosa. At this point there was also an iridocyclitis with hypopyon. The diagnosis was obtained in cooperation with an ophthalmologist.

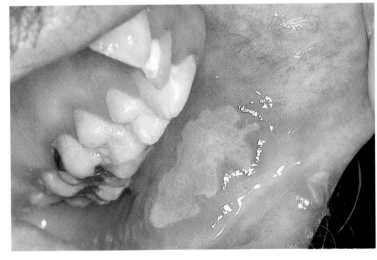

Fig. 12-14 Behçet's syndrome. Oral participation in the form of a painful giant aphtha of long duration on the cheek mucosa. In total there were six more aphthous lesions in the oral and oropharyngeal region. There were also ulcerations in the genital area. These bipolar aphthae gave clues to the diagnosis (referral to a dermatologist).

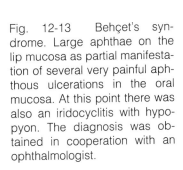

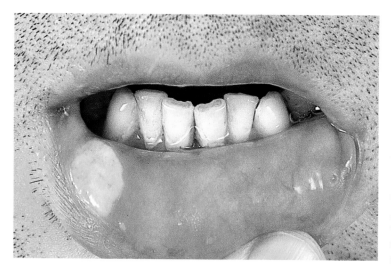

Fig. 12-15 Behçet's syndrome. As partial manifestations were several oral aphthae, among them these painful giant aphthae on the lip mucosa. There were also aphthous ulcerations on the scrotum and the inner upper thighs. Diagnosis was made with a dermatologist.

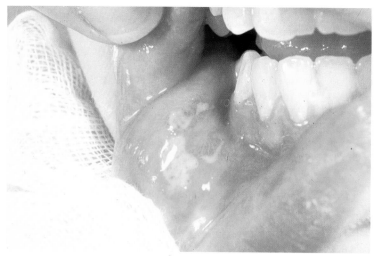

Fig. 12-16 Partial oral manifestation of chronic recurrent aphthosis (Touraine aphthosis), a recurrent aphthous ulceration on the lip mucosa. Developing aphthae can be seen in the marginal area of a regressing aphthous ulcer.

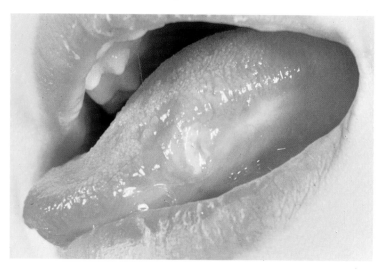

Fig. 12-17 Tongue findings in the patient seen in Fig. 12-16. Aphthous lesion on the lateral zone of the tongue with whitish, fibrinoid-covered ulcerations. The oral mucosal manifestations were preceded by gastrointestinal episodes (subileus). Vascular damage of probable autoimmune origin can be demonstrated histologically in all affected organs. Depending on the affected organ, it leads to typical localized symptoms.

Chapter 13

Clinical Aspects of Cysts of the Oral Cavity

Cysts of the jaw

Soft tissue cysts
  Mucoceles
    Mucocele of minor salivary glands
    Mucocele of the sublingual gland
  Dermoid cysts

Although they have varying etiologies, all true epithelial jaw cysts (as opposed to the rarer jaw pseudocysts) have similar pathognomonic signs: a thin or thick liquid content filling a cavity delimited by a wall of connective tissue lined by epithelium, and a specific growth pattern (slow expansion because of continuously or intermittently increasing inner pressure). The granular epithelial cells do not proliferate in an autonomous-neoplastic manner but multiply only to compensate for the increasing size of the cyst. Only the squamous cells show a deviant growth pattern.

By their nature, cysts have a different biologic behavior than that of hyperplasias and true growth. They are benign lesions; but superimposed malignant changes may sometimes occur in the cyst epithelium.

The clinical picture of the lesions of oral soft tissues is the main focus of this chapter. Development of cysts located in the jawbone is limited as exemplified in a few instances, in which these slow and painlessly growing structures overstep normal bone contour and visibly protrude into the oral cavity. A series of illustrations that outline the important findings for differential diagnosis is included for this purpose.

Cysts of the jaw

Cysts, which lie in inner bone, are often discovered by accident. The diagnosis rests on radiographic studies, eventually a biopsy, and on obligatory histologic examination after surgery.

If a large cyst leads to visible distention of the bone in the oral cavity, clinical findings can yield the first important indications for the tentative diagnosis. This is especially true if the cortical bone is very thin and can be deformed or disappears completely between the oral mucosa and the cyst so that the cyst is seen and felt under the mucous membrane like a firm ball (Figs. 13-1 to 13-4).

There are actually no suspicious changes to be looked for on inspection of the mucous membrane; rather, the location and shape of the lesion and, under some conditions, the changing color of its surface are important. The examples shown relate to odontogenic cysts and are limited to those most frequently encountered: radicular cysts (Fig. 13-1), eruption cysts (Fig. 13-2), and particular forms of follicular cysts.

Nonodontogenic cysts containing epithelial tissue exist independently of the tooth system as a result of embryonal jaw and facial development. They develop in the region of preexisting epithelial ridges and walls of the embryo's facial furrows and crevices from the remains of the epithelium.

The pathogenetic origin of these *dysontogenetic cysts* is not yet fully explained. These cysts include the rare midline mandibular cysts (Fig. 13-3), nasopalatine cysts, and incisive palatine cysts (Fig. 13-4). Differential diagnosis with other lesions of the same areas should be considered (Figs. 13-5 and 13.6).

Reference should be made to appropriate textbooks for further information about the systemic and clinical studies and therapy of the cysts in the jaw and facial regions.

Soft tissue cysts

Only those cysts of the soft tissues in the facial and throat region that have a close relation to the mucosa because of their submucosal location will be considered here. The lymphoepithelial system will not be considered.

These lesions, which are found in typical locations immediately accessible by inspection and palpation, must be differentiated from tumors.

Mucoceles

Mucoceles can be divided into *mucocele extravasation cysts* and *retention cysts* with regard to their mechanism of development and histomorphologic criteria. Their clinical picture is the same.

Secretion from the salivary glands can leak into the surrounding tissue and lead to a reactive inflammation with lymphoid infiltrate or to the formation of a cyst from rupture of the glands, particularly as a result of traumatic events on the excretory duct and the gland parenchyma. The extravasion cysts formed in this manner do not have any epithelial lining but are lined only by a flattened endothelial-type layer. They are the most frequent form of mucoceles of the oral mucosa.

Pure retention cysts are rare. They develop from a secretory obstruction in the excretory duct of the gland with subsequent dilation. It is thought today that the cause of the cysts is not so much complete obstruction but more an intermittent and partial closure of the duct. Retention cysts always contain real epithelium.

Mucocele of minor salivary glands (ICD-DA 527.61 [527.60])

In principle, the mucocele can occur in every location ot the mucous salivary glands and of the oral mucosa. By far the most frequent location for these cysts is the lower lip due to extravasation of glandular secretion in the periacinal tissue (particularly the vermilion of the lip border), which is subjected to a certain amount of microtrauma. On occasion the cysts are also found in the region of the upper lip, cheeks, and floor of the mouth.

The usually well-circumscribed, painless, soft, sometimes fluctuating lesions protrude through the thin mucous membrane cover in a semispherical manner and are light blue and translucent (Figs. 13-7 to 13-9). Most mucoceles do not grow larger than a pea. However, much larger mucous cysts are not unusual on the lower lip (Figs. 13-8 and 13-11). Differential diagnosis in relation to infectious swelling and especially tumors (Figs. 13-13 to 13-15) in general is not problematic.

Because of chronic mechanical irritations (parafunctional activity), a reactive hyperkeratosis of the covering mucous membrane epithelium can appear (Fig. 13-10). Home remedies of puncturing, biting, or application of caustic materials can lead to recurrence with scar formation or even to prolapse of portions of the gland (Figs. 13-11 and 13-12).

The tender wall of the cyst can burst as the result of minimal trauma, as for example, during eating. After the mucus-like content flows out, the border of the cyst is no longer clearly visible. Complete extirpation of the mucocele, the only manner in which recurrence can be prevented, is best accomplished with a filled cyst. It requires a subtle preparation technique because of the easily damaged cyst wall.

Mucocele of the sublingual gland (ICD-DA 527.61 [527.60])

These cysts, which are located in relation to the excretory system of the sublingual salivary gland are like a large copy of a mucocele. The cyst is filled with mucous saliva and on histologic examination is usually an extravasation cyst. Mucoceles of the sublingual gland lie, as a rule, paramedian and above the mylohyoid muscle in the frontal region of the sublingual plica, where they protrude from the mucous membrane of the floor of the mouth in a hemispherical manner (Fig. 13-16). Location on the inferior surface of the tongue is also possible (Fig. 13-17). Characteristic is its tight, fluctuating consistency and most often its blue translucent appearance. Because of its similarity in appearance with the blown-up guttural bubble of a frog, the purely descriptive term "ranula" (little frog) has been introduced for this superficial cyst.

In some instances, the mucocele can extend over the median plane to the other side so that the tongue is displaced and the frenum of the tongue impinges into the anterior wall of the mucocele, giving the impression of bilateral symmetrical cysts (Fig. 13-18). Displacement of the tongue can cause difficulty in swallowing.

The ranula generally develops after puberty but can occur in early childhood.

Sublingual infiltrate and abscesses, as well as swellings of the excretory duct of the submandibular gland following stone occlusion, should not be ruled out in differential diagnosis. Because of the often clear clinical findings, differentiation from dermoid cysts, lymphangioma, and pleomorphic adenoma is generally not a problem.

Therapeutically, only complete removal of the cyst leads to a lasting cure. Other procedures, such as marsupialization (wide exteriorization of the cyst cavity by wide fenestration with scarring of the overlying mucous membrane), are burdened with a high rate of recurrence and are therefore not suggested. Operative intervention must take into consideration the topographic relationship of the submandibular gland and lingual nerve to the excretory duct and the fact that the cyst wall is thin. The resulting technical difficulties must not be underestimated.

Dermoid cysts (ICD-DA 528.41)

Dermoid cysts develop from epithelial inclusions caused by disturban-ces in the region of the facial process of branchial arches during the complicated developmental process. Only rarely do they result from a traumatically limited lodging of the epithelium in the deep layers of tissue.

The lining of the dermoid cyst wall, which develops from the horny, squamous epithelium, contains, compared to the *epithelial inclusion cyst,* integumentary appendages (i.e., hair follicles, sebaceous and sweat glands). Because of this, the cyst lumen is often filled with foul-smelling sebaceous remnants and frequently with hair. Cysts that also show tissue of mesenchymal origin, such as bone and teeth, are called *teratomas.*

The origin explains the relative frequency of dermoid and epithelial inclusion cysts in the facial and throat regions. The preferred intraoral site is the floor of the mouth where the dermoid cysts lie either sublingually (above the mylohyoid muscle) or submentally (below the mylohyoid muscle). Dumbbell-shaped combination forms that pene-trate the muscle are possible.

The painless, progressively enlarging structure, which is sur-rounded by a thick layer of connective tissue, frequently occurs between 15 and 25 years of age but not later. The cysts exhibit a firm or doughy consistency. They reach a considerable size and can, with sublingual localization, push the tongue up to the palate and pharynx so that eating and speech are hindered (Figs. 13-19 and 13-20). For differential diagnostic purposes, there is no obvious change in color of the mucous membrane. The different consistency on palpation con-trasts with that of mucoceles of the sublingual gland. Therapy consists of complete surgical removal of the cysts.

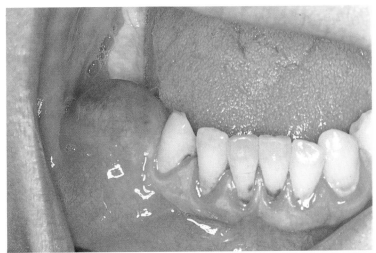

Fig. 13-1 Residual radicular cyst that protrudes into the oral cavity, left in the jaw after removal of tooth 47 (31). The bone between the mucous membrane and the cyst has already resorbed. The cyst lies under the mucous membrane like a firm ball.

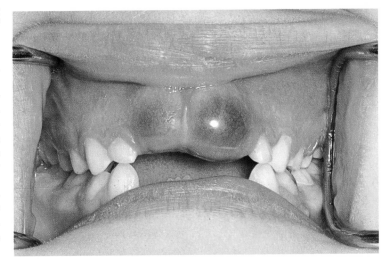

Fig. 13-2 Bluish, translucent eruption cysts in the region of teeth 21 and 11 (8 and 9) in an 8-year-old boy with delayed dentition. The eruption cyst is a cystically transformed dental follicle and therefore corresponds pathogenetically to follicular cysts. They are predominantly observed in primary teeth and more frequently in the canine region than in the incisor region. They are, as a rule, transitory findings in the pre-eruptive phase and disappear with tooth eruption. Only in unusual cases is surgical intervention necessary.

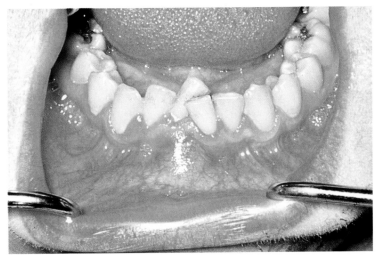

Fig. 13-3 A median mandibular cyst, which is unrelated to the tooth system, in a 24-year-old patient. Pressure from this very rare cyst lead to the displacement of the roots of the vital mandibular incisors (compensatory convergence of the crowns). Also, in the case of unsuspected clinical and radiographic cyst findings, verification of the clinical diagnosis by pathohistologic examination of the surgical specimen is necessary.

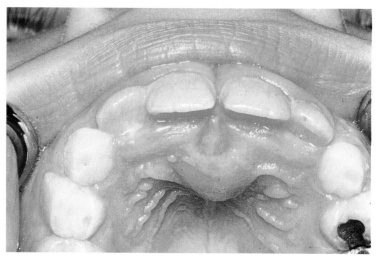

Fig. 13-4   A nasopalatine cyst in the region of the incisive papilla. It appears clinically as a firm median protrusion on the mucous membrane of the palate outside the bony structure. The duct cysts of the incisal canal, because of persisting epithelium of the embryonic nasopalatal space, are usually located further inside the incisive canal. Depending on location (toward the nose or toward the oral cavity), they are covered with respiratory or squamous epithelium.

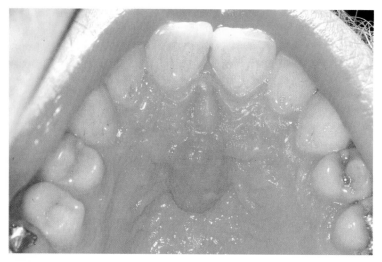

Fig. 13-5   Differential diagnosis of cysts in the region of the incisal papilla: large flat fibroma on the middle of the palate that is clearly set apart from the incisal papilla. Dysontogenetic cysts of this location (medial palatal cysts) are extremly rare findings.

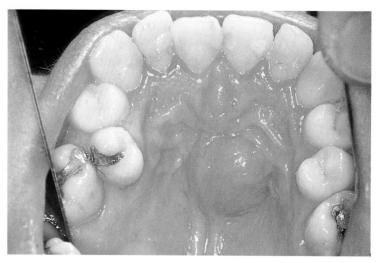

Fig. 13-6   Differential diagnosis of cysts in region of incisal papilla. Pleomorphic adenoma on the hard palate. This frequent tumor of the salivary glands, especially of the parotid gland, also occurs in minor salivary glands of the oral mucosa. In such cases, the most common position is the posterior portion of the hard palate, i.e., the transitional region of the hard palate and the soft palate (see chapter 20).

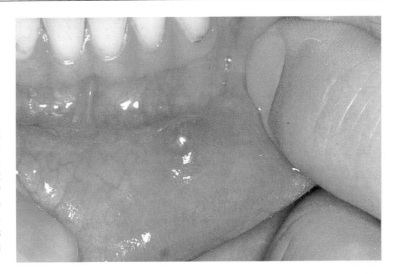

Fig. 13-7   Early clinically visible stage of a mucocele on the mucosa of the lower lip. As a rule, these are extravasation cysts. The preferred location on the lower lip is due to the fact that this region is affected by microtrauma. This may damage the excretory duct of small mixed mucous and serous glands with a discharge of secretion into the surrounding tissue.

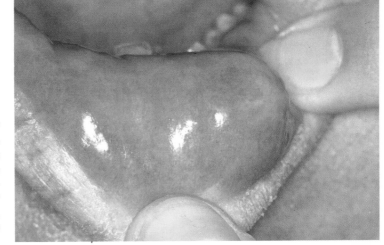

Fig. 13-8   Large mucocele of the lower lip. The painless, fluctuating mucous cyst gleams as a pale blue transparent mass through the thin mucous membrane. The faint scars already indicate multiple perforations, which were confirmed by the patient history.

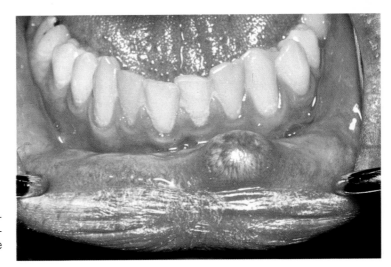

Fig. 13-9   Well-defined, hemispherical blue translucent mucocele of long duration in the lower lip.

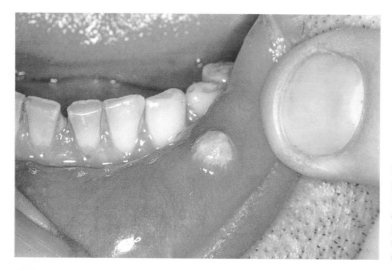

Fig. 13-10   Mucocele on the lower lip. The mucous membrane appearance indicates reactive hyperkeratosis in the protruding region because of mechanical-irritative influences (parafunctional activity).

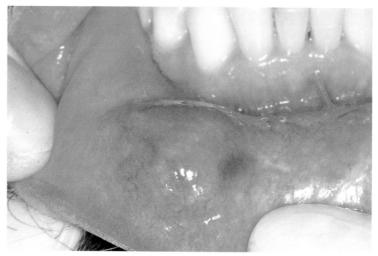

Fig. 13-11   Recurrence of mucocele on the lower lip. The treatment aim is complete extirpation of the intact cyst. If the lumen of the mucous cyst is opened accidentally, the extension of the mucocele can no longer be clearly established. In this case, surgery should be postponed until the cyst has filled again. Compromises in early surgery increase the likelihood of recurrence.

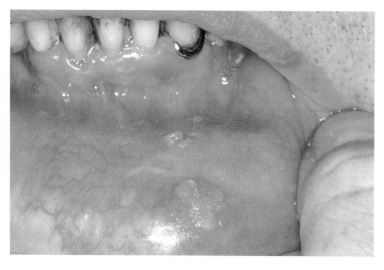

Fig. 13-12   The condition after repeated attempts of self-treatment by the puncturing and biting of a mucocele on the lower lip. These traumatic influences resulted in scar formation and prolapse of glandular parts of several small mucoserous salivary glands and persistent recurrences. The findings should not be confused with local epithelial hyperplasia (Heck's disease; see chapter 11).

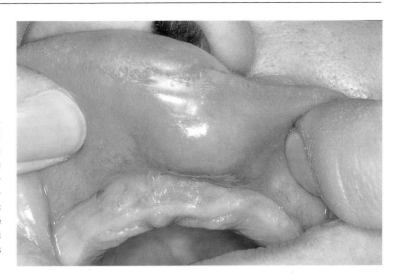

Fig. 13-13   Differential diagnosis of mucocele: localized
odontogenic abscess, starting
from the remaining root of tooth
21 (9). History in addition to clinical findings allow definite differentiation between pyogenic
infections and mucocele. The
clinical picture of pleomorphic
adenoma of the upper lip is
shown in Fig. 20-1.

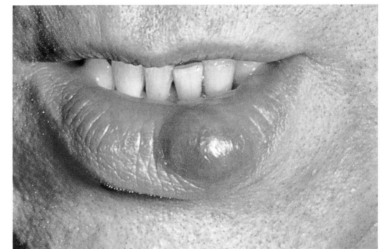

Fig. 13-14   Differential diagnosis of mucocele: heman-
gioma of the lower lip, which is
well delimited from its surroundings and is as large as a hazel-
nut. The patient noticed a slow
enlargement of the nonmalig-
nant growth over 10 years.

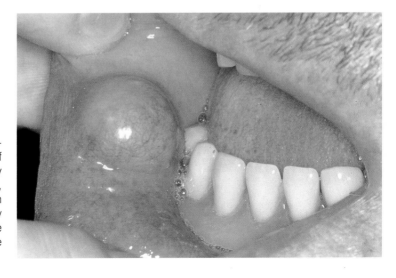

Fig. 13-15   Differential diagnosis of mucocele: lipoma of
lower lip. These benign, fatty
tumors, if superficially located,
can protrude into the mucosa in
a hemispherical manner. They
are soft and are not fixed to the
mucous membranes or to the
underlying tissue.

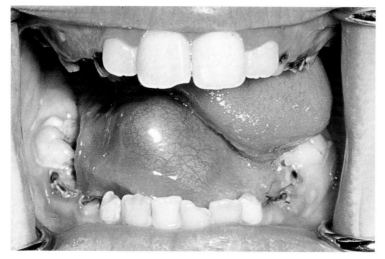

Fig. 13-16 Mucocele (ranula) of the floor of the mouth in a 9-year-old girl. Most often it is an extravasation cyst that is located close to the excretory duct system of the sublingual gland. Apart from the typical location (paramedian, above the mylohyoid muscle in the region of the sublingual fold), characteristic of this lesion are the tense, fluctuating consistency and the translucent blue color.

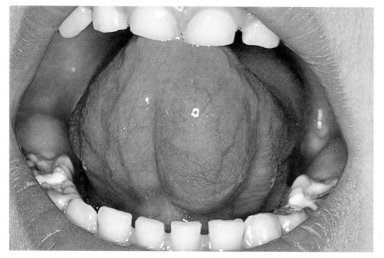

Fig. 13-17 Larger sublingual mucocele of firm, fluctuating consistency in a 6-year-old girl. Complete extirpation of the cyst, which is needed for definitive cure, requires sufficient surgical experience because of the thin wall of the cyst.

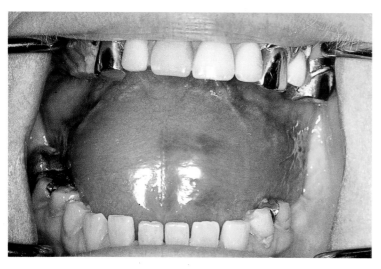

Fig. 13-18 Unusually large mucocele of the floor of the mouth that has grown over the median plane to the opposite side. The tongue is forced upward and dorsally. The patient finally sought medical attention because of difficulty in swallowing. Note the indentation in the cyst contour caused by the stretched frenum of the tongue. Palpation did not suggest a dermoid cyst, which must be ruled out in the differential diagnosis of this case. Surgical treatment must take into consideration the close topographic relationship of the cyst to the excretory duct of the submandibular gland and lingual nerve, among other factors.

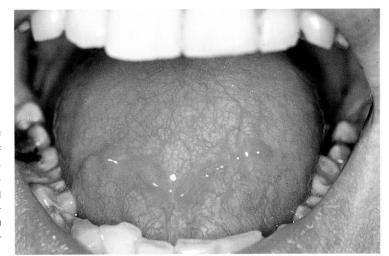

Fig. 13-19   Dermoid cyst of goose-egg size in the floor of the mouth. The 25-year-old unmotivated patient sought medical treatment only when eating and speaking became impaired because the tongue, which is not visible here, was displaced to the palate and pharynx.

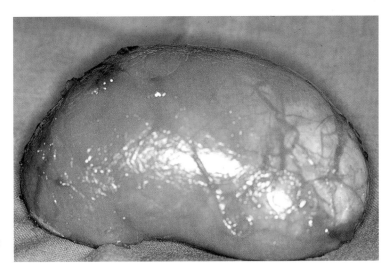

Fig. 13-20   Surgical specimen of dermoid cyst of Fig. 13-19.

Chapter 14

Different Forms of Epulis

Epulis granulomatosa

Epulis fibromatosa

Peripheral giant cell granuloma

Epulides with clinical features suggestive of neoplasms

Congenital epulis; congenital granular cell tumor

The term "epulis" means only a tissue formation located on the gingiva. Although this term is only topographic and therefore unsatisfactory, its use was decided on, after some consideration, for didactic purposes.

Epulides are circumscribed peripheral granulation masses of tissue on the gingiva or alveolar process. Corresponding to the respective predominant histologic pictures, they are classified according to histomorphologic criteria with explanatory adjectives.

With the exception of congenital epulis, which cannot be classified in this group because of nosologic considerations, we are concerned in the epulis group not with tumors capable of automatous growth, but with space-occupying lesions of *reactive (resorptive) inflammatory nature*. However, there is the tendency, particularly of the giant cell epulis, to recur, resulting in regional tissue destruction that can also involve bone (bone erosion).

The causal factors in the development of an epulis are local inflammation and mechanical irritation and a not clearly explained predispositon to abnormal tissue response. The opinion that the various epulis types are pathogenetically different from one another is still accepted. It has long been assumed that the different types of epulides were expressions of a uniform disease that could have varying differentiations and maturation levels. Some consider the different types of epulides as different and unrelated diseases and therefore advocate strict distinctions.

Apart from epulis granulomatosa, epulis fibromatosa, and giant cell epulis, some epulides show a clinical picture suggestive of neoplasm. It is difficult to separate these forms into a special group exclusively on the basis of clinical behavior, but the responsible dentist should keep in mind the possibility of epulides with more aggressive behavior.

Epulis granulomatosa (ICD-DA 210.43)

Epulis granulomatosa (Figs. 14-1 to 14-3) is a mass of inflammatory reactive granulation tissue, reddish to gray-purple, covered by epithelium. The lesion may have a broad, sometimes fungiform stalk extending from the alveolar process, or it may be dumbbell-shaped between two teeth. It has a soft, spongy consistency and bleeds easily after minor injury. The cause of the epulis granulomatosa is considered to be chronic local irritations of the gingiva (root remnants, sharp tooth corners, overhanging restorations and crowns, other traumatic irritations from abnormal dentition, or poorly placed prostheses).

Histologically one finds a nonspecific granulation tissue, rich in blood vessels. Some investigators consider this epulis a granulomatous form and a precursor to fibrous epulis.

The epulis that develops during pregnancy, epulis gravidarium, is usually an epulis granulomatosa. More discussion on changes of the gingiva under the influence of sex hormones will be presented in chapter 27.

We do not agree that epulis granulomatosa is identical to the pyogenic granuloma, as some have postulated. In our experience, a pyogenic granuloma is usually found in the region of the lips and tongue, seldom in other parts of the oral cavity, and has an ulcerated fibrin-covered surface, as opposed to the epulis granulomatosa (see chapter 21). Even in exceptional cases with other clinical similarities, the term "epulis" should be retained for lesions in the gingivoperiodontal area.

Epulis fibromatosa (ICD-DA 210.43)

Epulis fibromatosa (Figs. 14-4 to 14-6) is usually an inflammatory hyperplastic growth of hemispheric appearance with a broad base, sometimes with a stalk connected to the periodontal tissue. The center of the epulis is made up histologically of hypocellular, dense connective tissue composed of woven collagen fibers and with a relatively uniform histologic appearance. The structure, as compared to epulis granulomatosa, is more solid and hard, and it is pale to slightly red in color. The final stage can correspond clinically and histologically to that of a fibroma (Fig. 14-9), which, however, is very rare in this location. The epulis fibromatosa usually has no connection with the cortical bone of the alveolar process. As with the giant cell epulis, new bone formation may occasionally be seen in the core of the lesion (Figs. 14-7 and 14-8).

Epulis fibromatosa develops primarily as a reaction to the already mentioned irritation factors. It is considered by some as the maturation, healing stage of an epulis granulomatosa or a giant cell epulis. Histologically, transitional forms have been described. Pathogenetically, epulides and irritation fibromas are probably related (see chapters 22 and 33).

Peripheral giant cell granuloma (ICD-DA 523.83)

The epulis most frequently seen (better named peripheral giant cell granuloma) is also a hyperplastic reaction of connective tissue. The growth has characteristics of a chronic inflammatory lesion stimulated by irritation and with overgrowth of granulation tissue (reaction, resorptive granuloma). It also resembles a true benign tumor because of its relatively aggressive behavior (erosion of the limiting bone tissue, recurrence with incomplete removal).

The giant cell granuloma derived from gingivoperiodontal tissue (area of the interdental papillae) or from mucoperiosteal tissue shows a different clinical picture (Figs. 14-10 to 14-12). The consistency can be soft or hard, the surface tends to bleed, and it is smooth, spotty, or bumpy; the color has a reddish hue (that is, blue-red or rust brown).

The giant cell epulis is seen in childhood and young adults and more often in boys than girls. It mostly affects adults from the second to fourth decade, with more women afflicted than men. The preferential location is the vestibular region of the alveolar process of both jaws. Peripheral giant cell granuloma can also be present in edentulous areas of the alveolar process (Figs. 14-18 to 14-21). It is almost always possible to identify local irritative factors, such as chronic traumatic tissue damage or signs of smoldering chronic inflammation. In only a few cases is there no obvious clinical cause.

Peripheral giant cell granuloma frequently leads, as do other epulides, to resorptive damage of the adjacent bone, which can be seen on radiographs as an area of bone destruction under the base of the epulis or the disappearance of the interdental septum. This can cause mobility of the affected teeth.

The histologic picture involves typical characteristics of the giant cells (hence the name of the epulis): fibroblast proliferation, spindle cells, and macrophages loaded with hemosiderin.

Central giant cell granuloma is the intraosseous equivalent of peripheral giant cell granuloma. These forms can be distinguished from each other only by their location. The central giant cell granuloma must be differentiated from the giant cell tumor of bone (osteoclastoma), which occurs seldom if ever in the jaws. The differentiation is very difficult even from the histologic viewpoint and requires an experienced pathologist. Because epulides grow into the oral cavity, they can be easily injured during normal mastication. Consequently, there can be evidence of recent or old bleeding (Figs. 14-15 and 14-16), erosions and ulcerations (Figs. 14-1, 14-2, 14-4, 14-10, 14-12, 14-16 to 14-18), and leukoplakial changes (reactive hyperkeratoses), which make diagnosis more difficult.

Epulides with clinical features suggestive of neoplasms

Lesions arising from edentulous areas of the jaw must always be considered with great suspicion because clinically they cannot always be diffentiated from malignant neoplasia or metastasis (Figs. 14-17 to 14-21). The same is true clinically for some atypical epulides on the dentate alveolar process (Figs. 14-13 to 14-16). In all of these questionable cases the dentist should refer the patient for consultation.

Congenital epulis (ICD-DA 210.43); congenital granular cell tumor (ICD-M 9580/0)

The so-called congenital epulis has nothing to do with the forms of epulis described above with the exception of the location on the alveolar ridge. It is therefore discussed in this chapter only because of location.

Histologically, it is a variant granular cell tumor, which appears, however, exclusively in newborns (usually girls) and with typical location on the anterior alveolar ridge of the maxilla, and seldom on the mandible (congenital granular cell tumor).

Clinically the impressive growth consists of roundish to oval, sometimes multiple nodules, maximally 1 to 2 cm in diameter, that as a rule have a broad base growing from underlying tissue. The mucosal covering is intact (Figs. 14-22 and 14-23).

So far there is no agreement on histogenesis or formal classification of the granular cell tumors. The most accepted theory is that it is true tumor and not the final stage of a primary inflammatory-degenerative process. Based on new information, it is possible to discard the original idea of Abrikossoff that rhabdomyoblasts form the tumor matrix (therefore also the name myoblastoma). Currently the tumor is causally associated with Schwann's cells of peripheral nerves. The congenital granular tumor does not usually continue to grow after birth. Complete spontaneous regression within a month has often been reported, which we can confirm with one of our cases (Figs. 14-24 and 14-25). If the tumor persists, it should be removed. Recurrences and further involvement of the affected jaw are not to be expected. Disturbances of dental eruption are possible (Fig. 14-26).

Clinical therapy of clear-cut epulis cases

Epulides must be removed very carefully because of extension into healthy tissue. This requires operative revision of the underlying bone and—with considerable periodontal damage—removal of teeth involved in the lesion. Intact, well-preserved teeth can remain after elimination of the irritating factor.

In the case of a recurrence of the epulis, extraction is, however, necessary. Epulis fibromatosa, by experience, is the easiest to remove from bone. With the help of radiographs, surgical removal of an adequate rim of the involved bone is compulsory, because recurrences are otherwise unavoidable, particularly in giant cell epulis. Care of the wound is successfully performed using periodontal therapy. To confirm the clinical diagnosis of epulis, histologic examination of the surgical specimen is essential.

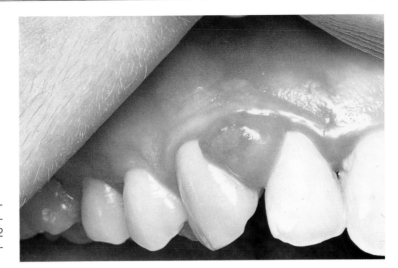

Fig. 14-1 Epulis granuloma-tosa with ulcerated surface, located between teeth 13 and 12 (6 and 7) in a 27-year-old woman.

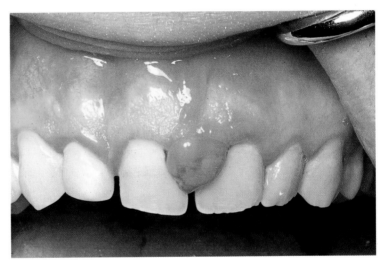

Fig. 14-2 Epulis granuloma-tosa between teeth 11 and 21 (8 and 9) in a 22-year-old man. Local cause: traumatic irritation resulting from malocclusion with excessive vertical overlap.

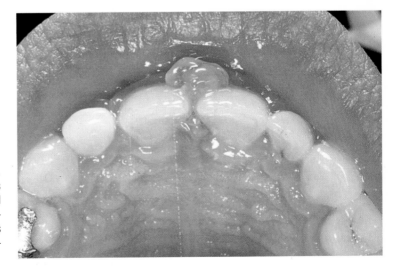

Fig. 14-3 The patient in Fig. 14-2. The relation of the epulis (pedunculated on the palatal side and growing toward the labial side) to the periodontium is clearly shown in this mirror photograph.

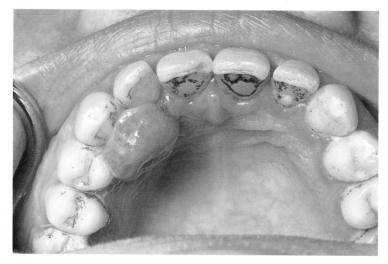

Fig. 14-4   Mushroomlike palatal, elevated epulis fibromatosa between teeth 13 and 12 (6 and 7) in a 35-year-old patient with traumatic occlusion.

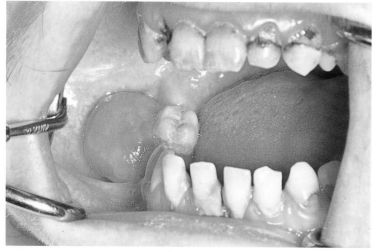

Fig.   14-5   Hemispherical growth on the alveolar process in the area of tooth 47 (31). The epulis fibromatosa with a broad base has been present for several years in this 51-year-old woman. Note the neglected dentition (smooth surface caries, marginal periodontitis with massive calculus formation and subgingival concretions).

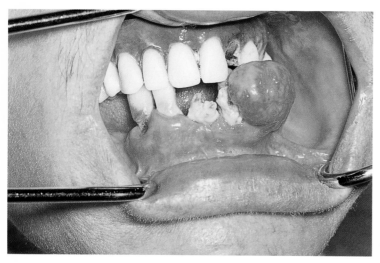

Fig. 14-6   Spherical pedunculated epulis fibromatosa situated on the alveolar process in the area of teeth 32 and 33 (21 and 22). Note the neglected dentition in the mandible. The 56-year-old woman had worn a defective rubber-based, complete maxillary denture for 18 years.

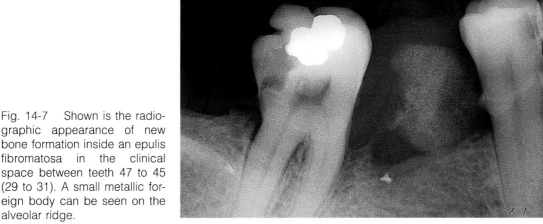

Fig. 14-7 Shown is the radiographic appearance of new bone formation inside an epulis fibromatosa in the clinical space between teeth 47 to 45 (29 to 31). A small metallic foreign body can be seen on the alveolar ridge.

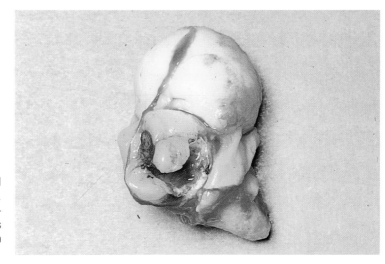

Fig. 14-8 Surgically removed specimen from patient in Fig. 14-7. It reveals the sessile connection of the spherical epulis with the periodontium of tooth 47 (31).

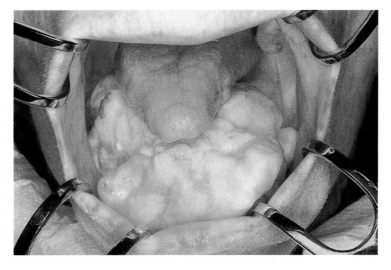

Fig. 14-9 Final condition of epulis fibromatosa—at this stage essentially a fibroma—present in the 71-year-old woman for the past 25 years but left untreated. The firm pale tumor, displacing the tongue dorsally, has a peduncular connection with the alveolar process in the area of the anterior teeth.

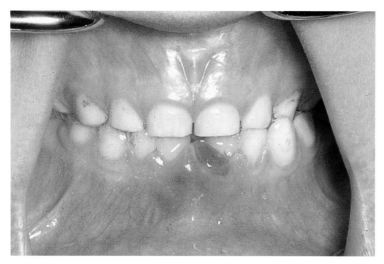

Fig. 14-10 Giant cell epulis with partial surface ulceration that led to bone resorption in the area of the interdental septum between teeth 81 and 71 (O to P), demonstrated radiographically in a 6-year-old boy.

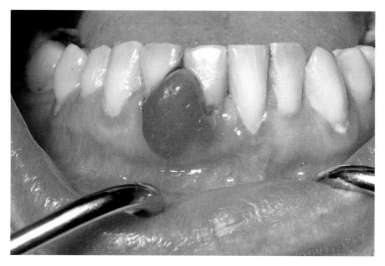

Fig. 14-11 Pea-sized, sessile giant cell granuloma of firm consistency in the area of teeth 42 and 41 (25 and 26) in a 34-year-old patient.

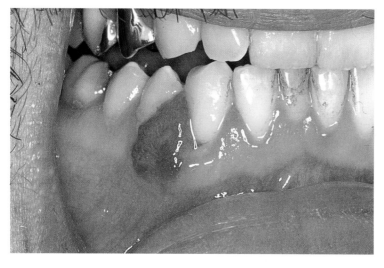

Fig. 14-12 Vestibular, broad-based peripheral giant cell granuloma in the area of teeth 44 and 43 (27 and 28) with ulcerated surface and tendency to bleed. The 35-year-old patient observed the size increase for 4 months.

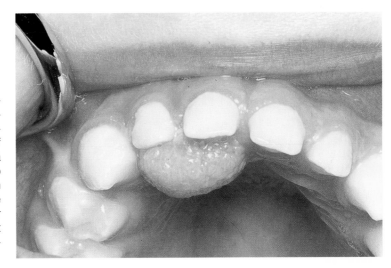

Fig. 14-13 Tumorlike condition with a finely nodulated surface and a firm consistency arising from the palatal area of teeth 52 and 51 (D and E) in a 5-year-old boy. According to his parents, this proliferation developed within a short time and was clinically suspect for that reason. Histologically it was found to be an epulis fibromatosa.

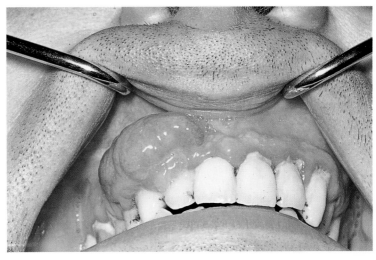

Fig. 14-14 According to this 31-year-old man, the spongy, painless, clinically atypical epulis on the right side of the maxilla developed within a few weeks. Examination of a biopsy specimen failed to confirm the suspected neoplasm with overlying inflammation but revealed the presence of an epulis fibrogranulomatosa.

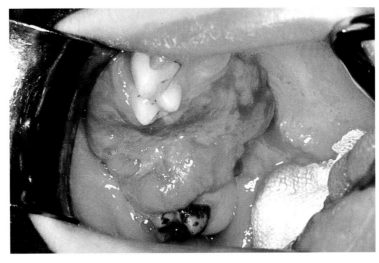

Fig. 14-15 Unusually voluminous epulis fibromatosa on the right maxilla in a 28-year-old woman. The firm mass with an ulcerated surface appeared clinically suspect and histologically was shown to be a fairly well-delimited epulis fibromatosa.

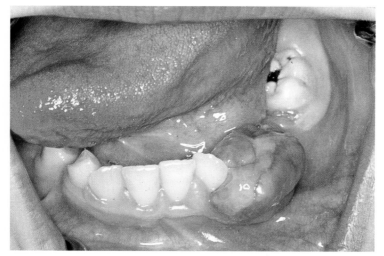

Fig. 14-16   Recurrence of a peripheral giant cell granuloma after incomplete enucleation in a 23-year-old woman in the areas of teeth 32, 33, and 34. The light-brown color is caused by the richness in blood vessels with remote episodes of bleeding. The surface is traumatized because of the occlusion. The bony alveolar process is eroded.

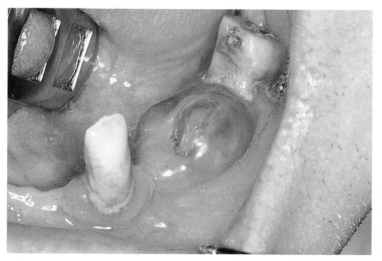

Fig. 14-17   This broad-based tumor growing on an edentulous alveolar process on the left mandible is a suspicious change in this 62-year-old patient. The extractions in the affected area took place 2 years earlier. In the last 3 months, the patient observed an increase in the size of the mass, which moved the molar distally. Histologic examination demonstrated peripheral giant cell granuloma.

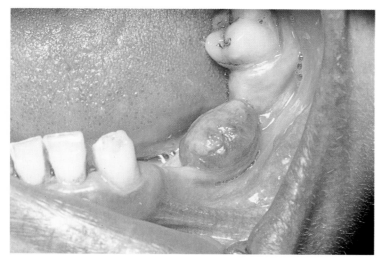

Fig. 14-18   Histologically confirmed, sessile giant cell epulis with ulcerated surface, localized on the edentulous alveolar ridge in a 50-year-old woman. Differential diagnosis should take into consideration a malignant neoplasm and especially metastasis, which often have similar clincial features.

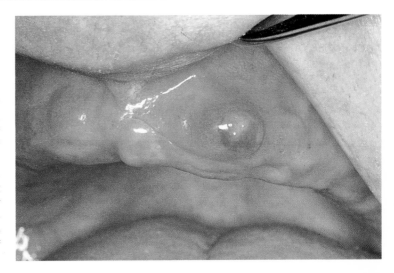

Fig. 14-19 Development of a new ulceration on the alveolar process of an edentulous maxilla in the vestibular region of tooth 23. The change took place 4 months after removal of a mobile tooth and change of the prosthesis to a complete denture. Histologically, it was found to be a peripheral giant cell granuloma. It was originally caused by irritation of the periodontal tissue, which in the meantime led to the loss of tooth 23 (11).

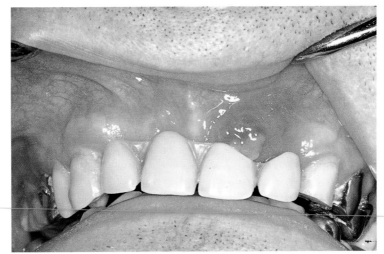

Fig. 14-20 Nodular change with ulcerated surface of the mucosa under a sharp border prosthesis of tooth 21 (9), which affected the alveolar process. Histologically, it was possible to diagnose a giant cell granuloma.

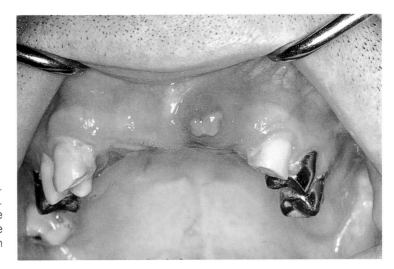

Fig. 14-21 The patient in Fig. 14-20 without the prosthesis. The finding is limited to the area of tooth 21 (9). A definite bone erosion was noticed on the radiograph.

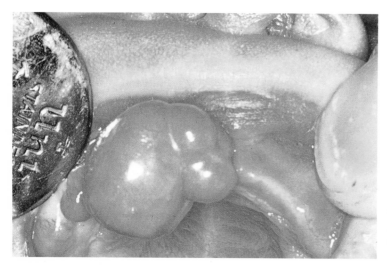

Fig. 14-22   Clinical finding interpreted as congenital epulis in a 3-day-old girl. The sessile, bulbous tumor of soft consistency, situated on the anterior alveolar ridge of the right side of the maxilla, was present at birth.

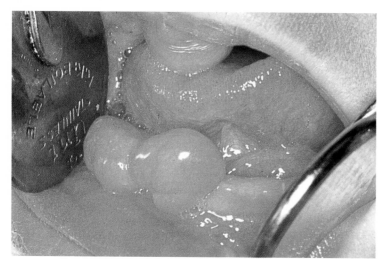

Fig. 14-23   The child in Fig. 14-22 at the time of examination. Two pea-sized tissue growths are also present on the alveolar ridge of the right side of the mandible. The so-called congenital epulis is usually solitary; however, occasionally several epulides can be present.

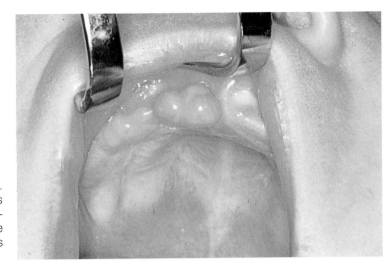

Fig. 14-24 The child in Figs. 14-22 and 14-23 three months after birth. Marked spontaneous regression is seen on the maxilla. Infant development is normal according to age.

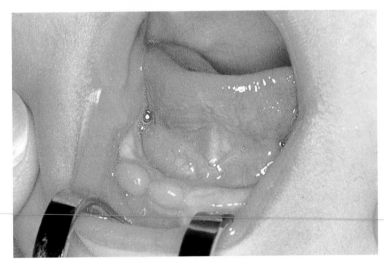

Fig. 14-25 The patient in the previous figures 3 months after birth. The nodules on the mandibular alveolar ridge have regressed markedly and spontaneously.

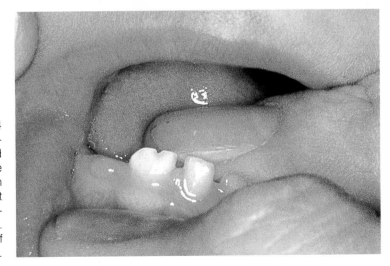

Fig. 14-26 The patient 14 months after birth. Only a lentil-sized protuberance remained of the "congenital epulis" on the maxilla. An abnormal tooth with bifid crown has appeared at the former site of the mesial nodule in the mandibular region. A rice grain-sized remnant of the distal nodule is still present.

Chapter 15

Gingival Fibromatosis

Gingival fibromatosis (ICD-DA 523.80)

Gingival fibromatosis often leads to strong, protruding, firm to hard, pale tissue overgrowths that affect the whole gingiva or a part of it. No satisfactory cause is known for this fibromatous growth, which histologically consists of an extensive deposit of collagen fibers in hypocellular tissue.

The generalized participation of the gingiva points to the involvement of an incompletely understood disturbance of the control of collagen formation. This is also the case for special forms of the proliferative change in relation to molars and tuberosity with bilateral, equal, and even symmetric localization.

The primary increase of fibrous tissue in the absence of obvious inflammation is considered by many investigators to be a hyperplastic overgrowth and not a true benign tumor. Differentiation of a fibrous hyperplasia from a fibroma is difficult and not always definitively possible in oral pathology (see chapter 22). The etiology of gingival fibromatosis continues to be unknown. There have been repeated attempts to find an underlying genetic predisposition.

The entire gingiva is thickened, hard, and protruding (Figs. 15-1 to 15-6). A tendency to bleed on touch or probing is usually not present. Oral hygiene is affected by the pseudopockets. Particularly in case of neglected oral care, the lesion can exhibit secondary inflammatory changes (Figs. 15-7 and 15-8). Inside the bulging, hard, fibrous growths only the occlusal surface of the crowns of the posterior teeth are seen. They can also be completely covered.

The fibromatous gingival changes are often present in the primary dentition. During puberty, they tend to grow more extensively and then, after jaw growth is completed, to come to a standstill. In the mixed dentition, there are often gaps in the dentition and eruption disturbances probably determined by the gingival abnormalities. Cases associated with excess hair (hypertrichosis) and/or condensation of the facial soft parts have been repeatedly reported. An underlying endocrinologic functional disturbance has not yet been convincingly proven.

Aside from its differential diagnosis with gingival hyperplasia of puberty (see chapter 27), iatrogenic fibrous gingival hyperplasia must primarily be considered (see chapter 31), because it presents similar clinical findings (Fig. 15-9). Therefore, there should always be a question concerning medications as a part of the medical history.

Obviously there are special forms of gingival fibromatosis such as the *so-called symmetric peripheral jaw fibromas.* In the maxilla, these usually start on the palatal side of the first molars and develop dorsally and toward the palate (Figs. 15-10, 15-11, and 15-13). In the mandible is a corresponding distolingual extension tendency (Fig. 15-12). Other information on symmetric and asymmetric peripheral jaw fibromas is given in chapter 22. There is no preventive therapy for gingival fibromatosis. To ensure undisturbed tooth eruption or in initiation of orthodontic treatment, periodontal surgery is advisable, and appropriate oral hygiene is also assumed.

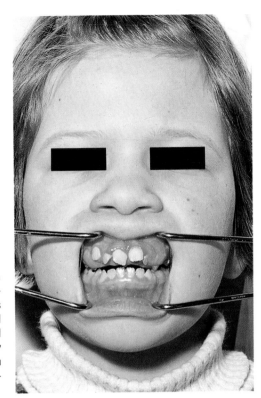

Fig. 15-1 Eleven-year-old girl with gingival fibromatosis without the associated symptoms such as thickening of the facial tissues, hypertrichosis, mental retardation, damage to sensory organs, and hypopigmentation usually described in the literature.

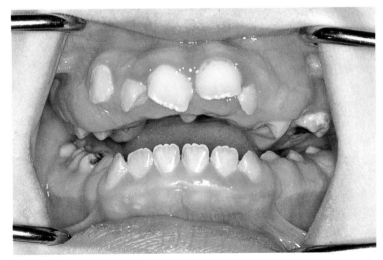

Fig. 15-2 Intraoral findings of the patient in Fig. 15-1 at the time of examination. Note the abnormal occlusal development caused by the increased fibromatous tissue (tooth displacement, eruption problems, open occlusal relationship).

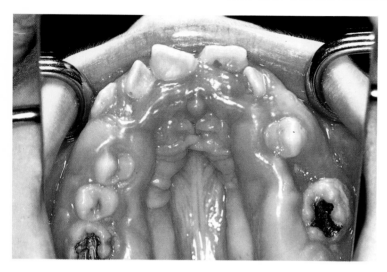

Fig. 15-3   The patient in Figs. 15-1 and 15-2 at the time of examination. Palatal appearance with arcade formation and fibromatous mucosal changes. In spite of the difficulty in maintaining oral hygiene, only few foci of inflammation are seen in the area of the pseudopockets.

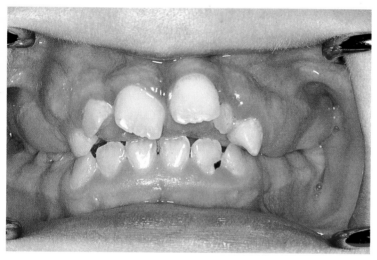

Fig. 15-4   The same patient 4 months later. The gingival fibromatosis changes have reached the occlusal surface and altered the occlusion. Periodontal surgery before initiation of orthodontic treatment is advisable. Motivation to excellent oral hygiene is important because of the possibility of recurrence.

Note

Puberty gingival hyperplasia
Main location is on the vestibular region of the maxillary anterior teeth, seldom on the mandible. The gingiva is usually normal posterior to the second premolars.

Medication-induced gingival fibromatosis
Findings similar to gingival fibromatosis. The gingiva of the anterior teeth is more often and more heavily affected. Positive medication history.

Gingival fibromatosis
Either the entire gingiva is affected or, as a special form, only the gingiva in the molar area is affected with typical palatal or lingual localization and predominantly symmetric distribution.

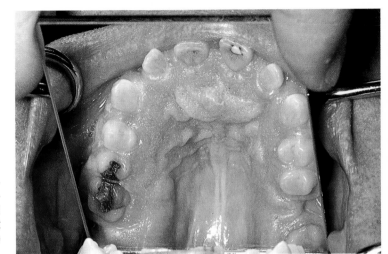

Fig. 15-5 Twenty-seven-year-old patient with gingival fibromatosis. There are pale, hard masses that have been present for 10 years according to the patient.

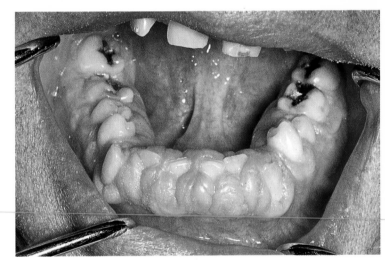

Fig. 15-6 The patient in Fig. 15-5 also at the time of examination. The hard fibromatosis without bleeding tendencies is clinically inflammation-free despite more difficult oral hygiene. It is particularly obvious in the area of the mandibular incisors. Diagnostically it must be differentiated from hydantoin gingival hyperplasia (medication history). Periodontal surgery is indicated.

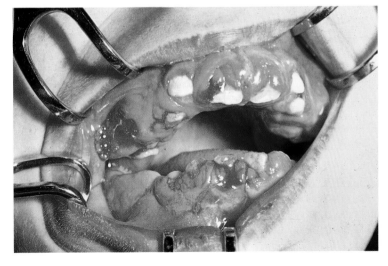

Fig. 15-7 Gingival fibromatosis in a 9-year-old child. The crowns of the teeth are almost completely overgrown by the large masses of fibromatous tissue, especially in the area of the posterior teeth. Modified clinical findings from secondary superimposed inflammations as consequence of poor oral hygiene.

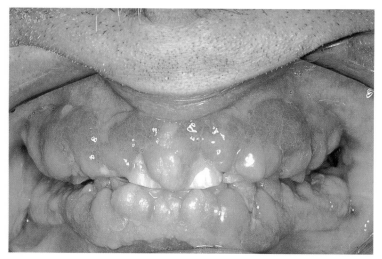

Fig. 15-8   Gingival fibromatosis, present for many years in a 35-year-old patient. Note the developing secondary inflammatory changes with the transition from the fibromatous changes of the gingiva to the movable mucosa. Systematic periodontal treatment with short recall periods is desirable.

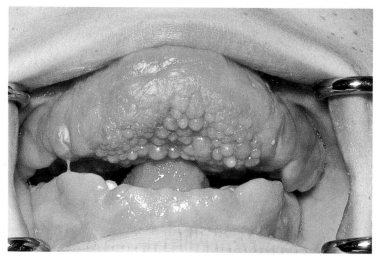

Fig. 15-9   Differential diagnosis of gingival fibromatosis: severe gingival hydantoin hyperplasia in a 14-year-old boy. The almost complete covering of the teeth by tissue masses allows only a selective occlusion. Therapy involves extensive periodontal surgery with short recall periods. A neurologist should be consulted about changes in the antiepileptic medication.

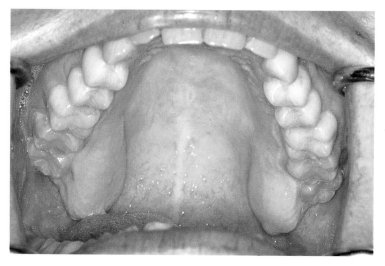

Fig. 15-10   Special form of gingival fibromatosis: so-called symmetric peripheral jaw fibroma in a 23-year-old patient. Note the tooth impressions of the antagonists predominantly in the molar region where there is localized, bilateral palatal tissue overgrowth.

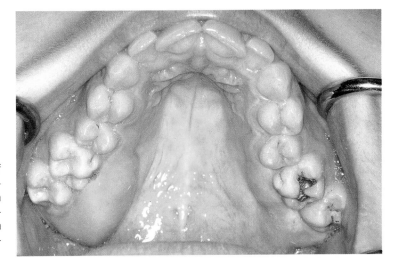

Fig. 15-11 Particular form of gingival fibromatosis in a 22-year-old patient. Particularly on the right maxilla there are extensive fibromatous changes in the molar area, again with typical palatal location.

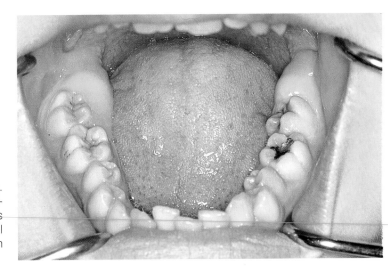

Fig. 15-12 The patient in Fig. 15-11 also at the time of examination. There are fibromatous tissue changes with distolingual extensions in the molar region of the mandible.

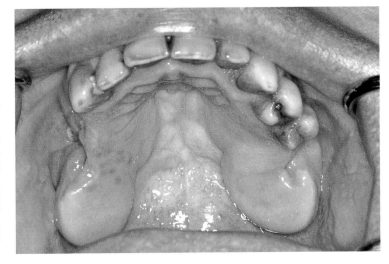

Fig. 15-13 Particular form of gingival fibromatosis with symmetric peripheral jaw fibroma in a 53-year-old patient. Appearance after removal of several posterior teeth in the areas involved by fibromatosis. This will require prosthetic treatment. As an additional finding there is an erosive herpes lesion on the right side.

Chapter 16

Lichen Planus of the Oral Mucosa

Reticular lichen planus

Variant forms
    Plaque-type lichen planus
    Erosive lichen planus
    Bullous lichen planus
    Atrophic lichen planus

Malignant transformation in oral lichen planus

Lichen planus of the oral mucosa should be given more importance in dental practice because more than half of all whitish oral epithelial changes are caused by lichen planus.

Because of the importance of this disease with its various and often misinterpreted appearances in the oral cavity, this chapter is devoted solely to lichen planus. Such treatment is also important because the definition of leukoplakia (i.e., white, not removable by wiping, not associated with a definite illness of the oral mucosa) given by the World Health Organization does not apply to lichen planus. The description and classification of leukoplakia is discussed in the next two chapters.

Lichen planus is a noncontagious inflammatory papular dermatosis with a chronic or subacute course. In this itching lichenoid skin disease (Fig. 16-1), there is—as examinations in the general patient population show—oral mucosal involvement in over 50% of cases. In 25% of cases only the oral mucosa is affected, hence the dentist plays an important diagnostic role. In addition to the typical basic form, there are special forms that exhibit their own therapeutic and prognostic problems.

Reticular lichen planus (ICD-DA 697.01)

Oral manifestations of reticular lichen planus are often discovered only accidentally by the dentist because they lack subjective complaints as opposed to the itching skin efflorescences. However, observant patients describe a feeling of decreased taste and increased rigidity of the affected area of the oral mucosa.

The characteristic clinical picture of reticular lichen planus of the oral mucosa is of whitish, nonremovable, stippled-like fine lines arranged in net-forming or fernlike branched patterns (Figs. 16-2 to 16-5) that sometimes are surrounded by a discrete erythematous border.

The delicate, white, slightly raised lines are called *Wickham's striae*; they are diagnostic of oral lichen planus. Definite preferred points of location are the middle and dorsal third of the cheek in 80% of cases. There are also findings in the vestibule of the posterior teeth, tongue, gingiva, palate, and lips.

Striae and net-forming changes rarely affect the gingiva (Figs. 16-6 and 16-7) and the lips (Figs. 16-11 to 16-13). Ring-form structures and foci in disk forms (Figs. 16-9 and 16-10) that result from enlargement of the filiform papillae appear in the area of the dorsum of the tongue as local variations.

Women are affected more often by an isolated lichen planus of the oral mucosa after 30 years of age.

Histologic findings are usually characteristic. Immediately sub-epithelially, there is a bandlike lymphocyte infiltrate (overwhelmingly T-lymphocytes) caused by the destruction of the basal cell layer and reaching into the epithelial layer. The stratum granulosum is prominent; there is hyperkeratosis and acanthosis. The irregular epithelial acanthosis leads to a picture of "toothsaw rete ridges."

The etiology of lichen planus as an inflamatory dermatosis continues to be unexplained. Viral causes, autoimmune phenomena, psychic trauma, and stress situations were and are discussed as possible factors over a genetically determined predisposition. A series of observations indicate that there is no definite proof that lichen planus is a purely psychosomatic disease. Also, speculations that metallic restorations in the oral cavity may have a causal relationship to lichen planus lack scientific basis.

It is a peculiarity of reticular lichen planus of the skin that mechanical irritation factors (scrubbing, itching) as well as chemical and medication agents induce the development of new efflorescences or intensify those present *(isomorphic irritation effect, Koebner's phenomenon).*

Isomorphic irritation effects on the oral mucosa are also possible in predisposed patients, where chemical factors may play a role. It is possible that the development of additional efflorescences induce transition to special forms or provoke them.

The basic form in a chronic course sometimes shows spontaneous remission. The longer the disease exists, the less likely there will be spontaneous healing. This is true particularly for lesions of the oral mucosa.

On the basis of the different etiologic hypotheses, different remedies have been used. Even today there is no effective treatment for reticular lichen planus of the oral mucosa. It is still true that the patient should be informed by an experienced person that the benign condition can worsen with constant useless therapeutic attempts. Irritating local factors should be removed or alleviated as far as possible, and regular preventive examinations should not be neglected. In fact, they are obligatory in the special forms.

Variant forms

Oral manifestations in almost half the cases of variant forms represent a transition from the original basic form. Other cases follow the initial presentation. It is possible to differentiate plaque type, erosive, bullous, and atrophic special forms based on the clinical picture.

Plaque-type lichen planus (ICD-DA 697.04)

This form can be recognized by its considerable epithelial thickening. It is also called the hypertrophic special form and can be distinguished by the heavy, flat plaques from the filigree motif of reticular lichen planus (Fig. 16-8). At first glance it resembles a homogeneous leukoplakia with typical Wickham's striae at least in the border zone. Preferential locations are the cheek and tongue. The plaquelike variation may derive from a further irritation of an already existing lichen planus. Also, the plaque-type variant occurs more frequently in smokers. Still unexplained is whether there is a possible combination of this lichen planus with a homogeneous leukoplakia.

Erosive lichen planus (ICD-DA 697.02)

The astute observer of oral lichen planus will in many cases discover erosive changes. The erosions or shallow ulcerations (Figs. 16-13 to 16-19) can be small and scattered or extended over large areas. Large ulcerations are more frequent in older persons and offer special differential diagnostic problems (Figs. 16-23 and 16-24). It is almost always possible to see at the border of the erosions or ulcerations a speckled coating that shows the original basic form (Figs. 16-15 and 16-16), and this is important for clinical diagnosis. Transition forms with atrophic findings can also be seen.

One difficult diagnostic task for the dentist is to differentiate an erosive lichen planus of the gingiva propria (Figs. 16-19 to 16-22) from desquamative gingivitis when there is absence of skin or mucosal findings. The clinical findings of both diseases can be so similar that differentiation can be made only by an immune fluorescence microscopic examination (biopsy, unfixed specimen). Further discussion of desquamative gingivitis is found in chapter 29.

Complaints regarding erosive lichen planus vary from patient to patient, including a feeling of a mucosal wound to severe pain that interferes with eating. Older person's health can be compromised by refusal to eat.

The need for and type of symptomatic treatment depend on the extent of the erosive findings. Irritative factors (isomorphic irritation effect) should be reduced. This includes eliminating all types of mouthwashes; particularly damaging are those with astringent additives or with an alcoholic base. Oral hygiene should be performed, but very gently. A continuous effective plaque removal must be instituted by use of a toothpaste with low surface tension. With the use of alkaline toothpastes it is sometimes possible to achieve some subjective improvement. Fixed prosthodontics can be initiated after rehabilitation of the periodontal condition and with continued plaque control.

If the erosions decrease under these conditions and recommendations, the patient can be motivated by recall for regular control with no other measures. After many years, there is healing with residual atrophic areas remaining in the portions of mucosa involved by disease.

In the case of refractory, circumscribed erosions, topical application of glucocorticoid (ointments, lozenges) over a limited time is shown to be effective. Topical anesthetics in the form of ointments, gels or lozenges may be indicated for pain reduction.

In conditions of isolated, small-surface erosions that have been present for months, surgical intervention (excision) can be performed. This will often heal the lesion. This procedure offers the possibility of histologic confirmation of the clinical diagnosis.

In large but single oral mucosal lesions of an erosive (bullous erosive) lichen planus, systemic therapy with glucocorticoid, sometimes in combination with immunosuppressive agents, may be indicated. This treatment belongs in the hands of the dermatologist. The risks of side effects demand continuous supervision of certain laboratory parameters.

Bullous lichen planus (ICD-DA 697.03)

The rare bullous variant of lichen planus results from a greater amount of inflammatory exudate in the subepithelial connective tissue, which leads to a circumscribed lifting of the epithelial surface with colliquation of the basal cell layer and consequent blister formation.

The blisters can have a diameter of few millimeters (Fig. 16-25) to several centimeters (Figs. 16-26 to 16-28). Because of the unavoidable microtraumas of the oral cavity and the macerating effect of saliva, the blister stage is short. At intraoral examination one usually finds erosions or fibrin-covered shallow ulcerations, at times with floating epithelial remnants of the blister top.

Although lichen-type efflorescences are usually demonstrable either on surrounding areas or an other areas of the oral mucosa, the skin, and/or in the genitoanal region, this special bullous form is usually misdiagnosed. Consultation with a dermatologist may be of help in reaching a diagnosis. In dubious cases, distinguishing these from blister-forming dermatoses requires use of other diagnostic measures, which can include excision biopsy.

Therapy is discussed in the section concerned with "erosive lichen planus."

Atrophic lichen planus (ICD-DA 697.02)

About 25% of all cases of lichen planus of the oral mucosa are considered atrophic special forms where combinations with erosive changes are often seen (erosive-atrophic form). Atrophic lichen planus is a condition that may continue for decades, especially those changes associated with active inflammatory reaction.

Clinically in the mucosa there are relatively well-limited, slightly depressed smooth areas (Figs. 16-29, 16-30, 16-32, and 16-33). In the bordering areas are usually Wickham's striae. Atrophy leads to papillary loss in the tongue (Figs. 16-34 to 16-36). As opposed to the clinical picture in the skin, in the oral mucosa there is rarely postinflammatory melanin pigmentations in the center of the lesion (Fig. 16-31). The atrophic area is easily traumatized with tendency for poorly healing tears and erosions.

During the long chronic course, many patients learn to avoid irritative and provoking factors.

The atrophic (erosive atrophic) form of lichen planus should be evaluated at regular intervals for the reasons stated in the next section.

Malignant transformation in oral lichen planus (ICD-M 8070/3)

The possibility of a malignant transformation in each dysplastic epithelial change of the oral cavity is not to be excluded (facultative precancerous conditions). For some diseases, it is possible to establish a correlation between the type of tissue change and the likelihood of secondary malignant changes (obligatory precancerous conditions).

Whether and how to identify and evaluate facultative and obligatory precancerous changes, with all the consequences for therapy and later care, is a matter of clinical judgment and opinion.

The possibility of a carcinomatous change on the base of an oral lichen planus has long been discussed. Opinions vary on whether erosive and atrophic variants of lichen planus offer an increased cancerogenous potential or whether a carcinoma together with a lichen planus of the oral cavity represents coincidental unrelated findings.

It is not clear whether long-term action of a cancerogenic agent increases the risk of malignant changes in lichen planus more than that in normal mucosa. In this context, it has already been discussed that some forms of treatment (now largely abandoned) may have contributed to the carcinoma formation (see Fig. 31-37). It is certain that erosive and atrophic special forms of lichen planus require regular and careful supervision at 3- to 6-month intervals. With the suspicion of cancer, inspection and palpation should be carried out as described in chapter 19.

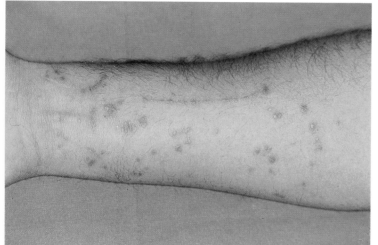

Fig. 16-1 Lichen planus of the skin. The typical primary efflorescence is the flat, polygonal, limited, shiny or dull, hard papules about the size of rice grains. As opposed to lichen planus of the oral cavity, with skin lesions there is itching. Preferred locations are the flexor surface of the forearm, hand, lower leg, skin covering the joints, and the genitoanal region. By itching and scrubbing, new lichen planus efflorescences can be induced (isomorphic irritation effect, Koebner's phenomenon).

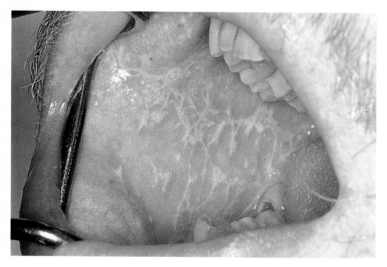

Fig. 16-2 Typical reticular type of a lichen planus at a typical location of the cheek mucosa. The netlike whitish epithelial changes are called Wickham's striae.

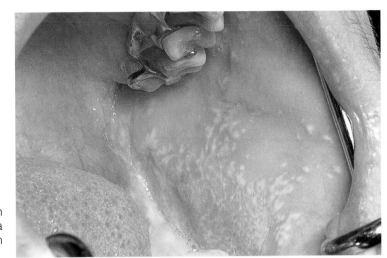

Fig. 16-3   Basic type of lichen planus of the cheek mucosa showing efflorescences with partial stippling.

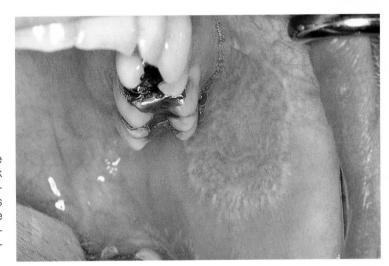

Fig. 16-4   Fernlike basic type of lichen planus of the cheek mucosa as the only manifestation of illness. The Wickham's striae are thicker in the middle of this change and are distinctly different from the compact field of a leukoplakia.

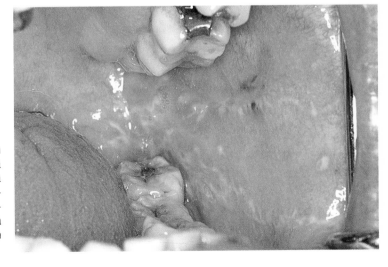

Fig. 16-5   Basic type of lichen planus of the cheek mucosa with small epithelial lesions as a consequence of a bite. This lichen lesion can be differentiated from a linea alba because a Wickham's stria can be seen in a caudal location.

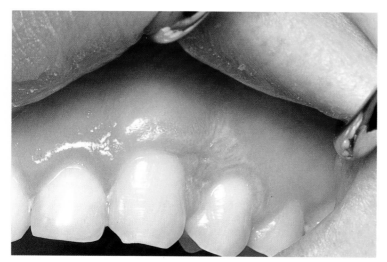

Fig. 16-6 Basic type of lichen planus of the attached gingiva in a 20-year-old patient studying for examinations; similar lesions were also seen in other parts of the oral mucosa (cheeks and tongue). Other changes decreased after the patient passed the examination (spontaneous remission) and with medication (containing mild sedatives).

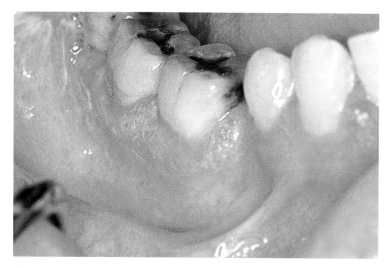

Fig. 16-7 Reticular basic form of a lichen planus, present for several years on the attached gingiva in the posterior tooth area.

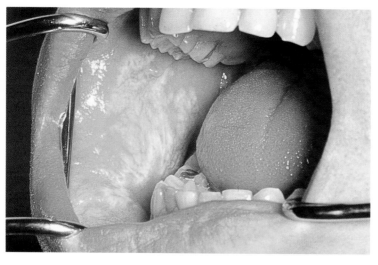

Fig. 16-8 Plaque-like variant of lichen planus of the cheek mucosa. Note the more plump lesions reminiscent of leukoplakia. The typical design of Wickham's striae in the border region usually allows for a definitive differentiation from a flat homogeneous leukoplakia.

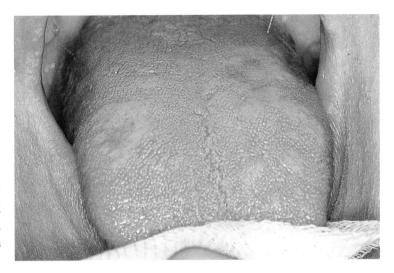

Fig. 16-9   Effect of location of a basic type of lichen planus in the tongue region. The predominantly ring-form and disklike lesions on the dorsum of the tongue are histologically identical to the typical lesions of lichen planus. They are usually present only in association with typical efflorescences in other areas at the same time, for example, on the cheek mucosa (intraoral preferred location).

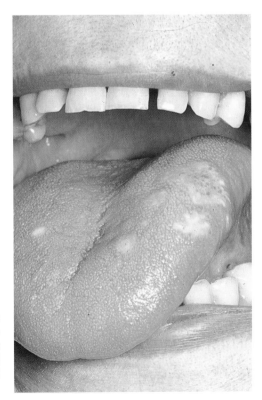

Fig. 16-10   Lichen planus on the dorsum of the tongue predominantly distributed as disk foci as a partial manifestation of lichen planus of the entire oral mucosa.

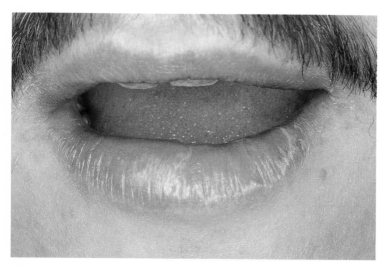

Fig. 16-11   Reticular lichen planus (basic type) of the lower lip.

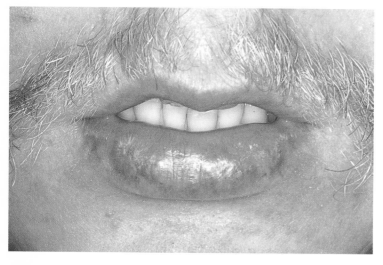

Fig. 16-12   Effect of location of basic type lichen planus on the lower lip with clearly evident erythematous border zone. The patient had other intraoral lichen foci as well as skin efflorescences in typical places (flexor surface of forearm).

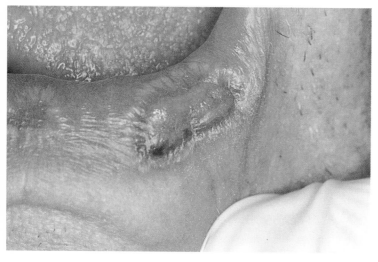

Fig. 16-13   Lichen planus of the lower lip with central fibrin-covered erosion-ulceration. A lichen focus on the lower lip (left border of photograph) is slightly raised above skin level. This erosive-ulcerous finding requires a careful evaluation for exclusion of a lip carcinoma, which in cases of doubt should be referred to a specialist by the dentist.

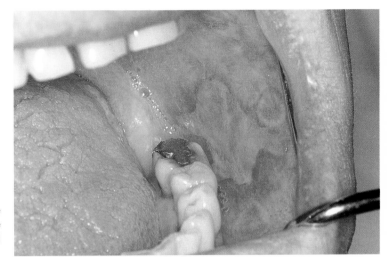

Fig. 16-14 Recent erosive form of lichen planus of the cheek mucosa in a 41-year-old patient.

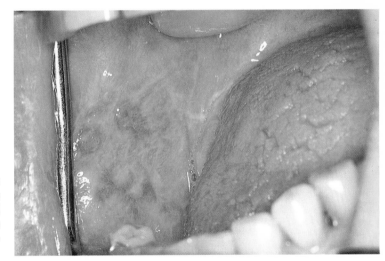

Fig. 16-15 Recent erosive form of lichen planus of the cheek mucosa in a 33-year-old patient. At the same time, there were skin changes in the preferred areas.

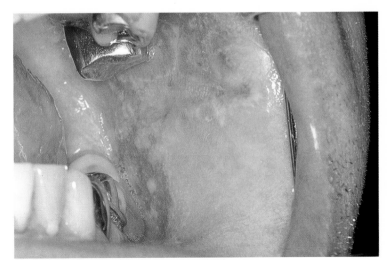

Fig. 16-16 Erosive lichen planus of the cheek mucosa with Wickham's striae predominantly on the periphery.

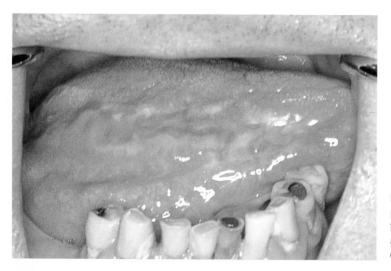

Fig. 16-17 Erosive lichen planus on the dorsum of the tongue in combination with flat atrophic areas caused by loss of papillae.

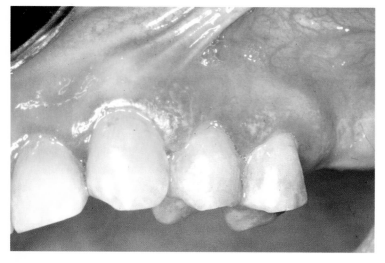

Fig. 16-18 Erosive lichen planus of the attached gingiva. Basic efflorescences predominate.

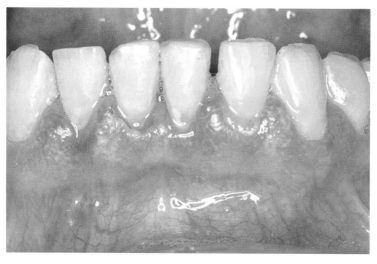

Fig. 16-19 Erosive lichen planus of the attached gingiva. The changes should not be confused with chronic gingivitis.

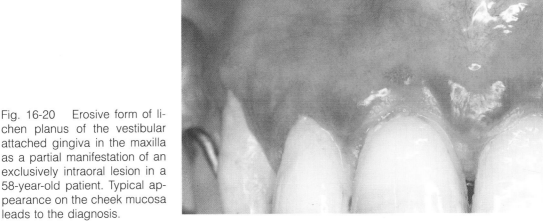

Fig. 16-20   Erosive form of lichen planus of the vestibular attached gingiva in the maxilla as a partial manifestation of an exclusively intraoral lesion in a 58-year-old patient. Typical appearance on the cheek mucosa leads to the diagnosis.

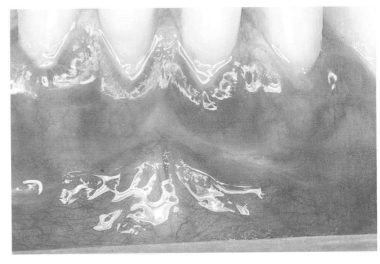

Fig. 16-21   The patient in Fig. 16-20 also at the time of examination. There were erosive changes as a partial manifestation of an oral lichen planus on the vestibular attached gingiva of the mandible. With appropriate oral hygiene (plaque control), the periodontal supporting tissue may be spared.

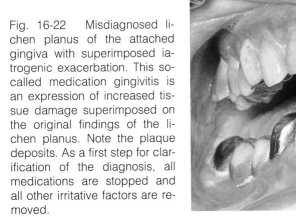
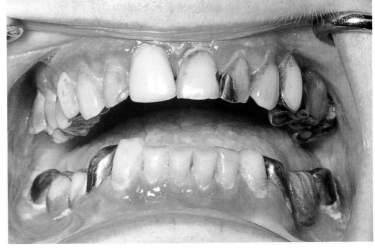

Fig. 16-22   Misdiagnosed lichen planus of the attached gingiva with superimposed iatrogenic exacerbation. This so-called medication gingivitis is an expression of increased tissue damage superimposed on the original findings of the lichen planus. Note the plaque deposits. As a first step for clarification of the diagnosis, all medications are stopped and all other irritative factors are removed.

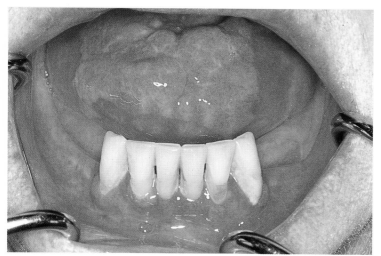

Fig. 16-23   Large lesion of the oral mucosa including foci of erosive lichen planus in a 62-year-old patient. Severe pain hampered the patient's ability to eat to such an extent that the use of topical anesthesia was recommended.

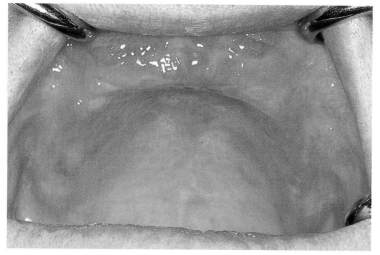

Fig. 16-24   Maxilla of the patient in Fig. 16-23. The diagnosis of this extensive finding requires additional histologic and immunofluorescent studies to exclude autoimmune diseases and bullous dermatoses. Therapeutically, there is a systemic gain under ambulatory conditions (skin clinic). The finding should not be confused with a prosthesis stomatitis (see chapter 33).

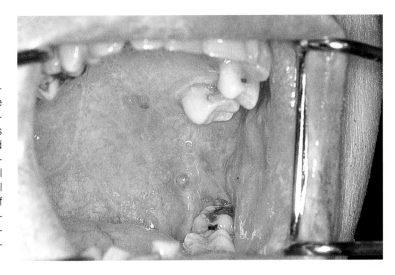

Fig. 16-25 Bullous efflores-cences of a lichen planus of the palatal mucosa and the retro-molar area. The blister stage is very short in the oral cavity and therefore can only rarely be ob-served. Sometimes there is still a floating rim of the residual blister cover at the border of the erosive changes. The dia-gnosis is facilitated by the con-comitant presence of typical li-chen lesions.

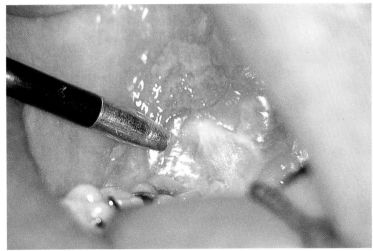

Fig. 16-26 Unusually large blister histologically confirmed as bullous lichen planus of the oral mucosa. An air blast failed to produce a blister when ap-plied to the mucosa adjacent to the lesion (negative Nikolsky's sign). More is presented on this in chapter 29, "Blister-forming diseases."

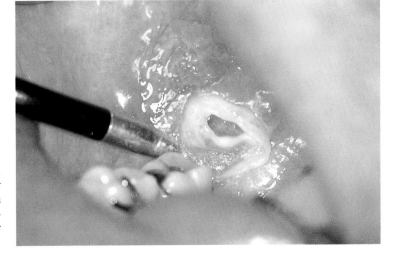

Fig. 16-27 The patient in Fig. 16-26. Under the torn blister cover, the fresh erosion is noticeable. In the area surroun-ding the blister there are other fibrin-covered areas of erosion.

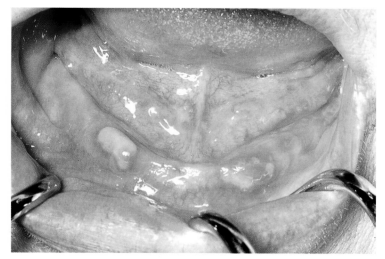

Fig. 16-28 Various stages of a bullous erosive lichen planus of the mucosa in the area of an edentulous mandibular alveolar process of a 75-year-old woman. The differential diagnostic separation from pemphigus vulgaris was facilitated through the typical netlike epithelial changes (basic type) of the cheek and palatal mucosa and confirmed through histologic examination.

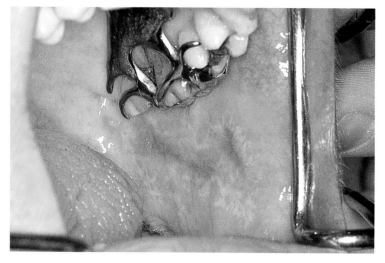

Fig. 16-29 Predominantly atrophic lichen planus of the cheek mucosa with distinct Wickam's striae on the border zone; it had existed for many years. In all erosive atrophic forms of lichen planus, there is a need for accurate, regular evaluation.

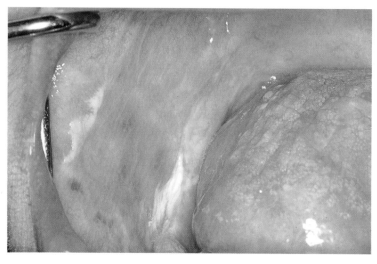

Fig. 16-30 Atrophic lichen planus depressed below the mucosa level with scattered erosive foci and an obvious keratotic border zone.

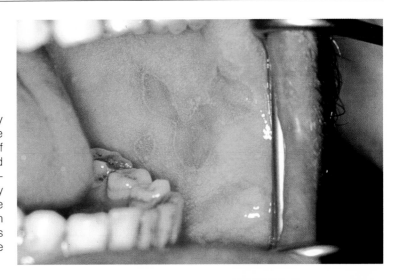

Fig. 16-31   Postinflammatory melanin pigmentation of the cheek mucosa in the area of lichen foci in a 25-year-old patient. As opposed to corresponding skin postinflammatory pigmentary alterations, these findings are rare in the mouth mucosa. Note the Wickham's striae in the border zone of the changes.

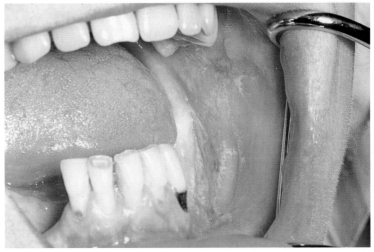

Fig. 16-32   Erosion stage of a lichen planus of the oral mucosa with atrophic zones that had been present for years. Removal of teeth with amalgam restorations did not lead to improvement. A removable prosthesis is problematic (isomorphic irritation effect) in these cases.

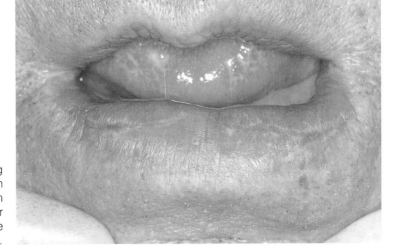

Fig. 16-33   Overwhelming atrophic change of lichen planus of the lower lip with Wickham's striae in the border zone and on the tip of the tongue in a 71-year-old woman.

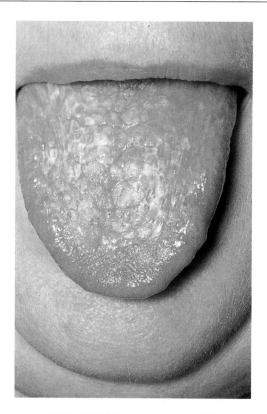

Fig. 16-34   Present is a large basic-type lichen planus on the dorsum of the tongue; on the left tongue border is an atrophic area with interspersed small, spotty erosions.

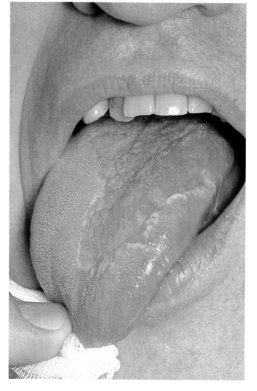

Fig. 16-35   Atrophic form of lichen planus on the dorsum of the tongue with partially erosive, partially atrophic areas; the lichen planus had been present for 1 year. At the same time were skin changes and atrophic fingernails in the 45-year-old patient. Precancerous leukoplakia should be considered; it can be excluded only histologically.

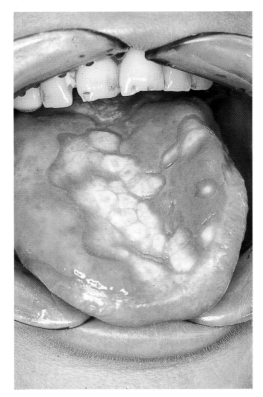

Fig. 16-36 In addition to the usual oral mucosal findings (erosive lichen planus of the cheek mucosa) there is a clinically suspicious lichen planus with massive plaquelike keratinization on an atrophic tongue surface (nearly complete loss of papillae). The histologic examination did not confirm the suspicion of cancer in the 66-year-old woman, but did confirm lichen planus without malignancy.

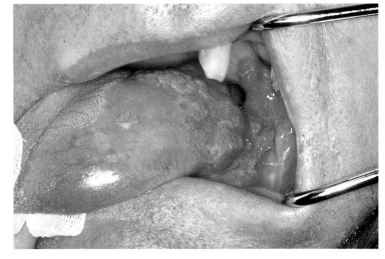

Fig. 16-37 Histologically confirmed squamous cell carcinoma over a partially bullous, partially atrophic lichen planus of the oral mucosa that has been present for 20 years. On the left posterior tongue border is a hard nodular infiltrate with extensive ulceration of the mucosa of the cheek and of the floor of the mouth. Note further the atrophic mucosal changes on the anterior part of the tongue. The lichen planus had been treated with ionizing radiation many years previously in this 66-year-old patient.

Chapter 17

Simple Leukoplakias

Frictional keratosis

Smoker's leukokeratosis

Leukoplakia of the oral mucosa

Since 1877, Schwimmer's concept of "leukoplakia" has been criticized and questioned, particularly as the cause of the misunderstanding that leukoplakia is always a precancerous lesion.

Leukoplakia is a purely descriptive clinical designation of a change that can be considered a special efflorescence of the mucosa. *By recommendation of the World Health Organization (WHO), a leukoplakia is understood to be a white spot of the mucosa not removable by wiping* that cannot be associated with any other disease.

If one follows this recommendation, leukoplakial changes that are symptoms of diseases of the oral cavity should not be classified as true leukoplakias. These symptomatic *"leukoplakias"* with a completely different etiology include the findings of inflammatory dermatosis (i.e., lichen planus, lupus erythematosus), of granulomatous mycosis, of specific infections (tuberculosis and syphilis) as well as cheilitis granulosatosum, and the glossitis of the Melkersson-Rosenthal syndrome. These are discussed elsewhere in this book. The same is true for certain leukoplakia-like conditions of the tongue that lack completely or in part clinical or true disease characteristics (among others, hairy tongue–see chapter 2).

In other cases we are concerned with an inherited disturbance of keratinization, which, as in Darier's disease, can have a hyperkeratotic manifestation on the oral mucosa and is predominantly of interest to the dermatologist. This is not discussed here except for the *white sponge nevus*, which is discussed in the text associated with Figs. 17-1 and 17-2.

Leukoplakias in the sense of the WHO definition can be divided into two groups according to clinical criteria (i.e., color and surface characteristics) that provide conclusions as to type and prognosis:

- Those classified as simple leukoplakias with pan-homogeneous form and a low malignancy rate
- Those prognostically unfavorable spotty leukoplakias (verrucous and erosive forms) that are discussed with their clinical findings in chapter 18

In relation to this classification there should be further subgrouping because histologically diagnosed simple leukoplakias, even if only in rare cases and after a long time, can change into a precancerous lesion and finally into cancer. Also, clinical appearance does not always correlate with histologic findings. Definite determination of the biologic potential of the lesion is not determined by the clinician from changes taking place on the surface of the leukoplakia but by the pathologist determining changes in the depths of the tissue. Even so, this classification has proven its value because its use represents an important orientation point in daily practice.

Simple leukoplakias clinically show a plain homogeneous surface that is mirror smooth to faintly dull. The impression of a white spot is produced by the keratinization and/or thickening of the mucosal epithelium, which loses the normal transparency. The color tone varies from milky-cloudy to opaque to resembling mother-of-pearl. Very discrete forms of simple leukoplakia are not palpable. Marked lesions raised over the mucosal level become palpable.

Histologically, simple leukoplakias are characteristically epithelial condensations with a hyperkeratotic surface layer as well as a thickening of the spinous cell layers (acanthoses). The keratinization of the mucosa can run a course similar to the physiologic occurrence on the skin of an orthokeratosis (cornification without nuclear remnants) or of a parakeratosis (cornification with nuclear remnants). The epithelial layers have a normal polarity. There is no epithelial atypia. Subepithelial lymphoplasmacellular infiltrate, if present at all, is scanty.

These simple leukoplakias make up about 50% of all oral leukoplakias. When their origin is not known or is insufficiently explained, the term used is idiopathic leukoplakia. Other investigators call these lesions leukoplakias in the strict sense of the word.

At this point, abandoning for didactic reasons the WHO classification, one should consider that idiopathic leukoplakias may regress if mechanically irritative factors or smoking habits are eliminated, or they may progress to mucosal lesions of greater severity if the stimuli are maintained for a long time.

Frictional keratosis (ICD-DA 528.78)

Under the classification frictional leukoplakias fall keratinizations of nonkeratinized mucosa or hyperkeratosis of normally cornified mucosal areas *(irritative hyperkeratosis)*, which are related in a pathogenetic manner to chronic trauma.

A long-acting mechanical stimulus on the oral mucosa can lead to keratinization in the same manner as production of a callus. This is also referred to as a *pachydermia* or as a white spot because a hyperkeratosis, particularly of the orthokeratotic type. The squamous epithelium presents a normal stratification and orientation. These focal irritative hyperkeratoses are frequently found in the oral cavity usually close to sharp tooth edges, unsuitable prostheses, defective support elements, or other similar problems (Figs. 17-3 to 17-7). As signs of mechanical failure or overstress, these are found not infrequently on the surface of the flabby ridge and irritation swellings (see chapter 22). They can also be the consequence of chronic cheek and lip chewing (see chapters 32 and 34).

Removal of the irritating factor causes frictional keratosis to regress. The regression should, however, be reevaluated with follow-up examinations, so that misinterpretation can be avoided and a carcinoma ruled out (see chapter 19).

Smoker's leukokeratosis (ICD-DA 528.72)

Another important example for the dentist is the leukoplakia caused by smoking irritation. Affected predominantly are heavy smokers, pipe smokers in particular. The cause is not so much thermal effect as the chemical stimulus of tobacco components.

Leukokeratosis of smokers presents typical and almost unmistakable findings on the palate. However, other regions of the oral cavity suffer similarly from the smoking habit (Figs. 17-8 to 17-12, 17-17 and 17-18). On the hard and sometimes soft palate, whitish hyperkeratotic epithelial changes of the oral cavity resemble a cobblestone pattern (Figs. 17-13 to 17-17). The openings of the inflamed, swollen minor salivary glands do not show keratinization. They rise distinctly as small, red points from surrounding thickened, whitish mucosa. Regions of the palatal mucosa that are prosthetically covered are spared from the leukokeratosis (see Figs. 33-27 and 33-35).

Reduced tobacco consumption by the patient or total cessation of smoking will make the changes disappear. According to current knowledge, the development of a cancer from a leukokeratotic lesion is unlikely. This finding is surprising, because smoking has been demonstrated to increase the cancer risk on the bronchial mucosa and on the lip mucosa.

Leukoplakia of the oral mucosa (ICD-DA 528.6X and 523.84)

The relevant clinical and histologic signs of leukoplakias of unknown cause have been discussed.

The characteristic signs of leukoplakia simplex of the flat homogeneous form appear clinically as flat or slightly raised, relatively small, white surface lesions that are sharply delimited from the surface of the normal mucosa. In particular conditions, the lesion surface may have a different appearance. In the retroangular cheek mucosa– which is a favorite point and is often bilaterally and symmetrically affected–as well as in the area of the cheek border line, which is also subjected to stress, there are occasionally distinct checkered leuko- plakias (Fig. 17-19). Because of the difficulty in the differential diag- nosis of these lesions, these findings are discussed together under "Mouth corner and leukoplakias" in chapter 34. On the dorsum of the tongue with sharply contoured and sometimes diffuse-appearing leukoplakias, papillary relief is lost. The tissue structure also has the checkered look of leukoplakia (Figs. 17-20 to 17-23). In the area of the base of the mouth, the leukoplakia surface is often wavy. It resembles the contour of a washboard or the surface of the ocean at low tide (Figs. 17-24 to 17-26). Simple leukoplakias of the gingiva apparently often spare the marginal region (Figs. 17-27 to 17-29).

Final remarks for the dentist

Patients with simple leukoplakias associated with trauma or irritation that regress after elimination of the suspected cause must be ex- amined at regular intervals. Checkups are necessary because even in the flat homogeneous form, the transition to precancerous leukoplakia can never be completely excluded, and a malignant transformation is possible in rare cases. The dentist should therefore carefully weigh whether he or she wants to assume the responsibility alone or feels that this responsibility is better transferred to a specialist or a clinic.

There is also the question of whether limited zones of simple leukoplakias should be removed in toto for preventive reasons. The experimental conservative treatment of large surfaces of simple leuko- plakias using high doses of vitamin A should be reserved for the specialist. The immediate concern of the dentist is to remove damag- ing, local irritating factors and to motivate the patient to improve oral hygiene procedures.

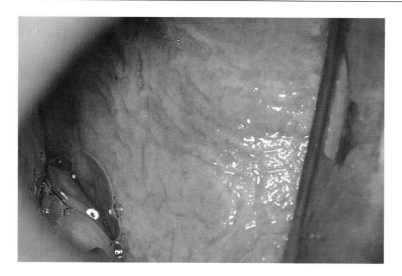

Fig. 17-1   Differential diagnosis of simple leukoplakia: white sponge nevus of the cheek mucosa, oral epithelial nevus, familial white-folded gingivostomatitis (ICD-DA 750.26). The white mucosal changes can be noted as irregularly contoured and not sharply delimited from the surrounding mucosa with extended folding of the surface. They were present on the mucosa of both cheeks and on the lateral surface of the lip mucosa in the 8-year-old girl. They had been noticed 4 years previously. After more than 2 years of observation, the findings remained unchanged.

Histologic evaluation revealed acanthosis, hyperkeratosis and, particularly in the prickle cell layer, many epithelial cells showing swelling and vacuolization of cytoplasm as well as by pyknotic nuclei (ballooned cells). The connective tissue was unaffected.

The wavelike, or striplike, focally wrinkled surface of the white sponge nevus represents a rare and benign disturbance of keratinization that is present at birth or appears in early childhood and parallels the growth and intensity of the developmental years.

Preferred locations are the cheek and lip mucosa as well as the attached gingiva. The often bilateral symmetric change can take place anywhere in the oral cavity. Extraoral manifestations on the mucosa of nose, esophagus, vagina, and anus have been reported.

The white mucosal nevus does not produce subjective symptoms; in severe desquamations, a rough feeling can develop. Higher lamellae and epithelial layers can easily be removed with a spatula or pliers without bleeding. Because of the lack of symptoms, the sponge nevus is usually recognized only by accident after several years of latency.

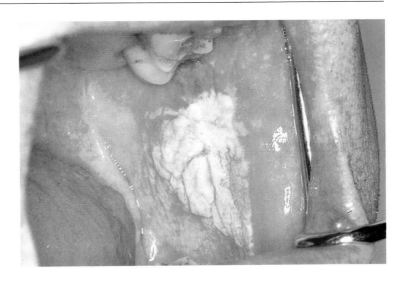

Fig. 17-2   Differential diagnosis of a simple leukoplakia: white sponge nevus of the cheek mucosa. The 32-year-old patient reported that the whitish spots were first seen during childhood by a pediatrician. The findings have been followed by the authors without any change and no patient complaints.

A familial accumulation of white, spongy nevus with autosomal-dominant transmission has been documented repeatedly. In this case, it could not be verified.

Differential diagnosis of all forms of oral leukoplakia from other leukoplakial manifestations of diseases of the oral mucosa is usually performed on the basis of the histologic findings and other criteria. According to the literature, because of their clinical characteristics and etiology, whitish, shiny leukoderma cannot be clinically or histologically differentiated with certainty from white sponge nevus when extensive.

The periodic recurrence of leukoderma and the older age of onset are reliable differentiation criteria. Another important differential diagnostic sign is *Candida* infection, confirmed by the demonstration of fungus and the presence of inflammation, as opposed to the white sponge nevus.

Therapy of the harmless keratinization is superfluous. Regular control during routine dental or medical examination is available. The real importance of the white sponge nevus must be kept in mind in differential diagnosis. If it is misdiagnosed, it can lead to years of undesirable or unsuccessful therapy.

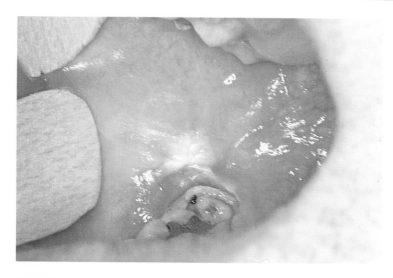

Fig. 17-3   Circumscribed leukoplakia (stress hyperkeratosis)
in the retromolar region of the
right side of the mandible as a
consequence of chronic mechanical irritation. The cause is
the sharp edge of carious tooth
48 (32).

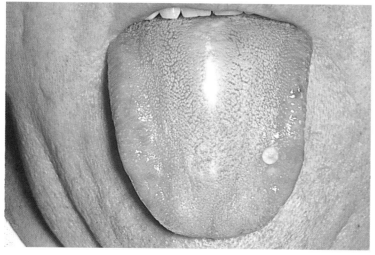

Fig. 17-4   Line-shaped leukoplakia as a result of a mechanical hyperkeratosis on the dorsal surface of the tongue in a
51-year-old man. A chronic mechanical irritation caused by a
projecting palatal connector
was present. A lentil-sized papilloma is seen as a secondary
finding.

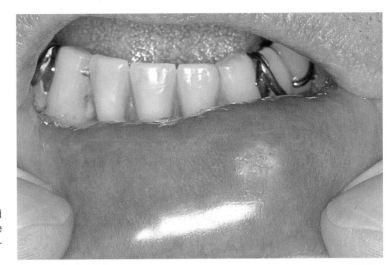

Fig. 17-5   Leukoplakia caused by mechanical irritation on the lower lip mucosa from prosthesis clamps.

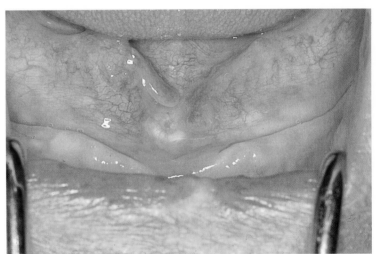

Fig. 17-6   Chronic prosthesis pressure point (ulcer) on the lingual side of the edentulous mandible with surrounding leukoplakia (mechanical hyperkeratosis). Note: after correction of the prosthesis corners, the finding is checked within 10 days –provided retention of the prosthesis is allowed–to avoid missing the diagnosis of a carcinomatous ulcer (see Fig. 19-36).

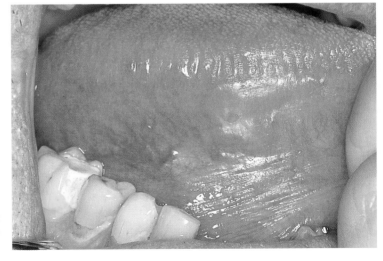

Fig. 17-7   Small chronic ulcer with surrounding leukoplakia on the right tongue border. Cause: long-acting mechanical irritation from a jagged tooth. Note: healing after the removal of the causative irritation factor (follow-up after 10 days) rules out the suspicion of a carcinomatous ulcer (see chapter 19).

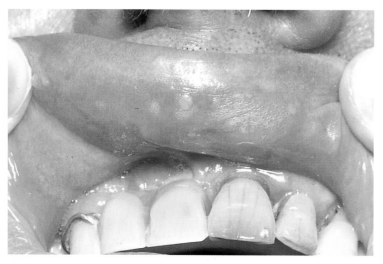

Fig. 17-8 Leukokeratosis of the upper lip mucosa of a cigarette smoker (cigarette smoker's lip). Note the typical irritation change caused on the lip where the cigarette is usually held.

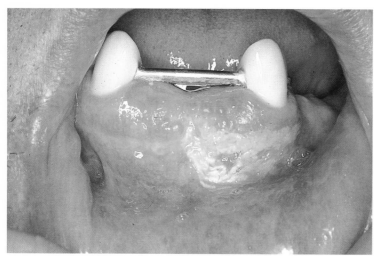

Fig. 17-9 Leukokeratosis of the vestibular mucosa in the anterior part of the mandible. The cigarette smoker (more than 40 cigarettes per day) usually used a cigarette holder, which directed the main smoke stream to this part of the mucosa. The prosthesis-covered mucosa is shielded from these changes, explaining the horizontal alveolar ridge border.

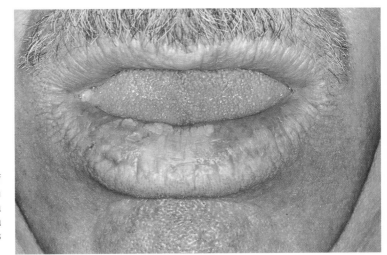

Fig. 17-10   Leukokeratosis of the lower lip in combination with a cheilitis actinica chronica (chronic light damage) of a heavy pipe smoker who works in road construction.

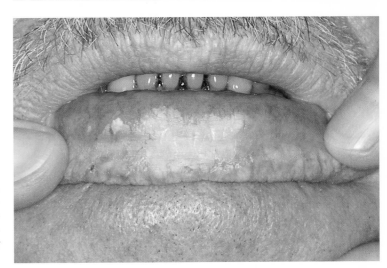

Fig. 17-11   The patient in Fig. 17-10 also at the time of examination. The contour of the irritation-caused leukoplakia is visible on the inside of the lower lip.

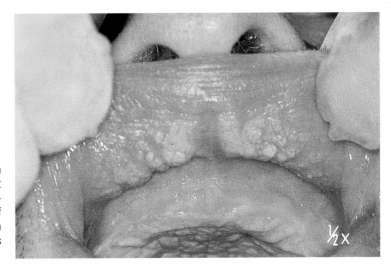

Fig. 17-12   The patient in Figs. 17-10 and 17-11 also at examination. There are papulous changes on the mucosa of the upper lip as an expression of a marked leukokeratosis from pipe smoking.

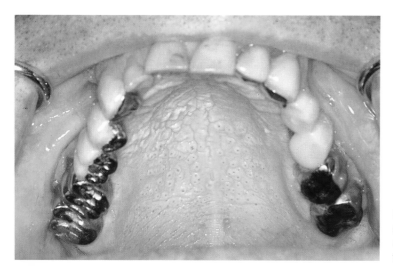

Fig. 17-13 Typical cobble-stonelike palatal mucosal findings of a smoker's leukokeratosis ("smoker's palate").

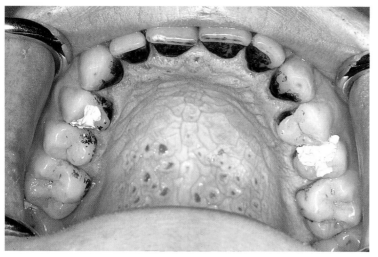

Fig. 17-14 Smoker's palate of a pipe smoker. The lesion is subdivided in fields. The inflamed enlarged excretory ducts of the minor salivary glands stand out as central red points inside the individual fields.

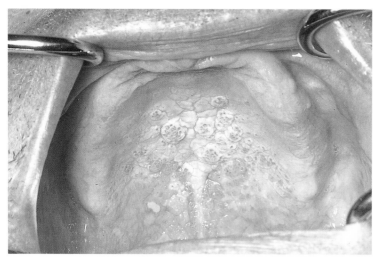

Fig. 17-15 Marked leukokeratosis of the palatal mucosa of a 70-year-old heavy pipe smoker. The complete maxillary prosthesis has not been in use for years. With such leukokeratotic findings, there is often relative mouth dryness.

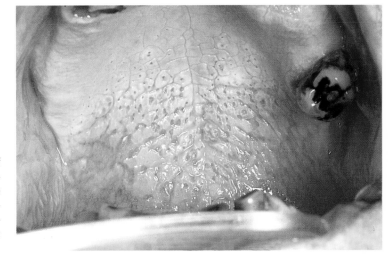

Fig. 17-16 Smoker's palate of a pipe smoker with characteristic leukokeratotic changes. The average daily tobacco consumption of the 56-year-old patient was 10 pipes and seven cigarettes.

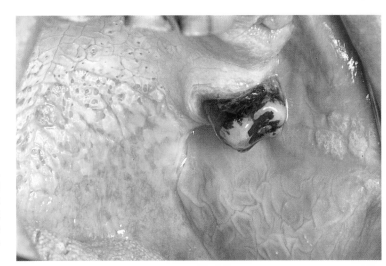

Fig. 17-17 The patient in Fig. 17-16 also at examination. The epithelium of the cheek mucosa appears as if covered by a milky veil (leukoderma). Note the distinct folding of the surface.

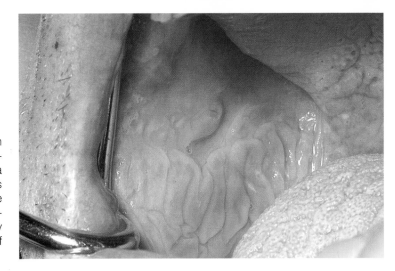

Fig. 17-18 The patient in Figs. 17-16 and 17-17 at examination. The specialized mucosa of the dorsum of the tongue is altered by leukokeratosis. The leukoderma of the cheek mucosa stands out prominently during maximal stretching of the cheek.

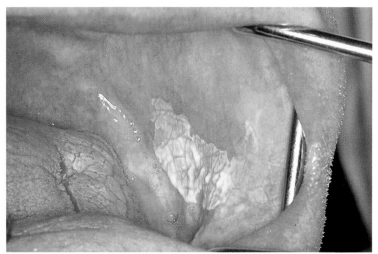

Fig. 17-19 Simple (homogeneous) idiopathic leukoplakia of
the cheek mucosa with distinct
checkerboard-like pattern. The
sharply delimited finding was
observed by the patient for 4
years and remained unchanged in form or extension under
clinical control over another 3
years.

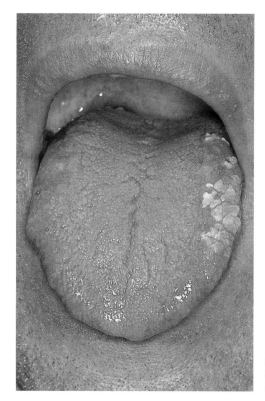

Fig. 17-20 Simple idiopathic
leukoplakia of 2 years' duration
on the left tongue border.

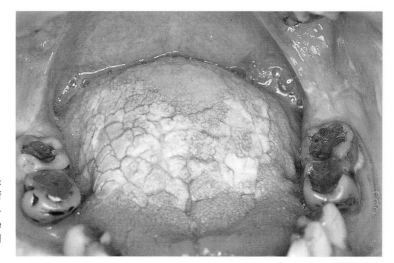

Fig. 17-21 Simple idiopathic leukoplakia of the dorsum of the tongue. The checkerboard-like pattern in this case is due to the presence of furrowed tongue.

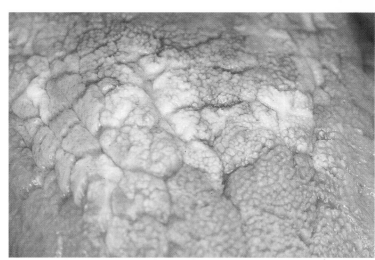

Fig. 17-22 Close-up of the tongue in Fig. 17-21. The simple leukoplakia leads frequently to findings of waviness on the dorsum of the tongue. The brittleness of the thickened epithelial surface facilitates rhagade formation, which can cause complaints.

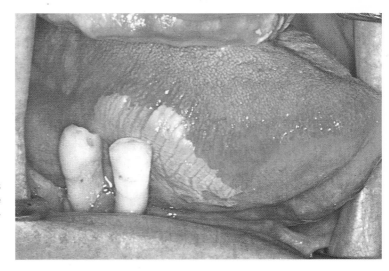

Fig. 17-23 Flat homogeneous leukoplakia on the right tongue border. (From Krüger E. Lehrbuch der chirurgischen Zahn-, Mund- und Kieferheilkunde, vol. 2. Berlin: Quintessenz, 1988.)

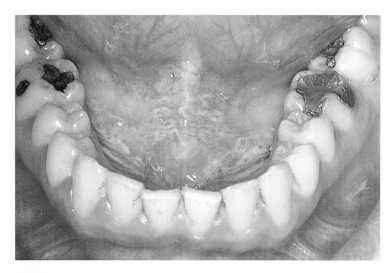

Fig. 17-24 Simple idiopathic leukoplakia; the floor of the mouth mucosa is a favorite location.

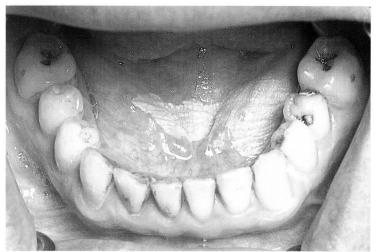

Fig. 17-25 Circumscribed leukoplakia on the floor of the mouth in a 37-year-old man. The mother-of-pearl-colored, leathery lesion, which resembles reptile skin and could not be removed by rubbing, existed unchanged in outline and extent for 3 years.

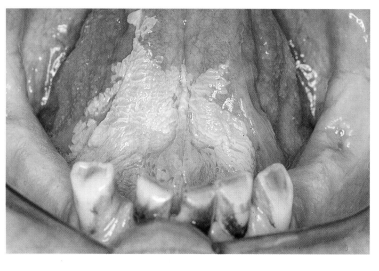

Fig. 17-26 Circumscribed, idiopathic leukoplakia of the base of the tongue and anterior part of the mouth. The 82-year-old woman stated that a nonpainful, large lesion had been present for 8 months. Another circumscribed leukoplakial area was found on the right cheek mucosa. Because of the lesion's tendency to spread, a virus typing was done with papilloma virus type 1 up to 41 hybridization and cross hybridization at the skin clinic of the University of Düsseldorf in the German Cancer Research Center in Heidelberg. There was no evidence of papilloma virus DNA. Histopathologic study after biopsy confirmed the existence of a leukoplakia without an epithelial dysplasia.

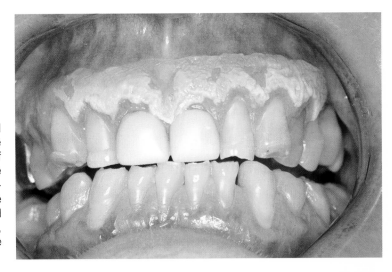

Fig. 17-27 Circumscribed leukoplakia strictly limited to the attached gingiva in the area of teeth 13 to 24 (6 to 12). The hyperkeratotic epithelial thickening has been in existence for 1 year, is sharply separated from the surrounding mucosa, and has spared most of the marginal gingiva.

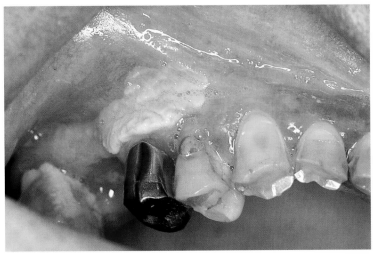

Fig. 17-28 Circumscribed leukoplakia with a massive keratin mass in the area of tooth 15 (4). The finding has been stationary for years. An excision in toto (therapeutic excision) is indicated. Histopathologic examination demonstrated an exophytic leukoplakia with a slight epithelial dysplasia.

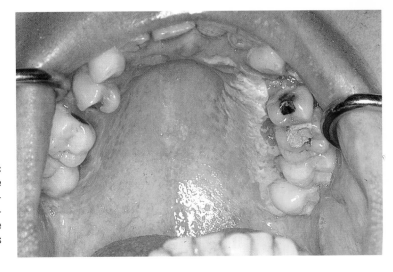

Fig. 17-29 Simple idiopathic leukoplakia of the gingiva close to the palatal mucosa. The nature of the lesion was determined by biopsy. In this case no epithelial dysplasia was found.

Chapter 18

Precancerous Leukoplakias

The fundamentals of leukoplakias are presented in chapter 17.

Precancerous leukoplakia is the most frequent precancerous lesion of the oral cavity. *Precancerous* is understood, in general, as a long-term morphologic change of tissue that – without being cancer – brings with it a significantly high cancer risk. In other words, in precancerous lesions there must be transformation after an interval of undetermined length into an invasive cancer. The average interval is 5 years. This time span is related to later statements regarding the frequency of malignant transformation. The eventual development of cancer is a statistical certainty. However, for any given patient, malignant transformation is only a possibility that must take into consideration the existence of all cofactors, such as the use of tobacco and alcohol consumption.

The frequency of malignant transformation of oral leukoplakia, in general, was overestimated in the past. Based on past and present data we cannot make a definite statement on the percentage of carcinomas that – measured against the total number of all oral cancers – developed from a precancerous leukoplakia. Based on present knowledge, most oral cavity carcinomas develop from original, inconspicuous mucosal precancerous lesions.

The origin of precancerous leukoplakia is covered here in a single chapter because in the precancerous stage active prophylaxis is possible, and therefore the development of carcinoma can be avoided. The dentist is very important in cancer prevention. This chapter describes the clinical aspect of changes that must be treated as suspicious precancerous lesions and should cause the dentist to refer the affected patients without delay.

Histologic and cytologic criteria confirm the clinical suspicion and the classification of the precancerous leukoplakia; help from an expert on biopsies is also necessary. Exfoliative cytology has not proven to be sufficient.

Histopathologic evaluation criteria

In histologic rating and prognostic evaluation, the demonstration of premalignant epithelial dysplasia in oral leukoplakias is the determining criterion. Epithelial dysplasias are described as a wide range of changes of the histologic pattern associated with cytologic abnormalities.

With detailed tissue abnormalities presented in the following table, it is possible to distinguish several levels that can be correlated with the clinical course and prognosis of precancerous leukoplakias. The risk of malignant transformation in relation to the severity of dysplasia is also presented in the table. Of particular clinical importance is the differentiation of intermediate and high-grade dysplasias in which the epithelial polarity is also disturbed. Only 10% of all clinical leukoplakias exhibit a high-grade dysplasia or a transition into a carcinoma in situ.

Dysplasia Criteria*

Grade	Signs	Frequency of transformation into carcinoma
Low	Basal cell hyperplasia Disturbance of basal cell polarity	3%
Intermediate	Basal cell hyperplasia Loss of basal cell polarity Marked cell pleomorphism Slight increase of mitotic rate Few dyskeratotic cells	4%
High	Basal cell hyperplasia Loss of basal cell polarity Marked cell pleomorphism Elevated mitotic rate Many dyskeratotic cells Full-thickness epithelial loss of polarity	43%
Transformation into carcinoma in situ	Histologic evidence of worsening dysplasia Loss of epithelial polarity No connective tissue invasion yet	

* According to *Burkhardt A., Maerker R.*, 1981, and *Seifert G., Burkhardt A.*, 1981.

In addition to the grade of dysplasia, there are other fine tissue changes to observe that are related to immunologic defense mechanisms and that influence the prognosis:

- The total number of lymphocytes and Langerhans' cells in the epithelium parallels the severity of the dysplasia and can be as high as five times the normal number.
- With the increase in severity of the dysplasia there is an increase in the cellular reaction in the subepithelial stroma with collection of immunocompetent cells (lymphocytes, plasma cells, macrophages) and increased immunoglobulin formation in the plasma cells.
- Thrush is present in about 10% of all leukoplakias (candidiasis). It increases in frequency with increased dysplasia and is demonstrable in leukoplakias with severe dysplasias in about 40% of cases. It is considered a risk indicator and a risk factor.

The quantitative measure of DNA content of the cell nucleus (DNA histogram) can improve the prognostic evaluation concerning the risk of malignant transformation.

Clinical appearance of precancerous leukoplakias

The *papillary-endophytic* or *verrucous-exophytic* precancerous leukoplakias (Fig. 18-3) appear clinically as *spotty (dotted)* mucosal changes. They can be divided into two forms according to color and surface appearance:

- Verrucous leukoplakia
- Erosive leukoplakia

Characteristic of the less spotty *verrucous leukoplakia* is the obviously abnormal, changed, rough surface with nodular warts or sometimes papillomalike lesions (Figs. 18-1 to 18-4, 18-6 to 18-10, 18-14, and 18-16). The verrucous leukoplakia makes up about 25% of all oral leukoplakias. Its transformation rate is less than that of the erosive form.

The often-encountered, not-well-delimited erosive leukoplakia as a rule shows a very irregular configuration and a heavily spotted surface where there are whitish areas interspersed with reddish, erosive lesions (Figs. 18-11 to 18-13, 18-15 and 18-17). The transformation rate is given as 38%.

Clinical signs of a threatening malignant transformation are:

- Increased inflammatory changes under the leukoplakia and/or in the adjacent mucosa
- Chronic candidiasis
- Worsening of epithelial changes with an increased tendency for keratinization and/or erosion

The clinical picture becomes more striking through these changes. The differential diagnosis between a precancerous leukoplakia and a *carcinoma in situ (intraepithelial carcinoma)* is not possible clinically because these early stages of cancer can be diagnosed by pathologic examination only when all criteria of carcinoma, with the exception of stromal invasion, are present. Carcinoma in situ is discussed in chapter 19.

Precancerous leukoplakia of the floor of the mouth and border of the tongue often undergoes malignant transformation. Other high-risk zones are the lower lip and cheek mucosa.

People over 50 years of age are among those affected, and males are at higher risk. With increased life expectancy, the frequency of transformation into cancer increases. The same risk factors that also affect the development of oral cavity cancers (smoking, alcohol consumption, lack of oral hygiene) facilitate the development of precancerous leukoplakias.

Reddish oral leukoplakias are rare and are called *erythroplakias* (ICD-DA 528.70). Analogous to leukoplakias is the clinically defined red spot that cannot be associated with any other disease. Erythroplakia located at the level of mucosa is usually a well-delimited dark red lesion with a finely granular surface (Fig. 18-18). The dark red color is caused by increased vascularity. Following mechanical irritation is slight bleeding. Mixed forms of leukoplakia/erythroplakia can occur. Microscopic evaluation uses dysplasia criteria because they are relevant to the divisions of leukoplakia. Histopathologically, erythroplakias correspond more often to a carcinoma in situ or even an invasive cancer (see chapter 19).

Final considerations for the dentist

A step-by-step approach should be used in diagnosis and treatment of leukoplakia-like lesions. First, there is mechanical irritation leukoplakia, possibly with a central erosive lesion, that requires elimination of all irritative factors. Differential diagnosis must also take into consideration manifestations on the oral mucosa of lichen planus in its erosive or erosive-atrophic forms; in cases of doubt, clarification is necessary.

If the clinical report indicates heavy colonization with *Candida albicans*, local antimycotic therapy should be introduced. After regression of the *Candida*-induced inflammation, in many cases there is reappearance of the original homogeneous leukoplakia.

If several different causes have been eliminated and if there is still a tendency for lesions to recur, all clinical findings must be considered precancerous – as opposed to simple leukoplakias – and must without exception be clarified with histologic studies. Small leukoplakia foci are removed *in toto* for this purpose. With large leukoplakias, an incisional biopsy is performed at a particularly suspicious area of the lesion.

If histologic examination determines there is no reason to suspect malignancy but rather epithelial dysplasia, the patient is seen for cancer prophylaxis at regular intervals. If during follow-up there is again suspicion of malignancy, another biopsy may become necessary.

Correct biopsy technique and follow-up with evaluation of lesion progression require much clinical experience.

Above all, the dentist must ensure that competent specialists perform the differential diagnosis and supervision of patients with precancerous leukoplakias.

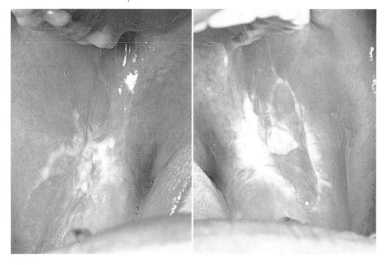

Fig. 18-1   Bilateral precancerous verruciform leukoplakia in the retromolar region in a 51-year-old man. In addition to plaque-like areas of milky opalescence, raised wartlike zones are present. Histologically there is no evidence of impending malignant changes of the epithelial layers.

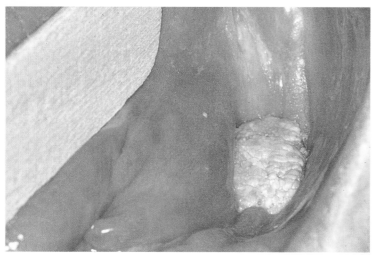

Fig. 18-2   Precancerous verruciform leukoplakia on the edentulous mandibular process of a 62-year-old woman. The excision of the wartlike formation in toto is indicated. Histologic findings: leukoplakia with intermediate-grade epithelial dysplasia. Careful supervision is needed because on other areas of the oral leukoplakia foci are present that are not yet clinically suspicious.

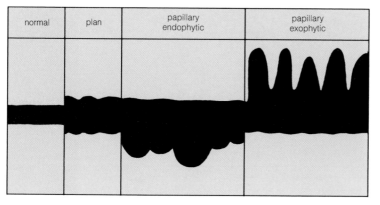

normal	plan	papillary endophytic	papillary exophytic

Fig. 18-3   Types of leukoplakias with tendency to show growth. In flat, homogeneous leukoplakia, the surface is smooth and the hyperplasia of the basal layer of the epithelium appears distinctly limited. In the papillary endophytic form, epithelial basal growth is directed downward whereas the papillomatous exophytic growth extends toward the lumen of the oral cavity. (From: Mittermayer C., Riede UN., Härle F.: Präkanzerose der Mundhöhle. Frankfurt: M Hoechst AG 1980:19.)

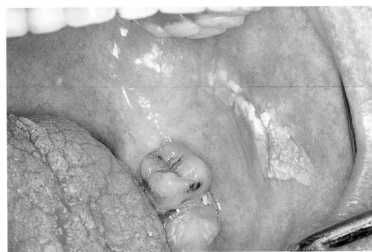

Fig. 18-4 Typical verrucous form of a precancerous leukoplakia of the cheek mucosa. The 68-year-old patient reported that he first noted the changes 2 years ago. Histologic examination: leukoplakia with low grade of epithelial dysplasia.

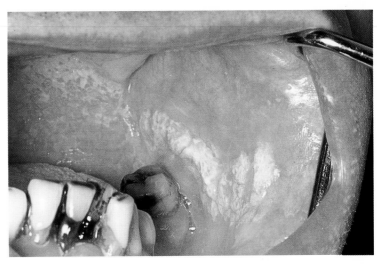

Fig. 18-5 Symmetrically distributed, faintly spotted, clinically precancerous, suspicious, large leukoplakia of the cheek mucosa with wartlike elevations. The 62-year-old patient was a heavy smoker (also note the leukokeratosis on the palate) and had neglected occlusal relationships (risk factors). After a drastic decrease in smoking and improved oral hygiene, the changes regressed.

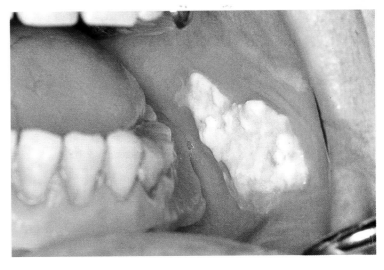

Fig. 18-6 Verrucous form of a precancerous leukoplakia of the cheek mucosa. Only after the appearance of massive hyperkeratosis did the 70-year-old woman seek medical help. The surrounding area of bumpy, lumpy leukoplakia is clinically without inflammation. Histologic evaluation of the in toto excised lesion: leukoplakia with intermediate to high-grade epithelial dysplasia.

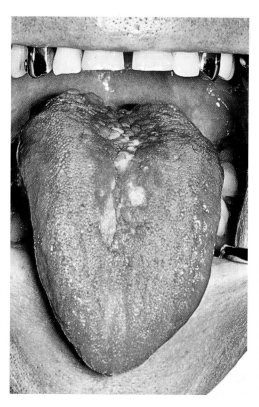

Fig. 18-7   Precancerous leukoplakia with palapable verrucous thickening that extends into the area of the median rhomboid glossitis on the dorsum of the tongue in a 45-year-old man. Histologic examination indicated a multifocal precancerous condition without malignancy.

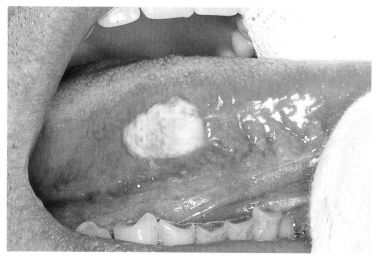

Fig. 18-8   Slablike elevated precancerous leukoplakia of verrucous type on the right tongue border of a 57-year-old woman. Histologic findings: leukoplakia with intermediate-grade epithelial dysplasias. These lesions are to be removed and evaluated in toto, because precancerous leukoplakias on the border of the tongue often contain a cancer.

Fig. 18-9   Large precancerous leukoplakia with a wrinkled, fissured surface on the lower lip of a 69-year-old woman.

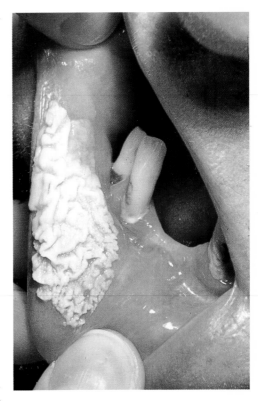

Fig. 18-10   Large, cauliflower-like precancerous leukoplakia of the cheek mucosa in a 50-year-old woman. The keratinized, white-red surface shows tooth impressions. With this type of finding, a biopsy with the aid of frozen sections is indicated in most cases. For example, the pathologist's report might read: "tissue of the left cheek measuring 3 × 2 × 0.5 cm oval biopsy piece with cauliflower-like rough whitish surface and central 1 × 1.5 cm measuring defects (after previous biopsy). The tissue is completely cut into sections. Microscopically, the tissue on the surface is covered by a thick layer of squamous epithelium. On average, the lesion is almost 3-mm thick. The papillae are greatly elongated. The epithelium tends to maintain its polarity. There are few individual dyskeratotic cells. At the base of the lesion is a bandlike lymphocytic infiltrate, and on the surface is a distinct hyperkeratosis. This is a leukoplakia with focal epithelial dysplasia. No areas suggestive or diagnostic of malignancy have been found. Stepwise cuts of the more abnormal area show foci of moderate dysplasia with bud-forming basal proliferations. In these areas the inflammatory infiltrate is more severe. The dysplasias in lesser development appear up to the surgical margin. There is no definitive evidence of malignancy. The patient should remain under observation." (Published with permission of Prof. Dr. W. Hort, formerly Director of Pathology of the Institute of Heinrich-Heine, University of Düsseldorf.)

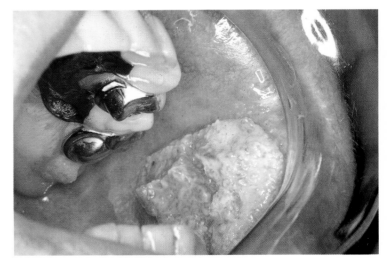

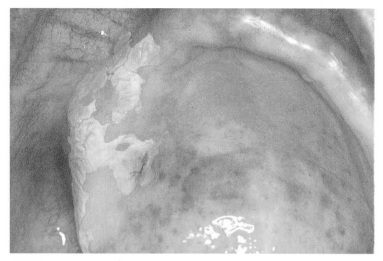

Fig. 18-11   Flat leukoplakia (with irregular pseudopod-like contour) in the area of the right edentulous maxilla; extensive occurrence on the vestibular side of the palate. An erosive lesion can be distinguished in the middle of the whitish change on the palate. A biopsy specimen was taken from this area. Pathologists findings: leukoplakia with single demonstrable focus of low-grade epithelial dysplasia.

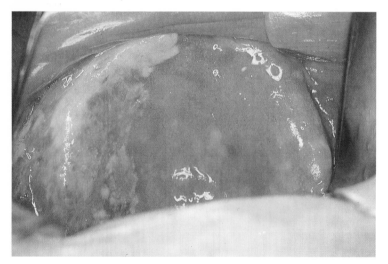

Fig. 18-12   In part flat, in part spotty *Candida*-infected leukoplakia in the area of the right edentulous maxilla. After antimycotic local treatment and improved prosthetic hygiene there was regression of the changes so that at the time there was no need to perform a biopsy of the extended homogeneous leukoplakia. Periodic follow-up examinations are indicated.

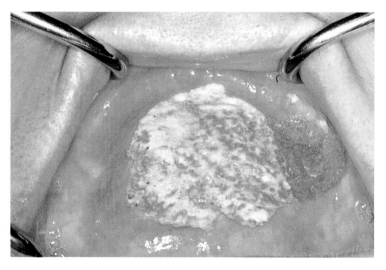

Fig. 18-13   Flat precancerous leukoplakia of the palatal mucosa covered with thrush colonization. The colorful clinical picture showing focal hyperkeratosis and foci of erosion is greatly suspect. The biopsy material removed in several areas showed a pathologic leukoplakia with intermediate to high–grade epithelial dysplasia as well as a demonstration of fungus threads. Complete surgical removal of the lesion is indicated as a prophylactic measure.

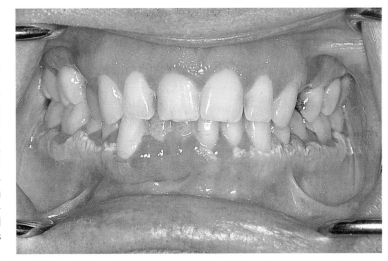

Fig. 18-14   Gingival manifestation of a multifocal leukoplakia of the oral mucosa. The mostly paramarginal change in several points was in small nodules. Pathologic evaluation of the biopsy specimen of the gingival leukoplakia revealed basal cell hyperplasia as an expression of a mild dysplasia. In such extensive findings (gingiva, cheek, palate, and tongue), medical treatment is justified.

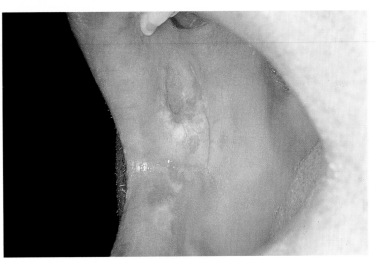

Fig. 18-15   Retroangular precancerous leukoplakia of the erosive type in a 43-year-old woman. These findings, particularly in the mechanically functional area of the angle of the mouth, are often clinically difficult to evaluate (see also "Angle of the mouth and leukoplakias" in chapter 34). Pathologic evaluation: leukoplakia with intermediate grade of epithelial dysplasia as well as additional traumatic tissue damage.

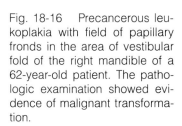
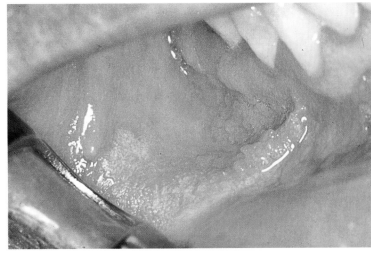

Fig. 18-16   Precancerous leukoplakia with field of papillary fronds in the area of vestibular fold of the right mandible of a 62-year-old patient. The pathologic examination showed evidence of malignant transformation.

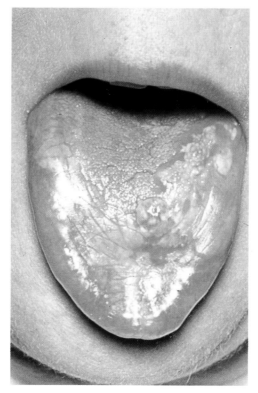

Fig. 18-17   Precancerous leukoplakia of the dorsum of the
tongue in a 49-year-old woman
who had a geographic tongue
since youth. On an atrophic
mucosa in the area of the tip of
the tongue are whitish leukopla-
kic plaques side by side with
isolated, palpable hyperkeratotic areas and circumscribed
erosive lesions. This patient was
examined 25 years previously
and the histologic diagnosis at
that time was: leukoplakia,
signs of Bowen's disease evident in some areas. According
to today's nomenclature, this
corresponds to a leukoplakia
with a high grade of epithelial
dysplasia and transition to a
carcinoma in situ.

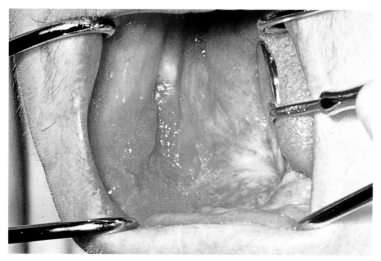

Fig. 18-18   This is clinically
considered a erythroplakia in
the area of the right edentulous
mandible and the bordering
cheek mucosa of a 67-year-old
woman. At the level of the mucosa are wet shimmering red
lesions with a finely granular
surface sharply separated from
the surrounding area. Histologic evaluation: unchanged, as
biopsy of 2 years ago, no evidence of malignant changes.

Chapter 19

Carcinomas of the Oral Cavity and the Lips

Carcinoma in situ

Oral mucosal carcinoma

Carcinoma of the lip

One of every four Germans at the present time must expect that during his or her life he or she will be a diagnosed with cancer.

Two of every three families have to face the fact that a member of the family has cancer.

One third of all patients can expect that they will be living 5 years after the diagnosis.

(From Flatten G. Prävention–Eine bewährte Strategie ärztlichen-Handelns Wiss Reihe des Zentralinstitutes für die Kassenärztliche Versorgung in der Bundesrepublik Deutschland, vol. 41. Köln: Deutscher Ärzte-Verlag, 1988: 64.)

Reliable statistics show that in the year 2000 every third European will have had a cancer during his or her life. Cancerphobia is a noticeable problem for certain individuals and their approach to cancer prevention. An understanding of this disease can only be reached with better information on the causal relation of and constructive motivation to change certain habits and behaviors. Acceptance of preventive measures and early recognition and early treatment of cancer could dispel some of the fear about the disease. According to *H. zur Hausen*, German Cancer Center, Heidelberg, cancer (or at least numerous neoplastic diseases) is, in principle, preventable and curable.

The realization of this goal in the medical office is possible only through a continuous and intense preventive strategy. As in the past, many patients with cancer do not seek treatment until the stage of advanced disease. Except for certain forms of skin cancer, this means that the diagnosis of cancer is a death sentence within the following 5 years for 50% of those affected.

The etiology of cancer is very complex and still not completely understood. It is a consequence of changes in genetic makeup of a body cell (monoclonal development) that have untoward influences. To this must be added that genetic factors, which more often suppress than activate, play a role in cancer genesis. The development of cancer is a process of many steps (many steps theory). The initiation phase through exogenous and endogeneous injuries follows the promotion phase, in which activation and endogenous suppressive events lead to the derailment of cell growth that eventually becomes uncontrolled.

Based on research in virology, the infectious origin of cancer is extensively discussed. It is calculated today that about 15% of worldwide human cancer forms can be associated with viral infections. This depends on a process involving multiple steps and involves a latency period of 20 to 50 years. Primary liver cancer (hepatocellular carcinoma) is certainly associated with hepatitis B virus infection. Other examples are the association of retroviruses with T-cell leukemias and the association of Epstein-Barr virus with Burkitt's lymphoma and nasopharyngeal carcinoma. The oncogenic potency recognized a few years ago in a series on human papillomavirus is the subject of intense research in many laboratories. Further discoveries in the field of virology and molecular biology will possibly provide new light on the pathogenesis of oral cavity cancers.

Malignant epithelial tumors called carcinomas are the most relevant and definitely most frequent malignant neoplasms of the oral cavity and perioral region. Because of the lack of barriers to infiltrating destructive growth, they destroy normal tissue. Metastasis by seeding of tumor takes place through lymphatic transport first to regional (submandibular, submental) lymph nodes, and then to the cervical and supraclavicular lymph nodes. Based on anatomically determined crossover phenomena of the lymph circulation, it is possible that (for carcinoma of the tongue in particular) the development of contralateral lymph node metastases are of great clinical importance. A hematogenous tumor spread (from the thoracic duct into the venous system and therefore into the lungs or through direct tumor invasion of smaller vessels) occurs only rarely.

Epidemiology and classification

Epidemiologic data on oral cancer are not a statistical end but an important instrument for evaluation of risk factors and for research in the manifestations of the course as well as the therapeutic possibility of cancer. They include information on age and sex distribution, city and country distribution, and social layering.

In general, cancer statistically holds second place for mortality, following cardiovascular diseases, but it is unfortunately on the rise.

The illness rate is determined by the prevalence and incidence. *Prevalence* gives the frequency, for example, of oral cancer in a definite population either related to a point in time (target date) or to a time limit. Oral carcinomas make up 1% to 5% of all cancers found in Europe (Germany, 1.5%; Ireland, 5%). Because of other risk factors, the prevalence in India is over 40%.

Incidence calculates the number of *new illnesses* in a defined population during a limited time. In Germany each year 270,000 persons are affected by a new cancer, of which 3,500 have oral cancers or cancers of the face.

In development of oral cancer—besides some systemic diseases—alcohol and tobacco use and poor oral hygiene compose a *triad of risk factors*. We do not have accurate data today, as we do for lung cancer, to determine the individual importance of each factor in the development of oral cancer.

It is proven today that pipe or cigarette smokers have a 3.7 times higher risk of lung cancer than nonsmokers (1 time risk). The more serious of the two is cigarette smoking. The risk of lung cancer increases with the increased number of daily inhalations of cigarette smoke and is 18.6 times with 11 to 20 cigarettes/day and as high as 31.6 times with 21 to 35 cigarettes/day as compared to nonsmokers. The double load of habitual use of alcohol and habitual smoking increases the incidence of oral, throat, and gastrointestinal tract cancers 20 to 40 times in relation to a nonsmoking and nondrinking individual.

In regard to sex distribution, men are still affected more frequently than women, particularly for lip and tongue carcinomas.

Cancer is a disease that, as a rule, appears only after the fiftieth year. Eighty percent of all patients with carcinoma in our specialty are between 50 and 80 years old. The average is in the sixth decade.

The clinical classification of carcinomas based on pre-, intra-, and postoperative findings today follows standard international rules. In view of the exchange of information among medical centers, the important and useful TNM staging system (T = tumor; N = node; M = metastasis) has been developed. Special points of the fourth edition (1987) of the updated classification are presented in Table 1 along with the UICC (Union Internationale Contre le Cancer) worldwide accepted definitions for carcinomas of the oral cavity and squamous cell carcinomas of the vermilion of the lip.

Table 1   TNM: Clinical classification

T – Primary tumor

TX	Primary tumor cannot be evaluated
T0	No basis for primary tumor
Tis	Carcinoma in situ
T1	Tumor 2 cm or smaller
T2	Tumor larger than 2 cm but not more than 4 cm at largest diameter
T3	Tumor larger than 4 cm at largest diameter
T4	*Lip:* tumor infiltrates neighboring structures such as cortical bone, tongue, or throat
	Oral cavity: tumor infiltrates neighboring structures such as cortical bone, skeletal muscle of the tongue, jaws, or skin

N – Regional lymph nodes

NX	Regional lymph nodes cannot be evaluated
N0	No regional lymph node metastasis
N1	Metastasis in solitary ipsilateral lymph nodes 3 cm or less in size
N2	Metastases in solitary ipsilateral lymph nodes larger than 3 cm but not more than 6 cm in size, or in multiple ipsilateral lymph nodes, none larger than 6 cm; or in bilateral or contralateral lymph nodes, none larger than 6 cm in extension
N2a	Metastasis in solitary ipsilateral lymph nodes larger than 3 cm, not more than 6 cm in extension
N2b	Metastases in multiple ipsilateral lymph nodes, none larger than 6 cm in extension
N2c	Metastases in bilateral or contralateral lymph nodes, none larger than 6 cm in extension
N3	Metastases in lymph nodes larger than 6 cm in extension

M – Distant metastasis

MX	Existence of distant metastases cannot be evaluated
M0	No distant metastasis
M1	Distant metastasis

The tumor formula, T1N1M0, indicates that the primary tumor is 2 cm or less at its largest diameter with a metastasis in a single lymph node on the side of a tumor and not larger than 3 cm at its greatest measurements without demonstrable metastasis at a distance.

The tumor formula allows further group division in stages (Table 2).

Table 2   Stage grouping

Stage 0	Tis	N0	M0
Stage I	T1	N0	M0
Stage II	T2	N0	M0
Stage III	T3	N0	M0
	T1	N1	M0
	T2	N1	M0
	T3	N1	M0
Stage IV	T4	N0, N1	M0
	each T	N2, N3	M0
	each T	each N	M1

When combined with the general health condition of the patient and the determination of the risk factors, these parameters form the basis of preoperative evaluation.

Clinical evaluation also uses the categories of the TNM system of the corresponding pathologic classification (pTNM). The well-differentiated squamous cell carcinoma is at present by far the most frequent form of cancer in the oral cavity. Nonkeratinizing squamous cell carcinoma is the term used to describe tumors lacking cornification but with the presence of intercellular bridges. This cancer, in which prickle cells predominate, is less differentiated and in its clinical behavior is considered more malignant than the keratinizing squamous cell carcinoma. The highest grade of nondifferentiation is shown by the undifferentiated (anaplastic) carcinoma with many atypical cells and mitoses. Its differentiation from sarcomas presents histologic problems that, thanks to progress in immunohistochemistry, can today be overcome. Carcinomas found in the oral cavity are classified according to their differentiation (histopathologic grading of the UICC-−see Table 3).

Table 3 **Histopathologic grading**

GX	Differentiation level cannot be determined
G1	Well differentiated
G2	Intermediate differentiation
G3	Poorly differentiated
G4	Anaplastic

The relevant diagnostic and therapy data should be stored in order to compare treatment results and to allow the development of prognostic criteria.

The survival rate of cancer patients, in general reported as a *5-year survival rate*, establishes important prognostic factors. There is no doubt that the size of the tumor at the beginning of treatment is important in the success of cancer therapy. The 1973 therapy study of the German-Austrian-Swiss work group for tumors of the jaw and face region (DOSAK) strikingly demonstrates that about 80% of patients with a primary tumor size T1, about 50% of patients with a primary tumor size T2, and less than 30% of patients with a primary tumor size T3 survived for 5 years. Overall 5-year survival/cure rates at the moment are about 20% to 40%.

As in the past, about 70% of patients seek treatment during tumor stages II and III. Those data indicate that all the efforts of medical and dental continuing education of the past 30 years, as well as intensive media efforts, practically did not improve the rate of early detection of oral cavity cancers, and that a large percentage of patients arrive too late for therapy. This takes into consideration that extensive therapy did not considerably improve survival. Nevertheless, quality of life for patients could be improved through further development of treatment methods.

What is needed is an early detection program for the oral cavity cancer in which the following points are to be considered:

- By directed prevention (see chapters 17 and 18), the development of carcinomas can be prevented.
- Precancerous and early stages of oral cavity cancer are certainly accessible to a clinical diagnosis of suspicion (preliminary diagnosis). For diagnosis of invasive cancer and therapies, specially equipped centers are available.
- The significance of risk factors (tobacco and alcohol use, poor oral hygiene) must be intensively explained to lay persons and in an easily understandable manner.

- Dentists are the first to examine 60% to 80% of all patients with an oral cavity cancer and have a great responsibility. To justify this trust, they must further their education and knowledge.

Basis for early dental diagnosis

As long as carcinomas are not hidden under a precancerous leukoplakia, tumoral growth and typical tissue destruction are macromorphologic signs of an early carcinoma of the oral mucosa.

In the otherwise variable clinical picture, two tumor types can be distinguished:

- The *endophytic ulcerative carcinoma* where, in a relatively early stage, there is the formation of craterlike ulceration through a central colliquation of the tumor tissue
- The *exophytic papillomatous (verrucous) carcinoma growing above the mucosal surface*, which often has a cauliflower-like appearance with granular surface and a distinctly recognizable appearance

The particular growth pattern of each tumor, whether endophytic or exophytic, tends to persist throughout the clinical course.

For early recognition of oral mucosal carcinoma, the oral cavity offers almost ideal conditions because all tumor findings are accessible to the eye and to palpation. Examination of the oral mucosa should be done with the same systematic approach and care used for examination of the dentition.

During inspection it is important to note the structural and/or superficial color changes (for example, ulcerations with raised borders, circumscribed thickening, atrophic mucosal areas, or wartlike formations). It is particularly necessary to observe the hidden areas of the oral cavity (floor of the mouth, dorsal border of the tongue, base of the tongue) because discrete pathologic findings can easily escape detection there.

Of great importance is palpation, which should follow inspection. Independent of the clinical appearance of a carcinoma, even for a small one, is the recognition that there is an increase of hard tissue in contrast to the surrounding mucosa. This is also the called "cancer-like" characteristic induration of the neoplastic tissue, which makes the transition from normal mucosa to the tumor very noticeable by palpation. Because with ulcerative carcinomas the wall-like border of the ulceration is made up of active growing tumor tissue (see Fig. 19-24), it is possible to feel thick-to-hard tissue on the ulcer base. Growths in the surrounding area can also be studied by palpation.

Another important examination step, to be used in cases of doubt, is comparison of a healthy side with the abnormal side (symmetric comparison).

Oral mucosal carcinomas generally are not painful. With the appearance of tissue necrosis, superimposed infection of the tumor is likely to occur and this can produce pain. Therefore, pain on pressure of palpation does not negate the presence of a tumor. Pain can result from the effects of the expanding tumor on the surrounding area (reduced ability to open the mouth, swallowing disturbance, irradiating neuralgic-like pain). Colliquating and necrotic oral mucosal carcinomas often have a characteristic smell.

Palpation of the submandibular and cervical lymph nodes is imperative in the event of tumor suspicion. Hard, matted lymph nodes are highly suspicious. Pressure pain in this area also does not negate the presence of a tumor. Additionally, the lack of enlarged lymph nodes is not evidence that metastasis has not taken place. The diagnosis can be difficult and requires great clinical experience.

Radiographs are not very useful for the early detection of oral cavity carcinomas, because the bone generally is only involved in advanced tumors (the destruction of the limiting bone manifests itself radiographically in a fuzzy limited clearing). Clinically there are other findings to consider to study tumors in deep tissue layers.

Although in this chapter we discuss only primary carcinomas of the oral mucosa and lips, for the sake of completeness, nonhealing extraction wounds with "granulations" growing out of the alveolus, as well as isolated loose teeth in an otherwise healthy dentition free of periodontal disease, may raise the suspicion of a growing deep tumor. In the posterior region of the maxilla, these changes are not uncommon as a consequence of carcinoma that destroys the alveolar bone and grows into the oral mucosa toward the oral cavity.

The dentist must be alert to *all* suspicious findings on the lip and the skin area of the perioral region. Special points to consider in this regard are discussed in the text and figures.

From experience, oral cavity carcinomas are often misinterpreted as chronic inflammatory lesions caused by mechanically irritative factors (e.g., at a prosthetic pressure point or at a so-called scrubbing point). A differential diagnosis problem not to be underestimated is a traumatic ulcer of long duration, the border of which is thickened because it has been infiltrated by chronic inflammatory cells and where surrounding mucosa shows leukoplakial changes. Based on the fast regeneration tendency of well-vascularized oral mucosa, these ulcerations generally heal in 8 to 14 days after removal of the irritating factor. If no healing occurs, there is always the possibility of a malignant lesion to consider, and further diagnostic studies with referral cannot be delayed. To give the dentist practical suggestions on the causative diagnosis, we have prepared a series of photographs of traumatic, inflamed ulcers to compare with the ulcerated carcinoma.

Information about the lesion provided by the patient is often unreliable, and patients' interpretations of nonmalignancy should not be accepted beforehand by the dentist. The dentist should rely on his or her own interpretation. Critical evaluation also depends on the observation of other health conditions.

Inspection, palpation, and in some cases the short time of development are cornerstones of early dental diagnosis. By making a tentative diagnosis of malignancy and immediately referring the patient, the dentist makes an extraordinarily important contribution in the area of early cancer detection. All other subsequent diagnostic and therapeutic measures belong in the hands of a specially equipped clinic. Because of the dangers of tumor cell spread, diagnostic difficulties, postoperative edema, and possible superinfection of the tumor, a biopsy should not be done in the dental office. The invasive diagnosis should be done by the person who will perform the tumor surgery, the accompanying oncologic therapy, and the follow-up.

Carcinoma in situ (ICD-DA 230.0); intraepithelial squamous carcinoma (ICD-DA 8070/2)

Carcinomas of the oral mucosa develop predominantly from an inconspicuous mucosal lesion. About 30% of oral cavity carcinomas develop over a previously existing mucosal change, of which precancerous leukoplakias are the most frequent conditions.

When all histomorphopathologic diagnostic criteria of a carcinoma (with exception of the invasive growth) are present, it is called a carcinoma in situ, that is, an intraepithelial carcinoma. It is highly probable that an invasive carcinoma with possibility of metastases will develop within 5 years. The diagnosis of carcinoma in situ can be made only by histologic examination. Differentiating a precancerous leukoplakia, a carcinoma in situ, and the early stages of an invasive carcinoma is not possible clinically.

The clinical appearance of a histologically proven intraepithelial carcinoma is shown in Figs. 19-1 to 19-6.

Certain conditions that were previously called Bowen's disease (ICD-DA 8081/2) now fall under carcinomas in situ. *Florid oral papillomatosis* can also be considered an in situ carcinoma.

Oral carcinoma, squamous cell carcinoma (ICD-M 8070/3), squamous cell carcinoma, keratinizing type (ICD-M 8071/3), verrucous carcinoma (ICD-M 8051/3)

Regarding the clinical conditions of oral mucosal carcinoma, it can simplistically be said that its malignancy also depends on its location in the oral cavity, that is, whether it increases from the front to the back, and from top down (hence, from anterior to posterior, and cranial to caudal).

Pictorial documentation can establish a certain arrangement depending on findings on the upper level, lateral spread, and lower level. The topographically codified location indicated in parenthesis (location key) represents the current international classification of malignant neoplasms.

Upper level

Carcinomas of the upper level can be divided further into:

- Carcinomas in the area of the upper alveolar process (ICD-O 143.0) and gingiva (ICD-O 143.9): see Figs. 19-8, 19-10 to 19-13, 19-18, 19-19, and 5-23 as well as differential diagnosis examples in Figs. 19-9 to 19-17 (primary jaw cavity carcinomas) and 19-14.
- Carcinomas in the area of the hard palate (ICD-O 145.2) and the soft palate (ICD-O 145.3): see Figs. 19-23, 19-25, 19-27, and 19-28 as well as the differential diagnostic examples of Figs. 19-15, 19-16, and 19-26.

Lateral spread

Carcinomas of the cheek mucosa (ICD-O 145.0) are shown in Figs. 19-7, 19-20, and 19-30; differential diagnosis examples here are shown in Figs. 19-34 and 19-35. Attention should also be given to chapter 34, "Problematic Angle of the Mouth."

Lower level

The carcinomas presented here can be further subdivided into:

- Carcinoma in the area of the mandibular alveolar process (ICD-O 143.1): see Figs. 19-21 and 19-22.
- Carcinoma of the retromolar region (ICD-O 145.6): see Figs. 19-20, 19-31 to 19-33.
- Carcinoma of the floor of the mouth (ICD-O 144): see Figs. 19-36 to 19-41.
- Carcinoma of the tongue: dorsum and border of the tongue in front of the vallate papillae–anterior two thirds (ICD-O 141.1, 141.2); base of the tongue–posterior third (ICD-O 141.0); and underside of the tongue (ICD-O 141.3)–see Figs. 19-41, 19-43 to 19-50 and all examples of differential diagnosis in Figs. 19-42, 19-51 to 19-56. In relation to the location of oral carcinomas, the following general points must be considered, especially with the clinical findings report and differential diagnosis.

Carcinoma of the gingiva in the early stages is often confused with hyperplastic ulcerative gingivitis. The lesion rapidly involves the alveolar process and therefore results in early bony destruction and loosening of the teeth. Preferred points *on the edentulous alveolar process* are those areas with chronic irritations (for example, a retromolar region).

Carcinomas of the palate mucosa develop preferentially on the transition area of the hard and soft palate. In this location, the differential diagnosis includes malignant tumors of the small palatine salivary glands (see chapter 20). In each case the dentist should be suspicious when a prosthesis that has been used without problems suddenly offers difficulties. On the other hand, it must be considered that patients with a prosthesis that has functioned for many years may not pay adequate attention to changes, particularly painless ones.

Carcinomas of the cheek mucosa are often preceded by precancerous leukoplakias. Pain and functional disturbances can occur very late in this area through infiltration of the neighboring structures. Thus there is the danger of a long undetected course.

Cancer of the floor of the mouth is one of the most malignant tumors of the oral cavity. The primary lesion on the anterior part of the floor of the mouth is often mistaken for a benign leukoplakial transformation or an inflamed ulcer in the area around the frenum of the tongue. Due to its fast rate of growth, it rapidly invades the dorsum and the body of the tongue or extends toward the central mandible. Bilateral lymph node metastases are not rare. In about two thirds of the carcinomas located in the posterior part of the floor of the mouth, metastases on the regional lymph nodes develop during the initial growth phase of the tumor. These cancers expand rapidly, particularly in the direction of the body of the tongue, base of the tongue, and arch of the palate (parapharyngeal space). Hence the omnious *palatal arch-tongue angle carcinoma* develops that is discovered too late. When jaw cramp is already present, the prognosis is very serious.

Carcinomas of the tongue are frequently found on the borders of the tongue and on the underside of the tongue, but they are rare at the tip of the tongue and anterior dorsum of the tongue. Recognizing carcinomas of the base of the tongue (dorsal third of the tongue) and of the pharynx requires a mirror technique. In cancer of the tongue there is a predominance of endophytic ulcerative growths. Corresponding to the complicated topography are different patterns of infiltration in the surrounding areas and of metastatic formation, which affects therapy and prognosis. A relatively early symptom of the extension of the tumor is the irradiation of pain toward the ear; a reduction of the mobility of the tongue as well as continuous pain are late signs. The peak incidence of the age curve for patients with tongue cancer is the fourth decade and thus is considerably earlier than oral carcinomas of other locations. The incidence of tongue cancer is dependent on life-style (drinking, smoking, use of spices, manner of food preparation, habits, oral hygiene), which is different in different parts of the world.

There is a problem of a completely different nature for dentists facing patients with tongue cancerphobia. Tongue cancer patients are more frequently men than women. The correct diagnosis, counseling, and supervision of these patients demand great clinical competence (see chapter 32).

Carcinoma of the lip (vermilion border) (ICD-O 140-0 and 140.1, ICD-M 8070/3)

Lip carcinoma is more frequent in older people, and here again men predominate (Figs. 19-57 to 19-59). The carcinomas start from the border of the vermilion of the lip, predominantly paramedian; about 90% are located in the lower lip.

In the development of the cancer, previous tissue damage plays a great role. Weather and light influences (UV irradiation) are responsible for early changes, especially in people who work outdoors. Repetitive mechanical, chemical, and thermal irritations (for example smoking) are important in this area too.

Lip carcinomas can start clinically as small lesions, initially appearing as flat ulcers or hyperkeratosis or as nodular thickenings, from which a hard infiltrate and then a larger ulcer usually covered with a crust develop. Corresponding to other endophytic or exophytic growths are different clinical findings (deep craterlike ulcerations with a wavelike, raised hard border and indurated surroundings; papillomatous cauliflower growth). With early (surgical) therapy, the prognosis is good, because lip carcinomas grow slowly and metastasize late.

Lip carcinomas are similar to skin carcinomas and mucosal carcinomas. The following should be reported:

Squamous cell carcinomas of the skin of the face appear predominantly in damaged skin areas (among others, burn scars and actinic, chemical, thermal, and inflammatory permanent injuries of the epidermis).

In relation to skin carcinomas, basal cell carcinomas (ICD-M 8090/3 NOS) characteristically grow on the skin of the elderly, infiltrating and destroying but not producing metastases. Single or multiple basal cell carcinomas originating in primary germ cells of the skin epithelium (pluripotent basal cells) do not have a common appearance. They can be divided clinically into different types (nodular, ulcerated = ulcus rodens; multicentric-superficial = atrophic-scarring; destroying = ulcus terebrans) from other special forms that will not be discussed here.

In general, therapeutic success depends on intervention at the right time. The surgical procedure allows histologic control of the borders and offers, as opposed to the findings after radiation therapy, favorable prospects for reconstruction. If, however, the slow-growing basal cell carcinoma remains untreated for several years and there is extensive involvement with destruction of soft tissue and bone, therapy will not be possible.

Because 90% of basal cell carcinomas appear on the skin of the face (particularly above the mouth: upper lip, eyelid, nose, nasolabial fold, cheek, forehead, neck, ear), the dentist should, during extraoral inspection, pay attention to suspicious skin changes in these areas (Figs. 19-60 to 19-62) and initiate appropriate referral for their treatment.

Final considerations for the dentist

Most patients with oral cavity cancer still seek treatment too late. Independent of the primary delay caused by the patient, there is a second loss of time during which the dentist/physician initiates appropriate steps. Delay of referral by the dentist or the physician is, in two thirds of cases, caused by incorrect diagnosis, followed by unwarranted therapy based on it.

Symptomatic treatment leads to aggravating mistakes and tragic loss of time. In addition to nonrecognition of the condition of the tumors for weeks and months, there are delays of up to 14 days despite the lack of therapeutic success and the suspicion of the tumor that should have taken place. When unclear ulcerations and infiltrations remain after removal of the suspected irritation (for example, sharp tooth corners in an ulcer of the border of the tongue), systematic control of the findings in short intervals should be omitted and further diagnostic procedures initiated. Malignancies growing from the depth of the dentulous alveolar process have been wrongly attributed to tooth mobility and tooth movement as well as nonhealing extraction wounds.

In tumors found under prostheses—usually considered to be caused by pressure—causes and effects are confused, and the prosthesis is continually adapted to the growing tumor.

In all cases of doubt, it is better to observe a developing ulcerative or proliferative tissue process over a few days with careful and critical regular control than to act with hasty symptomatic treatment of an uncertain differential diagnosis incorrectly conceived. In such cases, painting or rinsing and wide-spectrum antibiotics should not be used because they may confuse the clinical picture and give the dentist and patient a false sense of security. In all unclear findings, one should never persist in the working diagnosis but should always be willing to revise the decision if the course of the disease requires such a step.

Only exact documentation of findings allows for secure, sufficiently thoughtful support and with that the basis for the correct evaluation of the course of the disease. A photograph is of great help here.

Lack of concern, lack of self-criticism, and insecurity are avoidable impediments on the way to a correct diagnosis. In cases of doubt, a clinic equipped for consultation with neighboring specialities is called for. The dentist should not be afraid to obtain advice and early consultation from others regarding problematic-appearing ulcerations and proliferative tissue changes. It is better to make one referral too many than to have missed the right occasion.

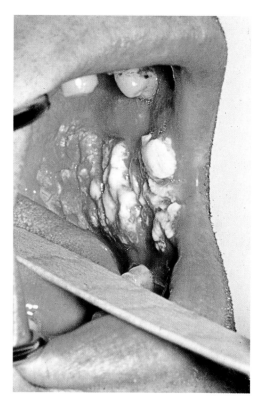

Fig. 19-1   Carcinoma in situ of the left cheek mucosa in a 55-year-old woman. Polymorphous mucosal findings with chalk-white, rugged elevations in the anterior part and more bedlike exophytic nodules on the posterior third of the cheek. An advanced precancerous lesion consistent with Bowen's disease was found on histologic examination. By today's terminology, this lesion is a carcinoma in situ (see chapter 18).

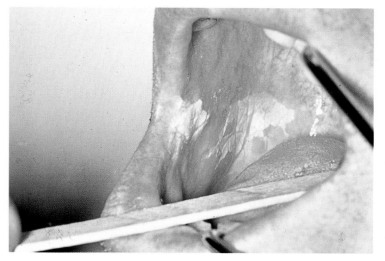

Fig. 19-2   The patient in Fig. 19-1 also at examination. There is a flat, homogeneous leukoplakia in the retroangular and middle region of the right cheek mucosa that was not considered histologically suspicious. The whitish spots were observed by the patient 3 years before. In the course of routine dental examination, a symmetric comparison should have provided an important early demonstration of a threatening change of the left mucosal side.

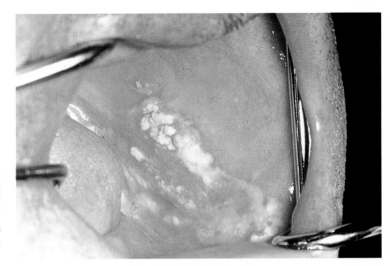

Fig. 19-3   Histologically confirmed carcinoma in situ with a clinical picture of severe, spotty leukoplakia of the cheek mucosa. On the other side was a soft flat homogeneous leukoplakia.

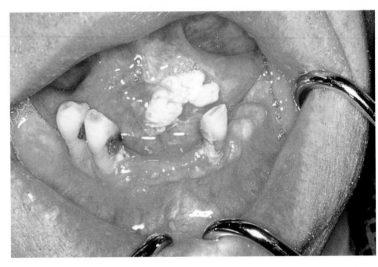

Fig. 19-4   Histologically confirmed carcinoma in situ on the anterior area of the floor of the mouth. Clinically there was a precancerous leukoplakia with chalk-white nodules that had been observed by the 65-year-old woman 2 years previously; valuable time was lost.

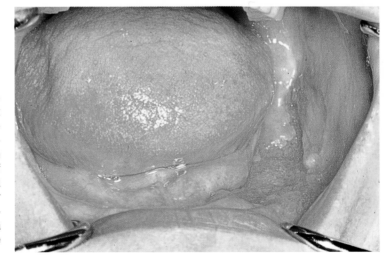

Fig. 19-5   This was considered a papillomatous change at the time in the area of the edentulous left mandible of a 61-year-old woman. The flat lesion depressed below the level of the healthy mucosa shows a fine corny surface with irregular borders. The suspicion of an invasive growing carcinoma could not be confirmed at the time of examination.

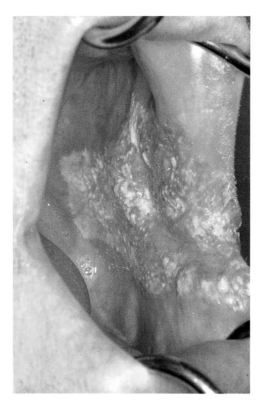

Fig. 19-6   Histologically confirmed carcinoma in situ (earlier denomination was Bowen's disease) of the cheek mucosa. According to the 65-year-old patient, the whitish areas had been there for over 10 years. Note the partly nodular, partly wartlike leukoplakia-like changes interspersed with erosive zones. The "polymorphous picture" of a leukoplakia should raise the clinical suspicion of a threatening change. Histologically there are not, as yet, signs of an invasive carcinoma.

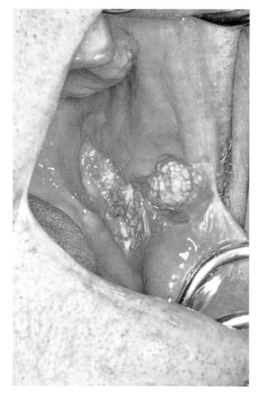

Fig. 19-7   Keratinized squamous cell carcinoma arising from a precancerous leukoplakia of the cheek mucosa in a 71-year-old patient. Note the ulcerated surface and the already visible wall-like hard raised border zone in the depth of the cheek musculature next to the wartlike leukoplakia area.

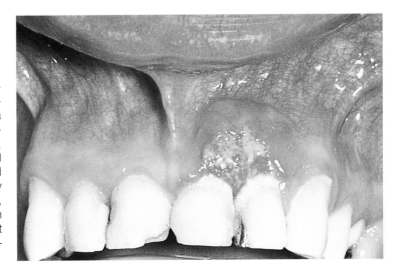

Fig. 19-8 Keratinized squamous call carcinoma on the alveolar process on the gingiva of teeth 21 and 22 (8, 9). According to the 39-year-old man, the lesion slowly spread toward the mucolabial fold and had been present for approximately 4 months. In this case, too, "gingival paintings" had been carried out before the patient was referred to a specialist (iatrogenic time loss).

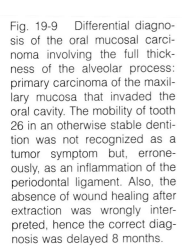
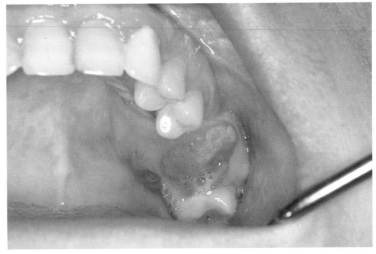

Fig. 19-9 Differential diagnosis of the oral mucosal carcinoma involving the full thickness of the alveolar process: primary carcinoma of the maxillary mucosa that invaded the oral cavity. The mobility of tooth 26 in an otherwise stable dentition was not recognized as a tumor symptom but, erroneously, as an inflammation of the periodontal ligament. Also, the absence of wound healing after extraction was wrongly interpreted, hence the correct diagnosis was delayed 8 months.

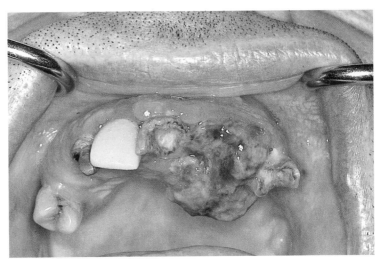

Fig. 19-10 Keratinized squamous cell carcinoma of the maxillary alveolar process with extensive necrosis. On the incorrect assumption of the presence of an epulis that induced tooth mobility, tooth 22 (9) was removed and part of the tumor excised in this 63-year-old patient. The mistaken diagnosis was followed by incorrect therapy and omission of the always-advisable histologic examination of the surgical specimen.

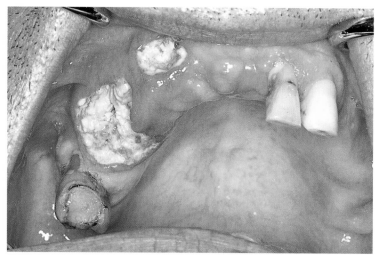

Fig. 19-11   Advanced endo-phytic keratinized squamous cell carcinoma on the edentulous maxillary alveolar process in the area of teeth 13 to 16 (3 to 6). The tumor was larger than 6 cm. According to the 54-year-old patient, the "tumor" had been present for 14 days. Time data given on previous histories are usually unreliable. Patients requiring oral hygiene or having mucosal-based prostheses often are careless and delay seeking medical advice until after the appearance of mucosal changes.

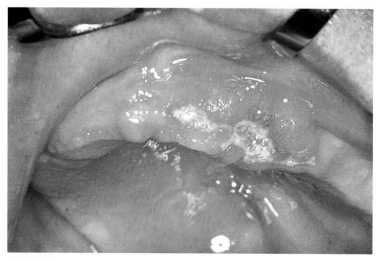

Fig. 19-12   Keratinizing squamous cell carcinoma of the edentulous alveolar process of the left side of the maxilla. Central bean-sized ulcer with actively growing, raised, firm margin surrounded by leukoplakia. The chronic mechanical irritation of the denture must be considered as a causative factor.

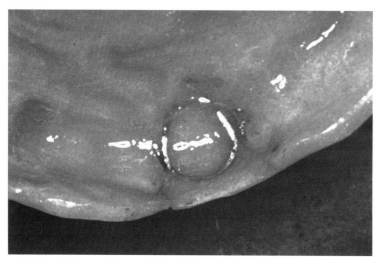

Fig. 19-13   Partial view of the complete maxillary denture of the patient in Fig. 19-13. The gold crown has been incorrectly inserted into the denture base, resulting in irritation from the sharp margin. The denture had been worn day and night. In individuals wearing prostheses, the tolerance toward changes in the prosthesis-bearing areas is always surprising.

Fig. 19-14 Differential diagnosis of ulcerated carcinoma of oral mucosa: mechanically conditioned ulcer (pressure point) in the area of mucosal fold of the edentulous maxilla caused by an ill-fitting prosthesis border. The ulcer of short duration shows an inflammatory hyperemic border zone with unremarkable palpation findings. With chronic pressure ulceration, the inflammatory infiltrate increases on the border of the ulcer. It feels hard, making the differential diagnosis with a carcinomatous ulcer difficult. Evaluation of the mucosal findings after correction of the prosthesis (in special cases, removal of the prosthesis until the control visit) is important and cannot be decided by the patient.

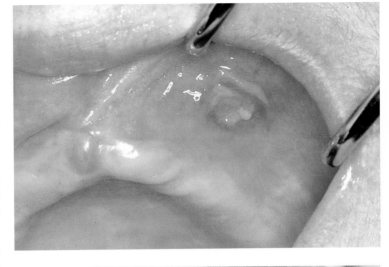

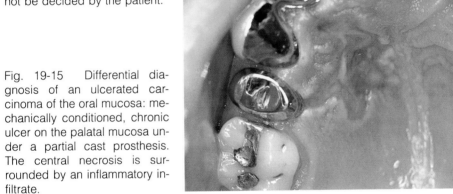

Fig. 19-15 Differential diagnosis of an ulcerated carcinoma of the oral mucosa: mechanically conditioned, chronic ulcer on the palatal mucosa under a partial cast prosthesis. The central necrosis is surrounded by an inflammatory infiltrate.

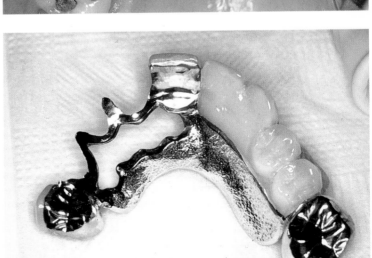

Fig. 19-16 The removable prosthesis of the patient in Fig. 19-15. The findings must clear up within 14 days without use of the prosthesis. If there is no healing of the ulceration within this time, other diagnostic measures should be initiated and the patient referred.

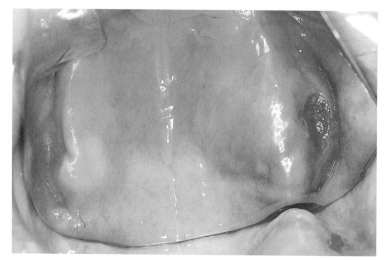

Fig. 19-17   Bulging in the tuberosity of the left edentulous maxilla due to extension into the oral cavity of a primary squamous cell carcinoma of the maxillary sinus. The prosthesis, which had been worn for years without problems, was adjusted with continuous removal of pressure spots. A symmetric comparison would have demonstrated early the need for radiographic evaluation. Carcinomas of the oral cavity are often diagnosed only in advanced stages. The prognosis is therefore much worse than with oral mucosa carcinomas.

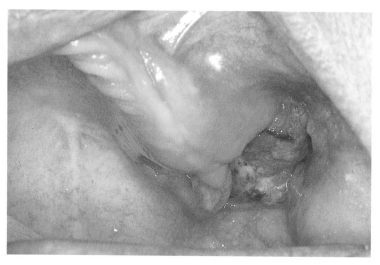

Fig. 19-18   Advanced keratinizing squamous cell carcinoma of the oral mucosa on the left tuberosity of an edentulous 58-year-old patient. The tumor involved the bone and advanced to the alar palatal pit (with subsequent reduction of mouth opening). With the predominantly endophytic growing cancer with large central necrosis, there had been a waste of almost 1 year of time.

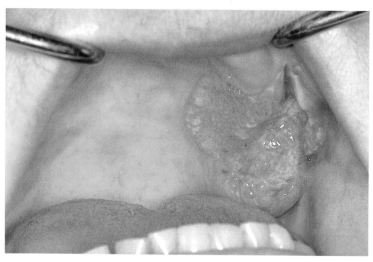

Fig. 19-19   Advanced, predominantly exophytic, squamous cell carcinoma of the oral mucosa on the left tuberosity. The prosthesis was incorrectly adjusted for the 68-year-old woman with shortening, rebasing, and border cuts. In this manner, diagnosis and therapy were delayed by months.

Fig. 19-20 Advanced keratinized squamous cell carcinoma in the retromolar region of the dentulous mandible. Tumor stage T3N0M0. The 42-year-old patient reported a feeling of tension on the mandibular left side followed by a more severe jaw spasm. The unbelievable time delay was due to unconscious denial. With the appearance of the necrosis was the unavoidable painful superimposed infection in the oral cavity. This inflammatory complication should not lead to a wrong diagnosis.

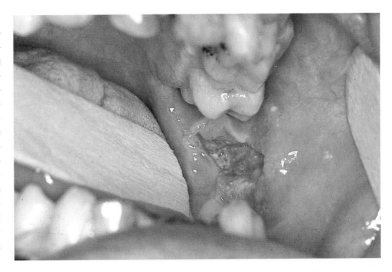

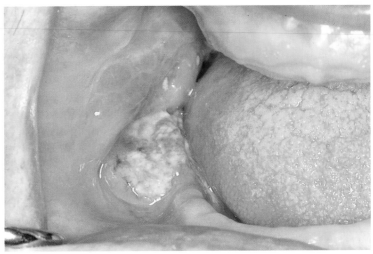

Fig. 19-21 Keratinized squamous cell carcinoma in the edentulous mandibular alveolar process. The 71-year-old woman had ignored the lesion for months. The tumor had already infiltrated the bone. The biopsy specimen confirmed the presence of an ipsilateral lymph node metastasis.

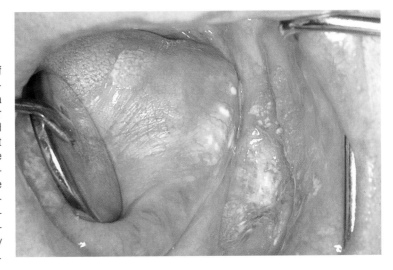

Fig. 19-22 Recurrence of squamous cell carcinoma arising from a leukoplakia in a 72-year-old woman. The tumor had been previously operated on elsewhere. At different points of the oral cavity were leukoplakias: in part flat homogeneous, in part verrucous. The region of the recidiva in the distal area of the edentulous mandibular alveolar process is characterized by the noticeably spotty, dotted mucosal change.

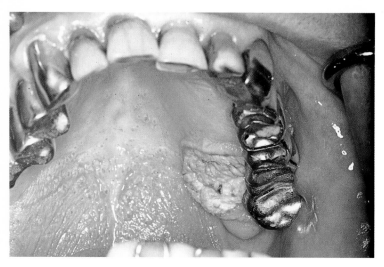

Fig. 19-23   Verrucous, well-differentiated, keratinizing squamous cell carcinoma of the mucosa of the hard palate. According to the 58-year-old pipe smoker, the change enlarged only slowly, which led him to think that it was due to a foreign body close to the fixed partial denture.

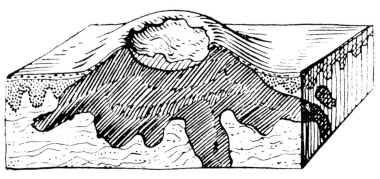

Fig. 19-24   Schematic representation of an ulcerated oral mucosal carcinoma. Typical for the oral mucosa carcinoma is the development of a central necrosis early in the growth of the tumor. There is a crater-forming ulcer with a raised, actively growing, damlike border. Further characteristics are induration of the tumor tissue ("crab hardening") and growth into surrounding structures.

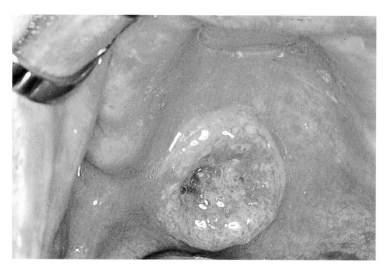

Fig. 19-25   Rapidly growing undifferentiated squamous cell carcinoma with central necrosis and damlike raised border on the palate of an 81-year-old patient.

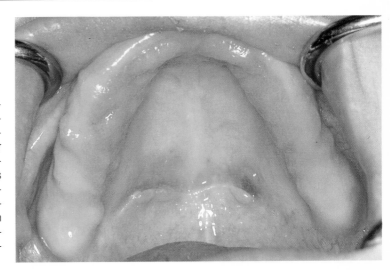

Fig. 19-26 Differential diagnosis of carcinoma in the palatal mucosa: prosthetic pressure spot near the posterior border of the denture. The situation was present for 3 weeks after placement of the prosthesis. The mechanically conditioned paramedian impression and ulceration are in spots surrounded by an inflammatory infiltrate.

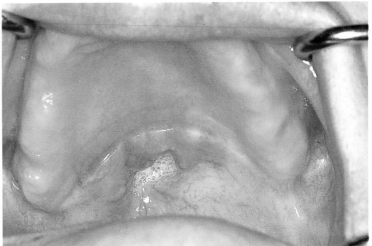

Fig. 19-27 Ulcerated squamous cell carcinoma on the soft palate of a 68-year-old woman. The impressions of the etching on the prosthesis base in the region of the Ah-line facilitates recognition of the extension of the tumor infiltration.

Fig. 19-28 Well-differentiated squamous cell carcinoma in the middle of the palate with large pressed out–appearing tissue defect. It is the result of a deep bone necrosis involving the periosteum. Differential diagnosis is with a lethal midline granuloma (see chapter 30; Figs. 30-18 and 30-19). Some weeks before, the 57-year-old patient had visited his dentist and requested an improvement of the prosthesis. The cause of the functional insufficiency of the prosthesis was not recognized at first and precious time for therapy was wasted in this manner.

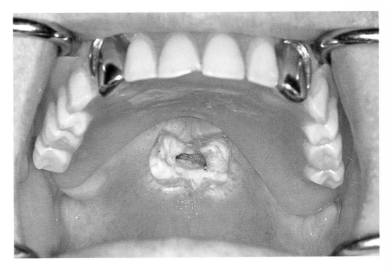

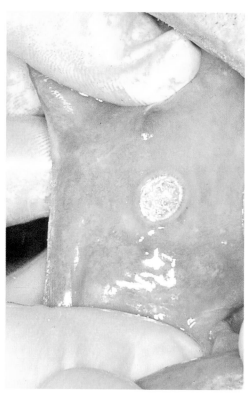

Fig. 19-29   Poorly differentiated nonkeratinizing squamous cell carcinoma of the cheek mucosa. According to the 69-year-old patient, a "vesicular" lesion had appeared in this area 2 months previously and had at first been "painted." This early stage of carcinoma of the oral mucosa clinically showed a circular protuberance with a raised indurated margin and a granular central surface.

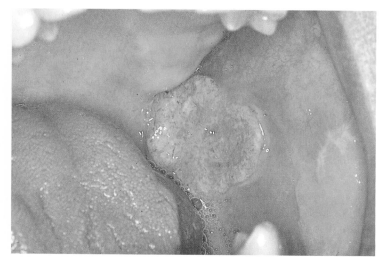

Fig. 19-30   Keratinizing infiltrating squamous cell carcinoma reaching to the area of the tuberosities and lateral wall of the throat in the cheek region of a 56-year-old woman. It had erroneously been associated with a removable prosthesis as a prosthetic pressure spot, and therapy had been delayed for weeks.

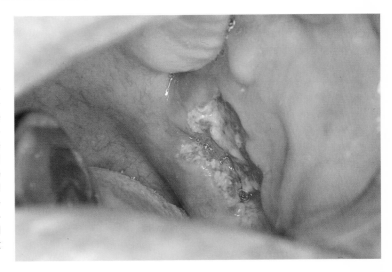

Fig. 19-31 Advanced squamous cell carcinoma of intermediate differentiation in the area of the left ascending ramus of the mandible. The 73-year-old patient had noticed the change 6 months before because of pain that started some time before (consequence of superimposed infection) and requested medical help. The tumor was verified at surgery: T4N3M0.

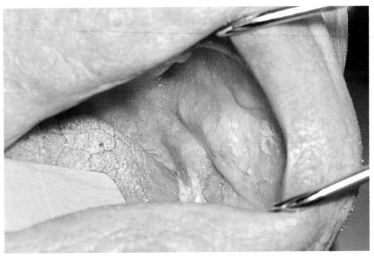

Fig. 19-32 Keratinized squamous cell carcinoma in the retromolar region of the edentulous mandible at the base of a large precancerous leukoplakia. The painless growth was nodular and hard. It had been treated as a pressure spot for 3 months in the 72-year-old patient.

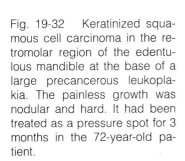

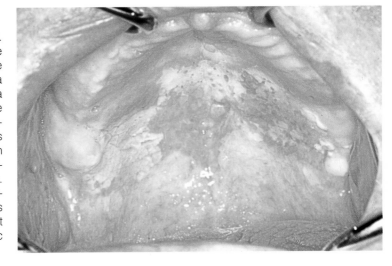

Fig. 19-33 The patient in Fig. 19-32 also at examination. The part leukoplakial, part erosive changes of the palatal mucosa are a partial manifestation of a multicentric leukoplakia of the oral mucosa. The clinical suspicion of a carcinomatous change also in the area shown here was not confirmed in several excision biopsy samples. This type of multicentric precancerous leukoplakia presents the professional with a difficult problem from the diagnostic and therapeutic points of view.

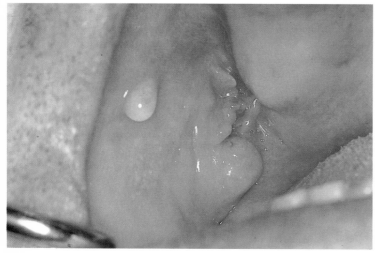

Fig. 19-34   Differential diagnosis of cheek mucosa carcinoma. Ragged prosthesis irritation hyperplasia of the cheek mucosa from damaging prosthesis border over long-standing proptosis buccalis (see chapter 22). The mechanically caused chronically inflamed tissue hyperplasia formed again after the correction of the prosthesis.

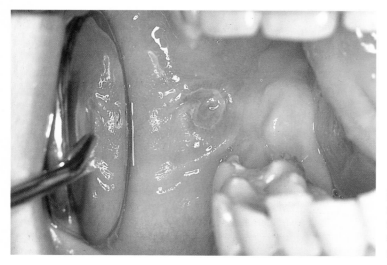

Fig. 19-35   Differential diagnosis to cheek mucosa carcinoma: traumatic mucosal ulceration (repeated bite damage) in new prosthesis wearer.

Special note

Each unexplained mucosal change must be considered cancerous until proven otherwise.

If an ulcer with a hard infiltrating border does not heal within 2 weeks after removal of possible local causes, refer the patient (cancer suspicion).

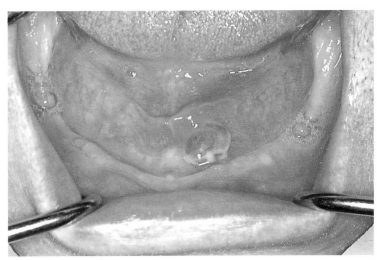

Fig. 19-36 Small, predominantly exophytic keratinizing squamous cell carcinoma in the glossoalveolar sulcus with massive superimposed inflammatory changes (increased vascularization on the left side of the floor of the mouth) in a 67-year-old patient.

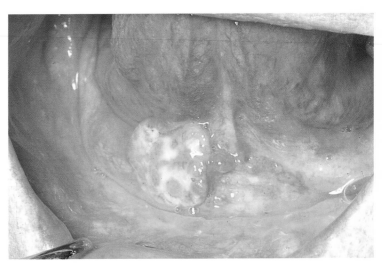

Fig. 19-37 Part poorly differentiated part low-grade keratinizing squamous cell carcinoma on the anterior floor of the mouth in a 77-year-old patient with arteriosclerosis. Nineteen years before, a vocal cord carcinoma had been successfully removed. About 2 years ago the patient, still a heavy smoker, noticed a persistent enlargement under the tongue, which caused him to seek out a doctor.

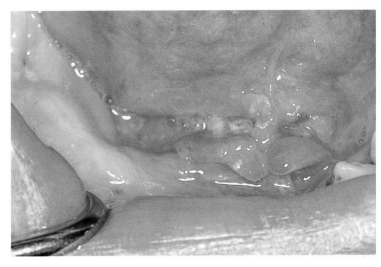

Fig. 19-38 Advanced low-grade keratinizing squamous cell carcinoma in glossoalveolar sulcus with marked tumor infiltration of the floor of the mouth. The patient is 62 years old with a history of alcoholism. There is already bilateral metastatic disease in the regional lymph nodes.

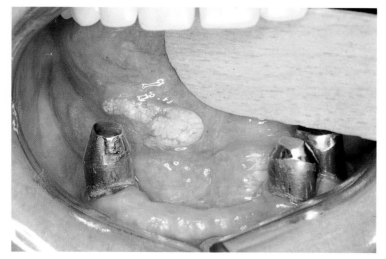

Fig. 19-39 Histologically confirmed keratinized squamous cell carcinoma with early stromal invasion: a precancerous leukoplakia of the floor of the mouth (leukoplakia carcinoma) in a 56-year-old woman. In the histologic preparation of the entire 2.5-cm-long mucosal change, an invasive carcinoma was found in the middle. The other parts of the specimen showed only slight epithelial dysplasia.

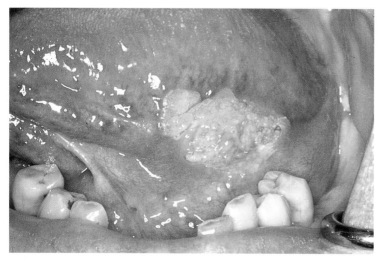

Fig. 19-40 Predominantly exophytic keratinized squamous cell carcinoma of intermediate differentiation at the base of an untreated long-standing precancerous leukoplakia of the floor of the mouth in a 65-year-old patient.

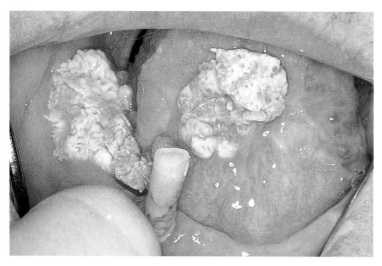

Fig. 19-41 Papillomatous keratinized squamous cell carcinoma of the oral mucosa in an 81-year-old woman. The cauliflower-like growth was localized under the tongue on the floor of the mouth and the alveolar process. There were submandibular lymph node metastases on both sides.

Fig. 19-42 Differential diagnosis of carcinoma of the border of the tongue: tongue tonsil in a 67-year-old patient. The tongue tonsil is located at the transition area of the dorsal tongue border between the floor of the mouth and the anterior palatal arch. The lymphatic tissue belonging to the Waldeyer's ring is made up of 40 to 90 lymphatic units whose different functional status provides different clinical appearances (swelling, reddening). The normal finding with its variations must be known by the dentist so that patients with cancerphobia can receive an appropriate explanation.

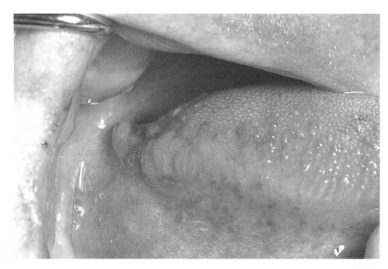

Fig. 19-43 Advanced keratinized squamous cell carcinoma originally from the dorsal border of the tongue with extensive keratinized tissue defects extending into the mouth floor, tongue border, and lateral pharynx wall in a 57-year-old patient.

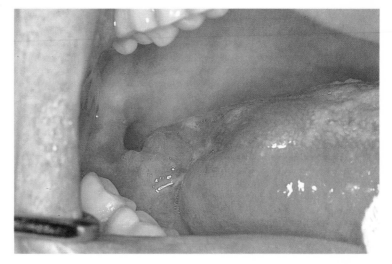

Fig. 19-44 Advanced intermediate-grade squamous cell carcinoma of the border of the tongue with nearby complete tumor infiltration of the left side of the tongue and floor of the mouth. The 51-year-old patient had noticed a hardening in the area of the left tongue border for 1½ years. The appearance of the enlarging tissue defect on the tongue as well as a distinct weight loss motivated—too late—the patient to visit the doctor.

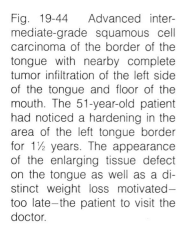
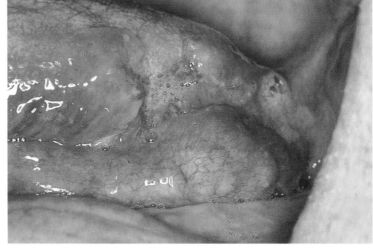

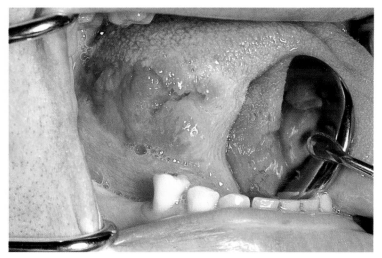

Fig. 19-45   Keratinized squamous cell carcinoma with central radiating necrosis on the tongue in a 40-year-old patient. At the time of evaluation, the complaint was a pain radiating from the ear, which first appeared 2 weeks before and had intensified in the last few days.

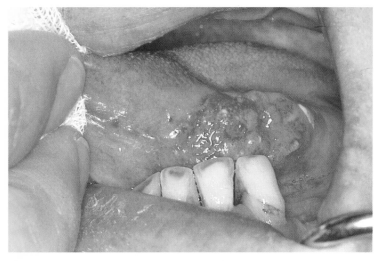

Fig. 19-46   Advanced, poorly differentiated squamous cell carcinoma of the tongue with crossover into the floor of the mouth. There was a regional lymph node metastasis on the tumor side. Tumor stage: T2N1M0. The 51-year-old patient apparently observed the lesion in this location only 4 weeks before. The factors predisposing to cancer were: smoking (30 cigarettes/day), relatively moderate but regular alcohol consumption, and bad oral hygiene.

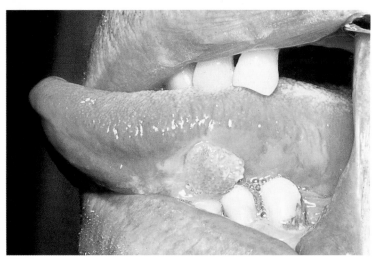

Fig. 19-47   Exophytic low-grade keratinized squamous cell carcinoma with wartlike surface on the ventral surface of the tongue. In this area, the 67-year-old patient had first noticed a somewhat painful, knotty induration 8 weeks previously. This lesion, which soon developed into a verruciform tissue mass, had initially been attributed by the dentist to a sharp tooth edge. Note the surrounding flat homogeneous leukoplakia.

Fig. 19-48 Keratinizing squamous cell carcinoma on the left tongue border on the bottom of a precancerous leukoplakia that had existed for many years. The 65-year-old patient reported (after more than 20 years of heavy smoking) oral mucosa "white spots" that had developed a few years before. For 1 year, there were uncharacteristic changes on the left tongue border and ventral side. On the dorsum of the tongue were circumscribed verrucous epithelial changes in the area of speckled leukoplakia. The carcinoma on the left side of the tongue was confirmed by histologic study.

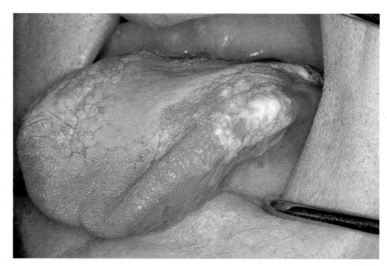

Fig. 19-49 Squamous cell carcinoma of the tongue: intermediate differentiation (ventral side of the tongue, border of the tongue on the left side) in a 64-year-old patient. Carcinoma with localization in the lower area of the oral cavity (alimentary gliding area) is often found in alcoholics (abuse with high-level-alcohol-content beverages), particularly in combination with smoking and poor oral hygiene (classic triad of cancer-predisposing factors).

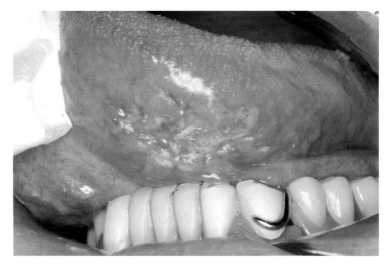

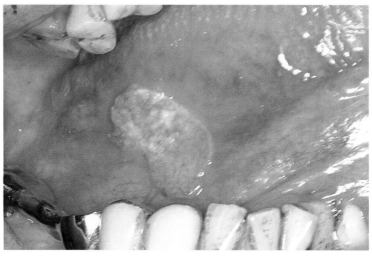

Fig. 19-50 Exophytic infiltrating intermediate differentiation squamous cell carcinoma on the ventral side of the tongue on the floor of the mouth in a 53-year-old patient. The clinical suspicion of a submandibular lymph node metastasis (palpable, hard matted lymph node on the tumor side) was histologically confirmed.

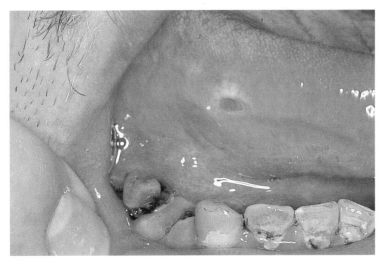

Fig. 19-51 Differential diagnosis of tongue carcinoma: chronic rubbing area on the right border of the tongue in a 47-year-old patient with neglected oral condition. The constant rubbing on the sharp corner of the deeply carious tooth 45 (29) caused a chronic ulceration with surrounding mechanically irritated leukoplakia. Once the local irritation factor has been removed, the finding must be controlled in a short time.

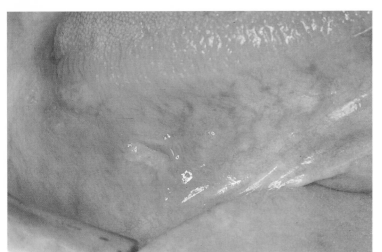

Fig. 19-52 Differential diagnosis of a carcinoma of the floor of the mouth: chronic inflamed ulceration of the oral mucosa in the transition to the base of the tongue in an edentulous 71-year-old woman. Because there was no improvement within 14 days after the dentist shortened the prosthesis, the patient was referred. In spite of the soft consistency of the change, a malignant transformation could not be clinically ruled out. Before any diagnostic intervention, the lesion healed spontaneously. Retrospectively, it was possible to make the diagnosis of solitary aphtha of the major type (see chapter 12).

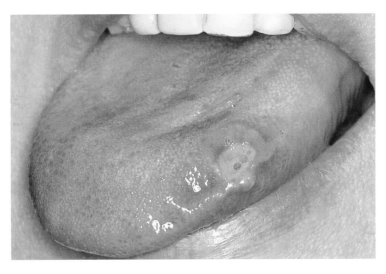

Fig. 19-53 Differential diagnosis of tongue carcinoma: fully developed stage of a solitary chronic recurring aphtha on the left border of the tongue. The base of the ulcer is covered with a slimy coating. The associated edema wrongfully gives the visual impression of a border dam.

Fig. 19-54 Differential diagnosis of a tongue carcinoma: traumatic ulcer on the left tongue border as a consequence of repeated self-inflicted wounds on a sharp tooth edge. The fibrin-covered boil shows an edematous swelling with tooth impression on the distal area. The lesion is unremarkable but painful to palpation. It caused a lymphadenitis of the associated submandibular lymph nodes and pain on swallowing.

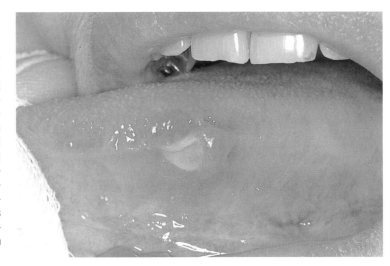

Fig. 19-55 The patient in Fig. 19-54 also at examination. The tongue in resting position shows the congruence of the ulceration with the sharp-edged tooth 36 (19).

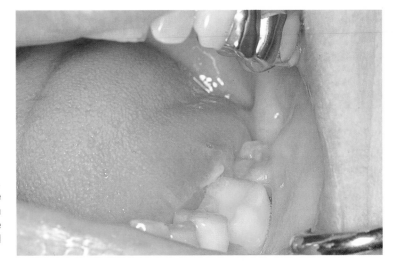

Fig. 19-56 The patient in Figs. 19-54 and 19-55 after 8 days. After the irritating tooth corner was smoothed, the mechanical-induced ulceration healed without local medication. A short interval control visit is unavoidable in this case. The patient cannot be trusted because after elimination of the irritative factor, a tumor may decrease in size as the inflammation decreases.

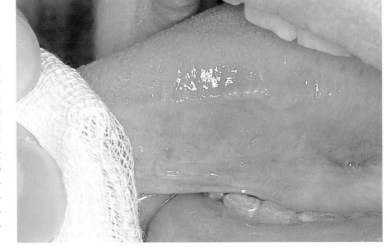

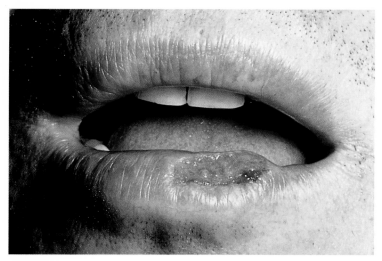

Fig. 19-57 Keratinizing squamous cell carcinoma of the lower lip in a 40-year-old patient. According to the patient, an ulcer had existed on the site for approximately 2 years without showing any tendency to heal. Note the raised, and to the palpating finger, firm, infiltrated border of the craterlike ulceration. Lip mobility is decreased.

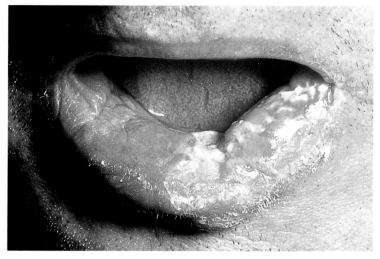

Fig. 19-58 Advanced keratinizing squamous cell carcinoma of the lower lip infiltrating the surrounding area in a 63-year-old patient. The vermilion of the lip is displaced by tumor infiltration. On the left lower lip mucosa are recognizable leukoplakial changes. The history dates back almost 2 decades; there was first an actinic cheilitis facilitated by UV irradiation (the patient worked outdoors as a farmer).

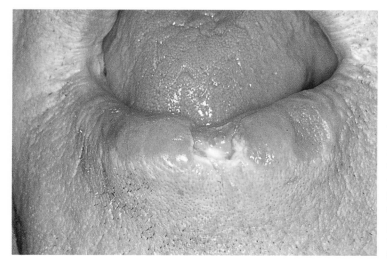

Fig. 19-59 Radiation therapy-resistant keratinized squamous cell carcinoma of the lower lip in a 65-year-old patient. In addition to a medially located craterlike ulcer, there is another flat carcinomatous lesion on the left side. After radiation, there was depigmentation and atrophy changes on the skin. Lip carcinoma should be treated surgically.

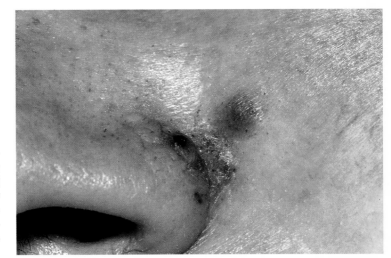

Fig. 19-60 Early partially pigmented basal cell carcinoma in a hidden location on the left side of the nose. Immediately adjacent is an elevated homogeneous brown-pigmented nevus cell nevus (compound nevus).

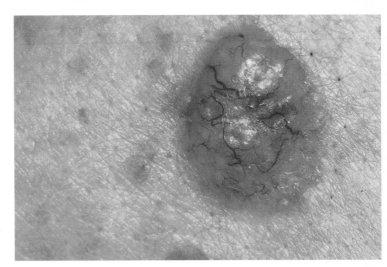

Fig. 19-61 Nodular basal cell carcinoma with typical clinical shiny translucent surface and numerous coiled telangiectasias. Palpable, firm, broad-based tumor.

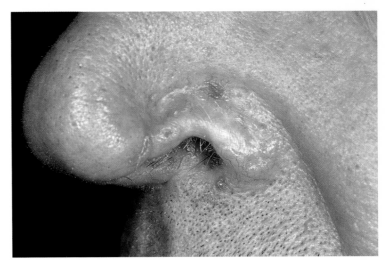

Fig. 19-62 Advanced basal cell carcinoma on the left side of the nose with deforming growth.

Chapter 20

Salivary Gland Tumors in the Oral Cavity

Adenomas
   Monomorphic adenoma
   Pleomorphic adenoma

Mucoepidermoid tumor (mucoepidermoid carcinoma)

Adenoid cystic carcinoma

Malignant mixed tumor

About 80% of tumors of the salivary glands are localized in the parotid gland; the rest are distributed in the small mixed salivary glands of the oral mucosa, the submandibular gland, and the sublingual gland.

The material discussed in this chapter is limited to a series of tumors originating in epithelium, that is, ectodermal gland parenchymas of the small seromucous, oral, salivary mucosal glands. The relatively rare neoplasms that originate in the interstitial connective tissue of the salivary glands or in the tissue that has migrated from the surrounding areas will not be discussed.

Microscopically, tumors of the salivary glands show a great variety of forms, which, however, is not apparent in their clinical appearance. Except for some rare cases, it is not possible based on the clinical findings to state the origin or the individual type of tumor due to absence of differentiating features. The clinical behavior for the whole group of salivary gland tumors cannot be characterized. Some dissociation between clinical behavior and histologic appearance of the tumor should also be considered. There are both benign and malignant forms of salivary gland tumors, which cannot be completely separated from each other.

One must start with the assumption that about 40% of all tumors of the small salivary glands are malignant. Of those that start out benign, it is known that each recurrence because of incomplete removal allows a locally aggressive growth to start. In the presence of uncertain clinical diagnosis, enucleation as an operative procedure should be avoided. It is important to completely remove the tumor during the first operative procedure. The dentist should therefore avoid any other treatment, possibly even with small circumscribed changes if the tumor is suspicious, and should refer the patient to a specialized clinic.

The dentist has the primary duty to consider the possibility of the presence of a salivary gland tumor during the differential diagnosis and should not confuse it with swellings of inflammatory origin (a cause of unnecessary incisions).

Because the palatal mucosa is a favorite location for intraoral salivary gland tumors, the dentist must pay attention to patients who wear a removable prosthesis so that cause and effect are not confused. Also, in cases of salivary gland tumors there is a danger of misdiagnosis by repeatedly adjusting an ill-fitting prosthesis because growth of the tumor continues.

Adenomas

Salivary gland adenomas derived from glandular epithelium and ductal epithelium can be divided into two groups.

Monomorphic adenomas, which are very rare in the oral cavity, are parenchyma-rich tumors. They show an epithelial arrangement similar to that of other glandular structures. In contrast, the tumors of the salivary glands that are more frequently found in the oral mucosa are the *pleomorphic adenomas,* a variety with "mixed" tissue pattern. Histologic characteristics are the neoplastic epithelial components, myxoid and cartilaginous-like stroma in different quantities, and varying proportions. Whereas monomorphic adenomas (Fig. 20-1) are benign tumors that do not or only seldom recur, pleomorphic adenomas (Figs. 20-2 to 20-7) can only be considered conditionally benign because of their high rate of clinical local recurrence.

Monomorphic adenoma (ICD-M 8146/0)

Monomorphic adenomas compose a group of slow and painlessly growing, usually well-encapsulated, benign tumors with a relatively uniform cell picture. The predominant epithelial component is arranged in islands with a distinct basal membrane separating it from the mature connective tissue stroma. Histologically there are solid, trabecular, tubular, acinar, and papillary cystic forms to differentiate.

Monomorphic adenomas of the small, seromucous, oral mucosal glands definitely are rare. Therefore, a detailed discussion of the individual special forms will not be presented. A variation, the basal cell adenoma (ICD-M 8147/0), appears primarily on the upper lip (Fig. 20-1). Finally, it must be remembered that clinical differential diagnosis among the different salivary gland tumors is impossible. Even the histomorphologic differentiation of monomorphic adenomas from pleomorphic adenomas can present difficulties.

Pleomorphic adenoma, mixed tumor (ICD-M 8940/0)

The pleomorphic adenoma is by far the most common tumor of the salivary glands, both of the large glands (about 90% of all cases are located in the parotid gland) and of the small heterocrine oral mucosal glands.

The old name of the lesion was "mixed tumor." This name calls attention to the many types of tissue found in this neoplasm, in which the epithelial parts are mixed with a metaplastic stroma with mucous myxoid and chondroid features. Quantities and distribution of these tissue components are extremely variable. The histologic picture varies within a tumor. The term "pleomorphic adenoma" is preferred today, to give recognition to the epithelial origin and the adenoma character of this complex tumor.

In minor salivary glands of the oral mucosa, pleomorphic adenomas predominate in the posterior area of the hard palate and particularly in the gland-rich transition zone to the soft palate (Figs. 20-2 to 20-6). They occur less frequently on the palatal arch, lips, tongue, and floor of the mouth. Affected patients usually are in the third decade of life.

Pleomorphic adenomas grow slowly and without symptoms for years. Intermittent phases, with a growth arrest, are not unusual. The tumors achieve walnut size or larger before they are subjected to therapy. On the palate they appear as hemispheric, painless growths usually of firm consistency. The bone underneath appears unaffected or slightly compressed on radiographs. On the basis of palpation, only the differentiation from cysts is, as a rule, nonproblematic. They have a smooth, unaffected, mucosa-covered surface, which sometimes is slightly bumpy (particularly in recurrence). The mucosa is not fixed to the underlying tumor. Ulcerations caused by mechanical factors are possible (Fig. 20-7). A connective tissue capsule that separates the tumor from the surrounding tissue is not always present. It can be partially or completely absent. There are also cases in which the tumor cell cords have grown through the capsule or have penetrated the capsule. Because of the high risk of recurrence, the pleomorphic adenoma is considered conditionally benign clinically, even though the histomorphologic findings may not always predict the future clinical course.

Intraoral pleomorphic adenomas should not be enucleated. They are to be resected with generous amounts of healthy tissue. In the area of the hard palate, the neighboring bone layer should also be removed. Incomplete removal leads to recurrence, which can be more aggressive locally. In rare cases, the malignant transformation of a pleomorphic adenoma is possible (see section on carcinoma in the pleomorphic adenoma).

Mucoepidermoid tumor (ICD-M 8430/0), mucoepidermoid carcinoma (ICD-M 8430/3)

The mucoepidermoid tumor is considered a malignant adenoma form with varying degrees of malignancy. Main locations are the large salivary glands with a predominance in the parotid gland. The neoplasm can also originate in the small salivary glands of the mucosa, preferentially in the palate and cheeks. Men are more affected than women, and both usually in the fifth or sixth decades of life.

Clinically the mucoepidermoid tumor is relatively well defined with a tightly elastic curvature or a thick nodule with a blurred border at palpation (Fig. 20-8). The surface may be smooth or bumpy. Histologically there are some glandular or cystic epithelial islands with mucous-producing cells and squamous cells with varying distribution and differentiation.

Mucoepidermoid tumors tend to have an infiltrative growth along the vessels and nerves and can develop metastases by hematogenous route and in far-removed lymph nodes (particularly in the liver and lungs). Differentiation of forms with a low and a high degree of malignancy is not possible. The histologic and cytologic findings often do not allow a reliable prognostic statement. Therefore the mucoepidermoid tumor must be considered like a carcinoma (mucoepidermoid carcinoma), with all the consequences of this for therapy (i.e., radiation of the surgical area).

Adenoid cystic carcinoma, cylindroma, cylindroid type of adenocarcinoma (ICD-M 8200/3)

The adenoid cystic carcinoma, which is inadequately characterized by the term *cylindroma,* is the most common malignant tumor of the small salivary glands (Figs. 20-9 to 20-11).

In comparison with other salivary gland carcinomas, the adenoid cystic carcinoma grows slowly initially, and size, consistency, apparent borders, and surface appearance are similar to the clinical appearance of an adenoma. Early on it shows, however, a definite treacherous tendency to extend and infiltrate via the perineural lymphatics and blood vessels, and after a time appears peripherally in healthy soft tissue—localizing in proximity to bone—and in the jawbone, with invasive progression. Even intraoperatively the extension of the tumor cannot be evaluated macroscopically, hence radiation of the surgical area is indicated.

Later in the clinical course the tumor ulcerates, frequently with the formation of a central crater (Fig. 20-11), as occurs in other types of carcinoma of the mucosa. With the passing of time (i.e., years), the behavior of the adenoid cystic carcinoma becomes more aggressive without major changes of the morphologic characteristics of the tumor. There is development of lymphatic and blood vessel metastasis. The remote metastases appear preferentially in the lung.

The short-term prognosis of the adenoid cystic carcinoma gives the false impression of a benign course as in other salivary gland carcinomas. Long-term prognosis is, however, poor because experience shows all types of therapy have little influence on the further course of the tumor and the future of the patient.

Malignant mixed tumor (ICD-M 8940/3)

Carcinomas in pleomorphic adenoma belong to the group of salivary gland carcinomas, which, according to their morphology and grade of differentiation, are divided into *adenocarcinomas, squamous cell carcinomas,* and *undifferentiated carcinomas.* They develop in older patients and behave as carcinomas of the oral mucosa.

The rare carcinomas arising in pleomorphic adenoma show peculiarities that differentiate them from primary salivary gland carcinomas on the basis of the patient's history but not from the clinical findings. Patients report that a nodule present for many years suddenly enlarged. It is calculated that the latency period before occurrence of a malignant transformation in a pleomorphic adenoma is 15 to 20 years. The original tumor does not become malignant as a whole but, according to the laws of cell autonomy, there is the appearance of a new malignant cell line which infiltrates and replaces the original adenoma.

In the parotid gland are deeply located tumors that escape clinical notice. The appearance of a facial paralysis is an alarming sign of malignancy. If the neoplasms originate in the small salivary glands, the malignancy becomes clinically suspect based on other criteria. Suspicious findings include the appearance of a nodular lesion or the sudden development of fast growth in an until-then-stationary untreated nodule. Indications of malignancy are also expansion of a blurred lesion border and irregularities of tumor shape as well as progressive growth and infiltrating and destructive expansion into the surrounding tissue. If the tumor appears at the mucous membrane surface, it forms an ulcer (Fig. 20-12) with the typical damlike raised border.

The basic treatment principles of carcinoma therapy are valid for salivary gland carcinomas.

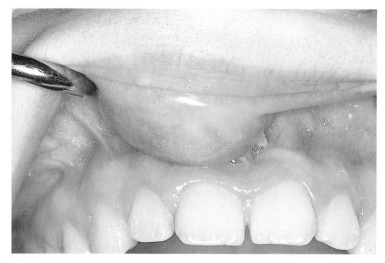

Fig. 20-1 Monomorphic adenoma in the upper lip of a 16-year-old girl. Histologic examination of this slowly growing, painless, well-encapsulated tumor demonstrated a basal cell adenoma that belongs to the group of monomorphic adenomas and is often seen in people over 60.

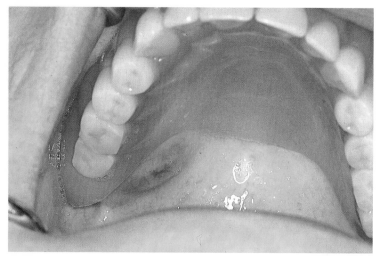

Fig. 20-2 Pleomorphic adenoma in the transition zone from hard to soft palate in a 63-year-old woman. While a new prosthetic device was being placed, the dentist noticed a growth that was painless at pressure and that was incorrectly diagnosed as inflammatory. After local medication treatment and incision, the patient was referred for further consultation.

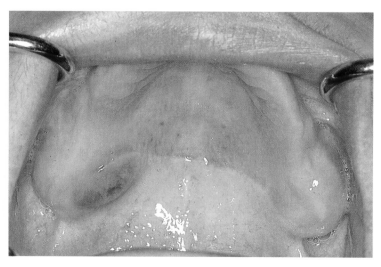

Fig. 20-3 The patient in Fig. 20-2 also at the time of examination. Removal of the complete prosthesis, which had already been shortened on the right posterior border, makes the incision more evident. The histologic picture corresponded to that of a pleomorphic adenoma.

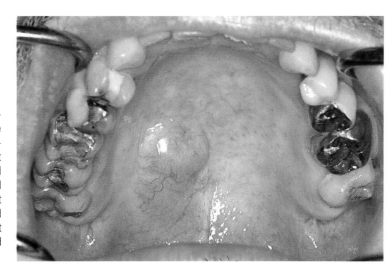

Fig. 20-4   Pleomorpic ade-noma in typical location on the hard palate of a 43-year-old pa-tient. The history indicated that on dental examination a hard painless condensation had been noticed for 4 years but was not considered to need treatment. After the patient moved, the new dentist referred the patient to the clinic.

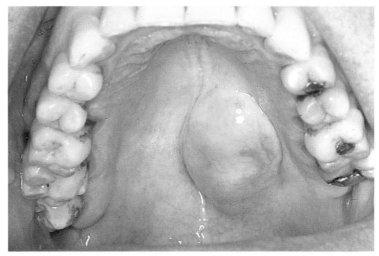

Fig. 20-5   Pleomorphic ade-noma of the palate. According to the 36-year-old patient, the tumor had grown without symp-toms over many years until it reached the present size. Pal-pation showed a firm growth well delimited from surrounding area with no pain on pressure.

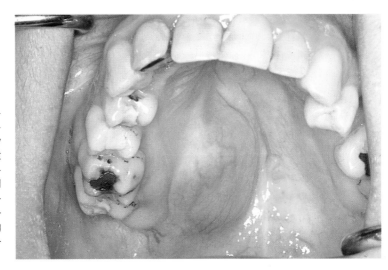

Fig. 20-6   Pleomorphic ade-noma on the palate of a 50-year-old woman. The salivary gland tumor in this patient showed a tight, elastic consis-tency. On the smooth mucosal surface, the blood vessel pat-tern becomes slightly accen-tuated. This type of finding should not be confused with in-flammatory swelling and cysts.

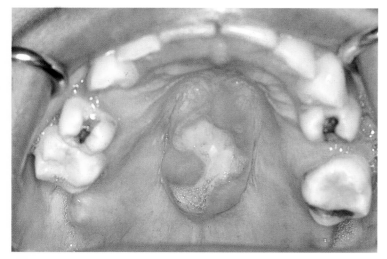

Fig. 20-7 Recurrence of a pleomorphic adenoma located on the hard palate in a 42-year-old woman. The tumor had been resected, obviously not completely, 4 years earlier. Incomplete removal often leads to recurrence. Even if there is no basis for malignancy in the histologic report, the recurrence of a pleomorphic adenoma is often more locally aggressive than the primary tumor.

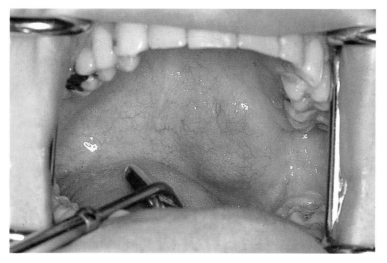

Fig. 20-8 Mucoepidermoid tumor (mucoepidermoid carcinoma) in a 28-year-old woman. The nodular lesion measures about 3 cm in diameter and is covered by an intact mucosa. It is located near the soft palate and is not well delimited on palpation. Note the obvious blood vessel pattern of the mucosa above the tumor. The mucoepidermoid tumor must be considered a carcinoma and therefore be treated aggressively.

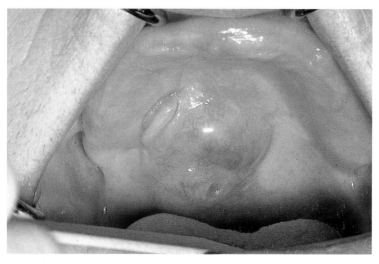

Fig. 20-9 Adenoid cystic carcinoma in the palate. The 65-year-old woman visited her dentist because of difficulties with the placement of the prosthesis. The dentist incorrectly suspected an inflammatory process and incised the growth. Shown is a large tumor in the transition zone between hard and soft palate with focal discoloration of the mucosa. The incision wound is still easily seen. In the dorsal area, the tumor has broken through and a lentil-sized ulceration has developed.

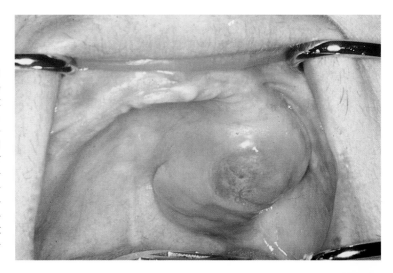

Fig. 20-10 Partially ulcerated adenoid cystic carcinoma the size of a hen's egg on the left side of the edentulous maxilla. The 64-year-old patient's history reveals her dentures had been repeatedly adjusted over the previous 2 years with misdiagnosis of the cause. The relatively slow-growing semi-malignant tumor frequently infiltrates the surrounding tissue at an early stage and requires radical surgery.

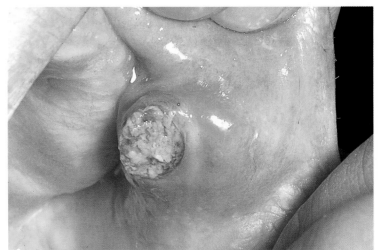

Fig. 20-11 A 72-year-old woman with an adenoid cystic carcinoma that invaded the oral cavity at the level of the cheek and that produced a large crater-forming mucosal defect. This most frequent malignant tumor of the small salivary glands can appear anywhere in the area of the oral mucosa containing salivary glands. Preferential localizations are the floor of the mouth or the cheeks. The adenoid cystic carcinoma can remain undetected for long periods or can be mistakenly considered a benign growth.

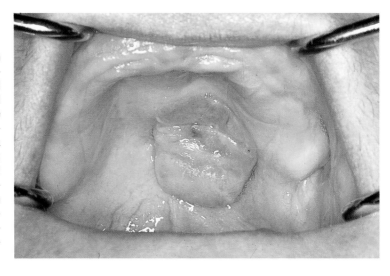

Fig. 20-12 Carcinoma in pleomorphic adenoma. The 61-year-old woman had observed the tumor for many years and informed the dentist that the pressure area from an old prosthesis had developed only a few weeks previously. During examination, the patient stated that after correction of the prosthesis everything was again in order. Histologic findings showed a carcinomatous transformation in pleomorphic adenoma.

Chapter 21

Malignant Melanomas

Malignant melanoma in Hutchinson's melanotic freckle

Acrolentiginous melanoma

Superficially spreading melanoma

Nodular melanoma

Nonclassifiable melanomas and special forms

Malignant melanomas are malignant tumors of the skin and mucosa. The particular problems associated with these tumors arise from the variability of their clinical courses. Melanoma cells differentiate from melanocytes that originate embryologically from the neural crest.

Many neoplasms of the pigment cell system are characterized by a two-phase growth pattern. In the first phase, the melanoma cells retain their epidermal location and they preferentially expand *horizontally (radial growth phase)*. This status, seen especially in lentigo maligna and superficially spreading melanomas, can extend for months, years, and even decades and can finally evolve into an aggressive *vertical* invasion (growth upwards and downward).

This change in biologic behavior of the melanoma is still not fully understood. There are no immunologically certain tumor markers that can provide an adequate explanation.

The classification of melanomas according to Clark (see page 427) is primarily related to the skin; it cannot be applied to the mucous membrane without modification (i.e., the acrolentiginous melanomas must be included).

Epidemiology

The incidence of melanomas has increased disturbingly over recent decades. For example, the number of new cases in Denmark, as recorded in the cancer registry, which has been in operation for a long period, rose from 1.1 per 100,000 population in 1943 to 5.7 per 100,000 in 1982. In Germany the incidence at present is 8 to 12 cases per 100,000 population, while in the southern United States it is twice as high; in Queensland, Australia the rate is two to three times of that in Germany. The incidence in Europe is expected to double in the next 10 to 20 years. The increase in occurrence is coupled with a shift of age distribution to younger age groups (20 to 40 years). Women are affected more frequently than men.

Approximately 8% of malignant melanomas of the head and neck region occur in the mucosa; about one half of these arise primarily in the oral cavity. Other statistics demonstrate that *oral melanomas* account for 0.5% to 1.5% of *all* melanomas. Strangely, oral melanomas account for 7.5% of melanomas in Japan. In contrast to oral mucosal carcinomas, with a site preference for the mandibular region of the oral cavity, three fourths of all primary melanomas are localized in the maxillary region (palate, cheek, and maxillary gingiva) (Figs. 21-2 to 21-6).

Etiology

In addition to a genetic disposition of whites and people with a light skin type, ultraviolet radiation from sunlight is a decisive exogenous factor. More recently, massive exposure to ultraviolet rays in tanning salons has been suggested as another possible factor in the increased frequency of melanomas.

The cumulative effects of lifelong exposure to ultraviolet light can lead to malignant melanomas in addition to epithelial neoplasms, e.g., basal cell and squamous cell carcinomas. Excessive exposure to ultraviolet light in childhood and youth (falling asleep in sunlight, sunburn requiring medical attention) favors the development of nodular and superficially spreading melanomas as a consequence of overstimulated cellular repair systems of the skin. In addition, chemical carcinogens such as aromatic and halogenated hydrocarbons are said to be important. The effect and importance of irradiation and exogenous factors for development of melanomas of the oral mucosa remain unclear.

Types of melanomas and their precursors

Based on morphologic and dynamic growth criteria, it is possible to differentiate four principal types of malignant melanomas; we prefer the classification system of Clark and Mitarbeitern (see Table below). Immunogenetic findings and variability of clinical course point to the possibility that these basic types may not correspond to separate and well-defined nosologic entities.

Classification of Principal Melanoma Types (from Clark and Mitarbeitern)

LMM	Lentigo maligna melanoma
ALM	Acrolentiginous melanoma
SEM	Superficially expanding melanoma
NM	Nodular melanoma

Unclassifiable melanomas and special forms

Melanomas can develop in clinically normal skin or mucosa or on the basis of precursor lesions of varying duration and varying degrees of risk factor for malignancy.

Particularly susceptible to melanomas are people with dysplastic nevi (see chapter 3) and congenital nevi (melanoma precursors). Large congenital nevi with a diameter of more than 20 cm at birth have a high risk of transformation. With time, melanomas develop in 2% to 6% of congenital nevi that have a diameter of less than 10 cm but more than 1.5 cm. For nevi of the oral cavity, no numbers are yet available concerning the frequency of malignant transformation.

Finally, all reports on the development of melanomas stress the following as suspicious clinical findings: irregularities of form, limit, and color; accelerated growth (ABCD rule: Asymmetry, Border, Color, Diameter).

Malignant melanoma in Hutchinson's melanotic freckle; lentigo maligna melanoma (ICD-M 8742/3)

The preinvasive precursor of this type of melanoma is associated with a decades-long history (average latent period is almost 15 years) of the symptoms of Hutchinson's melanotic freckle (ICD-M 8742/2). The malignancy is clinically characterized by relatively large, vitiliginous, brown to dark-brown macular lesions having an irregular border on sun-damaged, aged skin. For that reason, the condition is frequently seen on the faces of aged persons (Fig. 21-13; differential diagnosis in Figs. 21-14 and 21-15). It also appears within the dentist's purview; the oral mucosa may on rare occasion be the site of the precursor lesion (Fig. 21-1). Other criteria useful in differential diagnosis are noted in chapter 4 (see also Fig. 21-10).

Changes in the surface of the malignant melanoma in Hutchinson's melanotic freckle point to a progressive disease. Clinically, conversion to the malignant form manifests itself with the appearance of nodules and evidence of centrifugal growth. Xeroderma pigmentosum is a genetically determined form of this disease; the risk of the latter becoming malignant is 2,000 times greater than that of normal tissue.

Acrolentiginous melanoma (ICD-M 8720/3 NOS)

Acrolentiginous melanoma is a special form of malignant melanoma in Hutchinson's melanotic freckle. As its name indicates, it is found in the heavily cornified skin of the palmar-plantar region and in the nail (subungual) bed, i.e., not at sites particularly exposed to light.

Certain ethnic groups (blacks, Asians) that have a low incidence of melanoma develop this form almost exclusively.

Histologically, the presence of dendritic melanocytes should be characteristic of this type of melanoma. Some investigators, however, do not agree with the separate classification of this tumor. Approximately 5% of all cutaneous malignant melanomas are ascribed to this form. Recent studies indicate that many malignant melanomas of the oral mucosa, which is a site not exposed to light, may be classified in this category. Frequency of oral tumors as a percentage of this category is not available because of incomplete data.

Superficially spreading melanoma (ICD-M 8743/3)

The superficially spreading melanoma is the most frequent type of melanoma by far, accounting for 70% of cases. With a relatively brief history of only a few years, it is more frequently observed in the middle-aged individuals. The trunk and extremities are favored sites; manifestations in the facial region are not unusual.

The clinical appearance of superficial spreading melanoma of the skin is that of silver-dollar-sized, usually round-to-oval lesions having arched or polycyclic borders. In addition to the uneven brown to black-brown color, inflammatory reactions of the stroma may provide reddish nuances. The initially flat, horizontal growth becomes secondarily a nodular melanoma, at which point the surface of the tumor may also show nodule-like components. In advanced stages, depigmented, whitish areas are seen in regression zones so that ring- or kidney-shaped areas may be seen (so-called regression zones). In these areas, there is a prominent lymphoid infiltrate. Analogous intraoral findings have not been described. As the stromal invasion progresses, the prognosis worsens.

As on the skin, the rare nevus cell nevi and pigmented nevi of the oral mucosa are important in differential diagnosis, which should always include exogenous pigmentation, particularly amalgam tattoos.

Nodular melanoma (ICD-M 8721/3)

Nodular melanomas, accounting for nearly 20% of all cutaneous melanomas, manifest themselves practically without any precursor state. Pre-existing pigmented lesions can be demonstrated only rarely. Most often, the initial appearance is that of a vertically invasive tumor progression with a brief history of characteristic clinical symptoms (primarily exophytic or nodular endophytic growth with sharply defined lateral margins), substantiating the poor prognosis.

Nodular melanoma usually has a homogeneous black-brown color; it also is known as an infrequent special amelanotic form. Injuries occur easily to lesions of primarily exophytic growth. The resulting erosions and hemorrhage may lead to misdiagnosis with serious consequences.

All dark brown to bluish-black nodules seen on the oral mucosa should raise the suspicion of nodular melanoma. The differential diagnosis must particularly include Kaposi's sarcoma (see chapter 11; Figs. 11-68 to 11-70), thrombosed and sclerosed eruptive angioma (see chapter 22), glomus tumor (see chapter 22; Fig. 22-55), and nevi with nodular configuration. Visually, inflammatory granulation tissue may simulate the appearance of a melanoma because of repeated intralesional hemorrhage (Figs. 21-11 and 21-12).

Nonclassifiable melanomas and special forms

In addition to the four principal types, unclassifiable and special forms of melanomas exist (approximately 5% of all cases). These include amelanotic malignant melanoma, desmoplastic melanoma, malignant blue nevus, and familial melanomas. A number of mucosal melanomas, melanomas in and about the eye, and melanomas having unusual regression all fit in this category. Histomorphologic criteria distinguish other special forms.

Parameters important for the course of the disease

If precursor states are not recognized and removed, the window period for effective therapy of oral melanoma becomes even more limited than in carcinomas of the oral mucosa.

The unpredictability of malignant melanomas is underscored by the fact that they tend to have early regional metastases and lead to a general spread through lymphatics and blood vessels. The metastatic pattern includes satellites, in-transit, regional lymph nodes, and distant metastases. Satellite metastases are those appearing within 2 cm of the primary tumor (Fig. 21-3). Among the transit metastases are those of the skin or subcutaneous tissue, or those of the mucosa or submucosa, arising more than 2 cm from the primary tumor, before the first appearance of metastases in lymph nodes. The concept of regional lymph node metastases is self-explanatory. Distant metastases arise – especially in subcutaneous tissue – in the lung, the brain, and the liver, and occasionally in the oral submucosa (Figs. 21-7 and 21-8). Metastases may also appear as amelanotic forms (Figs. 21-3 and 21-9).

Various clinical staging groups are still used internationally in an effort to classify the anatomic forms and thus to obtain preoperative indications for determining a treatment plan appropriate to the state of the disease and the prognosis. Among others, this includes the TNM classification of the UICC (see chapter 19).

The clinical three-stage classification of the European Organization for Research on Treatment of Cancer (EORTC) is shown here as an example:

Stage I	Primary tumor
Stage II	Regional metastases
	a) satellites, in-transit
	b) lymph nodes
Stage III	Distant metastases

In addition to the clinical tumor stages, location and sex are important clinical factors in the course of the disease.

Prognostically important histopathologic parameters are, above all, *Breslow's maximum vertical tumor thickness* as well as the depth penetration of the tumor into the various layers of skin (level). Depth of penetration, as classified by Clark in 1967, dividing *penetration* into five levels, is an important measure, for example, in the pTNM classification system. Measurement of tumor thickness in accordance with *Breslow's* method is probably of great significance. The assumption, however, that malignant melanomas having a vertical diameter less than 0.75 mm are associated with very low or no risk of metastases must be interpreted with care. *Clark's* penetration concept today is 1.5 mm. These data refer primarily to melanomas of the skin.

The *level according to Clark* is presented on page 432, so that the dentist can properly interpret references to it in medical reports.

Level:
    I   Intraepidermal melanoma (melanoma in situ)
    II Infiltration of papillary derma
    II Melanoma extends to the border between papillary and reticular derma
    IV Infiltration of the reticular derma
    V   Infiltration of the subcutaneous tissue

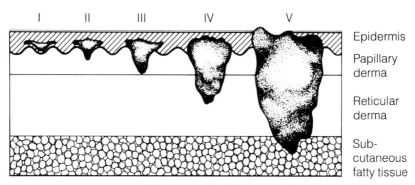

Levels according to Clark (penetration) with schematic representation. (From Kaufmann R, Weber L, Rodermund O-E. Kutane Melanome. Editiones Roche, 1989).

When the three-stage classification is used, the 5-year survival rate in stage 1 is 50% to 100%, depending on the tumor thickness and depth of penetration; when in-transit or lymph node metastases are present, the 5-year rate worsens to between 40% and less than 20%; and when lymphogenous or hematogenous distant metastases are found, the 5-year survival rate is zero, or 5% at best. These numbers document the dangerous nature of malignant melanomas.

Conclusions for the dentist

As in the past, treatment strategies for deeply invasive or already metastasized tumors today show little or no promise in terms of extending the patient's life. As statistics show, only early recognition and excision of the suspected melanoma in its very early or precursor stages decisively improves the chances of survival. The principle of watch and wait, as was applied to suspect lesions in the past, has been abandoned in favor of early, active treatment. There is unanimity that radical surgical excision with a wide margin into healthy tissue is the most effective and most promising form of treatment in these cases.

Because malignant melanomas of the oral mucosa have a particularly poor prognosis, because of delays in recognition and because no known therapy can overcome such delays, it is the dentist's duty to immediately refer patients for differential diagnosis, and treatment if necessary, if they show even one of the following changes:

- Indications of growth of pigmented spots (increase in surface area)
- Formation of elevations and other deviations in the surface relief of pigmented spots
- Irregularities in the color, such as unevenness, spottiness, and alterations in color intensity of pigmented spots
- Irregularities in the margins of pigmented spots (arched margins, steplike deviation at the margin)
- Erosions or ulcerations and/or hemorrhage in or about pigmented spots (usually found in advanced stages of melanoma)

Determining whether indications exist for prophylactic excision of a nevus or a lesion suspected of being a melanoma remains the responsibility of the specialist who is also, in the event of histologic demonstration of a melanoma, qualified to continue appropriate therapy.

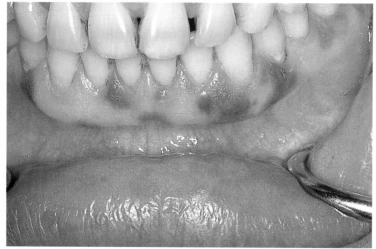

Fig. 21-1 Malignant melanoma in Hutchinson's melanotic freckle in the region of the vestibular gingiva of the anterior mandible of a 32-year-old woman. Note the nodular areas within the "pigmented spot." With this sort of finding, histomorphologic examination by excisional biopsy is required. Find additional differential diagnostic guidelines for melanin pigmentation in chapter 4.

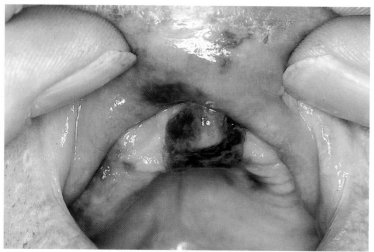

Fig. 21-2 Advanced malignant melanoma with lymphatic metastases distributed about the oral cavity and face in a 70-year-old man. The primary tumor was in the mucosa over the edentulous alveolar process in the center of the maxilla, thus explaining the bilateral spread of the metastases.

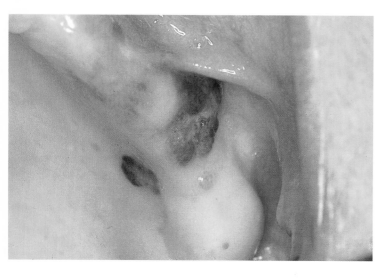

Fig. 21-3 Malignant melanoma on the edentulous alveolar process of the left side of the maxilla. The 68-year-old woman noted a bluish-black discoloration, which became elevated only 3 months earlier. Because of occasional bleeding and increase in size of the lesion, she sought treatment from a dentist, assuming the problem to be a pressure spot. Note the numerous variations in color and the irregular margin of the primary tumor elevated over the level of the mucosa. The partially amelanotic satellite metastases can be seen clearly together with the in-transit metastases to the hard palate.

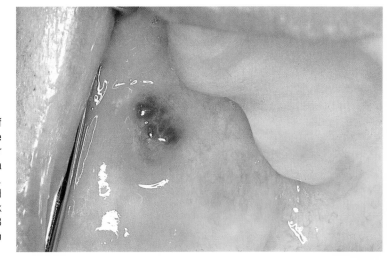

Fig. 21-4 Nodular type of malignant melanoma in the right cheek mucosa. The tumor must not be confused with a sclerosing eruptive angioma. The 64-year-old woman said that she had noted a "dark spot" for the first time only 8 weeks earlier; the spot then grew.

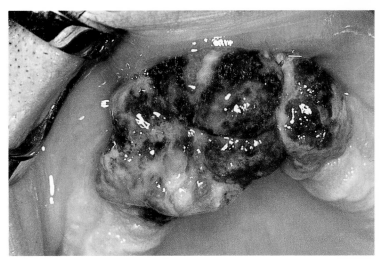

Fig. 21-5 Walnut-sized malignant melanoma in the anterior edentulous maxilla of a 71-year-old man. Uncertain descriptions by the patient indicated that it was a rapidly growing, nodular, blue-black, smooth-surfaced tumor with a tendency toward ulcerative disintegration. Distant metastases were found in the lung and brain at the time of admission; death occurred less than 6 months later.

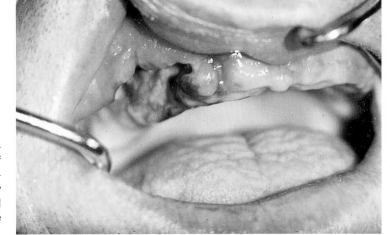

Fig. 21-6 Necrotic disintegrating malignant melanoma of the edentulous maxilla of a 61-year-old patient. The primary tumor within the oral cavity led to distant metastases on the skin and in internal organs.

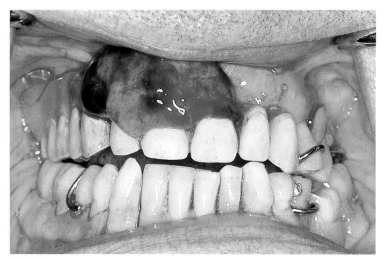

Fig. 21-7   Voluminous distant metastasis of a malignant melanoma in the edentulous anterior maxillary alveolar process, the site of the primary tumor being unknown. Occasionally, sites of primary malignant melanomas cannot be determined when distant metastases are present.

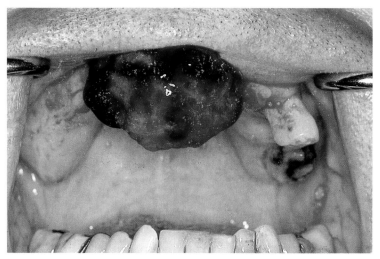

Fig. 21-8   The patient in Fig. 21-7 also at the time of examination. Removal of the partial denture shows the extent of the tumor. The erroneous initial impression was that of the so-called giant cell epulis (see chapter 14); the prosthesis was repeatedly adapted to the growing tumor by shortening several times during the surveillance period of several weeks. Note the checked, partially brown-black and partially reddish color of the metastasis.

Fig. 21-9   Amelanotic metastasis of a malignant melanoma in the posterior region of the left mandible of an 18-year-old woman. Misdiagnosis led to extraction a week earlier of the suddenly mobile tooth 36 (19). The tumor mass proliferating from the extraction site, together with bite injuries, is disintegrating. Biopsy examination demonstrated malignant melanoma. The patient's history indicated removal of an itching "wart" on the patient's back 10 weeks earlier. The wart, which was not examined histologically, corresponded to the primary tumor. The patient died a short time later from the consequences of brain metastases.

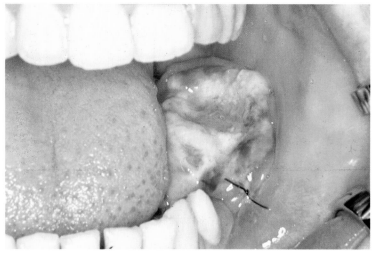

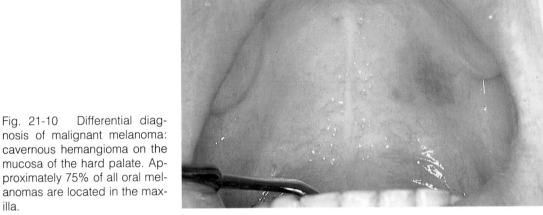

Fig. 21-10   Differential diagnosis of malignant melanoma: cavernous hemangioma on the mucosa of the hard palate. Approximately 75% of all oral melanomas are located in the maxilla.

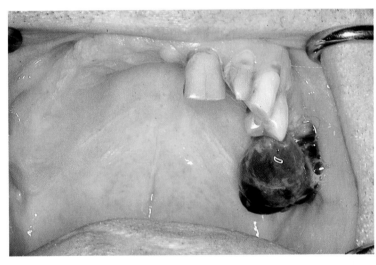

Fig. 21-11   Differential diagnosis of malignant melanoma: brown-black discoloration of inflamed granulation tissue at the extraction site of tooth 26 (14) arising from repeated hemorrhage into an untreated fistula tract between the oral cavity and the antrum. The lesion has the appearance of a melanoma.

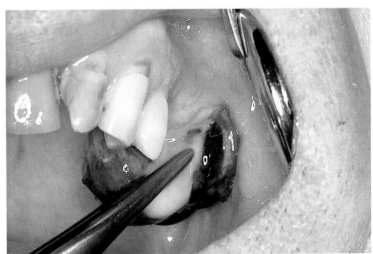

Fig. 21-12   The patient in Fig. 21-12 also at the time of examination. When probed, the antral empyema emptied.

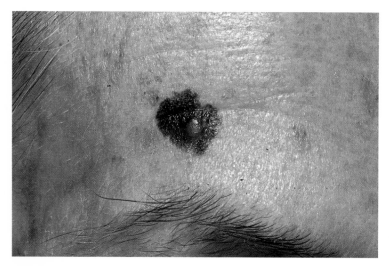

Fig. 21-13 Malignant melanoma in Hutchinson's freckle found supraorbitally at the right side of the forehead of a 70-year-old woman. Nodular invasive tumor component on the flat surface of a lentigo maligna melanoma. Maximum tumor thickness is 1.42 mm (Clark's level IV).

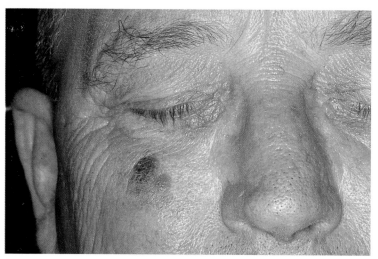

Fig. 21-14 Differential diagnosis of malignant melanoma: pigmented seborrheic wart of aging on the right cheek of a 74-year-old man.

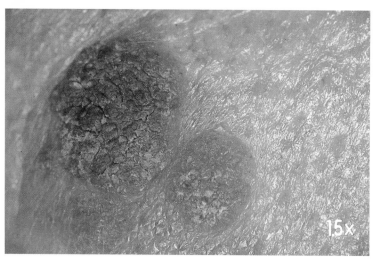

Fig. 21-15 The patient in Fig. 21-14. Enlargement of the pigmented seborrheic wart on actinic skin. Dentists frequently have the opportunity to observe the facial skin; they should learn to recognize visible lesions, to advise their patients, and when indicated refer them to relevant specialists.

Chapter 22

Circumscribed Hyperplasias and Benign Tumors

Circumscribed hyperplasias
Primary hyperplasias clinically inflammation free
 Gingival fibromatosis and localized enlargement
 Exostoses (torus palatinus, torus mandibularis)

Reactive hyperplasias as consequence of traumatic and in-
 flammatory irritation
  Proptosis of the lips, cheeks
  Denture hyperplasia
  Pyogenic granuloma
Benign tumors
 Fibroma
 Lipoma
 Hemangioma
 Glomus tumor
 Lymphangioma
 Papilloma
 Keratoacanthoma

Hyperplasias are limited excess tissue formation and represent an increase in tissue resulting from cell multiplication. In contrast, hypertrophy results from an increase in the volume of the cells, tissues, or organs that is independent of the number of cells. Hyperplasias, in contrast to true tumors, have no autonomic growth. Some hyperplasias exist entirely free of inflammation; in other forms, the proliferating tissue growth is a clear response to traumatic and inflammatory irritation.

Further, excess regeneration of tissue is possible in the course of wound healing. Reactive hyperplasias stop growing when the causative irritation is removed; these forms of hyperplasia are conditionally reversible.

Benign tumors must be differentiated from such hyperplasias. They react autonomously, i.e., are largely outside the systemic regulatory control of the organism. Such benign neoplasms have uniform typical cell characteristics and are exactly like the tissue from which they arise in terms of the degree of cell differentiation and metabolic requirements. They grow slowly and displace normal tissue by expansion, the surrounding tissue atrophying at the same time. The fibrous structures remain, so that certain types of tumors are enclosed in a connective tissue capsule. Benign tumors remain localized, have sharp demarcations from the surrounding healthy tissue, and do not metastasize. The concept of "benign," however, is a relative one, because even such tumors may be associated with life-threatening consequences if they occur, for example, in the brain. This aspect has no significance for benign tumors of the oral cavity.

Hyperplasias and benign tumors frequently occur in the mouth. Because of the special conditions that exist in the oral cavity, differentiation between a benign tumor arising from connective tissue and a fibrous hyperplasia arising from an inflammatory reaction is difficult for not only the clinician, but for the pathologist. This matter has already been described in chapters 14 (the various forms of epulis) and 15 (idiopathic fibrous gingival hyperplasia).

It is worthwhile to note that in some instances, malignant tumors can also have a clinical appearance similar to that of benign tumors or some form of hyperplasia. For this reason, histologic examination should be performed on all tissue removed in order to confirm the diagnosis, even when the tissue appears benign.

Circumscribed hyperplasias

In our specialty we can differentiate more on a clinical than a pathohistologic basis between hyperplasias that are primarily free of inflammation and have no apparent irritant as the cause, and those in which traumatic and inflammatory irritation is the cause of the exaggerated tissue reaction. The latter are reactive hyperplasias (i.e., caused by traumatic or inflammatory conditions).

Primary hyperplasias clinically inflammation-free

This group of hyperplasias can be included in those already described in chapter 15 (*idiopathic fibrous gingival hyperplasias; so-called symmetric peripheral jaw fibromas*).

Gingival fibromatosis and localized enlargement (ICD-DA 523.80)

The most significant clinical characteristic of this fixed overgrowth in the jaw is its often-symmetric arrangement at a typical point on both jaw halves. The lesion feels soft to cartilaginous, is usually pale red to pale pink, and is always covered by normal-appearing mucosa.

In the maxilla, the palatal molar and tuberosity region is affected (see Figs. 15-10, 15-11, and 15-13). From here, the peripheral jaw fibromas grow quite slowly toward the palate. They may grow to a monstrous size. In the mandible, the fibromatous changes, rich in collagen fibers, are usually lingual and distal to the last molar (Fig. 22-1; see Fig. 15-12). Occasionally the growth process is clearly greater on one side than the other, leading to a remarkably asymmetric appearance (Fig. 22-2). When tissue growth reaches the occlusal plane, changes in shape and surface from the effects of chewing are possible.

This gingival fibromatosis is believed to be a special form of idiopathic fibrous gingival hyperplasia.

Treatment consists of surgical excision of the fibroma, with the tissue near teeth being shaped as in gingivectomy.

Exostoses: torus palatinus (ICD-DA 826.83); torus mandibularis (ICD-DA 826.81)

Exostoses are excesses of bone formation. However, opinions still differ about whether these are true neoplasms. Exostoses, usually with a broad base, are located on the bone surface. The mucosa covering them is greatly stretched but normal in structure. Two variations occur in the oral cavity: *Torus palatinus,* situated in the center of the hard palate, with a flat to spindly, uneven, grapelike or completely irregular shape (Figs. 22-3 to 22-7), occurs in about 20% of the population.

Torus mandibularis, is situated on the lingual side of the mandible in the region of the canine and premolars. The exostoses in the mandible usually appear as multiple, horizontally arranged formations of varying size, unilaterally or bilaterally (Figs. 22-8 to 22-11).

Exostoses are not congenital. They develop slowly during life and reach their maximum size in the third decade. Surgical excision is often required before placement of a removable prosthesis.

Important in the differential diagnosis are multiple osteomas as a partial manifestation of *Gardner's syndrome* (Figs. 22-12 and 22-13). The typical triad of symptoms of this autosomal-dominant heritable disorder consists of multiple osteomas, especially of the facial and jaw bones, multiple adenomas of the intestinal tract with frequent conversion to adenocarcinoma, and multiple skin tumors (mainly fibromas). Supernumerary teeth also occur. Because the skeletal changes often become manifest in youth and are as a rule preceded by intestinal polyposis, the dentist can provide an important contribution to recognition of the condition by referring the patient to an internist when suspicion arises.

Also to be considered in the differential diagnosis are bony protuberances elicited by tumors of bone or cartilage (Fig. 22-14), and findings associated with fibrous dysplasia of bone (Fig. 22-15) and *Paget's disease* (Fig. 22-16). Each instance requires radiographic and histologic confirmation.

Reactive hyperplasias as consequence of traumatic and inflammatory irritation

In addition to the *epulides* already described in chapter 14 (see Fig. 22-20), this group includes *proptosis of the lips and cheeks* and *denture hyperplasia,* both reactive fibromatous lesions, and *pyogenic granuloma,* a reactive hemangiomatous lesion. *Inflammatory papillary hyperplasia of the palatal mucosa* is discussed in chapter 33.

Proptosis of the lips, cheeks

A form of reactive fibrous hyperplasia frequently found in the oral cavity is proptosis, with circumscribed outgrowth of soft tissue extending to the lumen in the region of the lips and cheeks. Such excessive tissue formations are seen congruent to edentulous spaces and poorly fitting fixed and removable restorations (Figs. 22-17 and 22-18). The pathogenesis is ascribed to a suction effect that is normal during the act of swallowing but excessive in connection with certain habits (see chapter 32). The surface may become secondarily hyperplastic or ulcerated as a result of mechanical irritation (e.g., cheek biting; Fig. 22-19), making the diagnosis more difficult. Unless the cause is eliminated, recurrence following surgical excision is inevitable.

Denture hyperplasia (ICD-DA 523.86)

Denture hyperplasias are especially likely to be found in patients who have worn a poorly fitting or otherwise faulty prosthesis for a long time. Mechanical stress resulting from anatomically incorrect or functionally inappropriate prostheses, including those with overextended or defective denture margins in the region of the movable mucosa, lead to local tissue destruction and traumatic ulceration. As the irritation continues on this inflamed mucosa, excess granulation tissue develops that later becomes this fibroma-like tissue. The process can lead to a wide variety of impressive clinical findings (Figs. 22-21 to 22-27). Denture hyperplasia is frequently associated with flabby ridges.

Surgical removal of the excess fibrous tissue, together with vestibuloplasty when indicated, promises to be successful in the long term only if appropriate prosthodontic therapy is also provided. Additional examples of prosthesis-induced alterations and hyperplasia in response to irritation, as may be explained in relation to other dental treatment, are described in chapter 33.

Pyogenic granuloma (ICD-DA 528.94)

Pyogenic granuloma is a reactive hemangiomatous lesion characterized by excess granulation tissue similar in appearance to capillary hemangioma because of its extensive vascular network. The "pyogenic granuloma" designation, although arising from the existence of granulocyte infiltration, is somewhat inappropriate because the condition is not of bacterial origin.

Pyogenic granuloma (granuloma telangiectaticum) develops quickly on the surface of a slight injury of the lip or tongue and, less frequently, on the cheek and other mucosal tissue. Initially it remains covered by a thin epithelial layer (Fig. 22-28); later, in the course of its relatively (by comparsion with that of hemangiomas) rapid growth, its surface ulcerates. Clinically, pyogenic granuloma appears as a soft, often pedunculated, pea-sized to bean-sized formation with a shiny, vividly red or fibrin-covered, ulcerated surface (Figs. 22-29 and 22-30). As a rule, it is not painful, but it bleeds at the slightest touch because of its rich vascularization.

Pyogenic granuloma can heal spontaneously or may form a fibroma-like nodule with scar formation. In persistent cases, excision is indicated.

It may appear on the gingiva as epulis of pregnancy (see chapter 27).

Benign tumors

Within the framework of oral mucosal diseases we feel compelled to describe only some examples of benign tumors of the oral soft tissues *(fibroma, lipoma, hemangioma, lymphangioma)* because the overlying mucosa with certain exceptions and in absence of complications remains unchanged. The situation is different in the case of benign epithelial tumors, among which we will consider papilloma and keratoacanthoma.

The reader requiring a more complete discussion of these topics is referred to textbooks of pathology and of oral and maxillofacial surgery; the latter also provide details of the principles of surgical treatment.

Fibroma (ICD-M 8810/0)

In contrast to the so-called irritation fibromas, which are reactive fibromatous lesions and not true tumors, fibromas are rare in the oral cavity and usually occur only in the elderly.

This well-circumscribed, broad-based, flat or pedunculated, benign connective tissue tumor of the oral soft tissues (Figs. 22-31 to 22-35) must be differentiated from fibromas of the jawbones (nonossifying fibroma, ossifying fibroma, aggressive desmoplastic fibroma), which present distinctly different problems in differential diagnosis and therapy and which are beyond the scope of this book.

Oral soft tissue fibromas grow very slowly and often stop growing after having reached a certain size. They are hard to soft *(hard fibroma, soft fibroma),* a quality that depends on the number and arrangement of the collagen fibers and the proportion of ground substance. Mixed forms with other tissue components are not rare (e.g., fibrolipoma, Fig. 22-36; fibromyxoma; osteofibroma).

The mucosa covering the fibroma that occurs on the cheek, tongue, palate, and gingiva is normal. When the tumor occurs on the cheek mucosa at the level of occlusion, hyperkeratosis or ulcerations may occur on the mucosal surface as a result of repeated traumatic irritation.

As a rule, excision of the fibroma is indicated, inasmuch as clinical differential diagnosis is not always sufficient to rule out other solid tumors, e.g., salivary gland tumors of the palate.

Lipoma (ICD-DA 214/X0, ICD-M 8850/0)

Lipomas, rare in the oral cavity compared to their occurrence in other body regions, ordinarily appear clinically after the age of 40. As submucous formations causing hemispherical elevations of the oral mucosa, they appear mainly on the cheek (Fig. 22-38), tongue, floor of the mouth, soft palate, and lips but may appear at any location in which fatty tissue is normally present. When the position is superficial, the benign fatty tissue tumor shines through the usually unaltered mucosa with a yellowish color (Fig. 22-39). The consistency of the usually solitary, connective tissue—encapsulated tumor is soft and may fluctuate on palpation (pseudo fluctuation). Its size ordinarily is a function of how long it has existed and permits estimation of the patient's reaction to it. Thus, monstrous growths may be seen (Fig. 22-39). In differential diagnosis, soft fibromas, soft tissue cysts, and lymphangiomas must be considered, especially when the floor of the mouth is involved. If fibrous or vascular tissue is present in large amount within the tumor, the tumor is called a lipofibroma or an angiolipoma. Lipomas are enucleated.

Hemangioma (ICD-DA 228.0); capillary hemangioma (ICD-M 9131/0); cavernous hemangioma (ICD-M 9121/0)

These tumors of the blood vessels, clearly benign despite their occasional infiltrating growth, have great clinical significance because of their relative frequency in the oral cavity and surrounding tissues, and because of the possibility of complications from hemorrhage, with which they are associated.

Most hemangiomas are congenital or develop soon after birth. They may be categorized as tumorlike malformations in the sense of *vascular hamartomas* (see flame-shaped nevus and blood vessel nevus in chapter 3; Fig. 22-51). Such hemangiomas grow initially as the body grows but often stop growing during the first year of life. Some then persist for life (e.g., the flame-shaped nevus), while others shrink over time. Which course the individual lesion will take is difficult to assess.

In addition to these, other hemangiomas appear initially in childhood and adulthood. Histologically, *capillary hemangiomas* (with narrow lumen, endothelium-lined capillary processes) are distinguished from *cavernous hemangiomas* (with a labyrinth of sinuslike blood-filled chambers having walls of flat endothelium). Intermediate and special forms also are known. Their clinical appearance varies (Figs. 22-40, 22-42 to 22-49). They may take on specific forms in the mucosa and skin, e.g., flame-shaped nevus, nodular elevations (planotuberous), nodal elevations (tuberonodous); in deep subcutaneous or subepithelial tissue layers, hemangiomas of greatly varying size occur.

The color of these blood vessel tumors, which appear in all regions of the oral cavity, depends on the degree to which they are filled and the position with respect to the surface. In general, capillary hemangiomas close to the surface are bright red; cavernous hemangiomas at this location are wine red to bluish red. Hemangiomas fade when pressure is applied with a glass spatula (Figs. 22-40 and 22-41).

Differential diagnosis includes Kaposi's sarcoma (see Figs. 11-68 and 11-69) and pyogenic granulomas (Figs. 22-29 and 22-30), varicosities (Fig. 22-49), and hematomas (Fig. 22-50). Hemangiomas, within the framework of angiomatoses, may be multicentric in the oral cavity and surrounding areas (Figs. 22-52 and 22-53).

Advising about therapy is demanding and requires many years of clinical experience. Competent consultants should judge whether a wait-and-see attitude is appropriate with respect to the possibility of spontaneous regression, or if active treatment (surgery or obliterating therapy; radiation treatment today is obsolete) is indicated.

The very rare *intraosseous (central) hemangioma* of the jaw, usually associated with angiomatous changes of the skin and mucosa, presents special problems. Hidden from clinical view, it manifests radiographically as a polycystic translucency or a honeycombed structural alteration. Tooth extractions performed because the lesion is not recognized can lead to life-threatening hemorrhages; deaths have been reported.

Glomus tumor (ICD-M 8711/0)

The glomus tumor, a benign blood vessel tumor, is related to the glomus organ, an encapsulated vascular tuft with arteriovenous anastomoses. The usually small tumor, which is structured like the glomus organ, is usually painful and is found predominantly in the region of the end arteries of fingers and toes, particularly under the nails. The tumor is quite rare in the oral cavity (Figs. 22-54 and 22-55).

Lymphangioma (ICD-DA 228.10); capillary lymphangioma (ICD-M 9171/0); cavernous lymphangioma (ICD-M 9172/0); cystic lymphangioma (ICD-M 9173/0)

Like the hemangiomas, the overwhelming proportion of lymphangiomas are congenital or appear clinically during the first 2 years of life. Subsequent growth may stop; regression as in the hemangiomas does not follow, however. Sites of predilection are the oral cavity, the face (parotid gland), the lateral neck region, and the axilla.

Histologically, these benign tumors of the lymph vessels are classified as *capillary lymphangiomas* (with netlike lymph vessel connections); *cavernous lymphangiomas* (with endothelium-lined, broad-chamber sinuses); and *cystic lymphangiomas* (with cystic expansion of the lymph vessels). The preferred oral sites of the most frequent, cavernous-cystic form are the anterior section of the dorsum and sides of the tongue; other sites include the lips, cheeks, and floor of the mouth.

Clinical signs range from cystic-papillary elevations having the appearance of frog spawn (Fig. 22-56) or sago grains; in the presence of small blood vessels these may appear reddish (Fig. 22-57). They also may appear as extensive, diffuse infiltrations of the soft tissue, including the muscles. The abnormal growth of the affected organs (e.g., macroglossia, macrocheilia) may lead to functional disturbances. Disfigurement of the face also is possible. In the oral cavity, traumatic changes may lead to incorrect diagnosis (Fig. 22-58).

Deep excision is required for cure. Limits are placed on this, however, by the need to spare anatomically important structures, so that in some instances only partial removal is possible.

Papilloma (ICD-M 8052/0)

The papilloma is the most frequent benign epithelial tumor of the oral mucosa. It occurs at all ages, with no significant predilection for either sex. Numerous small fronds of proliferating squamous epithelium and a scant vascularized stroma give this slowly growing neoplasm a villous, occasionally cauliflower-like appearance (Figs. 22-59 to 22-62). The color is white to gray.

The ordinarily pedunculated, more rarely broad-based papilloma is usually solitary, with a diameter of several millimeters. In extreme cases it can reach 1 cm or more (Fig. 22-63). Occasionally papillomas are arranged in multiple, bedlike groups. Tongue and palate are preferred sites, as are gingiva and lips. Any other localization is possible, however.

Warts and focal epithelial hyperplasia are included in the differential diagnosis; when the papilloma has a cauliflower-like surface, the initial stage of verrucous carcinoma must be considered. Excision is preferred in the healthy patient, because of a tendency to recur.

Keratoacanthoma (ICD-DA 701.10)

The keratoacanthoma is a benign epithelial neoplasm, although it is sometimes accompanied by signs of invasive growth. The keratoacanthoma arises in the form of a small, hemispherical nodule, grows with remarkable speed while forming a central invagination, and reaches its maximum growth, which may be several centimeters, after 1 or 2 months. In typical instances a central crater, filled with a keratinized mass, is formed. It has a bulging, indurated margin. Clinically and histologically, the appearance of the initial stage is largely similar to that of a prickle cell carcinoma. After persisting a few months, the tumor may undergo spontaneous regression and subsequent healing with residual scar.

The skin of the midface, including the lips, is a preferred site of keratoacanthomas (Fig. 22-64). Intraoral lessions also have been reported. Men over 60 have the highest rate of occurrence. Because of the great similarity between the keratoacanthoma and carcinoma, referral of the patient is always indicated. Instances of malignant degeneration are extremely rare (Fig. 22-65).

The example of the keratoacanthoma offers another demonstration of the manner in which the diagnosis is reached through the combination of patient history, clinical findings, and histopathologic examination, the clinical evaluation being particularly important in this case.

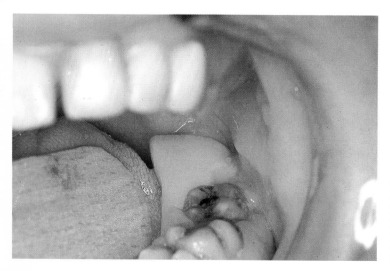

Fig. 22-1   Partial view of a peripheral jaw fibroma in the mandible. The clinically inflammation-free hyperplasia is at a typical site lingual and distal to the last molar.

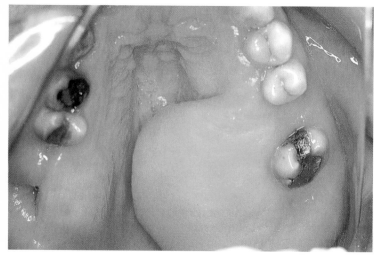

Fig. 22-2   Clearly asymmetric appearance of a so-called symmetric peripheral fibroma in the maxilla. The fibromatous tissue, growing slowly from the palatal gingival region of the molars, has crossed the midline on the left. Additional examples are discussed in relation to idiopathic fibrous gingival hyperplasia (see Figs. 15-10 to 15-13).

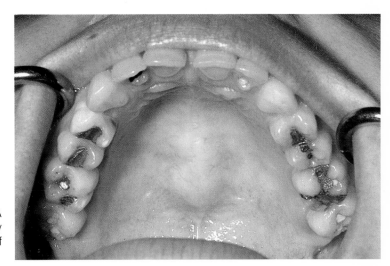

Fig. 22-3 Torus palatinus. A bone-hard bulge covered by normal mucosa in the region of the palatine suture.

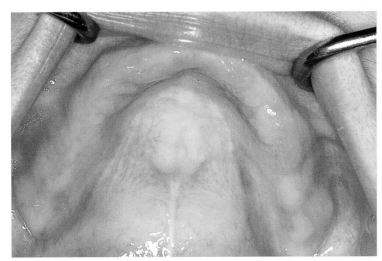

Fig. 22-4 Torus palatinus. As a corollary finding, pressure points are seen on the mucosa at the margin of the palate-free complete denture. Removal of the exostosis is indicated before placement of a mucosa-borne prosthesis.

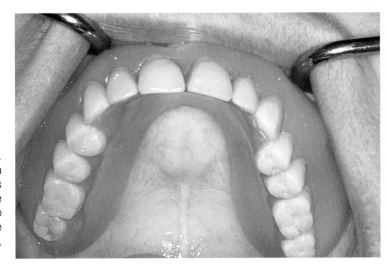

Fig. 22-5 The patient in Fig. 22-4 also at examination, with the denture in place. Deviations from the traditional shape of the denture base lead, as a rule, to early avoidable damage to the denture bed (see chapter 33, Figs. 33-27 and 33-28).

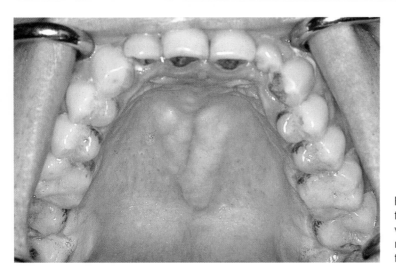

Fig. 22-6   Irregularly shaped torus palatinus. Exostoses develop very slowly and usually reach their maximum growth in the third decade of life.

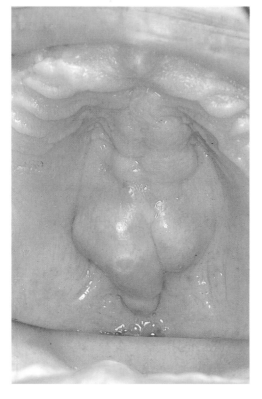

Fig. 22-7   Extreme form of torus palatinus. The irregularly shaped palatal exostosis has, at its top, a mucosal lesion caused by mechanical irritation.

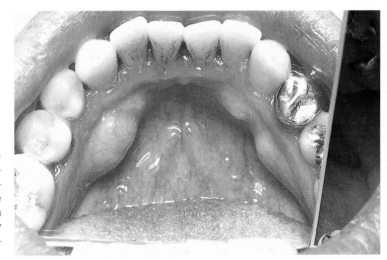

Fig. 22-8   Bilateral torus mandibularis. Such unilateral or bilateral growths are always located at the lingual surface of the mandible, just below the origin of the mylohyoid muscle; they are covered by stretched mucosa.

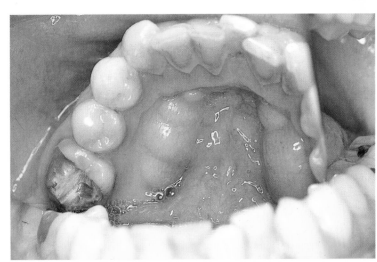

Fig. 22-9   Bilateral torus mandibularis in the form of a single lumpy, continuous exostosis. Surgical removal is usually indicated before placement of a mucosa-borne prosthesis.

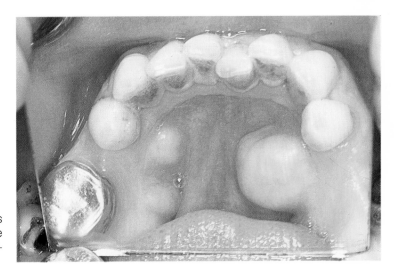

Fig. 22-10   Bilateral torus mandibularis with excessive overgrowth on the left side (mirror view).

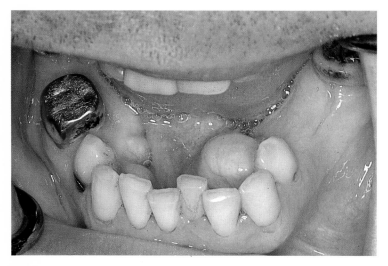

Fig. 22-11   Direct view of the patient in Fig. 22-10 at the time of examination. Differential diagnosis must eliminate malignant tumors of the bone in all instances of rapidly growing bony protuberances.

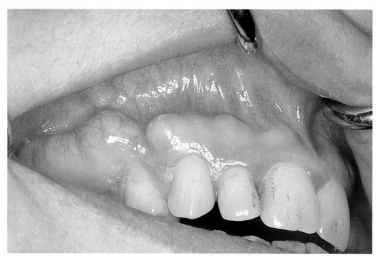

Fig. 22-12   Differential diagnosis of bony growths: multiple osteomas in the vestibular region of the maxillary alveolar process as a partial manifestation of Gardner's syndrome. Bones of the face and jaw are especially affected by these multiple osteomas.

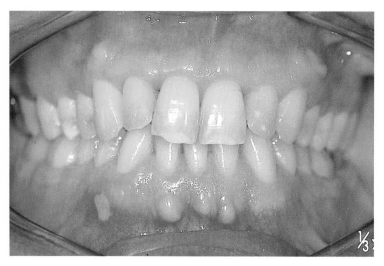

Fig. 22-13   Differential diagnosis of bony growth: multiple osteomas in the maxillary and mandibular alveolar processes. The bony changes precede formation of multiple adenomas of the intestinal tract, which are associated with a high risk of malignant transformation. Multiple skin tumors also are part of the syndrome. The dentist should refer the patient to an internal medicine specialist.

Fig. 22-14 Differential diagnosis of bony protuberances: periosteal (peripheral) osteoma on the vestibular side of the mandibular alveolar process near the first molar.

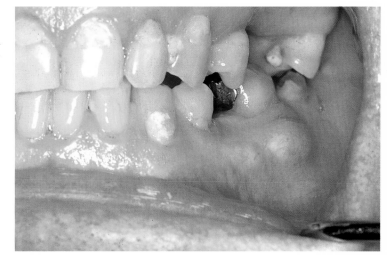

Fig. 22-15 Differential diagnosis of bony protuberances: distention of the right maxillary posterior tooth region caused by fibrous dysplasia (Jaffe-Lichtenstein syndrome) as monostotic form in a 16-year-old girl. This systemic bone disease affects only children and adolescents, particularly girls. The disease process stops after age 30; remissions are known. Diagnosis of this bony dysplasia (covered by intact mucosa) is made through clinical and radiographic findings (spotty homogenous shadowing) and histologic examination. When suspected, radiographic study of the entire skeletal system is indicated.

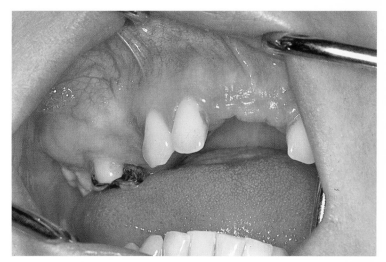

Fig. 22-16 Differential diagnosis of bony protuberances: Paget's disease as manifest in the edentulous mandible. This generalized chronically progressive osteopathy, which also appears in localized form, affects only the elderly, preferentially men. The condition leads to obvious enlargement of the facial skeleton, with intraoral bone alterations including malpositioning of teeth, occlusal disturbances, and thickening of the alveolar processes. Hypercementosis occurs regularly in the remaining dentition.

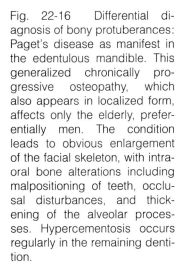
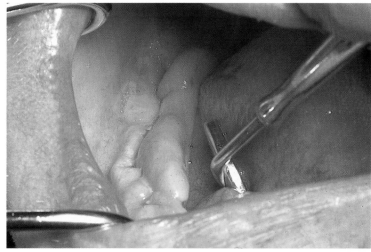

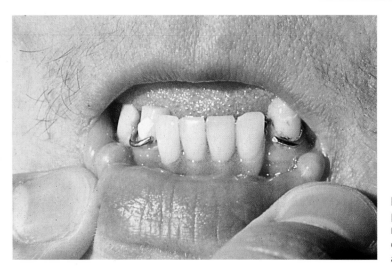

Fig. 22-17 Bilateral labial proptosis in congruence with a mucosa-borne sunken partial denture with clasps placed in an irritating position.

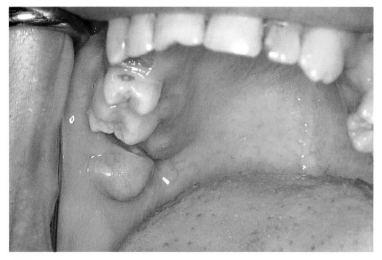

Fig. 22-18 Buccal proptosis. The circumscribed chronic ulceration was caused by the sharp edges of the distally carious maxillary right first molar.

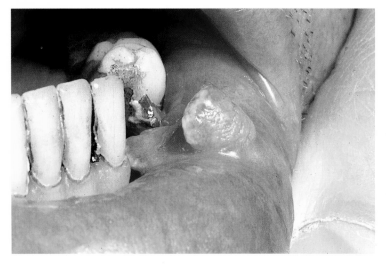

Fig. 22-19 Buccal proptosis. The advancing soft tissue largely fills the gap between the inadequate prosthesis and the root remnant of the posterior tooth. The mucosal surface shows stress hyperkeratosis and fibrin-covered ulceration as a consequence of mechanical irritation.

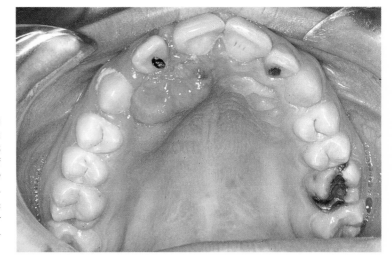

Fig. 22-20 Gingival irritation hyperplasia (fibrous epulis) in the region of teeth 12 and 13 (6, 7) as a consequence of traumatic irritation caused by abnormal occlusal development (deep bite with traumatic occlusion). See also chapter 14: The Various Forms of Epulis.

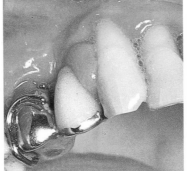
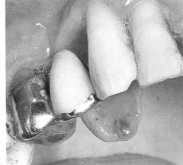

Fig. 22-21 Denture-induced lobular fibroma. In resting position, the pedunculated growth of the palate fills the space surrounding the distal pontic of tooth 14 (5) (picture at left) following removal of the partial denture and mobilization of the fibroma from its position (picture at the right).

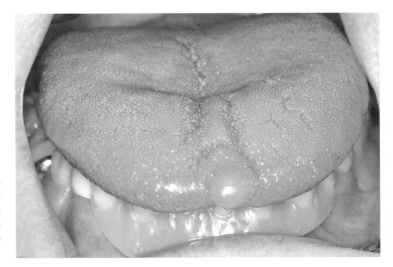

Fig. 22-22 Fibroma-like protruding stage of a fibrous hyperplasia at the tip of the tongue. Cause: traumatic irritation from the sharp edge of a prosthesis.

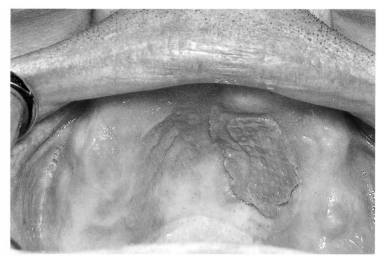

Fig. 22-23 Prosthetic irritation hyperplasia. The 67-year-old patient noted a painless, slow-growing formation on the palate over the course of 20 years. Because the maxillary complete denture was worn day and night for that period, the reactive tissue formation led to a congruent palatal impression.

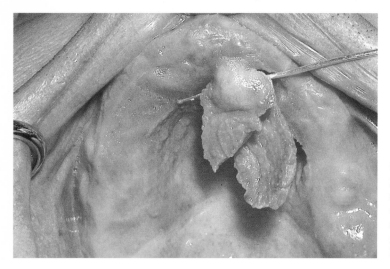

Fig. 22-24 Patient in Fig. 22-23 at examination. Elevation of the fibroma from the 7-mm-deep palatal impression makes clear its size, shape, and anterior narrow base. Other examples are found in chapter 33.

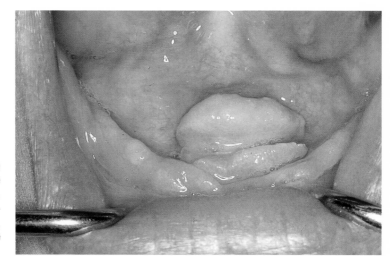

Fig. 22-25 Lobulated denture hyperplasia on the lingual side of the edentulous mandible. Cause: chronic traumatic irritation from an overextended, sharp denture border. Note the indentation.

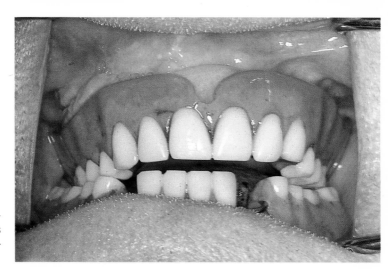

Fig. 22-26 Inadequate maxillary and mandibular prostheses worn for 15 years despite intervening tooth loss.

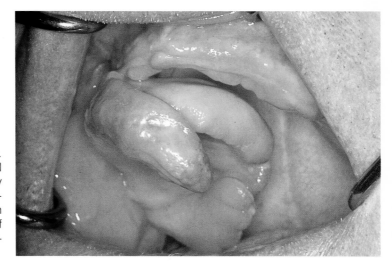

Fig. 22-27 Patient in Fig. 22-26 at examination. Removal of the poorly fitting maxillary prosthesis exposes several pedunculated fingerlike irritation fibromas as an expression of the monstrous denture hyperplasia.

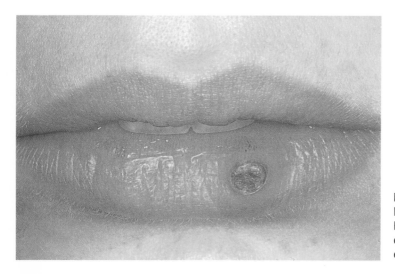

Fig. 22-28   Pyogenic granuloma in the vermilion of the lower lip. Early stage with a collarlike ulcer surrounded by epithelium.

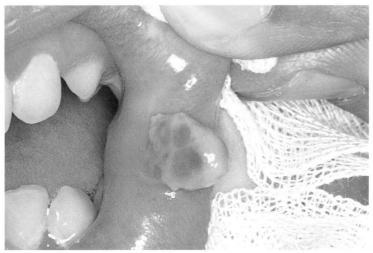

Fig. 22-29   Pyogenic granuloma. Completely developed stage of the reactive hemangiomatous lesion on lip mucosa. Note the vividly red, shiny surface in the center of the fibrin-covered ulcerations.

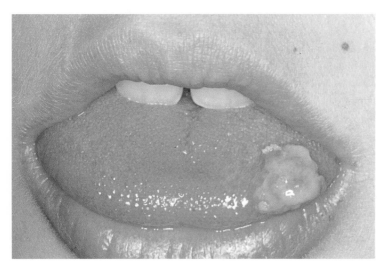

Fig. 22-30   Pyogenic granuloma. Completely developed stage on tongue with ulcerated, fibrin-covered surface.

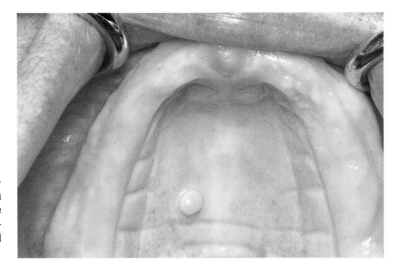

Fig. 22-31 Small, broad-based, elevated hard fibroma of the hard palate. The denture base shows reddish impressions arising from the etched denture.

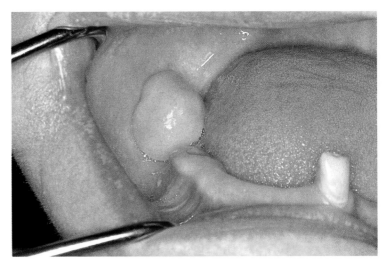

Fig. 22-32 Broad-based, firm fibroma in the retromolar space of the right side of the mandible.

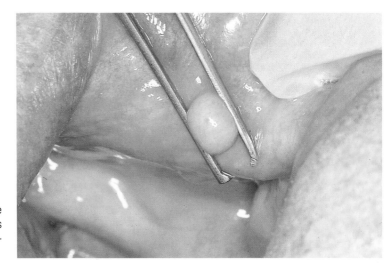

Fig. 22-33 Firm fibroma in the cheek. Forceps compression is intended to demonstrate consistency of the lesion.

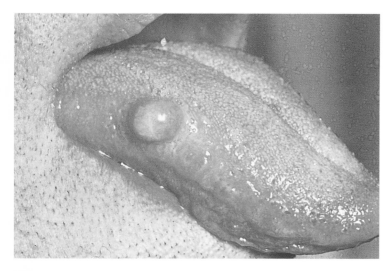

Fig. 22-34   Soft fibroma at the border of the tongue.

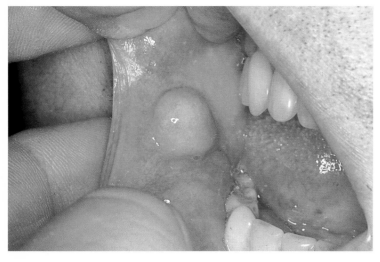

Fig. 22-35   Soft fibroma of the cheek. The tapering contour indicates a soft consistency, which is substantiated by palpation.

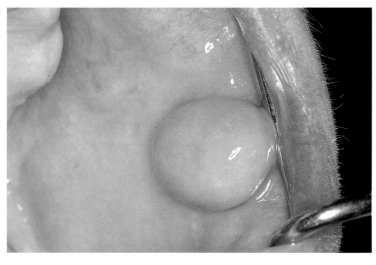

Fig. 22-36   Fibrolipoma of the cheek.

Fig. 22-37 Differential diagnosis of benign connective tissue tumors: peripheral giant cell tumor in the edentulous maxillary alveolar process (see also chapter 14). Signs of stress hyperkeratosis appear at the surface, together with a line-shaped pressure ulceration from the denture border. The denture was adapted several times to the growing granulation tissue mass by shortening at the borders.

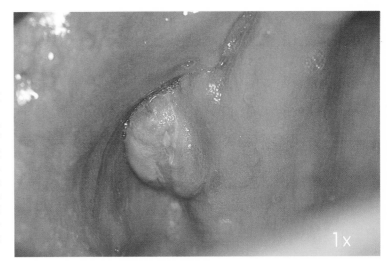

Fig. 22-38 Lipoma of the lower lip.

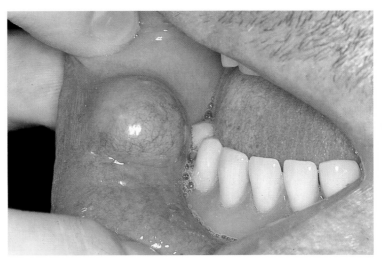

Fig. 22-39 Plum-sized lipoma of the floor of the mouth above the mylohyoid muscle in a 63-year-old man. The lesion, noted by the patient for 7 years, grew slowly and displaced the tongue dorsally. Only the altered appearance led the patient to seek medical advice.

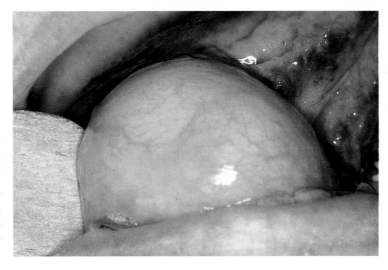

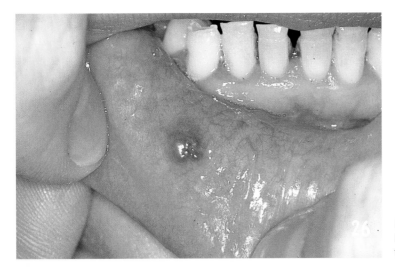

Fig. 22-40   Small cavernous hemangioma of the mucosa of the lower lip.

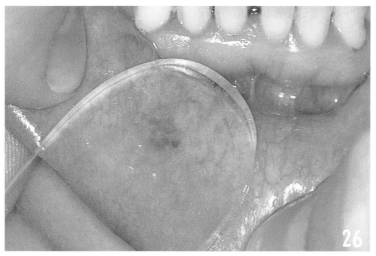

Fig. 22-41   The patient in Fig. 22-40 at examination. Pressure from a glass spatula leads to blanching of the hemangioma, located near the surface.

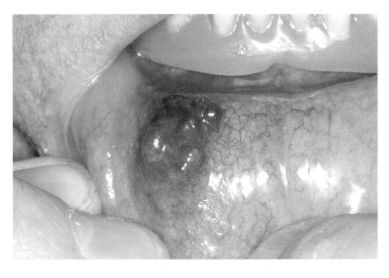

Fig. 22-42   Bulging nodular cavernous-type hemangioma of the mucosa of the lower lip. Hemorrhage will result from a minor injury.

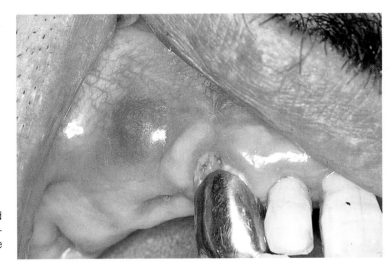

Fig. 22-43 Circumscribed planotuberous cavernous hemangioma of the vestibule of the right side of the maxilla.

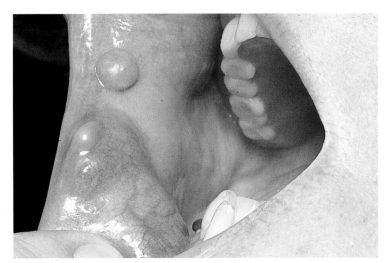

Fig. 22-44 Hemangioma of the right angle of the mouth. Two soft fibromas are seen in immediately adjacent tissue.

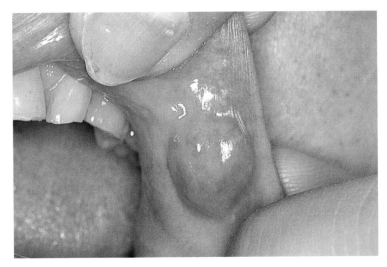

Fig. 22-45 Hemangioma of the left angle of the mouth.

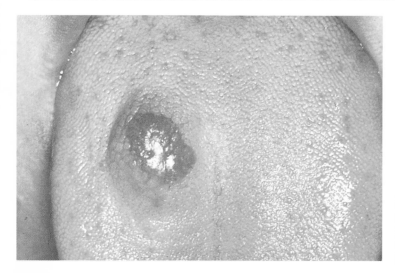

Fig. 22-46   Superficial hemangioma of the tongue. Hemangiomas often infiltrate into adjacent tissue but are nonetheless
benign.

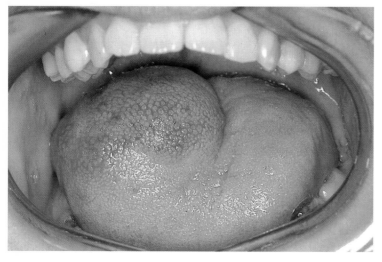

Fig. 22-47   Expansive hemangioma of the tongue.

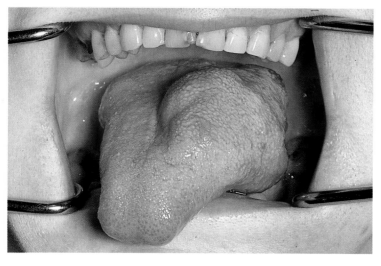

Fig. 22-48   Expansive hemangioma of the tongue.

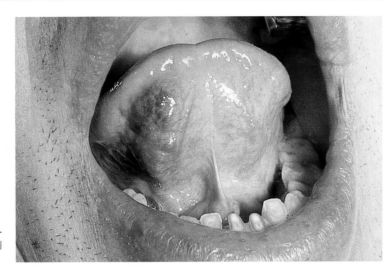

Fig. 22-49 Superficial cavernous hemangioma of the dorsal side of the tongue.

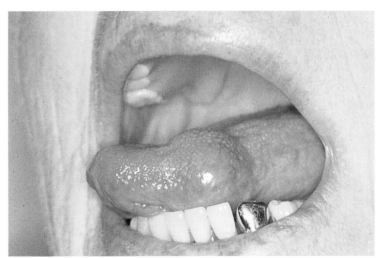

Fig. 22-50 Differential diagnosis of hemangioma: distended hematoma of the left side of the tongue in a 73-year-old woman with arteriosclerosis. Cause: the patient bit her tongue repeatedly (new mandibular denture), causing the hematoma.

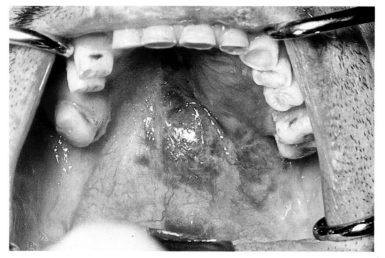

Fig. 22-51   Extensive cavernous hemangioma of the hard and soft palate with enormous enlargement of the left side of the jaw. It is one aspect of an angiomatous phakomatosis (see chapter 3). In dental surgical intervention of any type, extensive bleeding is likely so the dentist should regularly refer these patients.

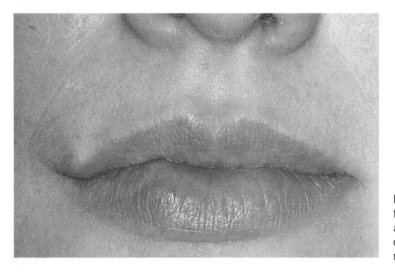

Fig. 22-52   Hemangioma on the right side of the lower lip and the angle of the mouth as one sign of congenital angiomatosis.

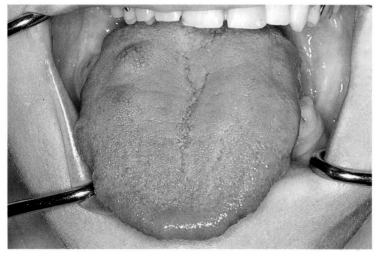

Fig. 22-53   The patient in Fig. 22-52, at the same examination. Additional circumscribed hemangiomas as seen on the tongue.

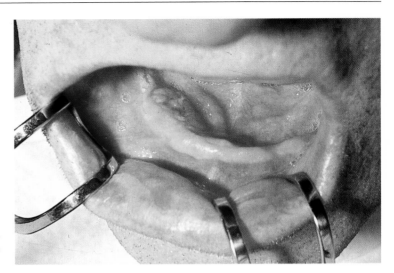

Fig. 22-54 Bean-sized glomus tumor on the right lingual side of the edentulous mandible. These benign neoplasms arising from the glomus organ are frequently painful.

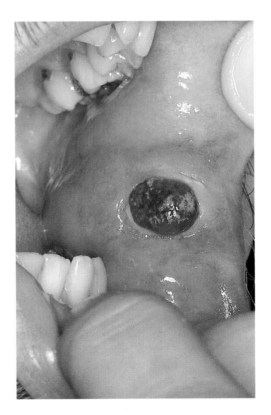

Fig. 22-55 Extraordinarily large glomus tumor of the right cheek.

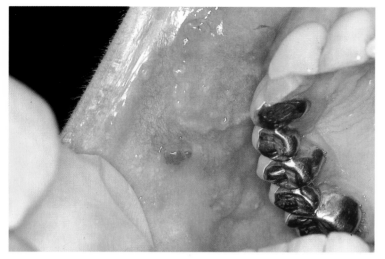

Fig. 22-56 A lymphangioma permeating the right cheek with frog spawn–like cystic-papillary elevations in the mucosa. Lymphangiomas, benign tumors of the lymph vessels, infiltrate as they grow. Removal by deep excision, therefore, may be problematic in some locations, even if the tumors are small.

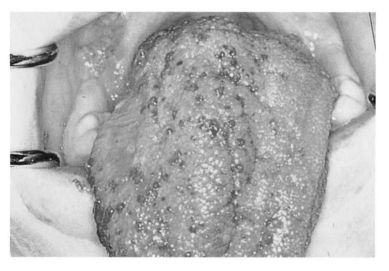

Fig. 22-57 Mixed (cavernous hemangioma and cavernous-cystic lymphangioma) vascular tumor of the tongue in a 9-year-old child led to unilateral macroglossia. Note the reddish sago grain–like elevations distributed over the back of the tongue.

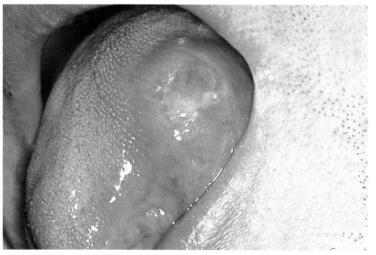

Fig. 22-58 Plum-sized lymphangioma deep in the tongue. According to the 19-year-old patient, the growth enlarged rapidly over a 3-month period. The flat ulceration at the left margin of the tongue is from chronic bite injuries due to tumor-related macroglossia.

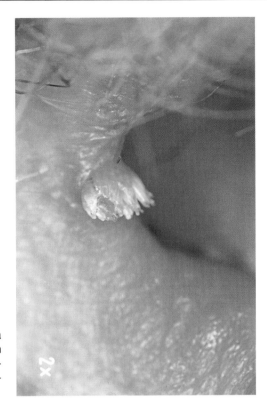

Fig. 22-59　Villous papilloma at the angle of the mouth. Each of the small projections is associated with its own scant vascularized stroma.

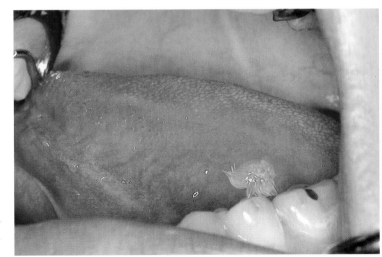

Fig. 22-60　Papilloma at the border of the tongue. Papillomas rarely grow endophytically into deep tissue (inverted papillomas).

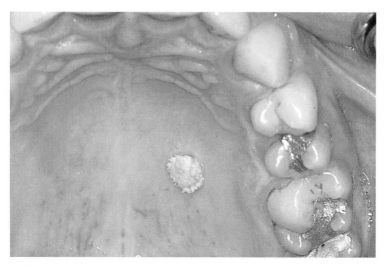

Fig. 22-61   Broad-based papilloma on the hard palate.

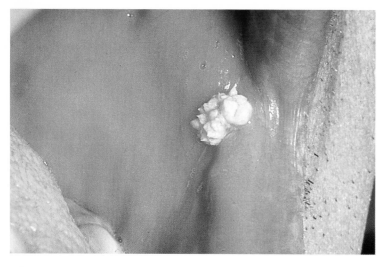

Fig. 22-62   Retroangularly located papilloma with wartlike structure in a 39-year-old patient. Differential diagnosis should include the initial stage of a verrucous carcinoma.

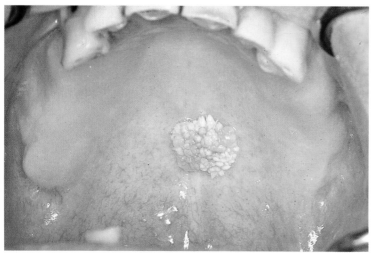

Fig. 22-63   Flat papilloma with patchy surface.

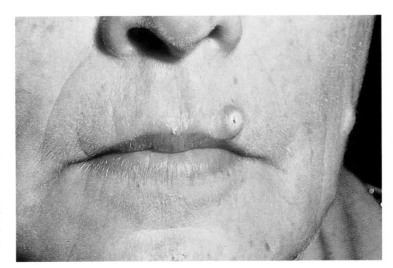

Fig. 22-64 Pea-sized kerato-acanthoma on the upper lip. Spherical nodule with central horny core. Despite their tendency to local invasive growth, keratoacanthomas are benign epithelial tumors. They occur particularly on the skin of the midface, and occasionally on the oral mucosa.

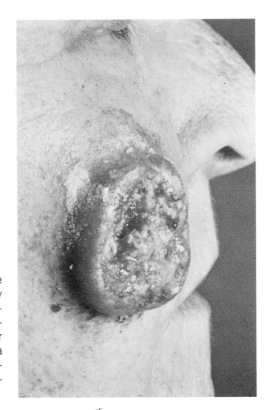

Fig. 22-65 Unusually large keratoacanthoma with partially extruded horny cover in a 65-year-old man. This keratoacanthoma, which recurred after surgical excision, underwent a rare transformation to a malignancy with lymph node metastases.

Chapter 23

Sarcomas and Non-Hodgkin's Lymphomas of the Oral Soft Tissue

Sarcomas of the oral soft tissue

Non-Hodgkin's lymphoma of the oral soft fibrous tissue

Sarcomas are malignant growths of the connective supportive tissue. Malignant neoplasms of the neuroectodermal peripheral nervous system are commonly assigned as sarcomas. The latter, as well as osteosarcomas and chondrosarcomas, are not considered here. The soft tissue sarcomas form a heterogeneous group histologically, and they also show great differences in their biologic behavior.

Among malignant diseases, sarcomas make up only a small fraction (1% to 2%). Their frequency in the mouth is so rare that the primary oral manifestation does not have epidemiologic significance. Nerverthe-less, or especially for this reason, sarcomas of the oral soft connective tissue deserve the special attention of dentists because they are often misjudged based on their clinical picture as tumors of another type or are confused with infectious processes. This applies equally to soft tissue sarcomas in the head and neck region.

The situation with *non-Hodgkin's lymphomas* is similar. Summarized under this generic term are all the malignant neoplasms, with the exception of malignant lymphogranulomas (Hodgkin's disease), which are derived from the cells of the lymphatic tissue with a different degree of maturation and differentiation. The non-Hodgkin's lymphomas are a very heterogeneous group. They differ not only cytogenetically and immunologically, but also in clinical picture, course, prognosis, and therapy. Because the oral cavity can be a primary or secondary location of manifestation, the dentist should have at least some basic knowledge about the nature and clinical symptoms of non-Hodgkin's lymphomas to be able to initially diagnose this malignant disease.

Sarcomas of the oral soft tissue

The soft tissue sarcoma previously mentioned that seldom occurs in the oral cavity can develop from connective tissue, fatty tissue, connective tissue of blood vessels, and muscle tissue. Corresponding to the originating tissue, the following forms of sarcoma can be differentiated (with other more detailed subgroups that will not be listed here):

Fibrous connective tissue	→ Fibrosarcoma (ICD-M 8810/3)
Fat tissue	→ Liposarcoma (ICD-M 8850/3)
Blood vessels	→ Angiosarcoma (ICD-M 9120/3)
Striated muscle (lips, tongue, cheek)	→ Rhabdomyosarcoma (ICD-M 8900/3)
Smooth muscle (vessels)	→ Leiomyosarcoma (ICD-M 8890/3)

For Kaposi's sarcoma, see chapter 11.

In the case of undifferentiated sarcomas, it was not possible with the earlier conventional method of morphologic diagnosis to determine its origin (tissue of origin) and thus to create a definite histogenetic classification. For this reason, differentiation was based, at any one time, on the predominating cell type, in small cell, round cell, spindle cell, and pleomorphic cell sarcomas. With the help of the tumor markers available today (monoclonal antibodies, especially against intermediate filaments), the possibilities of histomorphologic differential diagnosis have substantially broadened. In this way, for example, it can be established that a number of histogenetically different growths can hide with the appearance of a spindle-cell or polymorphic cell sarcoma.

In the early 1960s, *malignant fibrous histiocytoma* (ICD-M 8830/3), an independent form of tumor, took on an increased meaning. It is known today as the most frequently occurring soft tissue sarcoma of the adult years, but it can also occur in younger people. The histogenesis of this tumor, which can be divided into five histologic subtypes, is not yet clear. These forms of sarcoma show in part a histiocytic and in part a fibroblastic-like differentiation. For this reason, it has been proposed that these neoplasms develop from undifferentiated mesenchymal stem cells. They differ from the histologically similar fibrosarcoma and liposarcoma by their aggressive manner of invasion. An oral primary manifestation of malignant fibrous histiocytomas, similar to the tumors found in the extremities and retroperitoneal region, is apparently more frequent than once thought (Fig. 23-1).

According to their biologic behavior, the soft tissue sarcoma can be roughly divided into a low degree of malignancy and highly malignant forms. The *highly malignant undifferentiated sarcoma* grows rapidly and leads, in a high percentage of cases, to a hematogenous transport (first into the lungs, later into the liver, skeletal system, brain, and other organs), and has an unfavorable prognosis (5-year survival rate of under 30%). The *low-grade sarcoma* such as the well-differentiated fibrosarcoma, grows slowly, seldom metastasizes, and then only in an advanced stage, and has a relatively favorable prognosis (5-year survival rate of about 75%). In addition, there are forms with an intermediate grade of malignancy.

Histologic determination of the degree of malignancy (grading) is the most important factor of prognosis in regard to the tumor. Other important parameters for the prognosis are the size and depth of penetration of the tumors, their localization, the status of lymph nodes, and the age of the patient.

Soft tissue sarcomas of the oral cavity, which occur at every age, are most frequently localized on the alveolar process, palate, lips, tongue, and cheeks. When encountering areas of less resistance, the sarcoma of the oral soft tissue grows out of the depth into the oral cavity. The consistency is firm in cases of fiber-rich forms, soft in cases of undifferentiated cell sarcoma. As a rule, the mucous membrane stays smooth and undamaged over the bulging growth. Only in the further course of tumor growth, and significantly later than occurs with carcinoma of the oral cavity, do necrosis and ulceration develop on the lesion surface.

In the case of gingival localization, such as a malignant fibrous histiocytoma or a malignant hemangioendothelioma (ICD-M 9130/3; Fig. 23-2), there are also isolated epulis-like relatively early lesions, with necrotic, ulcerated changes developing in the mucous membrane. Depending on the aggressiveness of the sarcoma, the bone is attacked sooner or later and is eventually destroyed.

The oral cavity (alveolar process of the jaws, palate, and tongue) can also be the location of sarcoma metastasis (Fig. 23-3). The problem of early dental recognition is that the soft oral sarcoma is often mistaken for non-neoplastic fibrous tissue growth because of the intact covering mucous membrane. Especially serious are the cases in which swelling caused by the tumor is considered evidence of infection (infectious infiltrate, chronic abscess) and an intraoral incision for discharge is made in the growth, or a tooth located in the tumor is extracted (Fig. 23-4). Such instrumentation can cause the tumorous tissue to become infected, and the inevitable infection soon hides the disease process. Further, a possibility to be considered is an ulcerated, infected sarcoma in which the painful symptomatic infection, often accompanied by fever, can overlap and then dominate the clinical picture and can considerably delay the diagnosis of the underlying tumor.

Only those patients in whom the sarcoma is identified early in the clinical course have a good chance of recovery. To avoid misdiagnosis and the resulting loss of time with incorrect therapy—an error that can be crucial for the patient—the main points will be reviewed once again:

Even with clearly apparent, definite swellings (infiltrates) that are dependent on infection, the possibility of a tumor, which can be concealed, should never be ruled out initially. Whenever the normal dental procedures for treatment do not result in decreased inflammation within a few days, there should be suspicion of a tumor, and the patient should be referred elsewhere.

Treatment consists of radical surgical removal in the case of a mature sarcoma; in the case of immature forms, combinations of surgical, radiologic, or surgical cytostatic therapy are indicated.

Non-Hodgkin's lymphoma (NHL) of the oral soft fibrous tissue

Among the malignant lymphomas, *malignant lymphogranuloma (Hodgkin's disease)* occupies a nosologic position that is exceptional. It is briefly mentioned here to clarify the division of non-Hodgkin's lymphoma from the disease, which is malignant and which predominantly affects the lymphatic system.

Obvious clinical local symptoms of acute or asymptomatic beginning *Hodgkin's disease, malignant lymphogranuloma* (ICD-M 9650/3) are usually painless, firm swellings of cervical lymph nodes. These early palpable lymph nodes, which are located in the neck area in more than half the cases and with involvement, as a rule, of only one lymph node group, frequently precede by a long time systemic feeling of malaise with recurrent febrile episodes of undetermined nature. Frequently the patient complains about weight loss and itchy skin.

With increasing duration of the illness, a tendency for generalized involvement of the lymph nodes becomes apparent. The spleen is frequently involved. Involvement of other organs occurs through expansion of local parenchymal foci or by lymphogenic spread. When the course of this protean disease is advanced, it results finally in a diffuse involvement of nonlymphatic organs (lungs, skeletal system, liver, nervous system).

Hodgkin's disease can, in isolated instances, involve the oropharynx (lymphatic throat ring, tonsils). The few known occurrences are, however, uncharacteristic and rarely similar, and the oropharynx cannot be considered a pathognomonic location.

The diagnosis is confirmed through biopsy of the lymph node. Histologically identifiable and proven for Hodgkin's disease is the destruction of the normal lymph node architecture by a chronic pathologic granulomalike infiltrate with scattered, atypical mononuclear reticular cells (Hodgkin's cells) and/or multinucleated giant cells (Reed-Sternberg cells). According to histologic findings, it is possible to differentiate a lymphocyte-rich, nodular-sclerosing form, a mixed cell form, and a lymphocyte-poor form, which have different prognostic outlooks.

All other lymphomas differentiated histologically from the malignant lymphogranuloma are today designated non-Hodgkin's lymphomas.

This heterogeneous disease group was subdivided by classic pathology according to pure morphologic criteria into *reticulum cell sarcoma, lymphosarcoma (lymphocytic, lymphoblastic)* and *large follicular lymphoma (germinoblastoma, Brill-Symmers disease), including its generalized forms (among others, malignant reticulosis, leukosarcomatosis, paraleukoblastic leukemia).* This complex classification and terminology have always caused difficulties. Through progress in the field of lymphocyte research (immunophenotype standardization, molecular biology), knowledge of the cytologic origin, the functional characteristics, the degree of differentiation of the proliferating lymphatic cells, and, thereby, of the nature and the biologic relationship of these malignant lymphomas has considerably expanded. This increased knowledge has brought fundamental changes in the classification of lymphocytic lymphomas.

To better understand today's common system of classification for non-Hodgkin's lymphomas, there are several brief references to the development (see also the schematic diagrams of page 481) of the function of the lymphocyte:

Lymphocytes belong to the most differentiated cells of the human body. There are small, medium, and large cell forms with an average of 5 μm to 8 μm, 8 μm to 12 μm, and over 12 μm. Only about 4% of all lymphocytes are available in the peripheral blood. About 70% are found in the lymphatic organs (lymph nodes, spleen, thymus, tonsils, lymphatic tissue associated with the intestines); 10% are in the bone marrow and 15% in the remaining tissues.

Regarding the immune function of the lymphatic cell system, we must differentiate the *B-lymphocytes* (carriers of humoral immunity) and the *T-lymphocytes* (carriers of cell-mediated immunity).

The precursors of the B-lymphocytes originate in the bone marrow. Under the influence of a bursa-equivalent organ in the human (bone marrow?), they ripen to B-lymphocytes. These occupy the so-called "B" area in peripheral lymph organs, where they develop to antibody-producing and sensitizing cells after contact with antigen. The end result of development is either the differentiation into plasma cells that are not able to divide, or to memory cells (B_2-lymphocytes) as representatives of the immunologic memory. In this maturation, certain T-lymphocytes (helper cells) intervene by modulating the process.

The T-lymphocytes are stored temporarily in the thymus and are prepared there for their specific function. They then plant themselves in thymus-dependent "T" area peripheral lymph organs to take over various immunologic duties. T-cells that produce lymphokines are substantially involved in cellular immunity. Also, in the case of graft-host reaction, T-cells play an important role. Other T-lymphocytes regulate the immunologic activity of B-lymphocytes and other T-cells as helper or suppressor cells. Finally, there are T-lymphocytes, which, because of their cytotoxic cytolytic properties, can damage cells that are foreign to the body (so-called killer cells).

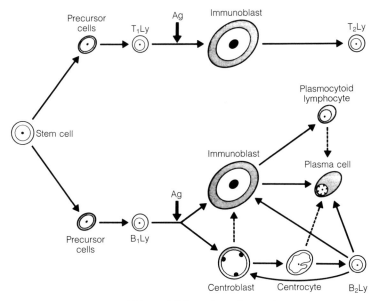

Simplified scheme of T- and B-lymphocyte system
Ag = antigen stimulation   Ly = lymphocyte
(From: *Lennert K, Feller AC.* Histopathologie der Non-Hodgkin-lymphome, ed 2.
Berlin. Springer, 1990:28.)

Rappaport differed from the traditional opinion on malignant lymphoma and in 1966 first classified the malignant diseases of the
lymphatic tissue according to *(1)* origin (lymphocytic, histiocytic,
mixed cells), *(2)* their degree of differentiation (well differentiated,
poorly differentiated, undifferentiated), and *(3)* their pattern of growth
(nodular, diffuse). In addition to many modifications of this classification, other suggestions for classification were made, among them, by
Dorfman in 1974, Lukes and Collins in 1975, and the World Health
Organization.

   In consideration of electromicroscopic, cytochemical, and immunologic criteria, in 1974 Lennert developed the so-called *Kiel
classification of non-Hodgkin's lymphomas.* It is the standard classification in Germany and several western European countries. Its clinical
and prognostic relevance was verified through numerous studies. The
Kiel classification of 1988 is given in Table 1. Because today we know
that nearly all non-Hodgkin's lymphomas are composed of B cells or T
cells, these malignant neoplasms are now classified as tumor of B- and
T-cell types. Subdivisions of non-Hodgkin's lymphoma into lower and
higher degrees of malignancy was retained, although it is hard to
apply in the case of T-cell lymphomas.

Table 1 Current Kiel classification of non-Hodgkin's lymphomas (from *Stansfeld AG, et al:* Updated Kiel classification for lymphomas. Lancet, February 6, 1988; 292–293).

B lymphocytes	T lymphocytes
Lymphomas of low degree of malignancy 　Lymphocytic 　　Chronic lymphocytic 　　leukemia and 　　prolymphocytic leukemia 　　Hairy cell leukemia 　Lymphoplasmacytic/lympho- 　plasmacytoid (immunocytoma) 　Plasmacytic 　Centroblastic/centrocytic 　　follicular ± diffuse 　　diffuse	Lymphomas of low degree of malignancy 　Lymphocytic 　　Chronic lymphocytic 　　leukemia and 　　prolymphocytic leukemia 　Small cell cerebriform mycosis 　fungoides, Sezary syndrome 　Lymphoepithelioid (Lennert's 　lymphoma) 　Angioimmunoblastic 　(ALLD, LgX) 　T-zone lymphoma 　Pleomorphic, small cell 　(HTLV-1 ±)
Lymphomas with higher malignancy 　Centroblastic 　Immunoblastic 　Large cell, anaplastic (Ki-1 +) 　Burkitt's lymphoma 　Lymphoblastic	Lymphomas with higher malignancy 　Pleomorphic, middle size and 　large cells (HTLV-1 ±) 　Immunoblastic (HTLV-1 ±) 　Large cell, anaplastic (Ki-1 +) 　Lymphoblastic
Rare types	Rare types

Detailed discussion of the various types of lymphomas is beyond the scope of this book. Details about the different types can be found in hematology and pathology textbooks. Following are some clinically important points to acquaint the dentist with the problems of non-Hodgkin's lymphomas.

Approximately 2% of all malignant neoplasms are non-Hodgkin's lymphomas. These occur in individuals of all ages but show a marked increase of incidence with increasing age. Generally *non-Hodgkin's lymphoma of lower degree of malignancy* consists of proliferating cells of more advanced differentiation. The primary clinical symptom is most often a gradual painless palpable increase in size of a single lymph node or a lymph node group with preferred localization in the neck, arm pit, or groin. Additional accompanying symptoms and general manifestations of the disease remain unnoticed for a long time. For this reason, the diagnosis can be obtained only histologically with an excision biopsy of a lymph node. Increase in number of circulating lymphocytes is the early symptom of the chronic lymphatic leukemias that are the most frequent (low grade) non-Hodgkin's lymphoproliferative disorder.

After a course of several years, generalization of the disease frequently occurs, with involvement of other lymph node groups and with participation of some internal organs (gastrointestinal, skeletal system, lung); an increase in the degree of malignancy may be observed at the same time. With the exception of chronic lymphatic leukemia, the staging classification is similar to that used for malignant lymphogranuloma (see Table 2).

The so-called *B-symptomas* (weight loss of more than 10% of body weight in the past 6 months, and/or temperature over 38°C and/or night sweats without other cause) are regarded as prognostically unfavorable signs.

Table 2   Classification of the Hodgkin's Disease Staging Classification Committee, Ann Arbor 1971

Stage I	Attack of a single anatomic lymph node region (I) or a single extralymphatic organ (I_E)
Stage II	Attack of two or more anatomic lymph node regions on the same side of the diaphragm (II) or localized attack on extralymphatic organs or tissues and one or more lymph node regions on the same side of the diaphragm (II_E)
Stage III	Attack of the lymph node region on both sides of the diaphragm (III), which can also be accompanied by spleen involvement (III_S) or a localized attack of extralymphatic regions (III_E) or both (III_{SE})
Stage IV	Diffuse or disseminated attack of one or more extralymphatic organs or fibers with or without lymph node attack.

Low-malignancy non-Hodgkin's lymphomas are, for example:

- *Chronic lymphatic leukemia:* chapter 26 describes, under "Leukemia," the most frequent leukemic form of older adults (about 25% of all non-Hodgkin's lymphomas).

- *Waldenström macroglobulinemia* (old nomenclature), which is considered today to be a special clinical variation (macroglobulinemia) of the morphologic cycle of the immunocytomas.
- *Mycosis fungoides* (ICD-M 9700/3), considered today as the most frequent T-cell lymphoma malignancy of the skin (Fig. 23-5).

Non-Hodgkin's lymphomas of high malignancy are identified by high proliferative activity of their cells (blasts) and clinically show features of rapidly progressive disease. They frequently begin acutely with rapidly enlarging, painful, firm lymph nodes (cervical, axial, inguinal, mediastinal), which most often involve multiple sites, so that the lesion remains circumscribed only for a short period of time. Symptoms may involve internal organs (gastrointestinal tract, spleen, liver) or the head and neck region (especially the nasal and throat regions but also the jaw and facial regions). In 20% to 25% of patients, the primary manifestation of the disease is an organ other than lymph nodes *(extranodal presentation).* The pathway of further spread varies from patient to patient.

Half of all patients with highly malignant non-Hodgkin's lymphoma complain at the time of first examination of systemic symptoms (B-symptomatic) that suggests an already advanced stage (III and IV).

In general, soft tissues of the oral cavity are rarely affected, but they are still an important primary or secondary location for the manifestation of an extranodal non-Hodgkin's lymphoma in which the high-grade forms dominate with a prognostically unfavorable tendency for generalization. The clinical picture of these lymphomas varies and is often uncharacteristic (see Figs. 23-6, 23-7, and 23-9), which explains the many cases of misdiagnosis.

They can appear on the hard palate as knotty growths with or without ulceration (Figs. 23-10 and 23-11), and can be confused with growths of the salivary glands. In the soft tissues of the oral cavity, which are covered by a mucous membrane lining, and on the tongue, the lymphomas are apparent earlier as soft-to-doughy swellings. Even gingival manifestations are possible in the form of diffuse necrotic and ulcerating penetrating proliferations, which can be clinically similar to hyperplastic gingivitis, acute exacerbating periodontal disease, or acute leukemia (Figs. 23-12 and 23-14 to 23-16).

Among the highly malignant non-Hodgkin's lymphoma with primary extranodal manifestation in the region of the oral soft tissue it is possible to find:

- *Malignant lymphoma, centroblastic type* (ICD-M 9632/3)
- *Malignant lymphoma, poorly differentiated* (ICD-M 9630/3)
- *Malignant lymphoma, immunoblastic type* (ICD-M 9612/3)

Most of the immunoblastic lymphomas correspond to the reticulum cell sarcoma of older nomenclature. A small portion of lesions referred to earlier as reticulum cell sarcoma is included with the centroblastic lymphomas.

Burkitt's lymphoma (ICD-M 9750/3) is recognized today as a separate type of lymphoma, because of its peculiar morphologic, immunophenotypic, and cytogenetic features. The disease appears predominantly in children and youths. The endemic type, which occurs in Central Africa, is consistently associated with the Epstein-Barr virus, whose genome can be demonstrated in every tumor cell. Predominant in the clinical picture is the rapid growth, which in 50% of cases occurs in the region of jaws and in 30% occurs in the gastrointestinal organs. In the case of the "non-African" type, which can be observed in the United States and Europe *(Burkitt-like lymphoma),* involvement of the face is not the rule (Figs. 23-17 and 23-18). Only 10% to 30% of jaws are affected whereas in 50% to 70% of cases there is abdominal involvement.

Non-Hodgkin's lymphoma is radiation sensitive and can also be treated by chemotherapy. Often, a combination of radiation therapy and cytostatic polychemotherapy is used. Prognosis depends on the type of lymphoma (relating to the classification), clinical stage at the time of diagnosis, location of the primary manifestation, and age and general condition of the patient.

The dentist can be considered the first link in the diagnostic chain with suspicion of nodal and extranodal lesions in the oral cavity and also in the head and neck region. When the condition is suspicious, treatment must be deferred and the patient immediately referred for interdisciplinary oncologic diagnosis and treatment.

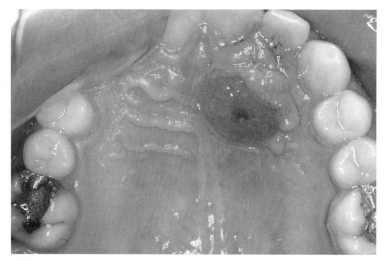

Fig. 23-1 Malignant fibrous histiocytoma in the anterior region of the hard palate of a 17-year-old patient. The sarcoma appeared clinically as a dome-like prominence contrasting in color with the surrounding tissue. According to the patient history, a red swelling was first noticed 3 weeks earlier, and it did not respond to antibiotic therapy. In differential diagnosis, tuberculous granuloma should be considered, among other possibilities.

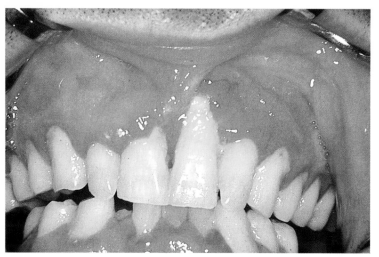

Fig. 23-2 Malignant hemangioendothelioma on the alveolar process in the region of teeth 11 and 21 (8 and 9) in a 43-year-old patient. A proliferation on the gingiva (area of mobile tooth 21), livid in color and repeatedly bleeding spontaneously, was attributed to traumatic occlusion resulting from an abnormal overbite. This lesion was repeatedly cauterized. At the time of examination a submandibular lymph node metastasis, the size of a hen's egg, was present together with the intraoral findings illustrated.

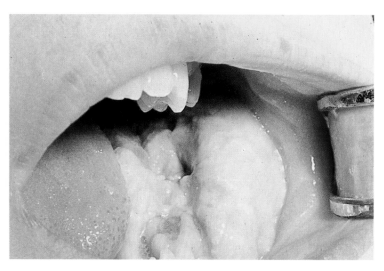

Fig. 23-3 Large metastasis of a spindle-cell sarcoma (no further classification) in the mandible of a 20-year-old woman. The primary tumor was located on a thigh. Sarcomas generally metastatize via the blood stream. The alveolar process, palate, and tongue are the main sites of metastasis in the oral cavity.

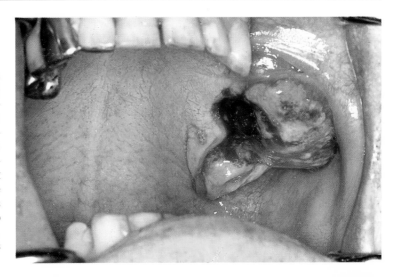

Fig. 23-4 Condition 12 days after extraction of tooth 26 (14) in a pre-existing growth of pleomorphic cell sarcoma, which had been misdiagnosed as inflammatory granulation tissue in the maxilla (without further analysis). The 45-year-old patient reported having noticed the cheek swelling only 2 months earlier. Remote metastases (to lung, liver, skeletal system, brain) were not present at this time.

Fig. 23-5 Surface type, plaque-stage skin infiltrate of a mycosis fungoides in the facial region. Some spots show initial tumor formation (transition from second to third stage). The disease (malignant T-cell lymphoma) shows a three-stage course over 10 to 15 years with unfavorable prognosis: in the premycotic phase there are nonspecific skin changes that are associated with itching and that resemble foci of subacute eczema. The second phase leads to bandlike lymphohistiocytic infiltrates and thickening of the foci with tendency to plaque formation. The third

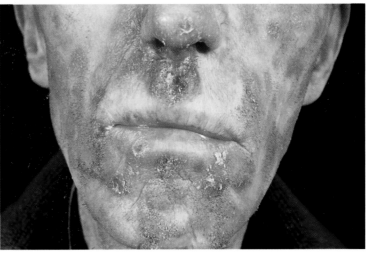

phase is characterized by nodular, mushroom growths that give the disease its name. The tumor phase shows the transformation to higher malignancy of the lymphoma with subsequent generalization ("immunologic oncogenesis"). Oral manifestations are rare and are almost exclusively found in the terminal phase of the disease.

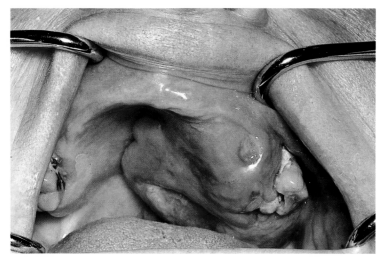

Fig. 23-6   Malignant non-Hodgkin's lymphoma ("lympho-sarcoma" in the old nomenclature) in the region of the left maxilla in a 79-year-old woman. The rapidly growing neoplasm growing into the oral cavity has already achieved a large volume and has passed the midline of the palate. It was first considered to be an inflammation. Radiographic examination showed advanced destruction of bordering bone structure.

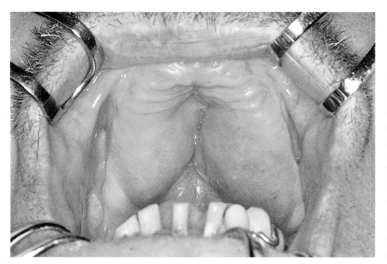

Fig. 23-7   Intraoral partial manifestation of a disseminated highly malignant non-Hodgkin's lymphoma ("lymphosarcoma" in the old nomenclature). Besides the noticeable soft enlargement of the palate that resembles symmetric fibroma, there are other manifestations in the area of the lymphatic border ring as well as generalized lymph node involvement. The mediastinal lymphoma led to a stridor with breathing.

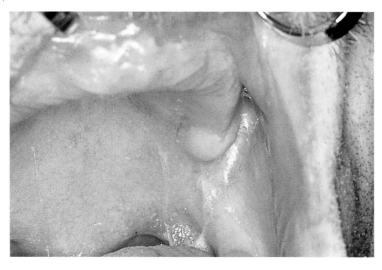

Fig. 23-8   The patient in Fig. 23-7 after irradiation therapy. In spite of temporary regression of the lymphoma on the palate, the prognosis in this advanced stage is poor.

Fig. 23-9 Highly malignant non-Hodgkin's lymphoma ("reticulum cell sarcoma" in the old nomenclature) on the border of the hard and soft palate. The 71-year-old patient had felt pain on the left maxilla for weeks. He visited his dentist only when his denture no longer "fit." The malignant neoplasm that was known as reticulum cell sarcoma corresponds in a high percentage of cases to the immunoblastic lymphoma of the Kiel classification. The others are predominantly classified as centroblastic lymphomas.

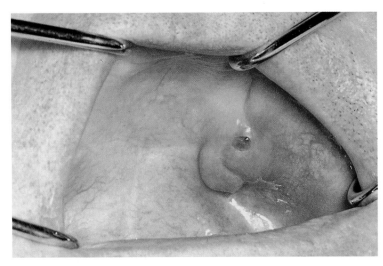

Fig. 23-10 Highly malignant non-Hodgkin's lymphoma of the immunoblastic type on the hard palate of a 65-year-old patient. Four weeks before the visit to the clinic, the patient first noticed a swelling in this area, which enlarged in the meantime. The lesion, fairly well delimited from the surrounding area, was hard, painful on pressure, and did not slide easily on the underlying structures.

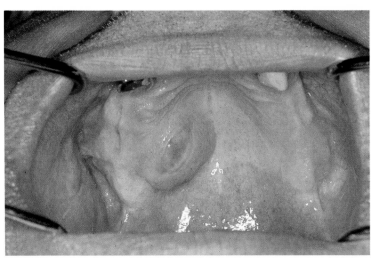

Fig. 23-11 The patient in Fig. 23-10, 10 days later, before beginning therapy. The rapidly evolving neoplasm, now with a superficial ulceration, documents the aggressiveness of this malignant non-Hodgkin's lymphoma.

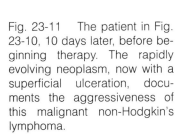

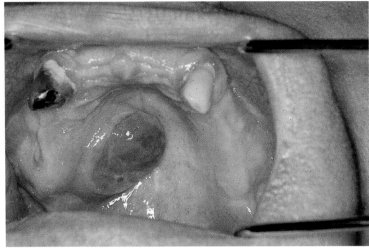

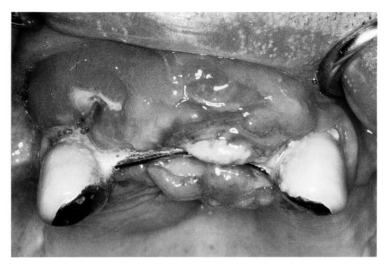

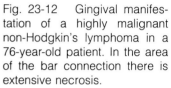

Fig. 23-12   Gingival manifestation of a highly malignant
non-Hodgkin's lymphoma in a
76-year-old patient. In the area
of the bar connection there is
extensive necrosis.

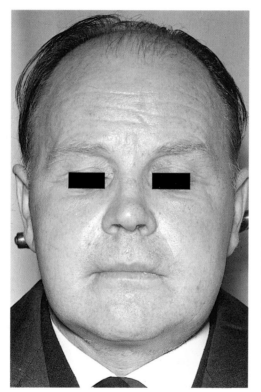

Fig. 23-13   Highly malignant
non-Hodgkin's lymphoma of
B-cell type in a 52-year-old patient. The patient's face demonstrates the compromised, febrile general condition at the
time of admission (10 days after start of the disease). The
disease, which originally was
diagnosed as a reticulosis (reti-
culosarcomatosis), was reclas-
sified. The malignant neoplasm
developed acutely, without prodromal phase within 3½ weeks
after the appearance of the first
clinically noticeable symptom in
the oral cavity, with the appearance of an increasing paralysis of the striated musculature
and peritonitis, followed by respiratory depression resulting
in death. Diagnosis could be
made only after death because
of the rapid disease course.
The autopsy showed diffuse infiltration in the stomach, kidneys, lungs, and bone marrow
of the spine with tumor, but no
obvious involvement of spleen
and liver.

Fig. 23-14 The patient in Fig. 23-13 also at the initial examination. Because of a painful-to-touch swelling over the apical regions of tooth 15 (4), the patient visited his dentist, who considered it an acute exacerbation of a chronic apical periodontitis and extracted the pulpless, sensitive-to-percussion tooth, together with tooth 17 (2). Both teeth were fixed partial denture abutments. Seven days after the intervention, a tumorlike enlargement, particularly in the area of the extraction wound, extended into the now-edentulous alveolar process with extensive central necrosis and the growth of nodular infiltrates in the surrounding area.

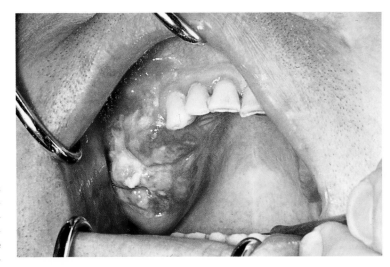

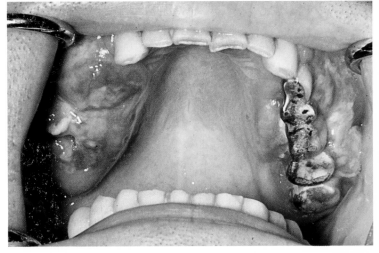

Fig. 23-15 The patient in Figs. 23-13 and 23-14 at the initial examination. In the untreated lateral tooth area of the left maxilla, there is tissue proliferation with necrotizing ulcerative mucosal changes. The bone structure is unaffected radiologically. The peripheral blood picture shows no evidence of an acute leukemia.

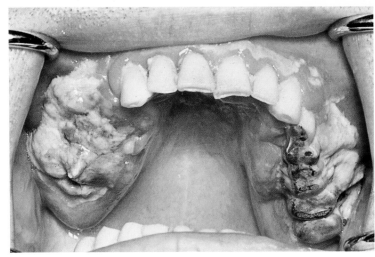

Fig. 23-16 The patient in Figs. 23-13 to 23-15 after 3 days. Dramatic worsening of the intraoral findings with distinct increase of tissue proliferation and rapidly enlarging necrotic areas. In the mandible were similar changes. At the same time, the worsening of the general condition of the patient was noticed.

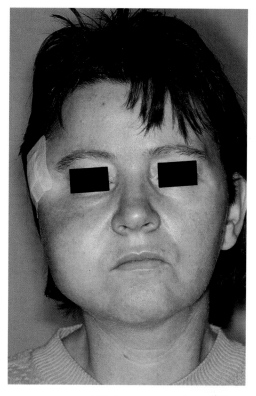

Fig. 23-17 Highly malignant non-Hodgkin's lymphoma of Burkitt type in a 43-year-old woman. After several weeks of uncharacteristic pain, a swelling was noticed in the area of the temple and cheek, which was treated with antibiotics without success. Upon hospitalization of the patient, there was the suspicion of a chronic infratemporal abscess related to the extraction of tooth 16 (3), which had taken place in the meantime. After intraoral and extraoral incision, there was emptying of inflammatory secretion. However, because the swelling did not decrease, even with additional antibiotic therapy, a malignancy was suspected.

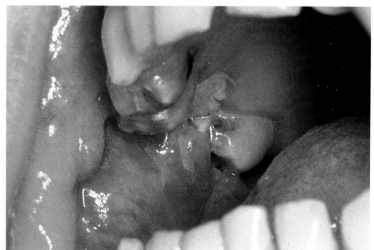

Fig. 23-18 The patient of Fig. 23-17 immediately before biopsy diagnosis. The intraoral finding shows that part of the highly malignant non-Hodgkin's lymphoma of the Burkitt type—as shown by computed tomography—had grown around the ramus of the mandible and was growing retromaxially with involvement of blood vessels intracranially in the middle skull groove as well as in the orbit and sphenoid sinus. Lymphomas of the Burkitt-type belong to those most rapidly growing (cell kinetics with a duplication time of 26 hours), but respond well to chemotherapy.

Chapter 24

Mucous Membrane Findings in Hematologic Diseases (Especially of the Erythropoietic and Leukopoietic Systems)

Diseases of the erythropoietic system
    Anemias
        Iron deficiency anemia
        Pernicious anemia
        Acquired hemolytic anemias
        Aplastic anemia
    Polycythemia vera
Diseases of the leukopoietic system
    Granulocytopenias
        Agranulocytosis
        Toxic neutropenia
        Special forms
    Leukemias
        Acute leukemia
        Chronic leukemia

Quantitative and qualitative disturbances of the red cell system are most often associated in the oral cavity with relatively uncharacteristic findings that seldom lead to a diagnosis. It is quite different with diseases of the white cell system. In the case of granulocytopenia, as well as in cases of agranulocytosis and (acute) leukemia, the early and clinically noticeable manifestations on the mucous membrane regularly serve as warning signals. In Germany, the annual number of new patients with symptoms of acute leukemia in the oral and pharyngeal region is of the same order as the incidence of other serious new conditions in the mouth and throat regions. The dentist therefore plays a very important role not only in the early recognition of oral cancer, but also in the preliminary diagnosis of acute leukemia and should in suspicious cases refer the patient to a specialist. General and specialized problems of this group of diseases are described.

For didactic purposes, chronic lymphatic leukemia will also be discussed under the leukemias even though today's knowledge classifies it with the low-grade non-Hodgkin's lymphomas. The remaining malignant diseases of the lymphatic system (lymphogranuloma and non-Hodgkin's lymphoma) are discussed in chapter 23. The changes in the oral mucosa caused by decrease and/or disturbance of platelet function—as long as they are not in pathogenetic association with leukemia—among the hemorrhagic diatheses are discussed in chapter 25.

Diseases of the erythropoietic system

Anemias

Every acute or chronic primary or secondary decrease in the number and/or the hemoglobin content of the red blood cells that deviates from the norm is designated as anemia. Anemia is not a diagnosis in the real sense. Rather, it is a symptom. Exact diagnostic clarification and classification is only possible via a hemogram and other laboratory tests, which provide information on the number of erythrocytes, the changes of their morphology, the color index (specifically the absolute hemoglobin content of the single erythrocyte (MCH), the average hemoglobin concentration (MCHC), the relation between the volume of erythrocytes and plasma volume (hematocrit value), and the volume of the single erythrocyte. At the same time they allow determination of the degree of severity of the anemia and provide indications of its original cause.

For the nonhematologist there is a wealth of different types of anemia differentiated by a variety of criteria (pathogenesis, morphology, hemoglobin content). Discussion of the numerous possible classifications must be omitted in this book. If the hemoglobin content of the individual erythrocyte is taken as a basis, then the major groups are the *hypochromic anemias* (in which the formation of the hemoglobin is more seriously disturbed than is that of the erythrocytes), the *hyper-*

chromic anemias (in which the formation of the erythrocytes is more seriously disturbed than is that of the hemoglobin, resulting in the increased color index), and the *normochromic anemias* (in which the erythrocytes and hemoglobin are decreased by the same amount). Examples of individual disease entities of these three groups are given.

The clinical picture of all types of anemia is determined by the degree of severity and duration of the disease. Frequent general symptoms in pronounced cases are pale skin color (the paleness also develops in the mucous membrane), difficulty in concentration, weakness, headaches, sleeplessness, a dazed state, ringing in the ears, faintness, and in certain situations paresthesia. As a result of hypoxia, other compensatory cardiovascular reactions can develop.

It is also important for the dentist to know that all chronic anemias can lead to atrophic findings of the mucous membrane as well as to regressive changes on the skin (brittleness, tendency to form tears and fissures).

Iron deficiency anemia (ICD-DA 280 and 280.X0)

The main group of the hypochromic anemias includes the widespread iron deficiency anemia. Hemoglobin formation, impaired by iron deficiency, is most often associated with changes in the volume of the erythrocytes (microcytic).

Frequent causes of iron deficiency are chronic blood loss (menorrhagias or metrorrhagias in young women and girls; chronic occult bleeding, especially in the stomach and intestinal regions in men and women of older age). Iron deficiency anemia can also occasionally be the result of disturbed iron absorption (for example, after total gastrectomy, in cases of reduced stomach secretion) or an increased demand for iron (in cases of pregnancy, infections, or tumors).

In addition to the typical general symptoms of anemia in serious cases there may be abnormal eating habits that are designated as "pica" (soil, clay, calcium). There may also be broken hair, dystrophy of the nails (koilonychia), fissures of the corners of the mouth (angular cheilitis), and a very painful glossitis (Fig. 24-1). A superficial infection follows the beginning of atrophy of the tongue papillae starting at the tip and the borders of the tongue (Fig. 24-2). Because—as in all mucous membranes—the mucosa of the esophagus also shows atrophic changes, there is characteristically painful, difficult swallowing (dysphagia) and esophageal and cardiospasms associated with a feeling of dryness and soreness in the oral cavity *(Plummer-Vinson syndrome)*.

Pernicious anemia (ICD-DA 281.0 and 281.00)

Pernicious anemia is a frequent hyperchromic form of anemia that is primarily a disease of aging. The symptom of burning tongue, of which many patients complain, can long precede changes in erythropoiesis, as well as disturbances of the nervous system (paresthesia), and can, after normalization of the hemogram, continue for months. Ailments in the region of the digestive system accompany the general symptoms. The red, flat tongue that is shown in textbooks *(Moeller-Hunter glossitis)* is not observed, because of the therapy for anemia administered by the family doctor. Empiric treatment before establishment of a diagnosis is a poor choice.

The blood count shows, in addition to hyperchromic anemia, a leukocytopenia and thrombocytopenia, as well as morphologic abnormalities of red cell precursors (megaloblasts) in the erythropoietic series; in serum, the vitamin B_{12} level is greatly reduced. Due to atrophic gastritis, stomach secretions are as a rule reduced (histamine refractory achylia).

Pernicious anemia is an *autoimmune disease*. Antibodies are almost regularly identifiable in pernicious disease against the parietal cells of the gastric mucous membrane. In two thirds of all cases, there are the antibodies against the vitamin B_{12} site of the intrinsic factor, and less frequently also against those of the vitamin B_{12} intrinsic factor complex. Simultaneously with the atrophic gastritis there are often associated disturbances and infection of the thyroid gland (thyrogastric autoimmune disease). Even after successful therapy for anemia, patients require long-term control because of the great possibility for development of stomach carcinoma.

Acquired hemolytic anemias (ICD-DA 283)

In addition to anemias caused by acute bleeding, the hemolytic anemias belong to the normochromic anemia group. They develop because of erythrocyte breakdown (decreased life span of the erythrocytes compared to the normal life span of 120 days), which is increased by the disease and which cannot be compensated by the increased red blood cell production in the bone marrow. Hemolytic anemias can be acute, chronic, or episodic. The reduction of erythrocytes often takes place extravascularly; intravenous hemolysis leads to hemoglobinuria. The hemolytic icterus, which develops in acute cases, is the result of increased hemoglobin metabolism, which results from increased disintegration of the red blood cells.

In contrast to the constitutionally inherited hemolytic anemias, which are caused by membrane, enzyme, or hemoglobin defects, in acquired forms normal erythrocytes are as a rule prematurely destroyed primarily through exogenous or endogenous influences. The acquired *autoimmune hemolytic anemias* (ICD-DA 283.0) can be caused by autoantibodies directed against the body's erythrocytes and occur in diseases of the lymphatic system and collagen diseases. They can also follow infectious diseases or occur even without recognizable cause. Other autoimmune hemolytic anemias are triggered by the formation of irregular isoantibodies against the blood antigens of the ABO and/or the Rh system. The hemolytic complications in *erythroblastosis fetalis* (ICD 773.0 and ICD-DA 520.80) are a well-known example of this and are caused by an underlying intolerance to blood within the Rh system (rhesus factor incompatibility) of the mother (Rh−) and the child (Rh+). The serious form of the disease (icterus gravis) is accompanied by a prominent toxic jaundice and disturbances of the central nervous system (kernicterus). If the child survives, the disease can leave marked, yellowish to greenish-brown stains on the teeth in the primary dentition with or without enamel hypoplasias (Fig. 24-3). The extent of discoloration and the structural damage of the tooth substance, which are similar to those caused by tetracycline, depend on the duration of the hemolytic icterus (see chapter 31, Fig. 31-51).

Toxic hemolytic anemias (ICD-DA 283.1 and 283.10) can arise from exogenous causes (chemical blood poisoning, industrial poisons, misuse of analgesics, especially with phenacetin-containing preparations, which are no longer legal) or endogenous causes (as result of serious extensive burns, serious kidney diseases with retention of substances that are usually eliminated in the urine−renal anemia), or even by bacterial infections. A special form of toxic hemolytic anemia due to exogenous causes is *lead anemia.* The basophilic stippling of the erythrocytes, which is characteristic of this disease, is a more important indication of poisoning than the lead lines, which are more often described but are in fact noticeable only on the marginal gingiva and only in extreme cases (see also chapter 4, Fig. 4-22).

Aplastic anemia (ICD-DA 284 and 284.VO)

The term aplastic anemia is commonly used clinically for either acute or chronic, *often acquired* diseases of the bone marrow that cause not only anemia but also leukocytopenia and thrombocytopenia because of a serious defect in blood formation. All the conditions that involve these three cell types and lead to corresponding diseases that show clinical function reduction *(symptom triad)* are more accurately identified as panmyelopathy, pancytopenia, panmyelophthisis, or most often as *aplastic syndrome.*

The clinical picture mirrors the seriousness of the quantitative and qualitative disturbances in blood formation due to the damage or failure of the bone marrow. After an insidious beginning, in clearly compromised patients there are increasing signs of anemia, with hemorrhagic diathesis, as well as an increased susceptibility to infection and inflammatory processes. There are often early manifestations in the oral cavity in the form of thrombocytopenic bleeding disorders (see chapter 25) and necrotizing ulcerative infectious processes. The findings become worse with advanced destruction of the bone marrow. Frequent causes of death are septic complications and brain hemorrhages. Survival time can be increased with the aid of therapy (immunosuppressive and other medical treatment; allogeneic bone marrow transplants).

A panmyelopathy with corresponding oral mucosal symptoms can secondarily be caused by ionized rays, cytostatic agents, chemical substances (such as benzene and its derivatives), other toxic influences (such as uremia in the case of kidney failure; Figs. 24-4 to 24-6), as well as displacement of the marrow due to neoplastic processes, such as leukemia, malignant lymphoma, plasmacytoma, or solid malignancies that have metastasized into the bone marrow. Presumably, autoimmunologic processes that are directed against the bone marrow cell also play a role. It is also well known that certain medications (some antibiotics, sulfonamide, analgesics, sedatives, and hydantoin derivatives) have a potentially damaging effect on the bone marrow, usually when taken in high doses or long term, but also in many cases after the first administration (idiosyncrasy).

Fanconi's anemia (ICD 284.0) belongs to the *rare hereditary panmyelopathies,* which are discussed in Fig. 24-7 as well as in chapter 5 (Figs. 25-4 and 25-5).

Conclusions for the dentist

The intraoral findings associated with anemia are relatively non-specific and often fail to raise the suspicion of the dentist. The dentist should, however, think of the possibility of such hematologic diseases when unclear symptoms such as a burning sensation of the tongue and/or infectious-atrophic mucous membrane changes exist that are not explained by any other disease or cause. In these cases, patients should be referred to an internist for exclusion of anemia.

Polycythemia vera (ICD-M 9950/1)

Polycythemia vera, which is part of the group of myeloproliferative disorders, is recognizable by the marked increase in the erythrocyte count (7 to 9 million more per microliter) in the blood *(erythrocytosis),* in combination with a clear increase of the thrombocytes and—not as frequently or as intensely—even of the leukocytes. At the same time, hypervolemia and hyperviscosity exist, resulting in microcirculation disturbances. The bone marrow shows increased proliferation of all the red blood cell precursors as well as increased granulocytopoieses.

The disease is rare and occurs most often in men between the ages of 40 and 70. It has an insidious onset and progression with non-specific systemic symptoms (headaches, vertigo, insomnia, depression). In one half of cases, patients complain of itchy skin, especially after a warm bath. The skin has a deep red color (Fig. 24-8) and a plethoric appearance.

In the mucous membrane the excess blood is more evident due to the cyanotic color. In the presence of marginal periodontitis or in other previously damaged mucous membranes, bleeding occurs that is spontaneous or due to minor causes.

The prognosis of the relatively benign polycythemia vera with optimal therapy is guarded, because of widespread complications such as spontaneous hemorrhages (in the gastrointestinal tract and urogenital system, among other areas) as well as, above all, the affinity for thrombotic episodes. The long-term prognosis is unfavorable because the disease can change into an acute leukemia or myelofibrosis with progressive bone marrow failure.

Because of modern therapy (venesection, radioactive phosphorus, cytostatic agents, interferon), survival time can be extended from the previous 3 to 5 years to 10 to 15 years.

From the hematologic point of view, differential diagnosis must separate the *secondary polycythemias,* in which peripheral blood and marrow hyperplasia is largely limited to the red blood cell series. These types of reactive polycythemias can be a result of compensatory adaptation to an external lack of oxygen (altitude adjustment) or internal lack of oxygen. Patients with cardiac abnormalities and right-left shunts (Fallot tetralogy among others; see Fig. 26-1) as well as patients with pulmonary insufficiency (e.g., lung emphysema, left side cardiac failure) belong to this group.

In differential diagnosis, the hematologist must also consider polycythemias that are based on an increased stimulation of the erythropoiesis and that can directly or indirectly be triggered by various diseases (among others, malignant kidney diseases).

Another example is Cushing's syndrome. The same effect is seen as a side effect of long-term systemic use of adrenocortical hormones.

Diseases of the leukopoietic system

Granulocytopenias

Agranulocytosis (ICD-DA 288.0 and 288.00)

Agranulocytosis is an acute disease caused by a sudden marked decrease of granulocytes in the peripheral blood due to toxic or allergic (drug) factors. Mucous membrane necrosis is pathognomonic in the sepsis-like clinical course.

Middle-aged patients, 80% of whom are women, are affected. Information on morbidity ranges from 2 to 25 million people/year. Estimates of incidence of drug-induced agranulocytosis for each category of drugs are equally divergent. The relatively greatest risk among the drugs are the thyroid depressants. The so-called Boston study calculated the frequency of untoward effects for metamizol, a drug found in many preparations (see table on page 519) and a potential cause of agranulocytosis, but it did not provide accurate data for the worldwide population.

The causal factor remains unclear in a relatively large number of cases (20% to 40%), hence it is possible that agranulocytosis can also be induced by substances in the environment or by food products.

With regard to the pathogenesis, an underlying factor is the sensitization of the individual to a hapten or antigen with production of an antibody. The antibody is highly specific, but cross reactions with chemically related substances are possible. Triggering of the allergic reaction is not dependent on the dose and only selectively affects the neurotrophilic granulocytes that fall from a value below 1,000/μL. On the other hand, the erythrocyte and platelet values are normal in the peripheral blood. In typical cases, the bone marrow shows a serious hypoplasia.

The body loses its cellular defense mechanism against infection because of the resulting granulocytopenia. It is also rendered susceptible to the saprophytic, facultative pathogens and pathogenic organisms of the environment. The invading pathogen always acts first on the bacteria-infested mucous membrane. With a suddenly occurring intense feeling of illness, fever, and chills, there is the appearance within 12 to 24 hours of necrosis and deep ulcerations with tendency to spread on the surface, especially in the mucous membrane near the pharynx (Figs. 24-10 and 24-11) and pharyngeal mucosa *(agranulocytotic angina)*. The patient, who looks febrile and cyanotic, complains of difficulty in swallowing and of sore throat. Every other previously damaged region of the mucous membrane can also be affected (Fig. 24-9). In the initial phase, the skin is only affected in areas with pre-existing damage.

Because erythropoiesis and megakaryopoiesis are not involved, signs of serious anemia and thrombocytopenia with bleeding diathesis are missing, whereas they are present in acute leukemia.

The infections soon spread to the mucous membranes of the respiratory and gastrointestinal tracts. Later the internal organs are included in the sepsis-like clinical picture. The complete clinical picture of allergic agranulocytosis develops in a period of hours up to a few days.

Even today agranulocytosis is a serious disease. Unidentified or untreated, it leads to septic manifestations (among others, pneumonia). In cases of suspicion, immediate referral for in-patient treatment is critical.

The most important measure is the immediate elimination of the medication that is considered to be triggering this response. Over and above that, treatment consists of quickly initiating antibiotic therapy together with supportive measures against infections and for the avoidance of secondary infections by hospitalization (if need be, in a sterile isolation unit—specifically in a laminar air-flow room). With modern treatment, mortality could be reduced to under 10%.

It is preventive as well as therapeutic to institute good oral hygiene habits. Chlorhexidine digluconate (in 0.1% solutions), used as a gargle, is considered to be a plaque-inhibiting medication. All other oral disinfectants are much less effective. When patients survive the critical phase of immunosuppression, the blood count improves with intensive therapy and so eventually do systemic conditions. The granulocyte counts increase after several weeks and finally reach normal values.

The most important rule is, and remains, the immediate and future discontinuation of the triggering agent, which is identified by a careful history of medications used. Renewed contact with the causative medication (also possible cross reactions) can result in recurrence. With each recurrence, the prognosis becomes poorer.

Conclusions for the dentist

The dentist must consider that with his or her own pharmaceutical prescriptions he or she can at times induce serious side effects. The table on page 519 gives pertinent information. With the large number of pharmaceuticals that can trigger agranulocytosis, dental prescriptions of combination prepations should be avoided when possible.

With the suspicion of an allergic agranulocytosis, an emergency exists, and it is important to act quickly. To secure the correct clinical diagnosis, the dentist should *immediately* refer the patient to a physician, so that the suspicion can be confirmed or ruled out by blood examination (CBC with differential blood count). According to the results of the examination, the physician will arrange required care. The dentist has fulfilled his or her responsibility to his or her patient with this procedure.

Toxic neutropenia (ICD-DA 288.02)

As opposed to allergic agranulocytosis, there is a definite relation between duration and amount of an applied substance in the case of toxic granulocytopenia. It is understandable that among pharmaceuticals, alkali substances and antimetabolites used in cytostatic therapy most often result in a toxic granulocytopenia. In addition, there are a number of other medications that can cause a granulocytopenia and are dose-dependent because of toxicity or other drug-specific characteristics. To these belong, in addition to others, chloramphenicol, certain thyroid depressants, antirheumatics, anticonvulsants, and sulfonamides. For this reason, with prescription of these medications, blood counts at regular intervals are recommended. Several other possible causes are the chemically related benzene substances and serious infectious diseases.

Directly affected in these cases (as opposed to the allergic agranulocytosis) is the bone marrow in which the granulopoiesis is toxically damaged. The peripheral blood count may remain unremarkable for a longer period of time. The myelotoxic process can spread later to the erythropoiesis and thrombopoiesis and can lead to a panmyelopathy.

Toxic granulocytopenia develops over a long period and clinically is most often insidious. Because of impaired body defenses and the consequent general symptoms, necroses and ulcerations can eventually develop on the mucous membrane and in the oropharynx (Fig. 24-12).

Special forms

The extremely rare cyclic neutropenia (ICD-DA 288.01) belongs to the special forms of granulocytopenia.

As the name indicates, the disease occurs periodically. In near regular intervals of 3 of 4 weeks, a granulocytopenia appears, whereby the neutrophils in the peripheral blood as well as the cells of the granulocytopoiesis in the bone marrow greatly decrease in number.

During the few days of the neutropenic phase, patients complain of weakness, lack of appetite, insomnia, and on occasion of headache and joint pain. Because of the weakened defense condition, infections of the skin and mucosa often occur and may be accompanied by mild febrile episodes and swelling of the lymph nodes. In the oral cavity, exacerbation of chronic gingivitis or marginal periodontitis as well as recurring ulcerations of the gingiva and/or the remaining mucous membrane (in several cases with the appearance of a stomatitis) are not uncommon. At times they are the only clinical indication of the disease.

The pathogenesis of this condition is still unknown; a hereditary predisposition is not ruled out, and a relation with fluctuations in the sex hormone levels is considered a possibility. Therapy to reduce recurrences is not available. The prognosis of cyclical neutropenia, which frequently manifests itself in childhood and possibly runs its course for years or decades, is generally favorable.

A group of granulocytopenias is based on inherited inadequate bone marrow. The clinical picture of this *group of constitutional granulocytopenias* is the *infantile genetic agranulocytosis* or *Kostmann disease* (ICD-DA 288.0).

In this disease, there is almost complete absence of granulocytes in the peripheral blood. Serious infections dominate the clinical picture and course of the disease and occur as early as immediately after birth. In the past, they often led to death during infancy or early childhood. With modern hematologic therapeutic methods (allogeneic bone marrow transplants, use of hematopoietic growth factors), the former poor prognosis life expectancy can be improved.

Intraorally, the disease results in serious periodontal damage, with episodic exacerbations, during the pimary (Fig. 24-13) and permanent dentition stages (Fig. 24-14a) with advanced alveolar bone destruction and mobility and loss of teeth (Fig. 24-14b).

Leukemias

Leukemias are serious diseases of the hematopoietic system in which the white blood cells are changed qualitatively and quantitatively with disturbed maturation and differentiation. Involvement of the red blood cells in the form of erythroleukemia, on the other hand, is considerably less frequent.

Leukemias are a heterogeneous group of diseases, whose etiologies are still largely unclear. The clinical symptoms, course of the disease, degree of maturity, and source of the cells allow differentiation of *acute (immature cells)* and *chronic (mature cells)* leukemia and *myeloid* and *lymphatic forms.* These main categories can be cytologically, cytochemically, and immunologically subdivided into more subtypes. Based on the concentration of leukemia cells in the peripheral blood, they can be further separated into leukemic and aleukemic forms. The term *myelodysplasia* is common today for preleukemic stages with subleukemic appearance in the bone marrow and most often peripheral pancytopenia.

Acute leukemias are especially important in preliminary dental diagnoses, because they may be clinically recognized very early by changes of the mucosa and especially of the gingiva.

Acute leukemia (ICD-M 9801/3)

Untreated acute leukemias, which can lead to death within a period of days to a few weeks, are characterized by the occurrence of abnormal, immature cells of the hematopoietic system ("blasts") in the bone marrow and peripheral blood. The liver, spleen, and lymph nodes can be affected by the spreading leukemic cells during the disease process. The disease can also involve other body tissues, such as the mediastinum, brain, or testis. Eventually all body tissues can be affected. The undifferentiated leukemia cells, contrary to mature normal cell populations, maintain their ability to proliferate. Because of a lengthened cell cycle loss of function, they have, however, a longer life expectancy as ripe, functional cells. In this manner, there is an increased accumulation of cells, first in the tissue of origin, the bone marrow, and later in other organs.

In Germany, approximately six of every 100,000 persons of every age group suffer from acute leukemia. The ratio between sexes is almost identical.

Based on the predominant cell population (stem line), it is possible in many cases to morphologically distinguish, sometimes with the aid of cytochemical special staining, *acute myeloid leukemia* (ICD-M 9861/3) from *acute lymphoblastic leukemia* (ICD-M 9821/3).

In retrospect, this rather primitive system of classification is of great practical value for therapy and therefore prognosis. Both forms differ in how they affect different ages: while acute myeloid leukemia (AML) appears mainly during adulthood, acute lymphatic leukemia (ALL) appears mainly during two age periods, first in children with a peak age between the second and sixth year, and then again, with rapidly increasing frequency, in middle and old age. In general, the prognosis is more favorable the younger the patient is at the time of onset.

Neither clinical picture of acute leukemic disease depicts a unified progression. They can be categorized in several subclasses that appear to have very different prognoses according to degrees of cell maturity and differentiation. In the case of myeloid forms, differentiation is made predominantly by cytologic and cytochemical methods (for example, using myeloperoxidase and esterase reactions), and in the case of the lymphatic forms, predominantly by immunologic methods.

According to the suggestion of the French-American-British Cooperation Group (FAB) of 1976, acute myeloid leukemia is categorized into seven subtypes, with subsequent additions.

FAB classification of acute myeloid leukemia

(According to Bennet JM et al. Proposals for the classification of the acute leukaemias. Br J Hematol 1976; 33: 451, with subsequent additions.)

FAB-M1   Undifferentiated myeloblastic leukemia
FAB-M2   Myeloblastic leukemia with maturation
FAB-M3   Promyelocytic leukemia
FAB-M4   Myelomonocytic leukemia
FAB-M5   Monocytic leukemia
FAB-M6   Erythroleukemia
FAB-M7   Acute megakaryoblastic leukemia

The very rare *erythroleukemia* is characterized by simultaneous accumulation of myeloblasts and pathologic erythrobasts in the bone marrow.

In *acute lymphatic leukemia*, it is possible to differentiate five subgroups with the help of immunologic surface markers. There are variations from the common B-, T- and O-type with different prognoses.

Grouped under *acute undifferentiated leukemia* (AUL) are those cases in which the cytochemical stains are negative. Immunologic typing, however, most often enables classification into the previously mentioned immunologic subtypes of ALL.

The details of the characteristics of differentiation can be found in reference books on clinical hematology. Disregarding further classifications, acute myeloid leukemias and acute lymphatic leukemias show a series of similarities in their clinical symptoms and in their course. A dependable differentiation according to clinical criteria is therefore generally not possible.

General symptoms of acute leukemia

Acute leukemias most often begin from a condition of good health with signs of a severe febrile infection, exhaustion, fatigue, head and joint pain, and a tendency to bleed. Because the proliferating leukemic cells in the bone marrow interfere with normal hemopoiesis, hampering the production of erythropoietic cells, normal granulopoiesis, and megakaryocytes ("displacement myelopathy"), there is the development of a pronounced *anemia* (obvious pallor; Figs. 24-15 and 24-31) and increasing *thrombocytopenia with thrombocytopenic affinity to bleeding*. Primary coagulation disturbances (with or without fibrolysis increase) ranging to disseminating intravascular coagulation occur regularly only in promyelocytic leukemia (FAB-M3).

As a result of the hemorrhagic diathesis of thrombocytopenia or thrombopathy, profuse bleeding from the mouth, nose, gastrointestinal tract, and urinary tract can occur and can be a warning sign. On the skin a serious tendency to bleed can occur, often as a purpura with petechiae or ecchymoses (Fig. 24-16). In the meantime, hematomas develop (Fig. 24-17). Oral mucosa findings are discussed later.

The decrease of mature, functioning leukocytes and the disturbances caused by this, above all, of cellular defense mechanisms, lead to a *decrease in systemic resistance*. This leads to infectious complications, especially with opportunistic organisms (Fig. 24-15). Persistent, sometimes high fever, which occurs in many patients even in the following course of the disease, is not always a result of the infection but can result from malignant cell proliferation.

Enlarged liver, spleen, and lymph nodes (regional, multiple, or generalized) are especially characteristic for chronic lymphatic leukemia, but these also occur in acute lymphatic forms. They can also occasionally appear in myeloid leukemia (Fig. 24-18), especially, however, in lymphoblastic crises of the chronic myelogenous leukemias (CML). The participation of other organs, such as the central nervous system, respiratory tract, mediastinum, cardiovascular system, or others, takes place with varying clinical symptoms that will not be discussed here.

Intraoral symptoms of acute leukemia

Especially in myelomonocytic and monocytic forms of acute leukemia (FAB-M4 and M5), changes in the oral mucosa, especially in the gingiva, occur almost regularly and often even in early stages. The *premorbid conditions of the dentition* next to the morphologic and physiologic peculiarities of the oral cavity are the decisive factors in these frequent and early oral manifestations. The changes are substantially influenced by chronic infectious occurrences that were present before the outbreak of the disease (e.g., gingivitis or marginal periodontitis), by poor oral hygiene (microbial plaque), and/or by other local stimuli. In addition, there are other microtraumas unavoidable in the oral cavity.
  The main signs to be observed are:

- *Necrosis, ulcerations*
  (low resistance syndrome)
- *Swelling of the gingival tissue*
  (proliferative leukemic infiltrate)
- *Hemorrhaging*
  (thrombocytopenic or, rarer, plasmatic hemorrhagic diathesis)

With fewer mature functional leukocytes there is an increasing immune deficiency (acquired weakening of the immune system as in AIDS, caused, however, by tumor and not infection). Microorganisms of the oral cavity can penetrate deeper and be unhindered, especially on the previously damaged areas of the mucous membrane. In this manner, advanced *necrosis and ulcerations* of the gingiva and the remaining mucous membrane, which often occur without recognizable defense reactions, can be explained (Figs. 24-19 to 24-25). Even with a properly structured epithelial covering layer, necrosis in the deeper tissue layers with little or no cellular reaction can be detected histologically. An additional damaging effect is attributed to thrombosis of the small blood vessels with ensuing infarction. They are explained as a consequence of capillary occlusion caused by large, rigid leukemia cells (especially myeloblasts in "leukostatic syndrome"). Frequently, after decrease in immunity, candidiasis of the oral cavity results as an opportunistic infection (also see chapter 10, Figs. 10-7 to 10-9).

Another major oral sign is the *proliferation of the gingival tissue* (Figs. 24-27 to 24-38, 24-41). It is an expression of the leukemic cell infiltrate, especially proliferations in the subepithelial connective tissue, and it develops in adults mainly in myelomonocytic and monocytic leukemia. The tissue proliferation, which increases in volume with relative speed, is doughy or spongy and has a tendency, in some cases, to early necrotic disintegration, even in the form of hemorrhagic necrosis (Figs. 24-33, 24-34, and 24-42).

In the case of monocytic leukemia, gingival changes occasionally show an obvious purple color. In acute lymphatic leukemia of childhood, accompanying symptoms of the gingiva and marginal periodontium are rarer. This may be because of the lack of local irritative factors and chronic infectious alterations in this group. Because in children we are usually dealing with an acute lymphatic leukemia, leukemic enlargement of the lymph nodes of the throat is almost always present.

The leukemic proliferation of the gingival tissue should, in our opinion, not be designated as hyperplasia. This name designates excess formation, which therefore is reactively controlled rather than fundamentally uncontrolled autonomous cell proliferation or infiltrate.

As a result of *hemorrhagic diatheses*, variable hemorrhagic symptoms are possible in the oral cavity. They can present as discrete petechial signs of bleeding, ecchymosis, hemorrhagic gingivitis, hemorrhagic tissue necrosis, subepithelial hematomas, or profuse spontaneous hemorrhages (Figs. 24-25, 24-32 to 24-34, and 24-36 to 24-42).

These different main intraoral symptoms, which occur in changing combinations, should always be evaluated together with the patient's general appearance. Also, it must be remembered that findings in the oral cavity are variable according to the type and form of the leukemia, the degree of immunosuppression, and the patient's age. The severity of the lesion depends in part on the pre-existing gingival and periodontal conditions.

No gingival, periodontal, and oral mucosal findings are pathognomonic for a certain form of leukemia. In general, acute leukemia in adults is more often accompanied by intraoral manifestations and leads to substantially more serious changes in the oral cavity than does chronic leukemia.

Brief comments on diagnosis, therapy, and prognosis

In the presence of one or more of the previously mentioned warning signs, a hematologic examination is to be performed. In typical cases, the peripheral blood count shows, in addition to the signs of anemia and thrombocytopenia, immature leukemic cells, and mature granulocytes and lymphocytes next to each other *("leukemic hiatus")*. The total number of leukocytes can be normal, increased, or decreased.

The *diagnosis* of a leukemia is obtained by examination of the bone marrow (in the past, sternal puncture with marrow aspirate allowed only cytologic diagnosis; today punctures of the posterior iliac crest with "Yamshidi needles" yield bone marrow cores for histologic and cytologic studies). If blasts form 30% or more of marrow cells, the presence of acute leukemia is confirmed. The bone marrow can be so infiltrated with leukemia cells ("speedy cell sowing") that almost no cells of the normal hematopoietic marrow hematopoiesis are found. Further differentiation of the acute leukemia into subtypes, which is important for prognostic and therapeutic reasons, follows with cytochemical (ALM) and immunologic methods (ALL).

Differential diagnosis of acute myeloid leukemia includes, from the hematologic point of view, a later stage of preleukemic condition as myelodysplasia, especially with aleukemic forms of leukemia. Also to be considered are agranulocytoses, aplastic anemia (panmyelopathies), and infections causing bone marrow aplasia (such as brucellosis or leishmaniasis). In the case of acute lymphatic leukemia, differential diagnosis of high-grade non-Hodgkin's lymphoma with bone marrow involvement must be taken into consideration, especially with young patients, as should lymphotrophic viral infections (such as infectious mononucleosis).

Considerable progress has been made in the last few years in the *therapy* of acute leukemia. With early diagnosis and consequent therapy, these diseases have a significantly better prognosis than previously. The goal of induction therapy, consolidation therapy, and remission-obtaining therapy in clinics specializing in hematologic oncology emphasizes treatment leading to destruction of leukemic cells to achieve normalization of the hematopoietic system and permanent cure. With supportive measures (substitution of blood and blood plasma products, reverse isolation, antibiotic therapy), it is possible to cure up to 80% of children with acute lymphatic leukemia and up to 50% of those with acute myeloid leukemia with the aid of aggressive cytostatic polychemotherapy—partly in combination with radiation therapy and, if need be, with bone marrow transplants.

The prognosis of acute leukemia in adults has been substantially less favorable until now. Even though a high percentage of patients could be brought into complete remission, about 80% of the cases result in recurrence within 5 years. Only with the establishment of new costly methods, such as allogeneic bone marrow transplants (until now, predominantly from donor relatives but recently even from strangers). When there are no suitable relatives or unrelated donors, patients are given a chance of cure with autologous bone marrow transplants (with cytogenetically conserved bone marrow of the patient) together with blood stem cell transfusion.

Further therapeutic additions are evolving with the development of methods based on the use of monoclonal antibodies or on interventions in cell metabolism to selectively eliminate the leukemic cell clone. In this way, a justified hope exists that an even larger number of leukemia patients will be helped in the future.

With intensive oncologic therapy, local findings in the oral cavity normally improve. The additional local dental therapy should therefore be limited to the elimination or decrease of local irritative factors. Because of the existing bleeding tendency and the danger of infections, tissue trauma is to be avoided wherever possible.

Aggressive leukemia therapy is understandably burdened by considerable side effects. In dentistry, serious dystrophic periodontal changes are often observed even as early as in the primary dentition of children. Also, bone marrow depression may result from long-term therapy with cytostatically effective antimetabolites (Fig. 24-23). Ulcerations of the oral mucosa can also occur as a result of toxic drug effects.

Conclusions for the dentist

The extraordinary importance of the dentist for the continued improvement of the therapeutic results in these most serious diseases lies in the early tentative diagnosis of an acute leukemia and in the prompt referral for clarification.

Unfortunately, experience shows that under the guise of a febrile inflammation on the oral mucosa, acute inflammation precursors can be misinterpreted as a local condition, such as ulcerations or acute necrotized ulcerative gingivostomatitis. Consequently, considerable time is sometimes lost because of hesitation to refer the patient. When local treatment fails and a lesion progresses even under antibiotic therapy, a systemic disease should be suspected.

When two or three intraoral cardinal symptoms (see page 508) are demonstrable, there should be immediate suspicion of an acute leukemia. This tentative diagnosis must be ruled out or confirmed by an immediate hematologic examination!

To prevent the loss of valuable time for treatment of the patient, the dentist should, when in doubt, refrain from starting a symptomatic therapy on the assumption of attaining a diagnosis. Instead, a prompt hematologic clarification is indicated. For patients with leukemia, a tooth extracted due to incorrect diagnosis may mean the acute danger of bleeding to death. Such an extraction could also lead to sepsis because of invasion of pathogens into the blood stream in the patient whose defenses are extremely low ("acquired immunodepression").

With careful examination and critical interpretation of findings, in combination with the general symptoms, a tentative diagnosis of acute leukemia can be made. Intraoral manifestations of this condition appear to be as common as extraoral symptoms. By prompting hospital admission of the patient with suspicious conditions, the dentist can provide a decisive contribution to early recognition and successful therapy of acute leukemia.

Chronic leukemia (ICD-M 9803/3)

In the preliminary diagnosis of chronic leukemia, input from the dentist is less important than with acute leukemia. The description of this disease is therefore brief. Compared to acute leukemia, chronic leukemia shows only a slowly progressing clinical course of a disease with, most often, insidious onset and morphologically continuing maturation of the leukemic cells. One can differentiate chronic myelogenous and chronic lymphatic leukemia according to the involved cell population.

Chronic myelogenous leukemia (CML; ICD-M 9863/3), which is included in the group of chronic-myeloproliferative diseases, occurs overwhelmingly in adults with a peak at late middle age. The individual's general well-being can remain unaffected for a long time or be only slightly compromised. The disease is often discovered accidently after a routine blood test. The results show a leukocytosis with all maturation stages of the granulocytopoiesis ("pathologic deviation to the left"). In most patients, an acquired chromosomal anomaly of the bone marrow and blood cells is apparent *(Philadelphia chromosome)*. A clinical warning sign is the frequently seen considerable enlargement of the spleen. The liver can also be obviously enlarged. In the further course, foci of myeloid cell proliferation can develop in many organs, with increasing anemia and, in the early stage, thrombocytosis, and later thrombocytopenia with bleeding tendency.

After an average of 3 to 5 years, the disease changes to an accelerated and later acute phase with the appearance of acute myeloid leukemia (Fig. 24-28, *acute blastic crisis*). This blastic crisis kills most patients within a few months. All earlier concepts of treatment have been unable to improve life expectancy. Only the introduction of allogeneic bone marrow transplants has recently provided a chance for cure of CML patients. In the initial treatment stages, therapy with interferon is gaining importance.

Chronic lymphoid leukemia (CLL; ICD-M 9823/3) must be differentiated from other similar diseases such as hairy cell leukemia and prolymphocytic leukemia. It shows a unified clinical picture. It is grouped with the low-grade non-Hodgkin's lymphomas. The clinical indicating signs of these lymphomas are discussed in chapter 23.

This generalized disease of the lymphatic system occurs mainly in older individuals (over 50 years) and predominantly in men. It is characterized by the accumulation of small, often mature-appearing lymphatic cells in the lymph nodes, blood, bone marrow, and parenchymatous organs. In over 95% of patients, the proliferating lymphocytes belong to the B-cell type, and the disease correspondingly leads to an antibody deficiency syndrome with gradual decreasing gamma globulin fractions in the serum electrophoresis. T-cell malignancy is demonstrated in only in a small percentage of cases. This latter form may also affect young patients. Leukemic skin infiltrates can develop from this disease form, which can disfigure the face *("facies leontina").*

Clinical symptoms and the course of the disease can vary. Usually with insidious beginnings, chronic lymphatic leukemia can progress over years without significant impairment of the patient's general condition. Only with increasing participation of the lymphatic and parenchymatous organs and with increasing involvement of the bone marrow does the general condition gradually worsen. Anemia and thrombocytopenia occur as an expression of a displacement myelopathy. In other cases with relatively rapid progression, there is early generalized lymph node swelling, enlargement of the spleen, and diffuse bone marrow infiltrates with corresponding general symptoms. Between these two extremes are transition forms of the disease progression.

Chronic lymphatic leukemia leads to defects in the immune system with disturbances, above all, of the humoral defense mechanism because of hypogammaglobulemia in the B-cell disease. Because of progressive weakening of defenses, herpes zoster with a tendency to generalization can develop. Itching and unspecific changes in the skin (chronic eczema, pyodermia) are not unusual associated symptoms. In the oral cavity, because of the extensive corticosteroid treatment, there is frequently occurrence of typical thrush films.

In many cases the diagnosis can be made from the complete blood cell count because of the characteristic peripheral lymphocytosis. Other studies are required to distinguish the lymphoproliferative disease from other low-grade non-Hodgkin's lymphomas and to determine the immunologic type of the neoplastic cells. Therapeutically, because of the relatively favorable prognosis of the disease, the frequently older age of patients, and the limited therapeutic possibilities of cytostatic treatment, waiting is often indicated. Cytotoxic drugs should be started as late as possible and then only with caution because a full remission with normalization of all disease findings has not yet been achieved. The prognosis of the chronic lymphatic leukemia, which only seldom goes into a terminal blastic crisis, is in general more favorable than that with chronic myelogenous leukemia.

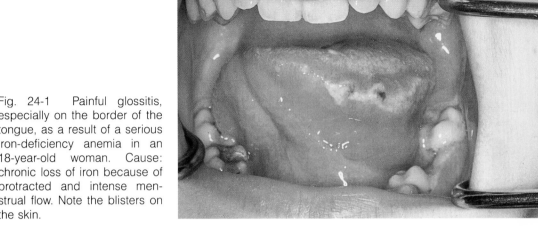

Fig. 24-1 Painful glossitis, especially on the border of the tongue, as a result of a serious iron-deficiency anemia in an 18-year-old woman. Cause: chronic loss of iron because of protracted and intense menstrual flow. Note the blisters on the skin.

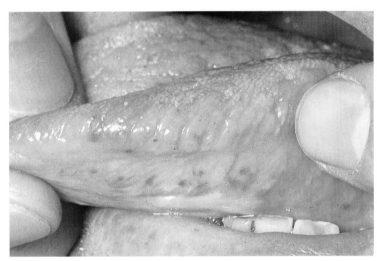

Fig. 24-2 Atrophic glossitis in a case of iron-deficiency anemia in a 62-year-old man. From the border of the tongue onward is an early papillary atrophy. Cause: disturbed resorption of iron after total stomach resection. In addition, the patient was undernourished due to alcoholism.

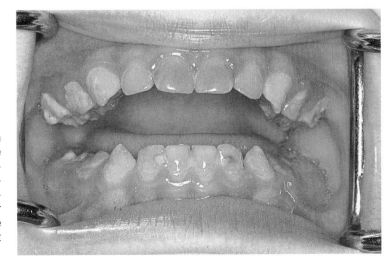

Fig. 24-3 Tooth discoloration with enamel hypoplasia in the primary dentition of a 4-year-old child. Cause: fetal erythroblastosis from rhesus factor incompatibility between mother and child. Postnatally, there was a serious kernicterus that caused cerebral damage.

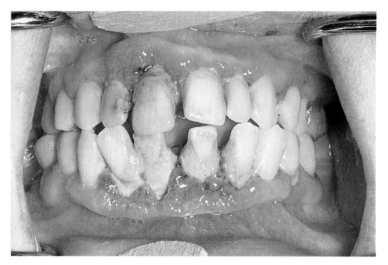

Fig. 24-4   Oral cavity findings of aplastic anemia in a 33-year-old woman. The panmyelopathy was caused by toxic damage to the bone marrow, as result of uremia, among other reasons.

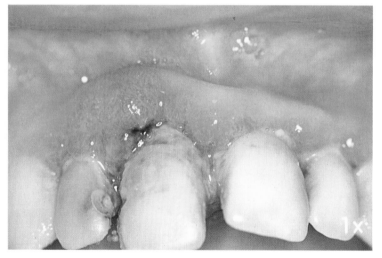

Fig. 24-5   The patient in Fig. 24-4 at the same examination. There is soft granulation tissue on the pale oral mucosa in the previously badly damaged periodontal region of the maxillary anterior teeth. There is a tendency to bleeding and necrosis because of the combined thrombocytopenia and granulocytopenia.

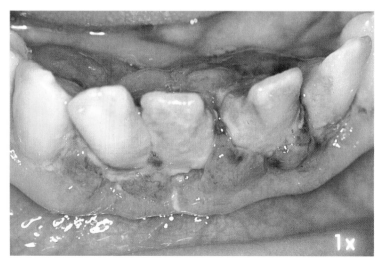

Fig. 24-6   The patient in Figs. 24-4 and 24-5 at the same examination. The detailed picture of the mandibular anterior region illustrates especially marked gingival changes caused by aplastic anemia. Extensive previous periodontal damage exists because of the grossly neglected oral hygiene.

Fig. 24-7 Gingivoperiodontal changes in a 16-year-old girl with Fanconi's anemia. This is a familiar special infantile form of panmyelopathy, which clinically shows progressing anemia, hemorrhagic diathesis of the thrombocytopenic type, and intercurrent infections between the fifth and tenth years. It is often associated with congenital anomalies (abnormal pigmentation, skeletal malformations, growth disturbances). With regular blood transfusions, the clinical picture can, despite the unfavorable prognosis, be compensated over the years. The changes appearing in the form of serious juvenile marginal periodontitis document the effects of pancytopenia.

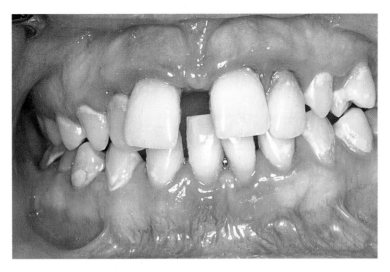

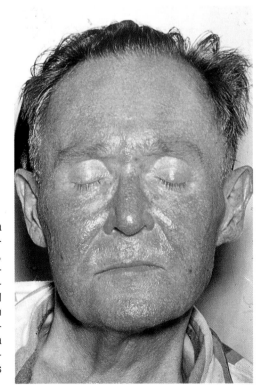

Fig. 24-8 Polycythemia rubra in a 59-year-old man. He complained of lasting headaches, dizziness, and painful circulatory disturbances in the extremities. In addition to the typical skin findings in the facial region (plethoric color with many telangiectasias), the oral mucosa is cyanotic red due to an excessive amount of blood. It was also prone to bleeding.

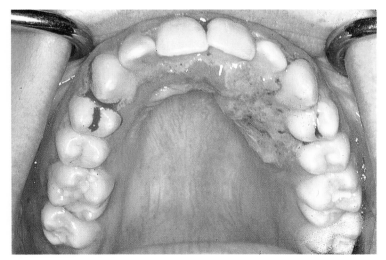

Fig. 24-9   Early oral manifestations of allergic agranulocytosis in a 26-year-old patient. The superficial ulceration of the mucous membrane of the hard palate, which is surrounded by a reactive marginal zone, developed within 48 hours with fever and chills. The papillary bleeding in the interdental region of teeth 14 and 13 (5 and 6) is due to injury. Triggering medication: phenylbutazone.

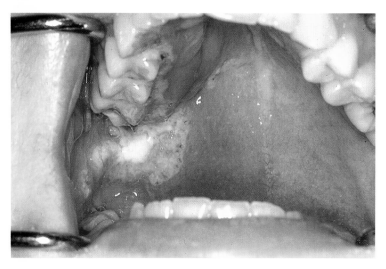

Fig. 24-10   Extensive mucous membrane necrosis with ulceration in the region of the hard and soft palate as a partial manifestation of allergic agranulocytosis in a 40-year-old patient. The palatal gingiva of the posterior teeth is included in the necrotizing ulcerative changes. Further ulcerations were present in the pharynx (sore throat). Triggering medication: a barbiturate.

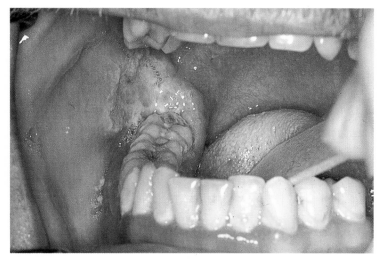

Fig. 24-11   Extensive necrotic ulcerations in the retromolar and cheek regions as an oral manifestation of allergic agranulocytosis in a 34-year-old patient. The condition shown is 36 hours after initial onset of fever and chills. The diagnosis was reached after a differential blood count. The triggering medication could not, in this case, be determined with certainty.

Important agranulocytosis-triggering medications in dentistry are shown at right. This grouping is not comprehensive. Many old and new medications have these rare, undesirable drug-induced effects. Explanations are given for each drug in the package circulars, the specialty information, or the *Physician's Desk Reference.*

Analgesics, antiphlogistics, antirheumatics
Pyrazolon derivatives, such as metamizol; oxyphenbutazone, phenylbutazone, and others; phenacetin; paracetamol

Antibiotics, chemotherapeutic agents
Antibiotics: penicillin, streptomycin, tetracycline, vancomycin, cephalosporin, and others
Chemotherapeutic agents: sulfonamide; other chemotherapeutic agents, e.g., metronidazol

Hypnotics, psychopharmacologic agents, anticonvulsants
barbiturates
chlorpromazine, and other tricyclic psychopharmacologic agents; hydantoin derivatives

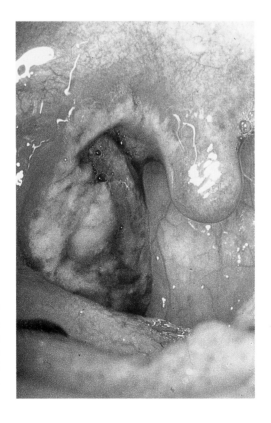

Fig. 24-12   Manifestation of toxic granulocytopenia in the right-side tonsillar bed with the appearance of a pseudodiphtherial angina in a 57-year-old patient. Cause: myelotoxic effect of cytostatic therapy.

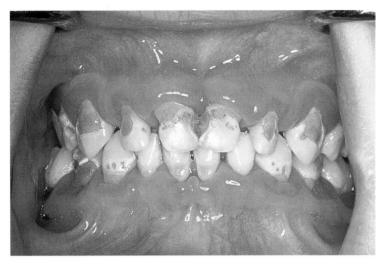

Fig. 24-13   Dental findings in a 4-year-old boy with agranulocytosis infantilis hereditaria of the Kostmann type. The inherited disease is characterized by the almost complete lack of granulocytes in the peripheral blood. At the age of 6 months was the first development of relapsing pyodermas, abscesses and tonsillitis together with high fever, which made long-term antibiotic therapy necessary and which receded slowly. Because of the defective cellular defenses, there is deep marginal periodontitis in the primary dentition. Note also the extensive cervical caries.

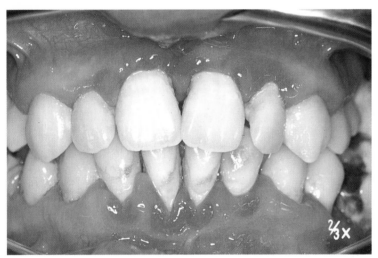

Fig. 24-14a   The patient of Fig. 24-13 at 17 years of age. Despite regularly administered gammaglobulin (at 4-week intervals) there is now, as before, increased susceptibility to infections and infectious processes. The intraoral findings show a deep marginal periodontitis with acute attacks and rapid progression in the dentition of a juvenile. After the extraction of a mandibular molar, a parapharyngeal abscess occurred. With modern therapeutic methods (allogeneic bone marrow transplants, administration of hematopoietic growth factors), the prognosis of patients with this disease has improved considerably in the last 5 years.

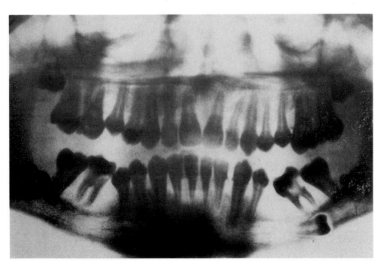

Fig. 24-14b   Radiographic findings of the adolescent in Fig. 24-14a at the same examination.

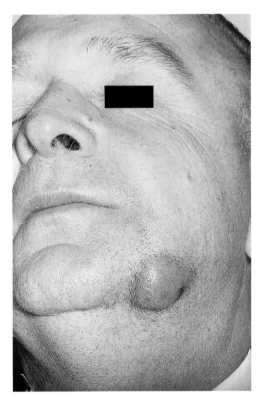

Fig. 24-15   Obvious blister on the facial skin (as a sign of anemia) and a subcutaneous abscess lying over the edge of the mandible (as a sign of decreased body defenses) in a 64-year-old patient with acute myelogenous leukemia. The subcutaneous abscess, which is not of dental origin, developed despite protective antibiotic therapy after an insignificant injury to the skin during shaving.

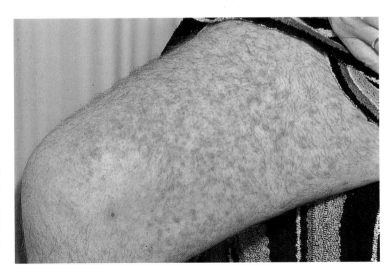

Fig. 24-16   Petechia and ecchymoses with the appearance of purpura in the skin of the upper thigh. Cause: bleeding diathesis of the thrombocytopenic type in the case of acute myeloblastic leukemia (displacement effect).

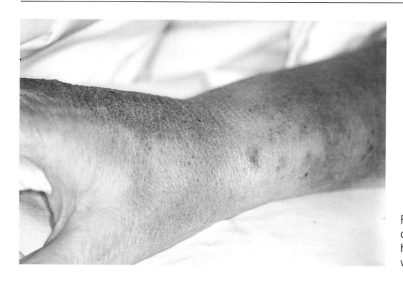

Fig. 24-17 Skin hemorrhage on the forearm and back of the hand of a 65-year-old patient with promyelocytic leukemia.

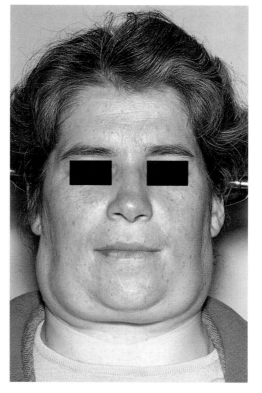

Fig. 24-18 Considerable bilateral enlargement of cervical and submandibular lymph nodes in a 62-year-old patient with acute myelogenous leukemia. These findings are typical for chronic lymphatic leukemia; enlarged but softer lymph nodes may also occur in acute lymphatic leukemia and, occasionally, as here, in myeloid leukemia.

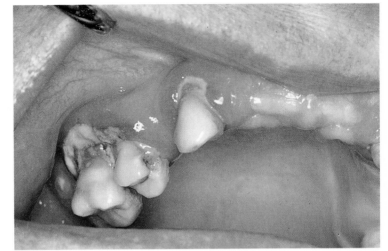

Fig. 24-19   The patient in Fig. 24-18 at the time of examination. Periodontal necrosis and ulceration in the previously damaged remaining maxillary teeth as an initial oral manifestation (low resistance syndrome).

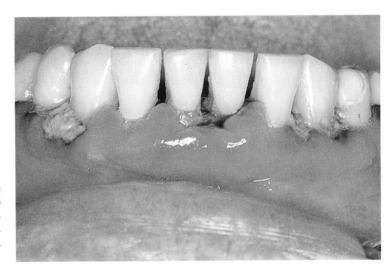

Fig. 24-20   The patient in Figs. 24-18 and 24-19 at the same examination. These changes are also found in the mandible in the form of acute necrotizing ulcerative gingivitis.

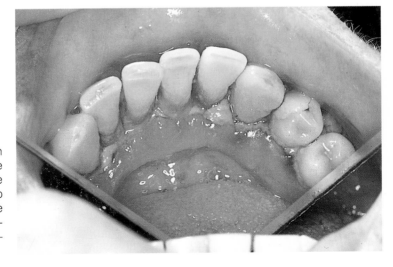

Fig. 24-21   The patient in Figs. 24-18 to 24-20 at the same examination. View of the mandible (mirror image) also demonstrates the extent of the infection with necrosis and ulcerations of the periodontal tissues.

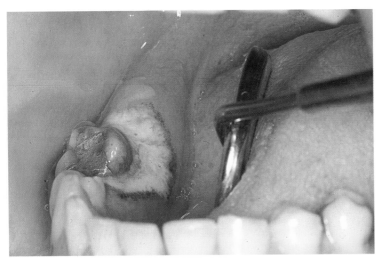

Fig. 24-22 Localized necrosis of the mucous membrane with tendency to spread on the alveolar process in the region of tooth 46 (30). This is a low-resistance syndrome in a 33-year-old patient with acute myeloid leukemia.

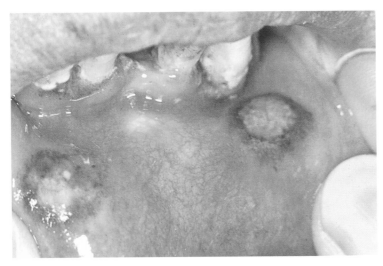

Fig. 24-23 Ulcerative gingivostomatitis (low-resistance syndrome) as primary oral manifestation of acute myeloblastic leukemia. During a febrile systemic condition, numerous short-lived ulcerations appeared on the oral and pharyngeal mucous membrane in this 63-year-old patient. Localized necrotizing ulcerated infectious processes with a surface spreading tendency were also found on the cheeks, gingiva, tongue, tonsils, and back of the pharynx as well as on the mucous membrane of the lower lip (where the lesions are partially confluent with the considerable microbial coating of the remaining teeth).

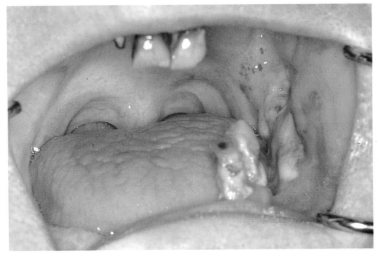

Fig. 24-24 Advanced and extensive soft tissue necrosis in the cheek region in a 73-year-old patient with acute lymphatic leukemia. Notice the petechial bleeding of the mucous membrane in the region of tissue damage (i.e., diagnostic combination of intraoral symptoms indicating acute leukemia).

Fig. 24-25 Acute myelogenous leukemia in a 28-year-old patient who died within the year. Serious, acute necrotizing ulcerous lesions of periodontal tissues with spontaneous bleeding. Shown is the situation immediately before the diagnosis by the internist. During the preceding 3 weeks, there had been warning oral symptoms in the form of spontaneous, recurring hemorrhaging of the gingiva and progressing necrotizing ulcerative gingivitis, which did not improve with local dental treatment (i.e., diagnostic combination of two or three cardinal symptoms in acute leukemia). The changes in the mucous membrane were related to progressive weakness, fatigue, pallor, and a general feeling of malaise associated with fever. The diagnostic workup was initiated by the dentist.

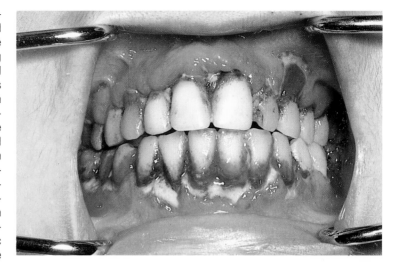

Fig. 24-26 The patient in Fig. 24-25 two weeks later. There is temporary improvement of the intraoral findings with intensive antileukemic therapy and accompanying local dental treatment.

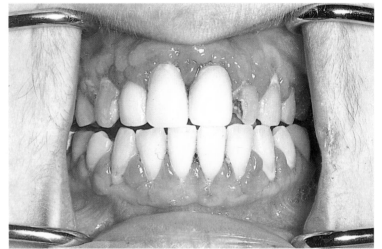

Fig. 24-27 Leukemic infiltrate in the region of the last remaining tooth 13 (6) considerably damaged by periodontal disease in the maxilla of a 67-year-old patient with myelomonocytic leukemia. Note that the mucous membrane of the edentulous alveolar process is free of leukemic infiltrate.

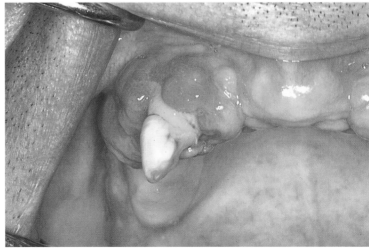

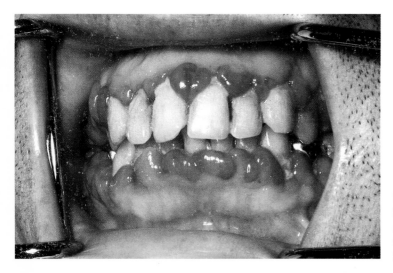

Fig. 24-28   Leukemic infiltrate in the gingiva of a 38-year-old patient with chronic myelogenous leukemia during the initial phase of an acute blastic crisis.

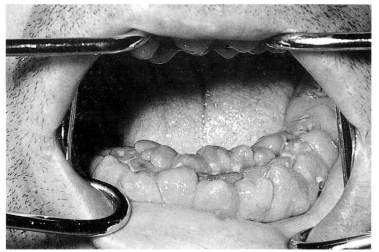

Fig. 24-29   Findings in the oral cavity of a 46-year-old patient with acute myeloid leukemia from which the patient died 3 weeks later. This massive proliferation of gingival tissue developed within 14 days and was associated with febrile episodes and progressive deterioration of the patient's general well-being. The leukemic infiltrates have nearly overgrown the teeth.

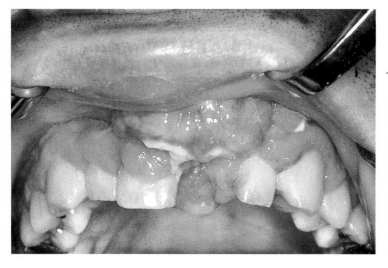

Fig. 24-30   Intraoral primary manifestation of acute myeloid leukemia in a 30-year-old patient. Two days earlier, tooth 21 (9) was removed because of an incorrect diagnosis of marginal periodontitis. Nodular masses and infiltrates with focal ulcerations are found in the region of the extraction wound. The suspicion of leukemia was confirmed by hematologic examination.

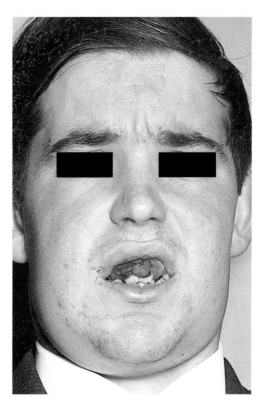

Fig. 24-31 Acute undifferentiated leukemia in a 17-year-old patient. The patient, who for several weeks complained of fatigue, weakness, and fever, only 14 days earlier noticed swelling of the gums, which increased rapidly and bled more frequently. Shown is the face of the febrile patient with swelling, especially pronounced on the right side, of the submandibular lymph nodes, as well as marked infiltrates of the gingival tissue in the visible region of the maxillary anterior teeth. Closing the mouth without tension is no longer possible. At this time, the diagnosis was yet not confirmed by a blood count.

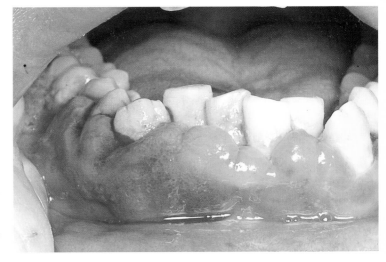

Fig. 24-32 The patient in Fig. 24-31 at the same examination. There is a pronounced doughy tissue proliferation in the region of the vestibular gingiva of the mandible. Ulcerations are present in the depth of the pseudopockets and bleed spontaneously. The findings should not be confused with simple gingival hyperplasia.

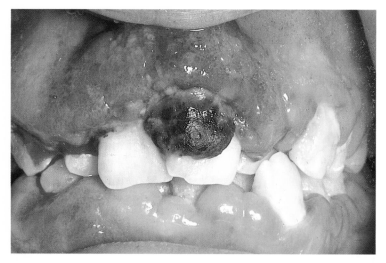

Fig. 24-33 The patient in Figs. 24-31 to 24-32 at the same examination. The massive gingival tissue proliferation in the region of teeth 11 and 21 (8 and 9) shows areas of hemorrhagic necrosis which, together with bleeding tendency, swelling of regional lymph nodes, and the suspicious general symptoms, suggest acute leukemia.

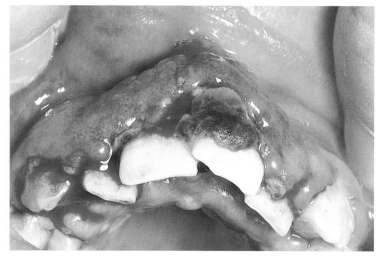

Fig. 24-34 The patient in Figs. 24-31 to 24-33 at the same examination. The view of the maxillary anterior teeth illustrates the extent of the changes with the cardinal intraoral symptoms of acute leukemia: gingival tissue proliferation (leukemic infiltrates) and necrotic ulcerations (as a sign of hemorrhagic diathesis of the thrombocytopenic type).

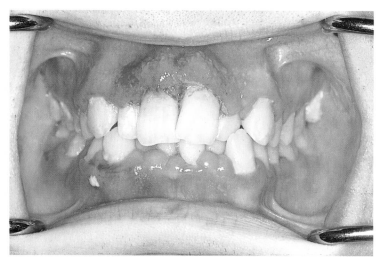

Fig. 24-35 The patient in Figs. 24-31 to 24-34, 14 days later. Temporary improvement of the oral cavity findings after the start of intensive antileukemic therapy and accompanying local dental treatment.

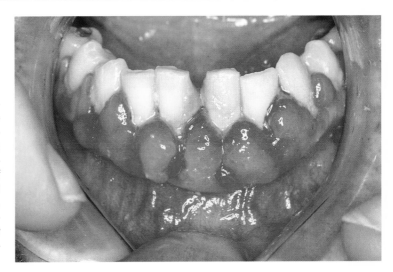

Fig. 24-36 Generalized gingival tissue proliferation accompanied by spontaneous bleeding in a 43-year-old patient with monocytic leukemia (i.e., diagnostic combination of two of the three cardinal intraoral symptoms in acute leukemia). The gingival changes in monocytic leukemia occasionally show—as here—an obvious purple color.

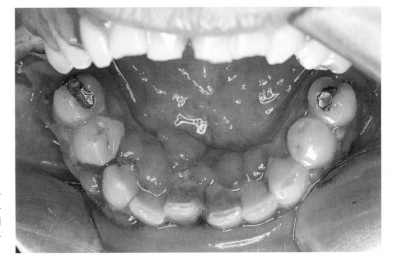

Fig. 24-37 The patient in Fig. 24-36 at the same examination. The view of the mandible (mirror view) documents that leukemic infiltrates also developed on the lingual side of the gingiva.

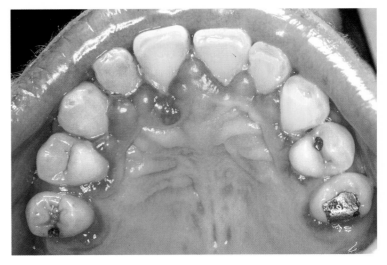

Fig. 24-38 The patient in Figs. 24-36 and 24-37 at the same examination. The view of the palate shows relatively mild infiltrates in the region of the palatal gingiva with obvious bleeding and signs of infection.

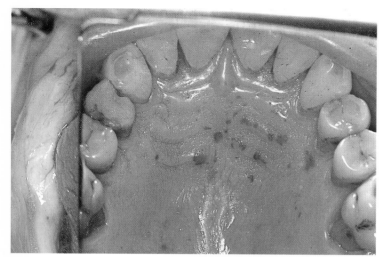

Fig. 24-39   Petechial bleeding on the mucous membrane of the hard palate as a partial manifestation of chronic myelogenous leukemia in a 49-year-old patient. Signs of bleeding of this type can be attributed to a number of different causes and require, in every instance, prompt hematologic examination.

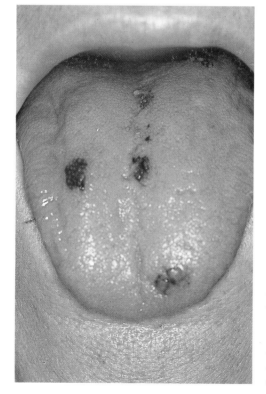

Fig. 24-40   Thrombocytopenic bleeding in the form of petechiae and ecchymoses on the dorsum of the tongue in a 55-year-old patient with acute myeloid leukemia. The bleeding diathesis of the thrombocytopenic type in acute leukemia is traced to the replacement of normal hematopoietic tissue in the bone marrow with proliferating leukemic cells (displacement effect). In chronic leukemia, the toxic effect caused by cell breakdown, which disturbs a normal thrombopoiesis, is also important.

Fig. 24-41 First clinically tangible manifestation of an acute myeloid leukemia in a 42-year-old patient. In the interdental papillary region of the mandibular anterior teeth are discrete petechial hemorrhagic foci, which change to gingival bleeding on the right side. In the region of tooth 26 (30), a remainder of the root is present and a leukemic infiltrate has formed (i.e., diagnostic guide combination of two of three cardinal intraoral symptoms of acute leukemia). Note that the changes, especially in the region of the mucous membrane with pre-existing damage, are extensive.

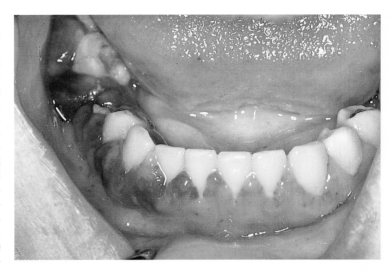

Fig. 24-42 Intraoral bleeding signs of a thrombocytopenic hemorrhagic diathesis in a 69-year-old patient with acute lymphoblastic leukemia. In the neighboring region of the last remaining tooth 24 (12), hemorrhagic necrosis is present. There are several subepithelial hemorrhages on the palatal mucosa.

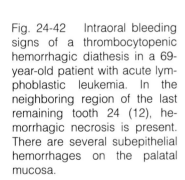

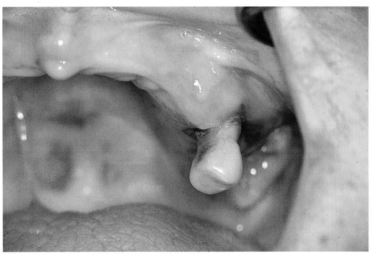

Fig. 24-43 Severe dystrophic periodontal findings in a 2½-year-old child in the terminal phase of an acute leukemia. Shown is the condition after a long-term polychemotherapy which, as expected, led to bone marrow depression.

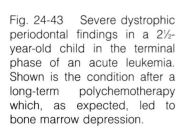

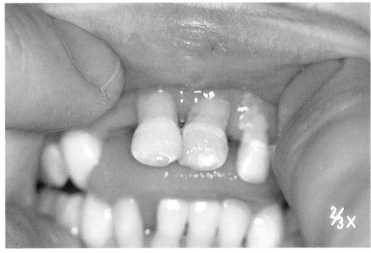

Oral Mucosal Symptoms in Hemorrhagic Diatheses

Thrombocytic-related hemorrhagic diatheses (thrombocytic disorders)
    Congenital thrombopathic diatheses
    Acquired thrombocytic diatheses

Plasma-related hemorrhagic diatheses (coagulation disorders)
    Congenital coagulation disorders
    Acquired coagulation disorders

Vascular-related hemorrhagic diatheses (vascular defects)
    Congenital vascular defects
    Acquired vascular defects

The cascading course of physiologic hemostasis (which cannot be discussed in detail here) rests on a complex interaction of the blood vessels, the platelets, and the coagulation system. Each lack, functional defect, or excess of one of the participating hemostatic components can cause bleeding problems.

Under the symptomatic collective term of "hemorrhagic disorders" is a combination of disease conditions that are very different etiopathologically but that can be recognized by an abnormal tendency for bleeding. They can be divided according to type of coagulation disturbance into thrombocytic, plasmatic, or vascular systems. The corresponding terms "thrombopathic," "coagulopathic," and "vasculopathic" are also used. Independent of the type of disturbance, the hemorrhagic disorders are further divided into congenital or acquired.

Hemorrhagic disorders may be independent diseases but may also be part of systemic diseases. In many cases, the diagnosis is first made because of suspicious bleeding of the mucosa.

To appreciate the diagnostic value of mucosal bleeding as a precursor of hemorrhagic disorders, it seems appropriate to present a basic explanation of the most frequent bleeding phenomenon in dentistry, namely, gingival bleeding.

Gingival bleeding even today is considered an indication of systemic disease among the laity. For the dentist, it is typically an associated symptom of inflammatory conditions in the marginal periodontium. Bleeding is an expression of permeability changes, which take place through bacterial action (microbial plaque) and which primarily affect the terminal ends of the circulatory system. Bleeding occurs primarily in the papillae and the gingival col as well as on the margins of the periodontium and the oral mucosa.

Mühlemann in 1978 tried to establish the relation between the intensity of the gingival inflammation and gingival bleeding and to establish an index (papilla bleeding index). The evaluation is made by gently probing the gingival sulcus (i.e., the gingival pocket) with a blunt probe, starting on the distal end of the sulcus and progressing toward the mesial end, or in the gingival pocket at the base of the papilla moving toward the point. The findings are divided into four grades to allow objective comparisons of the course of the inflammation of the (marginal) gingiva on the bleeding symptoms.

Papilla bleeding index according to Mühlemann

Grade 0 = no bleeding
Grade 1 = first appearing only at bleeding site
Grade 2 = appearing at several isolated bleeding sites or at a single isolated
            bleeding spot
Grade 3 = the interdental triangle fills with blood shortly after probing
Grade 4 = profuse bleeding with probing; blood flows immediately in the marginal sulcus

---

For most gingival bleeding sites, the cause of local irritation may be poor oral hygiene, carious defects, subgingival concretions, or restorations in need of improvement or that should be removed to control the periodontal disease. With appropriate local therapy and elimination of local irritation factors, gingival bleeding disappears as long as the patient cleans and cares properly for his or her teeth and gingiva.

If there is papillary bleeding of grades 3 and 4 not adequately explained by local causes, or if there is bleeding without inflammatory changes in the rest of the oral mucosa, the dentist must continue the differential diagnosis.

In relation to hemorrhagic disorders, symptomatic bleeding of the oral mucosa can take place spontaneously just as in other organs and tissues, that is, without apparent cause or as a consequence of slight mechanical stimuli. Because microtraumas are unavoidable in the oral cavity, the dentist may be the first to notice an as yet unrecognized hemorrhagic disorder.

The discrepancy between the local condition and the appearance, and in some instances duration of the bleeding, is evident. The experienced professional will include the overall appearance of the patient and the type of complaints in the findings.

It is particularly important to have an in-depth patient history. With suspicion of a hemorrhagic disorder it is often possible to evaluate the history to diagnose the bleeding disorder (thrombocytic, plasmatic, or vascular). The family history regarding the existence of congenital or acquired abnormalities allows definite conclusions. The individual's history should, in retrospect, lead to the consideration of an acquired disorder and should positively include a detailed medication and allergy history. For definitive diagnosis, it is necessary to determine whether an increased bleeding tendency was present before the initiation of a systemic disease.

From the large number of congenital and acquired thrombocytic, plasmatic, and vascular coagulation disturbances, examples important for the dental office will be discussed in this chapter.

Thrombocytic-related hemorrhagic diatheses (thrombocytic disorders)

Thrombocytic hemorrhagic disorders originate from reduction of the platelets *(thrombocytopenia)* or a functional disturbance of the blood platelets *(thrombocytopathy)*. These quantitative and qualitative thrombocytic defects are among the most frequent of all bleeding disorders; the acquired forms predominate—among them the thrombocytopenias. These diseases result in increased bleeding time with normal functions of the plasmatic coagulation factors. Capillary resistance and the retraction of blood clots are pathologically altered.

For an exact differential diagnosis, the platelet number and the results of different thrombocytic functions allow further differentiation of the disease. It is therefore possible to determine the depression of the thrombocytic function caused by disease, for example by medications with aggregation hindering effects (salicylates) and from congenital disturbances (i. e., Willebrand-Jürgens syndrome). The examinations require specialized laboratory procedures.

Thrombocytopenias predominantly manifest on the skin and mucosa as petechial bleeding, sometimes as purpura. In some cases, the presence of a single petechia–or in other cases dispersed discrete petechias–on the oral mucosa is the only sign of a thrombocytopenia, particularly if the skin does not show signs of bleeding (Figs. 25-1 to 25-3). These extravasations are the consequence of reduced numbers of platelets and thus decreased immediate sealing of capillary walls. In the area of previously damaged inflamed gingiva, profuse bleeding is possible (Fig. 25-5). Sometimes there is development of hemorrhagic gingivitis (Fig. 25-6).

Congenital thrombocytic diatheses

In the rare hereditary thrombocytic disturbances (e. g., *hereditary thrombasthenias*, ICD-DA 287.10), there is a retraction enzyme defect with biochemical changes in the normal number of platelets present. Besides petechial bleeding on the skin and mucosa in this disease, there is widespread skin bleeding and hematoma formation after only slight tissue trauma. In addition, *Fanconi's anemia* (ICD 284.0) as a familial infantile special form of aplastic anemia (panmyelopathy), which was discussed in chapter 24, should also be considered. Other indications of this disease are described in the legends of Figs. 25-4 and 25-5.

Acquired thrombocytic diatheses

Primary thrombocytopenia (ICD-DA 287.3 and 287.30)

Primary thrombocytopenia is understood to be thrombocytopenia with no exogenous cause or motivating disease. It is attributed to autoimmune conditions. There is a reduction of platelet numbers by increased platelet turnover. Bleeding time is usually distinctly increased but plasmatic coagulation parameters are unchanged.

Primary acute thrombocytopenia (idiopathic thrombocytopenic purpura), and often the recurring thrombocytopenia with a chronic course, are frequent causes of thrombocytopenia. Bleeding of the oral mucosa can be the first diagnostic sign of this disease (Figs. 25-1 to 25-3) and can lead to severe bleeding, particularly in the gastrointestinal and urogenital systems.

Secondary thrombocytopenia (ICD-DA 287.4 and 287.40)

In children of preschool and school ages, infectious diseases such as influenza, chickenpox, German measles, measles, and scarlet fever are the most frequent cause of acute thrombocytopenias. Postinfectious or parainfectious reduction of the platelet number is associated with toxic and allergic phenomena. The findings vary from a silent course to a serious conditon with skin, mucosal, and internal organ bleeding. Thrombocytopenias can appear *after inoculations* against poliomyelitis, smallpox, and tetanus. They can also appear as allergic reactions to the ingestion of certain *foods* (nuts, eggs, milk, fish, meat). Added materials, such as haptenes, form a full antigen with the platelets. The antigen-antibody reaction destroys thrombocytes.

Bleeding damage caused by *impaired platelet production* can be observed as a consequence of toxic bone marrow damage by chemical substances, cytostatics, and ionizing radiation as well as after bone marrow replacement in the case of malignant tumors and leukemias (Fig. 25-6; see also chapter 24).

Of great primary practical importance for the dentist are *medication-induced* thrombocytic coagulation disturbances, which make up 25% of all cases. Antibiotics, sulfonamides, oral antidiabetics, quinine, antipyretics, and particularly analgesics may lead in some cases to platelet damage with thrombocytopenia and/or thrombocytopathy (Figs. 25-7 and 25-8).

The effects of acetylsalicylic acid are well known as platelet-aggregation hinderers in low doses. This property is useful therapeutically. Salicylates are extensively used as a prophylactic agent in thromboembolic complications and for secondary prophylaxis of myocardial infarcts. After discontinuation of the medication there is an increased tendency to bleed for up to 8 days for which no antidote is available.

Plasma-related hemorrhagic diatheses (coagulation disorders)

In coagulation disorders, the cause of bleeding is not due to cellular blood elements but to the lack of, or anomaly of, coagulation factors in the plasma. Depending on the level of abnormality of the disease (residual activity of the factors), there may be severe and life-threatening bleeding for unexplained or minimal causes. Indicative are surface skin bleeding and extensive intramuscular hematomas after insignificant injuries.

Congenital factor VIII disorder (ICD-DA 286.0 and 286.00); congenital factor IX disorder (ICD-DA 286.1 and 286.10)

Of the congenital coagulation defects, lack of factor VIII (i. e., antihemophilic factor A) in hemophilia A and lack of factor IX (i. e., antihemophilic factor B) in hemophilia B are known to the dentist for the bleeding problems they cause. The X-chromosomal recessive hereditary hemophilia affects 1 in 10,000 individuals. The relative frequency of hemophilia A in relation to the clinically indistinguishable hemophilia B is 5:1.

The genetic severity of hemophilia must be determined in a special clinic. Here the patients receive certificates. Depending on the activity of factor VIII or IX, severe hemophilia (residual activity, 0% to 1%), hemophilia of intermediate severity (residual activity, 1% to 5%), mild hemophilia (residual activity, 5% to 15%) and subhemophilia (residual activity, 15% to 35% or—substitution ability—up to 70%) are differentiated. Particularly noticeable are patients with severe and moderately severe hemophilia and "bleeding joints" (hemarthrosis), which result from recurrent bleeding in the joints. Hemorrhages in the oral cavity appear after the smallest mucosal injury (Fig. 25-9). The appearance of these oral hemorrhages is codetermined by the influence of the saliva. The initial coagulation, later coagulum, destructive action and the contact area of blood/saliva with a thinner superficial fibrillar mesh, allows a voluminous pseudocoagulate to develop from which there can be many days of bleeding (Fig. 25-10). The bleeding can also occur in the tissue and a life-threatening volume increase, for example of the floor of the mouth, can develop. Petechiae are not a clinical feature. In the cases of subhemophilia there can be severe postoperative bleeding complications.

In general, a clinical dental-surgical intervention should be performed only in a hospital setting by an person experienced with children as well as adults with hemophilia A or B.

von Willebrand's disease (ICD-DA 286.4 and 286.40)

The autosomal-dominant hereditary von Willebrand's disease belongs to the most common congenital hemorrhagic diasthases. The severe bleeding depends on an impaired factor VIII synthesis combined with a factor VIII-associated protein defect. The combinations of possibilities are shown in the table on page 548.

The clinical symptoms are based on the degree of abnormality of the coagulation diagnostic laboratory parameters as well as large interindividual and intraindividual variations. Normal laboratory findings of a single examination (partial thromboplastin time, factor VIII, factor VIII-associated protein, and von Willebrand's factor) do not preclude the existence of von Willebrand's disease. With a strongly suspicious clinical and familial history, the patient should undergo several coagulation analyses.

Clinical findings correspond to a mixture form of hemorrhagic diatheses. On one hand there is skin and mucosal bleeding, which is similar to a thrombocytic or vascular coagulation disturbance (Fig. 25-11). On the other hand, in severe cases there are bleeding symptoms consistent with factor deficiency (e. g., spontaneous bleedings, increased post-traumatic bleeding; Fig. 25-12). Clinically there are also mute forms that appear only under the influence of pain killers (particularly salicylic acid derivatives). In cases of doubt, this is a reason for reduction of daily use of salicylate analgesics.

There are other autosomal, hereditary coagulation problems due to congenital deficiencies of other factors, but because of their rarity they will not be discussed here.

Acquired coagulation disorders

With the entrance into the blood of active proteolytic substances that dissolve and use up coagulation factors and platelet complexes, bleeding complications develop. Coagulation diatheses (defibrinization syndrome) are not considered because the diseases they are based on usually do not have immediate import for dental practice.

Among acquired coagulation diatheses, the dentist must first consider *prothrombin synthesis disturbances* as well as *acquired coagulation factor deficiency* (ICD 286.7)–the consequence of liver parenchyma damage and chronic gastrointestinal disease with poor digestion or malabsorption syndrome. The clinical bleeding symptoms appear in the skin and mucosa after mechanical stimuli. The danger of subsequent bleeding depends on the intensity of liver damage. In liver cirrhosis, thrombocytic petechial bleeding is possible.

For plasmatic hemorrhagic diatheses, it is desirable to normalize the blood coagulation using *appropriate therapy that may include anticoagulants*. Because the patient has an appropriate certificate, he or she brings the diagnosis with him or her. The conditions the dentist must take into consideration to perform dental surgical interventions in "marrow-damaged" patients are discussed in books on oral surgery.

In high-risk patients with a depressed marrow, the coagulation status should be evaluated preoperatively. After sucessful intervention, it should be monitored for the need for appropriate therapy that may even include temporary heparin administration to avoid the development of thromboses, infarcts, or embolisms. The level of desirable "heparin protection" depends on the clinical situation in regard to postoperative bleeding potential and the actual coagulation status, and it should be done in cooperation with the specialist.

The possible interaction between coumarin and other medications should be considered. An increase of anticoagulant action results from certain analgesics (salicylate acid derivatives, pyrazolone derivatives) and all antibiotics that affect the controlling mechanisms of the intestinal bacteria that influence vitamin K synthesis, to name the most important medications of the dental armamentarium. For a decrease of anticoagulation effect, that is, for a decrease of the prothrombin time, there are the barbiturates, corticosteroids, relaxants, ganglion blockers, and psychopharmaceuticals, among others, that allow stabilization of the patient. In the realm of indicated medications, the dentist must consider drug interactions and consult with the treating physician.

Vascular-related hemorrhagic diatheses (vascular defects)

Vascular bleeding problems result from blood vessel changes that allow increased passage through the vessel wall (permeability disturbance). As with the other hemorrhagic diatheses, there are congenital and acquired diseases.

Congenital vascular defects

Hereditary hemorrhagic telangiectasia (ICD-DA 448.00)

In this autosomal-dominant hereditary vascular anomaly, there is abnormal enlargement of the terminal blood vessels (arterioles, arterial and venous capillaries) of the skin, mucosa, and internal organs. Clinically one finds small, enlarged, and serpentine vessels with purpura red, red-violet, or more bluish nodular enlargements of the blood vessel walls. These multiple telangiectasias increase in number with age. Spontaneously or after mild trauma, blood vessel ruptures appear that can result in severe or moderately severe, quietly profuse bleeding of the mucosa (most frequently in the nose—Fig. 25-16—but also in the oral cavity and gastrointestinal and urinary tracts).

Diagnosis depends on the demonstration of characteristic vessel changes of the skin (face, extremities) and particularly the lip and oral mucosa. They appear preferentially on the vermilion of the lip (Figs. 25-13 and 25-16) and lip mucosa (Figs. 25-14 and 25-17) and in the anterior portion of the tongue (Figs. 25-16 and 25-17); they can also appear on the cheek and palatal mucosa (Fig. 25-18). Telangiectasias are often first reported in the accurate discussion of family history.

Telangiectasias pale under the pressure of a glass spatula (Fig. 25-15) as do vessel enlargements in infectious conditions (erythemas). However, a blood vessel that is losing blood does not disappear under the pressure of a glass spatula.

Acquired vascular defects

Among hemorrhagic diatheses a classical example of an acquired vascular conditioned is *scurvy (C-hypovitaminosis)*, for which early gingival bleeding is a typical symptom. Today, this disease is no longer of importance.

Among the acquired vascular wall defects in children and adolescents, *allergic purpura* (ICD 287.0) plays a major role in this age group. It is caused by an antigen-antibody-reaction of hemolytic streptococci or, more rarely, to albumin-containing foods or medications. It consists of vascular damage of the endothelium. Because of the consequent blood extravasation, there is the development on the skin (symmetric and the lower extremities) of a vascular purpura with a varied exanthematic picture. The vascular purpura is made up of numerous petechiae that are not determined by the thrombocytopenia (number and function of the platelets; also, the plasma-containing coagulation parameters are generally not altered). In addition to the skin symptoms, there can be the development of painful joint swelling and internal bleeding (kidney/urinary tracts, gastrointestinal tract). Bleeding in the oral mucosa is rare.

In adulthood, apart from *diabetic vasculopathy*, and particularly in women because of the many medications taken during the menstrual period, untoward drug reactions must be considered *(medication-conditioned immune-reaction vascular purpura*; Fig. 25-19).

It should be mentioned here that with the menstrual bleeding only few changes of coagulation are noticeable. Surgical dental treatment can therefore take place during menstrual bleeding. In patients with an additional medication load (e. g., analgesics–take medication history), bleeding can be intensified.

In older persons, there are primarily *arteriosclerotic* and *degenerative* vascular changes. They can also occur in the oral mucosa due to increased vessel fragility and can cause bleeding (Figs. 25-20 and 25-21) and postoperative bleeding complications.

Final considerations for the dentist

If the carefully recorded patient history points to the possibility of bleeding in the oral mucosa or skin with a suspicion of hemorrhagic diathesis, there should be a hematologic evaluation that includes plasmatic coagulation parameters and platelet and vascular function tests before each dental intervention. This means referral to a physician for the elimination, or explanation and classification, of the suspected hemorrhagic diatheses.

Based on a correct diagnosis, it is now possible to provide therapy recommendations for each patient. In patients with hemophilia or with coagulation problems that can lead to life-threatening bleeding, the coagulation functions should be evaluated before each intervention in the dental practice. These patients should be referred to a specialized clinic for treatment.

If there is a suspicion that there may be an increased bleeding tendency and there is already a known hemorrhagic diathesis, a complete perioperative coagulation analysis must be performed. Patients with congenital hemorrhagic diatheses have, as a rule, a "blood certificate" with exact information of the type of bleeding problem and the need for substitution therapy. Special clinics, blood banks, and special laboratories stock the corresponding products. The preparations have been clear of hepatitis B, hepatitis C (non-A non-B) and HIV since 1985.

In each case the dentist must determine if there is a decrease of bleeding risk because of previous therapy and if the anticipated problems of the local bleeding allow for the planned treatment to be done as ambulatory care. Careful and responsible dental treatment of the patient with hemorrhagic diatheses is necessary to avoid bleeding complications during and after the dental intervention. The dentist should always supervise threatening bleeding and in emergency situations use local therapeutic possibilities.

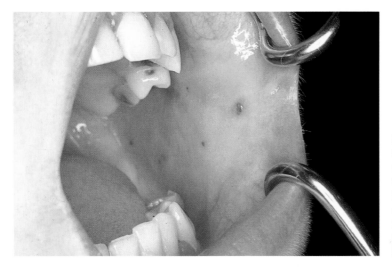

Fig. 25-1 Single petechia spread over a large area of the cheek mucosa in a 34-year-old woman. These discrete signs of bleeding were the only clinical demonstration of a long-standing but unrecognized idiopathic primary thrombocytopenia in the absence of skin findings.

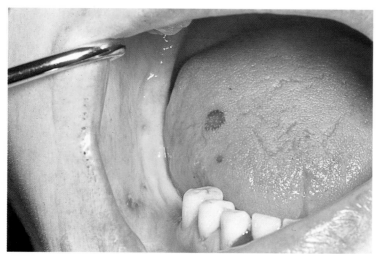

Fig. 25-2 Petechiae on the tongue and buccal mucosa in a previously unrecognized idiopathic thrombocytopenia in a 42-year-old man. The skin area of the corner of the mouth also shows several punctiform hemorrhages.

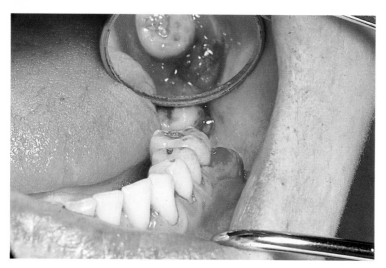

Fig. 25-3 The patient in Fig. 25-2 at the same examination. Old and new hemorrhages are seen contralaterally in the marginal region of periodontally damaged molars. One must beware of extractions. This patient's bleeding time was increased to 31 minutes. Referral is required.

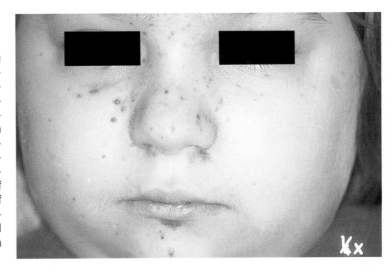

Fig. 25-4 Petechial bleeding on the facial skin of an 8-year-old child with Fanconi's anemia. This condition is a hereditary disturbance of the blood-forming bone marrow, which leads to a chronic pancytopenia (macrocytic anemia, granulo-cytopenia, and thrombocytopenia) and anomalies of the skeletal system (with lack of growth, microcephaly) and pigmentation disturbances as well as underdeveloped genitalia and mental retardation.

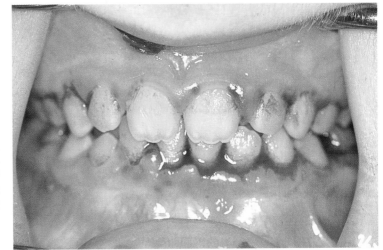

Fig. 25-5 The child in Fig. 25-4 at the same examination. Profuse spontaneous bleeding of the gingiva. The platelet count was 1000/µm. The clinical symptoms of this disease, which has a poor prognosis, manifest in early childhood.

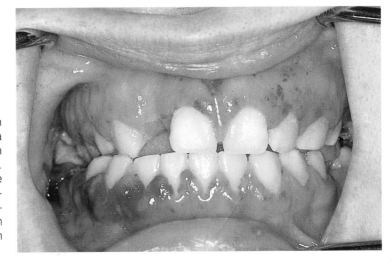

Fig. 25-6 Gingival bleeding in a secondary thrombocytopenia in a 42-year-old woman with acute myelogenous leukemia. There are numerous discrete petechiae on the vestibular gingiva of both jaws. A hemorrhagic gingivitis has developed in the mandible. (More details can be found in chapter 24.)

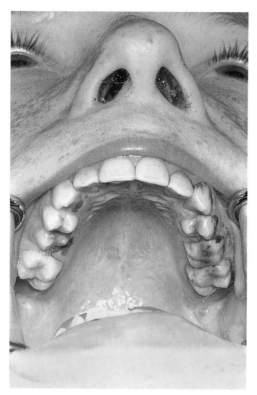

Fig. 25-7 This serious allergic thrombocytopenia, type II with thrombocytopathy in a 12-year-old boy was drug-induced. Spontaneous gingival hemorrhages were caused by prescribed medication. In the maxilla was development of spontaneous gingival bleeding. Recurring epistaxis and severe renal bleeding led to a life-threatening anemia.

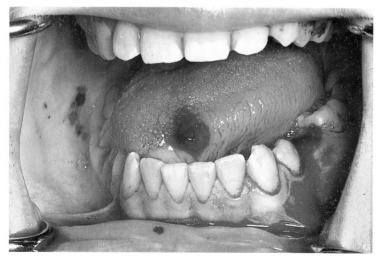

Fig. 25-8 The patient in Fig. 25-7 at the same examination. Bleeding lasted for days after insignificant tongue injury while eating. The mucosa near the root remnants of tooth 75 (K) also shows continued bleeding for a considerable time without coagulation. Note the petechiae on the buccal and labial mucosa, which can also be noticed on the skin of the face in Fig. 25-7.

Fig. 25-9 Previously unrecognized mild form of hemophilia A in a 2-year-old child. Hemorrhage after a minor injury to the tongue (during a meal) that had been present for 10 days, was not controllable with outpatient treatment. The diagnostic clue was found in the mother's family history and confirmed by hematologic examination, which is always essential. It demonstrated which of the X-chromosome-recessive forms was present (in this case deficiency of antihemophilic globulin, factor VIII or IX) and also provided explanation of the genetic grade of the coagulation defect (residual activity of the factor).

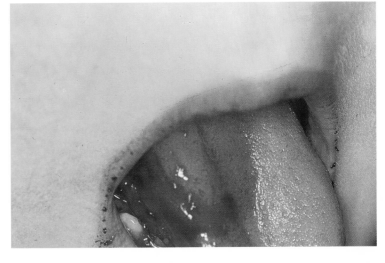

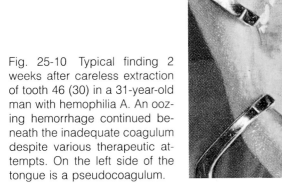

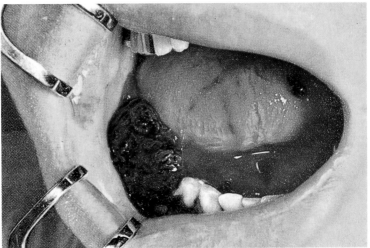

Fig. 25-10 Typical finding 2 weeks after careless extraction of tooth 46 (30) in a 31-year-old man with hemophilia A. An oozing hemorrhage continued beneath the inadequate coagulum despite various therapeutic attempts. On the left side of the tongue is a pseudocoagulum.

Special note

Even small dental surgical interventions in patients with severe and moderate forms of congenital or acquired coagulation disturbances should be performed in a hospital environment. Therefore, refer such patients to specialized clinics.

Division of von Willebrand's disease by the European Thrombosis Research Organization according to the nomenclature of the International Committee of Thrombosis and Hemostasis.

Type	Bleeding time	F VIII: C	F VIIIR: AG	F VIIIR: WF (RCF)
I	Increased	Reduced	Reduced	Reduced
II	Increased	Normal-to-reduced	Normal-to-reduced	Reduced
III	Increased	Normal	Reduced	Reduced
IV	Normal-to-reduced	Reduced	Reduced	Reduced

Abbreviation key:
F VIII: C
   = factor VIII coagulation activity
F VIIIR: AG
   = factor VIII = associated antigen
F VIIIR: WF (RCF)
   = ristocetin-cofactor activity

(Ristocetin is a glycopeptide antibiotic that leads to aggregation of normal platelets in the presence of normal plasma. In patients with von Willebrand's disease, this property is reduced or absent.)

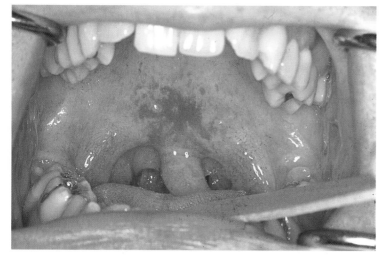

Fig. 25-11 Mucosal bleeding on the soft palate in a 31-year-old woman with von Willebrand's disease. The cause was an insignificant injury during eating.

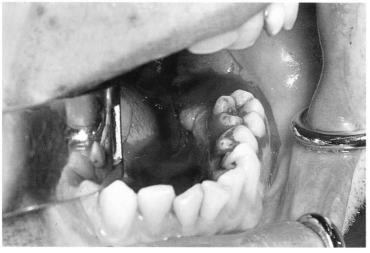

Fig. 25-12 Heavy and continuing bleeding could not be stopped for a long time under ambulatory conditions after an easy extraction of tooth 37 (18) in a 38-year-old man with von Willebrand's disease. In severe forms of the disease, the bleeding symptoms are similar to the coagulation disorders appearing in hemophilia.

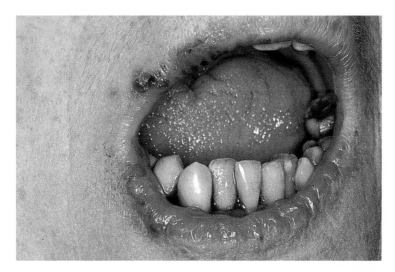

Fig. 25-13 Typical appearance of telangiectases in the lip region of a 57-year-old woman with Osler's disease. The telangiectases due to an abnormal enlargement of the capillaries increase during life in number and size. They are located here primarily on the vermilion of the lips. Note the symptoms of repeated bleeding.

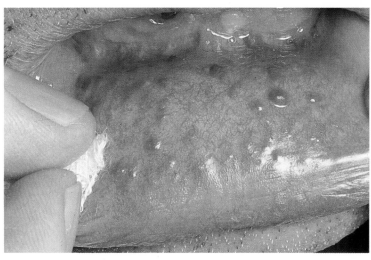

Fig. 25-14 The patient in Fig. 25-14 at the same examination. There are numerous telangiectases the size of pinheads in part also forming small red-violet nodules on the mandibular mucosa. Such oral manifestations, when taken together with the family history, are often a first and decisive indication of the existence of a hereditary hemorrhagic telangiectasia.

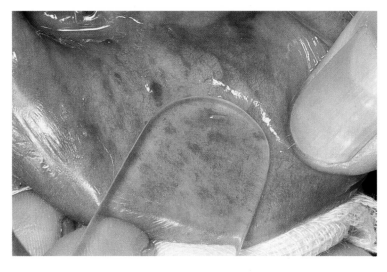

Fig. 25-15 The patient in Figs. 25-13 and 25-14 at the same examination. Under pressure with a glass spatula, the telangiectases pale, as also occurs in inflammatory blood vessel enlargement (erythemas). In contrast, blood that left the vessels does not disappear under the glass spatula.

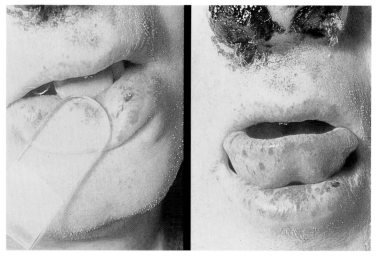

Fig. 25-16 Osler's disease with extended hemorrhagic telangiectases on the labial and lingual mucosa. Observe the partially encrusted tampon, inserted because of spontaneous epistaxis, and the anemic appearance of the skin. The autosomal-dominant hereditary vascular defect of the terminal vessels permits blood vessel rupture spontaneously or after slight trauma. There can be mucosal bleeding that is severe, profuse, and difficult to stop, most frequently in the nose but also in the oral cavity, stomach, intestine, and urinary system. In these patients telangiectases disappear when pressure is applied with a glass spatula.

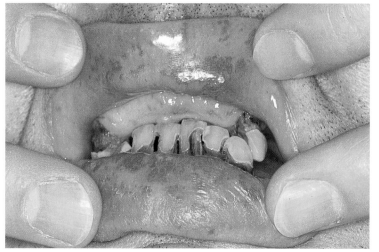

Fig. 25-17 Bleeding diathesis due to telangiectases on the mucosa of the upper and lower lip in a 36-year-old man with Osler's disease. Secondary local irritative factors–as here, teeth destroyed by deep caries and microbial plaque–can interfere with healing in these conditions. Also note the telangiectases on the tongue mucosa.

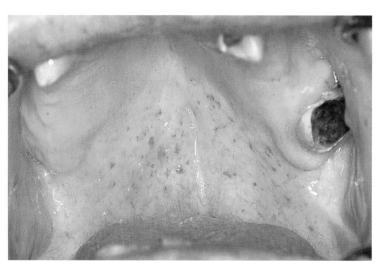

Fig. 25-18 The patient in Fig. 25-17 at initial examination. There were also numerous telangiectases on the mucosa of the soft palate.

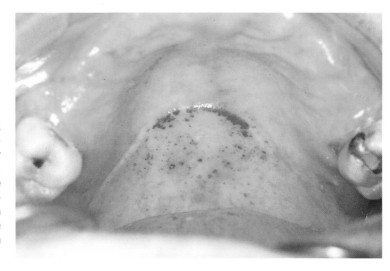

Fig. 25-19 Vascular purpura on the palatal mucosa of a 56-year-old woman with poorly controlled adult-onset diabetes. The petechiae, which can be traced to the diabetic angiopathy, are particularly extensive in the dorsal border zone of the maxillary prosthesis (not shown here).

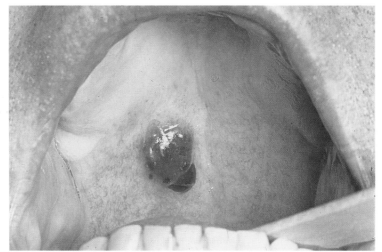

Fig. 25-20 Coin-sized, spontaneously recurring ecchymosis at the transitional zone of the hard and soft palate in a 67-year-old patient. The probable causes in this instance are the degenerative changes of the vascular walls and surrounding connective tissue. A causal connection with the complete maxillary denture was unlikely because the prosthesis had not been worn at the time this lesion appeared.

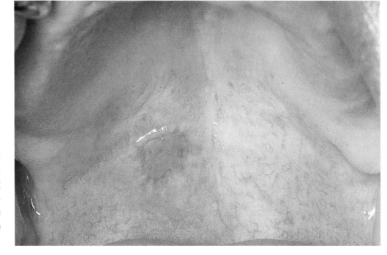

Fig. 25-21 The patient in Fig. 25-20, eight days later—healing stage of the erosion with marginal bullae remnants. Without knowledge of the patient's history, a secondary efflorescence of vesiculobullous disease should be considered.

Chapter 26

Oral Mucous Membrane Lesions in Selected Internal Diseases

Cardiovascular diseases
  Tetralogy of Fallot
  Occlusive arterial disease

Diabetes mellitus

Gastrointestinal diseases
  Malnutrition
  Maldigestion/malabsorption syndromes
  Chronic liver diseases
  Ulcerative colitis
  Crohn's disease

Amyloidosis

At some stage, internal diseases result in changes of the gingiva (including the marginal periodontium) and other parts of the oral mucosa. In this chapter, oral and perioral manifestations of some major chronic internal diseases are discussed. As a rule, the effects of the associated syndromes on the oral mucosa are of subordinate significance because the basic disease is known to most patients and information about it is provided at the time of history taking. Still, knowledge of clinical findings and symptoms in the oral cavity and perioral region is important for the dentist, because it reminds him or her of the importance of major illness in the considerations of indications and prognosis of dental therapy.

Cardiovascular diseases

The problems of patients with cardiovascular diseases are known to the dentist because of the need for avoidance of some therapies. As in all other tissues and organs, the vital maintenance and undisturbed function of the oral mucosa requires both qualitative and quantitative circulation of the blood. Oxygen content of the blood of less than 6.7% by volume eads clinically to cyanosis. This relation can be demonstrated in cases of congenital cardiovascular anomalies and when similar findings are observed with acquired heart, circulatory, and pulmonary diseases.

Arterial occlusive diseases are frequent complications primarily as arteriosclerotic changes. They may lead to ischemic necrosis that is sometimes observed on the oral mucosa.

Tetralogy of Fallot (ICD-DA 745.2 and 745.20)

Congenital heart defects with or without cyanosis are found in about 0.8% of newborns; many of them present a tetralogy of Fallot. This is a congenital quadruple cardiac defect comprising pulmonary stenosis, a high ventricular septal defect, a dextroposition of the aorta, and hypertrophy of the right ventricle. A description of the pressure and shunt relation that can be demonstrated precisely with heart catheterization will not be given here.

Pulmonary stenosis causes decreased circulation with resulting reduced O_2 saturation of the blood in the lungs. The oxygen deficiency and therefore the fairly severe reduction of oxygenated hemoglobin in the capillaries causes a high level of cyanosis in the newborn. This is particularly noticeable on the nails and vermilion of the lips and on the face (Fig. 26-1). Other typical changes are the "drum beater fingers" and "hour glass nails" (Fig. 26-2), which were known to Hippocrates as consequences of the "blue disease." With the associated reactive polycthemia, there is increased risk of thrombotic and embolic complications. The chronic hypoxia results in a severe developmental delay in these children. There is an extreme persistent weakness because of dyspnea in those most seriously affected. Mental retardation is generally not present. There is also a clinically noticeable cyanosis on the mucosa. The bluish gingiva (Fig. 26-3) is edematous and shows a significant increased number of subepithelial vessels. This increased vascularity is the expression of an attempt of the circulatory system to develop an adequate blood circulation, and in this manner to compensate for the oxygen deficiency.

Because of the generalized reduced performance of the children, there is also reduced oral hygiene. Therefore, it is not surprising that the previously damaged tissue develops early gingivoperiodontal inflammation. After successful heart surgery, the number of gingival blood vessels returns to normal. With planned hygiene is the improvement of the gingivoperiodontal changes.

Transposition of the large vessels results in a permanent cyanosis (Figs. 26-4 and 26-5).

Occlusive arterial disease (ICD 444)

Eighty percent of all arterial occlusive diseases are the consequence of arteriosclerosis. The most important and most frequent disease of the arterial vessel system has a chronic course and progresses in several stages. The disease changes begin with the deposit of lipids in the smooth musculature of the vessels (striated fatty deposition). There is hardening and increased rigidity of the blood vessel wall with loss of elasticity and increased reduction of the lumen of the vessel. In long-term stenosis of the vessel, there are many general and specific organ complications. The complete closure of an artery (obliteration) produces ischemic necrosis or gangrene of the affected organ. The best-known examples of stenosis and closure in the heart vessels are coronary heart disease and consequent heart infarcts. The effect of the vessel closure depends on the location of the occlusion, the speed of the development of the pre-existing collateral circulation, and the total situation of the circulatory system.

Ischemic necrosis of the oral mucosa is very rare and then only with the sudden occlusion of a previously severely damaged arteriosclerotic vessel in the presence of abnormal collateral circulation (Figs. 26-6 and 26-7). From a differential diagnostic viewpoint, an ischemic necrosis caused by cranial arteritis (giant cell arteritis) should be considered (see chapter 30, Fig. 30-14).

Finally, it is of interest to the dentist during therapy for coronary heart disease and hypertension that the calcium antagonist nifedipin—one of the most-used medications—can cause fibrous gingival hyperplasias (Fig. 26-8).

Diabetes mellitus (ICD-DA 250 and 250.VO)

Diabetes mellitus is a hereditary chronic metabolic disease based on an absolute (type I) or relative (type II) insulin deficiency. Environmental influences affect the rate of manifestation. Currently in Germany about 2.5% to 3% of the population is affected by diabetes mellitus. It is assumed that the number of individuals genetically susceptible without clinical illness is about equal. It must be calculated that the prevalence rate will continue to increase to the year 2000 when every twelfth inhabitant will suffer from the disease. Unquestionably, there is a need for increased diagnostic evaluation in which the dentist also takes part.

Obesity reduces the quality of life and finally decreases life expectancy due to disease. There is a need for more intense prevention programs (with improved life-style of the patient) and directed therapy (modifications of metabolism) with the aim of renormalizing the metabolism. The assistance of the dentist is also possible.

According to the suggestion of the World Health Organization in 1980, diabetes can be divided into:

- Type I—insulin-deficient diabetes ("juvenile diabetes")
- Type II—insulin-dependent diabetes ("adult-onset diabetes")
    II a without excessive weight
    II b with excessive weight
- Pathologic glucose tolerance (IGT) (in extraparenchymal-endocrine disease)
- Pregnancy diabetes
- Other forms of diabetes
    Disturbance of insulin receptors (genetic defects, receptor-autoantibodies).
    Medication-derived disturbances (e. g., from glucocorticoids, other exogenous introduced hormones, or other medications, such as benzothiadiazine derivatives).

Discussed here are only type I diabetes (IDDM: insulin-dependent diabetes mellitus) and type II diabetes (NIDDM: noninsulin-dependent diabetes mellitus).

Patients with *type I diabetes* represent only 10% of the total number of diabetes cases. The disease is recognized through the absolute lack of insulin in the labile metabolism with a tendency to ketoacidosis and diabetic angiopathy. The disease appears primarily in children and young adults but can manifest itself at all ages. Triggering factors are, among others, viral infections (coxsackie B virus, mumps virus, German measles). According to current knowledge, the actual disease onset depends on the genetically determined autoimmune disease. Insulin cell antibodies (ICA), insulin antibody (IAA), and antibodies against membrane proteins of B cells (anti 64 KD-protein) are often traceable in the early phase of the diseases. The serologic findings run parallel to a selective decrease of the insulin-producing B cells.

Early clinical symptoms of the metabolic changes (metabolic syndrome) are an increased thirst with increased fluid consumption (polydipsia), increased urine output (polyuria), loss of weight in spite of increased appetite (polyphagia), and generalized weakness and fatigue. These are caused by constant elevation of blood sugar (hyperglycemia), sugar elimination in the urine (glucosuria), and the disturbance of mineral and water metabolism.

Type I diabetes often manifests acutely with signs of ketoacidosis (increased appearance of ketones in blood and urine) and also in the form of a diabetic coma. The insulin-deficient diabetic is almost always a thin asthenic youth requiring insulin administration (i. e., *insulin-dependent diabetic*) for compensation of the metabolic disturbances.

In the nine of 10 diabetics with *type II diabetes*, the manifestations appear only after the fortieth year of life (adult-onset diabetes or maturity onset diabetes). Superimposed on familial cofactors are excessive eating and exercise deficiency as cofactors favoring the onset of disease. Most patients are overweight. The rapid increase of incidence of the disease in western industrial nations resulted in the thesis that this is a disease of the "well-off."

In contrast to type I diabetes, there is a relative metabolic activity. The insulin concentration in the blood can be normal because usually there is only a slight deficit of insulin. After glucose loading there is absence of the first phase of insulin increase. As a sign of a partial insulin insufficiency, onset of pancreatic insulin secretion is delayed (so-called secretion rigidity). There is at first a decrease of sensitivity of the tissue receptors (peripheral insulin resistance) to insulin. Because insulin secretion is still present, there is no development of ketoacidosis in about 50% of individuals but hypertension is noticeable.

Type II diabetes usually has an insidious onset. The glucosuria remains undetected for a long time despite the availability of easy test strips for demonstration of urinary sugar.

- The normal level of fasting blood sugar is 60 to 100 mg/dL.
- Pathologic or reduced glucose resistance defines a metabolic condition in which—in case of absent clinical symptoms—fasting blood sugar level is between 100 and 130 mg/dL and the blood sugar values 2 hours after oral glucose load are between 120 and 200 mg/dL.
- In a manifest diabetes, fasting blood sugar values are over 130 mg/dL and blood sugar values 2 hours after oral glucose load are over 200 mg/dL. Blood glucose concentration over 160 mg/dL leads to an increase of sugar loss in the urine (glucosuria).
- In badly controlled diabetes mellitus, blood sugar values are distinctly increased.
- Microalbuminuria appears as an early sign of an initiating microangiopathy.
- Glycosylated hemoglobin HbA or HbA1c are indispensable parameters for the retrospective long-term control of diabetes mellitus (6 to 8 weeks).

Adult-onset diabetes is treated by a regulation of the life-style to weight reduction through diet (diabetic diet as basis of all therapeutic measures), physical exercise, and in some cases eventually oral antidiabetic drug or insulin *(not insulin obligatory diabetes)*.

The diabetic coma (ketoacidotic coma in type I diabetes, hyperosmotic coma in type II diabetes) is the most severe incident of diabetic metabolic damage. The breakdown of metabolism is started by an intercurrent infection as well as omission or inadequate therapy due to lack of compliance. Currently less than 1% of all diabetic patients die of a diabetic coma.

Course and prognosis of diabetes mellitus depends on the blood vessel changes (generalized microangiopathy with resulting early appearance of retinopathy, glomerulosclerosis, severely evolving arteriosclerosis of the coronary, pelvic, and cerebral arteries) and hypertension. The longer the disease is present, the more difficult metabolism is to control and therefore the sooner diseases occur.

Life expectancy of each diabetic individual is decreased proportionally to the degree of metabolism alteration. In type I diabetics it is on average 10 years below normal life expectancy. The most frequent cause of death is heart infarct and kidney failure. Other manifestations of late diabetic syndrome are apoplectic insult, diabetic polyneuropathy (functional damage of the peripheral and central nervous system), diabetic foot, and diabetic cataract. Diabetes mellitus is the most frequent cause of blindness in the western world. As a consequence of microvasculatory retinopathies, about 2% of diabetic patients become blind 10 years after onset of the disease and about 10% in a 25- to 30-year diabetic course.

These short descriptions show the importance of prevention, early recognition of diabetes, conscientious adherence to the diabetic regimen, the faithful following of therapeutic measures, and regular follow-up examinations.

Almost every third diabetic patient shows accompanying skin changes which, however, are not diagnostically significant. Itching can be localized at the beginning and, for example, be limited to the genital area. Later, there is formation of multilocular irritation papillae which are scratched open and heal with difficulty. The predisposition to pyoderma (furunculosis) and dermatomycoses (among others, thrush) documents the increased tendency for infection. Changes in pigmentation are less noticeable and characteristic for the basic disease.

There are also oral cavity signs of increased inflammatory reaction associated with the metabolic syndrome of diabetes mellitus. It is not uncommon to observe multiple periodontal abscesses (Figs. 26-9 and 26-10), disturbances in wound healing after extractions and operative procedures (Fig. 26-13), persisting ulcerations (Figs. 26-12 and 26-14), and cheilitis of the corner of the mouth (see chapter 34, Fig. 34-29). In this phase of the disease there are frequent complaints of dryness of the mouth and reports of (peri)oral polyneuritis. In later courses of the diabetes mellitus onset, recurring candidiasis is possible on the oral mucosa–particularly in patients wearing prostheses and who have inadequate oral hygiene.

In the long run, there is also the development of atrophic changes on the papillary relief of the tongue with symptoms of glossodynia. All of these findings and symptoms are not specific for diabetes mellitus. Dryness of the lips and oral mucosa as well as halitosis with acetone smell are generally present only in seriously ill hospitalized patients.

The question of the causal relation between diabetes mellitus and the formation of a high-grade marginal periodontopathy is discussed in the literature. It is certain that there is no diabetic marginal periodontal disease nor any gingivitis or periodontitis in diabetes mellitus. Extension and progress of inflammatory periodontal disease depends greatly on oral hygiene. Even a severe noncontrolled diabetes will not cause periodontal damage with excellent oral care; on the other hand, even optimal conditions of metabolism will not reduce the damage that is possible with poor oral hygiene (plaque accumulation) and other marginal irritation. As shown in Fig. 26-11, lack of oral hygiene leads to plaque-conditioned inflammatory events, which are facilitated by diabetes mellitus. With increased duration of the disease, and the appearance of late complications due to blood vessel changes, there is an increase in the influence of metabolic changes on the course and intensity of the periodontal disease.

Periodontal conditions and consciousness of oral hygiene at the time of the discovery of the diabetes mellitus allow an important prognostic statement on the long-range maintenance of the teeth.

Final comments for the dentist

The dentist may be confronted with problems of differential diagnosis particularly with the child-juvenile patient in whom appearance of marginal periodontitis may lead to tooth mobility or recurrence of multiple pocket formations. In these cases, referral is indicated to exclude diabetes mellitus.

In the presence of an existing type I diabetes, the dentist should contact the treating physician before operative measures to be certain that there is a well-balanced metabolism. Patients who follow their diet, use insulin consistently, and have balanced blood sugar values can undergo ambulatory office dental-surgical treatment without problems. If there are complications in a diabetic patient, or the appearance of a local infection, jaw trismus, or lack of proper nourishment leading to a change in metabolic values, dental surgical intervention should be delayed until the attending physician ensures that there are no contraindications. If the treatment cannot be postponed, the patient should be transferred to the appropriate clinic for treatment (with medical consultation).

In the dental treatment of type II diabetes, in many cases preexisting associated diseases such as arteriosclerosis of the large vessels and coronary arteries (coronary disease), hypertension, and nephropathy merit consideration. The dentist must also consider that inflammatory processes of the oral cavity are not only a consequence of metabolic changes but that they also may facilitate or contribute to a latent diabetes. Therefore, oral prophylaxis and treatment of intraoral conditions should be performed in collaboration with the treating physician.

Gastrointestinal diseases

In the past, the oral mucosa was considered the mirror of internal conditions and the tongue in particular a diagnostic instrument for internal and external signs. In traditional Chinese medicine, an attempt was made to construct a lawlike relation between the total organism with organic disease and the location and type of tongue changes. This concept is no longer considered valid. The oral cavity is the beginning of the digestive process, but it has been considerably overrated in its significance as a diagnostic window of gastrointestinal disease. The classification of oral and perioral changes should be taken with reservations because only seldom can it be used for diagnostic purposes for stomach and intestinal diseases.

Exceptions are the oral and perioral pigmentations in the *Peutz-Jeghers syndrome* (see chapter 4), the multiple jaw osteomas in *Gardner's syndrome* (see chapter 22), and the oral mucosal manifestation in *Crohn's disease*, which can be early and guiding symptoms of the intestinal disease and will be discussed later.

The Plummer-Vinson syndrome discussed in chapter 24 as a consequence of an absolute or histamine refractory anacidity of the stomach (achlorhydria) is only seldom worth noticing. More frequent are dysphagias of a functional nature, which may cause the suspicion of a neoplasm of the esophagus, a suspicion that must be eliminated.

The coexistence of typical gastritis and ulceration signs in the oral cavity (i. e., spotty red spots on the soft palate, circumscribed papillary atrophies on the dorsum of the tongue, indicating apapillosis areata linguae) can at first be erroneously interpreted (Fig. 26-15) and should be abandoned completely for diagnostic purposes. Association of a marginal periodontopathy with subacidic or anacidic disturbances of the stomach in the patient history are not currently proven.

Malnutrition (ICD-DA 260-269)

A short-term *nutritional deficiency* is generally without major consequences because the body has reserves for up to 6 weeks, depending on circumstances. In children and youths, malnutrition of longer duration may lead to growth and development disturbances as well as to an increased susceptibility to infection.

In persistent *undernourishment*, the body continuously receives protein, carbohydrates, vitamins, and minerals in reduced amounts. The energy balance is possibly below the minimum required for subsistence level. According to reports from WHO, the most important nutrition-dependent deficiency diseases in developing countries are the nutrition-related diseases and the endemic struma due to the low protein calorie level (real hunger) together with lack of vitamin A. Individuals with *qualitative malnutrition* receive the necessary calories but not always the necessary protein, vitamins, and trace elements, that is, food intake is sufficient but is incorrectly balanced.

Finally, in abnormal nutrition there is also *caloric-excessive nutrition*, which can lead to fat deposition, development of type II diabetes and through it other diseases (for example, hypertonia, reduction of longevity).

In a healthy society, the appearance of nutritional-conditioned vitamin deficiency is greatly exaggerated by the laity. Classic scurvy as an early sign of lack of vitamin C is extremely rare. Other vitamin and mineral deficiencies can develop only when there has been long-term unbalanced nutrition. Latent deficiency of several vitamins can take place in old people living alone and with alcoholics.

A model disease that is informative and in which the effect of malnutrition can be noticed in the oral cavity is *anorexia nervosa* (ICD 307.1). This disease, which appears almost exclusively in pubescent girls and young women, is caused by abnormal psychic control and leads to food denial. Without psychiatric treatment, it has a mortality rate of 5% to 10%. The oral mucosa shows a general atrophy and paleness (as a sign of anemia) with a definite tendency to the development of rhagades. Inadequate oral hygiene leads to gingivoperiodontal changes. With frequent vomiting, as occurs with bulimia, is acid damage to tooth enamel occurs.

A frequent cause of deficient nutrition is extreme alcoholism. With the exception of the Islamic world, alcohol in its different forms is widely accepted as a drug. In excessive use, there are consequences *(alcoholism)* for the health of the individual and his or her social environment (family, society, profession). Data from the United States show that the average population receives about 5% of caloric needs from alcohol. One fourth of the male population consumes between 5% to 10% and another fourth over 10% of the desirable caloric intake with "empty" alcohol calories (1 g of ethanol delivers 7.1 kcal, a bottle of wine about 700 kcal). One kcal corresponds to 4.2 kJ (kilojoule). Habitual drinkers get 50% or more of their daily calories from drinks with high alcohol content. Toxic side effects include gastritis and enteritis as well as damage to the liver and pancreas with consequent malnutrition. In the alcoholic, the deficient nutrition is worsened by the fact that vitamins and minerals in particular are available in only very small quantities in alcohol.

Alcoholics often show glassy atrophic changes on the oral mucosa, in which the papillae relief of the tongue is decreased. The damaged tissue allows development of a secondary, usually circumscribed inflammation (Fig. 26-16). Surface erosions are frequently seen (Fig. 26-17). The patients usually complain of tongue and mucosal burning sensation because of the local tissue changes caused by the alcohol or by neuropathies. Oral hygiene is usually neglected. As stated in chapter 19, chronic consumption of highly concentrated alcoholic beverages is a risk factor for the development of cancer of the oral cavity, in particular on the lower part (tongue, floor of the mouth) and probably also of esophageal carcinoma.

Maldigestion syndrome; malabsorption syndrome (ICD-DA 579)

Malabsorption syndrome is a complex deficiency syndrome in which inadequate nutrition is caused by inadequate absorption of the nutritional materials from the intestine. The malabsorption can also be a disturbance of the digestion (maldigestion) resulting from deficiency of the digestive enzymes in chronic pancreatic insufficiency, liver disease (bile), other diseases, and postoperative conditions (stomach resection, small intestine resection). They can also be a consequence of disturbed resorption *(malabsorption)* due to damage to the resorption epithelium by inflammation and neoplastic diseases of the intestine, amyloidosis, celiac sprue, or alcoholism. Disturbances in the transport of resorbed materials, for example in congenital enzymatic conditions, can also be causes. The severity of deficiency depends also on the gravity of the basic disease.

Clinical symptoms include weight loss, abdominal complaints (such as flatulence, meteorism, diarrhea), decrease of activity, increased rate of infections, paleness (anemia), and skin and mucosal changes. The oral mucosa becomes atrophic, which can be clearly recognized in the disappearance of the tongue papillae (Fig. 26-18), and associated inflammatory signs. In the area of the corner of the mouth is frequently the formation of hard rhagades. In time, there is the development of glossitis or stomatitis. Gingivoperiodontal inflammatory events are influenced in their intensity by premorbid occlusal conditions and the quality of oral hygiene. The treatment of malabsorption consists in the therapy of the basic condition, such as the dietetic condition (gluten-free diet), oral or parenteral ingestion of vitamins, minerals, and enzymes. An example is the malabsorption due to zinc deficiency. Zinc is needed for biosynthesis and function of enzymes (as carboanhydrase, alcohol dehydrogenase, lactate dehydrogenase) and protein (such as insulin) and is therefore an element needed for life.

In the very rare disease *acrodermatitis enteropathica* (ICD-DA 686.8) there is a genetically determined gastrointestinal zinc resorption disturbance. As a consequence of the secondary zinc deficiency there is development of dermatitis in the mucocutaneous areas (mouth, nose, genitoanal region) and on the fingers and toes in the form of infected, red, and pus-oozing lesions (Fig. 26-19), followed by development of scales and atrophy of the skin. The clinical appearance resembles severe psoriasis. Nails and nail beds are altered in an inflamed-dystrophic manner. Hair loss can occur as can loss of the nails. Daily intake of zinc as zinc sulfate leads to total remission of the disease.

Chronic liver diseases (ICD 571)

Liver insufficiency is based on a more or less severe failure of liver cell function. The level of parenchymal loss and the degree of intrahepatic circulation damage can be determined in general by consequent clinical appearances. Because the liver is the central organ for metabolism, there are multiple severe disturbances in albumin content, hormonal metabolism, water content, and kidney function. Causes, classification, and course of chronic liver diseases will not be considered here.

In HBsAg-positive acute hepatitis and HBeAg-positive chronic hepatitis, there is also the possibility of transmissible infection. Dentists should follow proper infection control procedure when treating these patients.

Liver cirrhosis can sometimes proceed clinically without complaints. When complaints appear, they are noncharacteristic and include symptoms such fatigue, lack of performance, lack of appetite, nausea, inability to tolerate fats, feeling of fullness, itchiness, meteorism, and diarrhea.

In addition to a gynecomastia, this disease often involves skin changes that are in the dentist's purview. The skin vessels show small arterial telangiectases, which are primarily noticeable in the face, neck, chest, and dorsum of the hands as *spider nevus* (ICD 448). These characteristic lesions are also referred to as *liver stars*. In the center is a red pinhead-sized raised area. The lesions correspond to an enlargement of arterioles; from the center there is a centrifugal radiation of many fine blood vessels (Fig. 26-20). Other findings are palmar erythemas, white nails, and changes of the hair. The papillary relief of the tongue is often atrophic; the reddish flat dorsum of the tongue can shine like varnish (Fig. 26-18). The lips too can appear varnished (Fig. 26-22).

Liver disease is accompanied by many hematologic disturbances, in part of complex nature (coagulation problems due to disturbed synthesis of the coagulation factors in the liver, among others). When planninig and performing therapy, the dentist must realize that frequently sudden complications can appear in patients with several liver diseases (Fig. 26-21).

Ulcerative colitis (ICD-DA 555.1 and 555.10)

Ulcerative colitis is a recurring, chronic inflammatory condition of the colon that can appear with different degrees of severity (light, moderate, acute). Typical clinical symptoms are bloody diarrhea, abdominal pain, fever, weight loss, and anemia. Ulcerative colitis starts with a superficial inflammatory infiltration of the intestinal mucosa followed by crypt abscesses and extensive ulcerations.

In the reparative phase there is the development of pseudopolyps, scar shrinkage, and stenosis, which can cause complications. In a very severe course, the oral mucosa can also show inflammatory changes (Fig. 26-24). In a course of long duration and with extensive involvement, carcinomatous changes are possible. The causes are considered to be genetic, immunologic, and alimentary factors, as well as viral and bacterial infections.

Crohn's disease (ICD-DA 550.0 and 555.00)

Crohn's disease is an inflammatory granulomatous disease of unknown etiology that primarily affects the lower ileum but often too the colon and more proximal segments of the intestinal tract. The disease starts insidiously and usually manifests itself in people under 30 years of age. The inflammation, which starts with diarrhea, abdominal pain, and frequently colic as well as fever, affects the whole intestinal wall (transmural) and is usually segmentally limited and associated with changes of the mesenteric lymph vessel system. There is formation of ulcerations, fistulas, and necrosis with consequent formation of scar shrinkage and fibrosis. The disease leads to a malabsorption syndrome and may be a cause of amyloidosis. The histologic picture is made up of noncaseating epithelioid and giant cell type granulomas as well as lymphoplasmacellular infiltrates.

Systemic manifestations, in the form of a polyarthritis, among others, can develop and indicate an autoimmune process. Therapeutic improvement of Crohn's disease with corticosteroid and immunosuppressive agents allows for such an interpretation. While earlier hypotheses on the origin of the disease included genetic and exogenous factors, the discovery that there was decreased activity of the T-lymphocytes (suppressor cells) has led to the current suggestion of an insufficiency of the granulocyte system based on functional disturbances of the neutrophil granulocytes.

The oral mucosa is involved in 10% of cases, and according to the literature, there are some cases in which it was the first site of involvement. After an initial edematous phase is the development of signs of granulomatous inflammation, particularly on the mucosa of the cheeks but also in the vestibular area and mucosa of the lips with and without ulceration (Figs. 25-26 to 25-27). The changes—which are histologically similar to those in the intestine—resemble that of a chronic bite wound or an irritation hyperplasia. The lips can be swollen and thickened, and the appearance of granulomatous cheilitis resembles the lesion of Melkersson-Rosenthal syndrome. An association of both diseases is not impossible according to present knowledge.

Amyloidosis (ICD-DA 277.3 and 277.30)

Amyloidosis represents a group of conditions in which there is accumulation of fibrillar protein as amyloid in the ground substance of the connective tissue. The name amyloid rests on the staining of the pathologic proteinaceous deposits similar to the staining reactions of starch ("amylum"). Protein amyloids are bound to reticular and collagen fibers.

Clinical presentations differ and their severity depends on the organs that are involved and on the amount of amyloid deposited. If there is no demonstrable underlying disease, the condition is termed *primary amyloidosis*. The light chain amyloid deposited in this type of amyloidosis can be generalized or localized. In the generalized form, there are amyloid deposits in the heart, lungs, skin, tongue, gastrointestinal tract, and kidneys, and the tongue is often an early site for manifestation. Limited localizations, for example in only the heart or tongue, are also possible. The tongue acquires a spotty, hard consistency, with frequent swelling and enlargement (Fig. 26-23). As a consequence of macroglossia, there is difficulty in eating, swallowing, and talking.

In discussing treatment of the tongue, the dentist should also think of the possibility of an amyloidosis and request a diagnostic confirmation (via biopsy).

Secondary amyloidosis (inflammation-associated amyloidosis) develops particularly in consequence of chronic inflammatory diseases (e. g., tuberculosis), chronic inflammation of long duration with tissue destruction of different areas (such as polyarthritis, ulcerative colitis, Crohn's disease, and sprue), as well as malignant neoplasms. With the exception of myeloma-associated amyloidosis, which has the same amyloid protein as primary amyloidosis, the secondary forms show a nonimmunoglobulin protein amyloid. The amyloid deposits develop in the reticulum network and basal membrane of the larger parenchymal organs as well as in the arterial vessels and capillaries and can involve all other organs. Usually there are associated abnormalities of the serum gammaglobulins.

Myeloma-associated amyloidosis has the poorest prognosis among these diseases. The prognosis with renal and cardiac participation is poor.

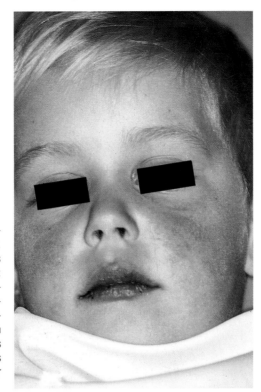

Fig. 26-1   Face of an 8-year-old child with tetralogy of Fallot. This complex heart disease is made up of four symptoms: pulmonary stenosis, high ventricular septal defect, aorta transposed to the right, and hypertrophy of the right ventricle. In children, body development is delayed. Noticeable cyanosis develops a few weeks after birth.

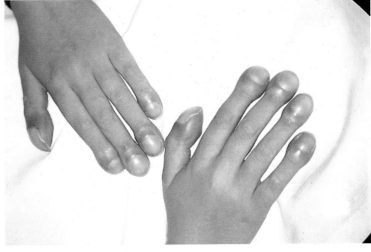

Fig. 26-2   "Drum player fingers" and "hour glass nails" of the patient in Fig. 26-1 at the same examination. The body tries—as in acquired pulmonary diseases (bronchiectasis, lung emphysema)—to compensate for the chronically reduced metabolic oxygen supply of the tissue through hyperplasia of capillary vessels as well as polycythemia.

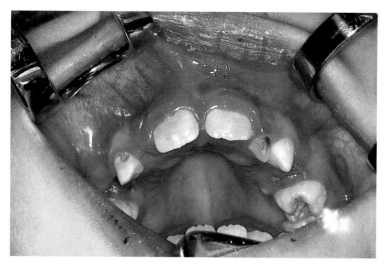

Fig. 26-3   Intraoral findings in the patient in Figs. 26-1 and 26-2 at the same examination. The cyanotic oral mucosa shows a vascular pattern. The gingiva is edematous; the dentition delayed. Lack of oral hygiene leads to smooth surface caries (among others, on tooth 53/C).

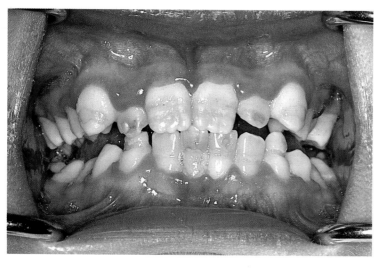

Fig. 26-4   Face and hands of a 10-year-old girl with transposition of the large vessels. In this developmental disease of the heart, the large vessels start in the wrong ventricle; the aorta starts in the venous right chamber of the heart, the pulmonary artery from the arterial left chamber of the heart. There can be a high degree of cyanosis at birth. The children have problems in the first years of life. Note the bluish discoloration of the fingers tips. Notice too the "drum player" fingers. The psychic and bodily development in these children is normal.

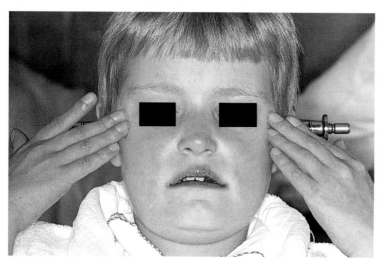

Fig. 26-5   The girl in Fig. 26-4 at same examination. The oral mucosa is cyanotic and the gingiva is edematous and thickened. Around the mandibular anterior teeth are already signs of periodontal damage. The postnatal disturbances in calcium-phosphate metabolism from gastrointestinal and pulmonary infection and their treatment can be seen on the permanent teeth in the form of enamel and dentin abnormalities.

Fig. 26-6 Ischemic necrosis (infarct) on the periosteal fixed oral mucosa. The 63-year-old patient (under medical treatment for several years for arteriosclerosis with hypertension and coronary heart disease) noted suddenly during the night a dull pain in the right side of the mandible and a triangular peculiar discoloration of the edentulous alveolar process the next morning. Shown are the findings 4 days after the episode. A sharply limited wedge of nonpainful necrosis affected the mucosa-periosteum due to arteriovenous obstruction.

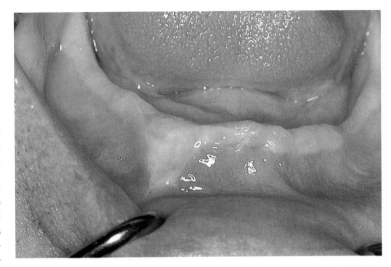

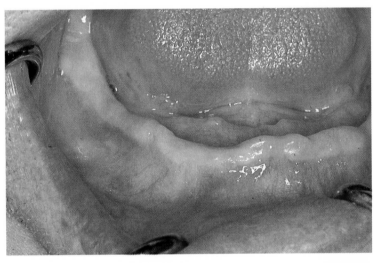

Fig. 26-7 The patient in Fig. 26-7 7 weeks later. As a permanent consequence of the infarct, there was a trough-shaped substance loss on the alveolar ridge. The extremely rare occurrence of an infarct on the oral mucosa can be explained only by a sudden obstruction of an arteriosclerotic vessel with an already pathologically altered collateral circulation.

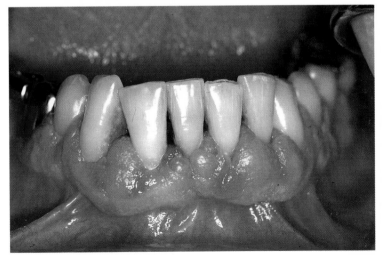

Fig. 26-8 Fibrous gingival hyperplasia as an undesirable side effect of nifedipine. Calcium antagonists are drugs that prevent entrance of calcium into the cells through so-called slow calcium channels. These are channels that open during cell excitation. Therefore, calcium-antagonists are useful in the treatment of high blood pressure and coronary heart disease. After the medication is discontinued, the fibrous gingival hyperplasia will regress.

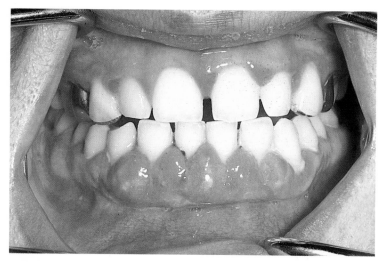

Fig. 26-9   Marginal periodontitis with multiple pocket developments in a 21-year-old insulin-dependent patient (type I diabetes). The poor metabolism (increased glucosuria) increases susceptibility to inflammation and facilitates the development of these findings, which are similar to those of pyoderma. Of major importance for the progression of the inflammation of the dental disease is the quality of oral hygiene.

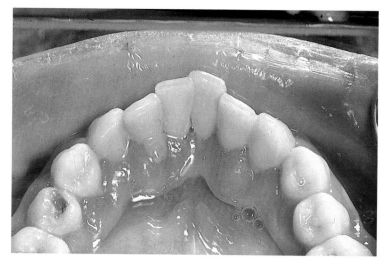

Fig. 26-10   Multiple periodontal abscesses on the lingual side of the mandibular anterior teeth in a 19-year-old insulin-dependent diabetic. The poor oral hygiene (plaque accumulation) and other marginal irritation factors, more than the disease itself, determined the extent and progress of the periodontal damage.

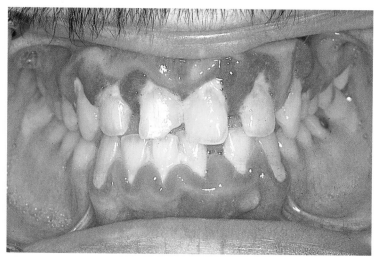

Fig. 26-11   Marginal periodontitis in a 23-year-old insulin-dependent diabetic patient who lacked understanding of the need for cooperation in the treatment of the metabolic disease and in the need for oral hygiene. Quantification of glycosylated hemoglobin HbA1 or HbA1c gives the information on the blood sugar level retrospectively for 6 to 8 weeks and, therefore, of the quality of the metabolism and the compliance of the patient.

Fig. 26-12 Gingival findings in a 45-year-old man with previously undetected type II diabetes. The ulceration near of tooth 32 (10) (which requires extraction) had been present for 8 days and was progressing despite local therapeutic measures. This lesion was the indication for a general medical examination, during which the diabetes was discovered. The severe periodontal damage was the first complaint reported.

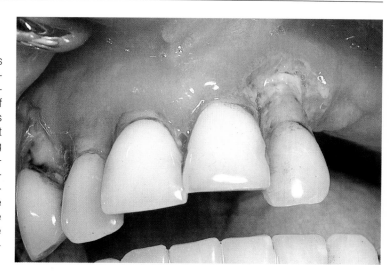

Fig. 26-13 Wound healing disturbance in existence for 3 weeks in a 52-year-old long-term diabetic after surgical removal of palatally impacted tooth 23 (6). In poorly controlled diabetes, wound healing delays are frequent. For this reason, preoperative metabolic normalizing is important. The patient already had complications of late diabetes (hypertension, coronary heart disease, circulatory disturbances in the foot).

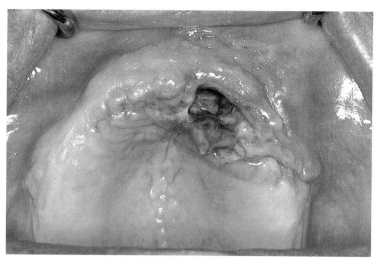

Fig. 26-14 Findings in maturity-onset diabetes. The 63-year-old prematurely aged patient had been referred for suspicion of lip cancer. The lower lip ulceration had been present for several weeks. Examination by the internist disclosed undiagnosed type II diabetes, which had already caused severe blood vessel changes. With treatment for the diabetes, the ulceration healed. Note the border areas of the ulceration, which are partially scarred, partially leukoplakial.

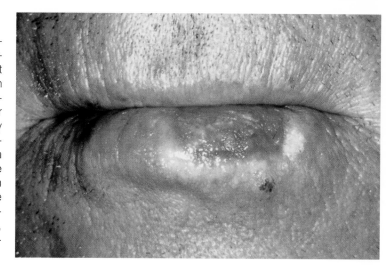

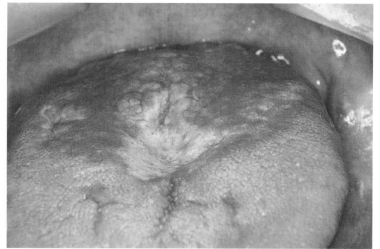

Fig. 26-15   This lesion was incorrectly diagnosed as a sign of gastritis (atrophic glossitis) in a 67-year-old woman. In the dorsal third of the dorsum of the tongue is recognizable "papillary loss," but these areas are not the accompanying symptoms of stomach disease. The changes are due to an erosive atrophic lichen planus. The earlier association of oral mucosa symptoms with gastritis and stomach ulcers is considered obsolete.

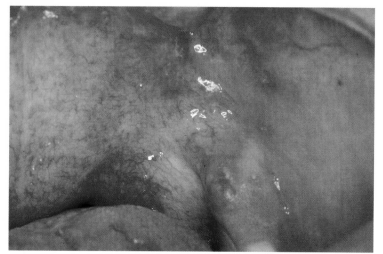

Fig. 26-16   Slowly healing erosions of an atrophic change of the oral mucosa in a 48-year-old alcoholic with chronic pancreatitis and early liver cirrhosis. The atrophic oral mucosa is not able to sustain normal physiologic stress. The increased vulnerability and delayed healing lead to uncharacteristic burning sensations. Tongue and mucosal burning can also be consequences of alcoholic neuropathies.

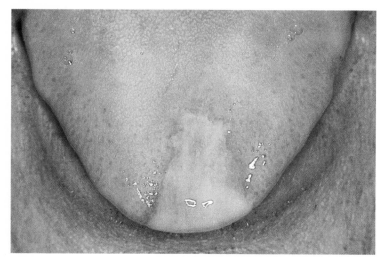

Fig. 26-17   Tongue findings in a 54-year-old alcoholic with deficient nutrition, chronic gastritis, and liver cirrhosis. The tongue surface shows atrophic changes, as do the other mucosal areas. A sheetlike erosion is evident in the area of the tip of the tongue where there was pain for a long time (alcoholic neuropathy).

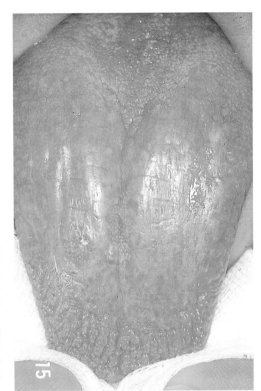

Fig. 26-18   Tongue findings in malabsorption syndrome. The 60-year-old woman had a history of stomach and gallbladder surgery and was under medical treatment for continuous diarrhea. Due to malabsorption, there was a large surface of the tongue with disappearance of the papillae. The tongue shows an atrophic change on a smooth dry surface.

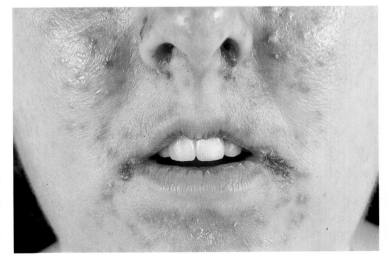

Fig. 26-19   Facial manifestation of acrodermatitis enteropathica with spotty erythema formation. There are pustule formations and rhagades in the corner of the mouth. The cause of the disease is a secondary zinc deficiency due to a genetically determined zinc resorption disturbance.

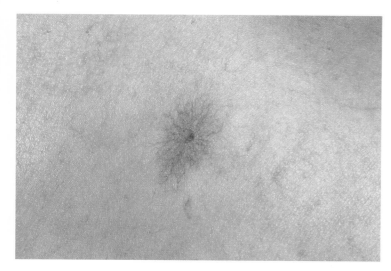

Fig. 26-20   Main finding in the face of patient with liver cirrhosis. In the thin-appearing skin are many fine blood vessel enlargements ("blotting paper skin"). In the center of the picture is a small arterial telangiectasis with the appearance of many small spiderlike vessels. The spider nevi can enlarge and become numerous in liver cirrhosis and chronic hepatitis and are the so-called liver stars.

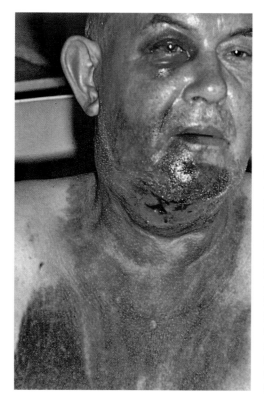

Fig. 26-21   Extensive hematoma in the soft tissues of the face, neck, and chest of a 62-year-old man following a submandibular abscess incision. This complication was caused by a multifactorial disease. The overweight patient had hypertension and severe vascular damage as a consequence of inadequately controlled maturity-onset diabetes. There was also fatty liver and an undiagnosed cirrhotic liver with consequent liver insufficiency and subsequent hemorrhagic diathesis.

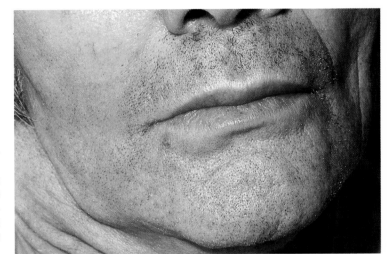

Fig. 26-22 Lip and skin findings in liver cirrhosis. The thin, dirty-looking, yellowish skin shows telangiectases. The "glossy lips" correspond to intraoral findings of a smooth tongue and are an expression of atrophic changes.

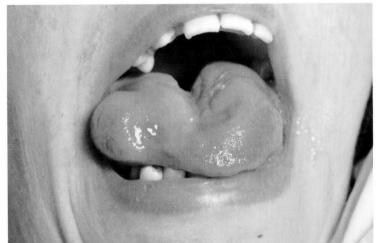

Fig. 26-23 Macroglossia in a 40-year-old woman with primary amyloidosis. Where there is no demonstrable basic disease, amyloidosis can be generalized or localized. In the first case the tongue is frequently an early manifestation site; in the second instance any of a number of organs may be affected. The fatty-looking induration of the tongue due to amyloid deposits appears as a tumorlike growth and complicates eating, talking, and swallowing.

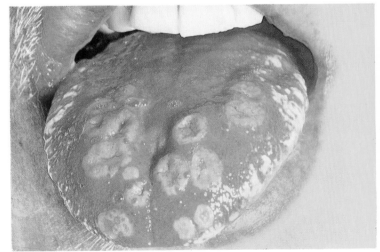

Fig. 26-24 Multiple craterlike ulcerations on the tongue as concomitant symptoms of ulcerative colitis with fatal course in an 18-year-old patient.

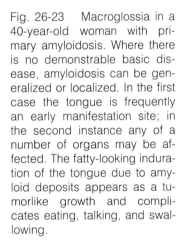

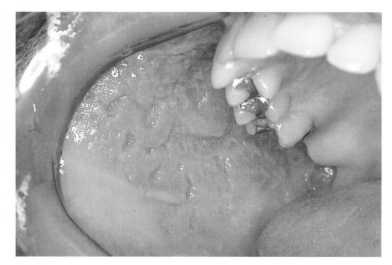

Fig. 26-25 Hyperplastic granulomatous cheek mucosal change in a 28-year-old patient with Crohn's disease. In this chronic recurrent inflammatory, granulomatous intestinal disease, up to 10% of patients show oral manifestations.

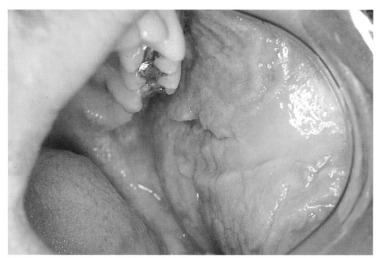

Fig. 26-26 The patient in Fig. 26-25 at the time of examination. On the left cheek mucosa there is also corresponding thickening of the furrow formation. This often leads to a cobblestone appearance. Sometimes there are painful ulcerations. Oral accompanying symptoms are most frequent in the area of the cheek mucosa, vestibulum, and lips.

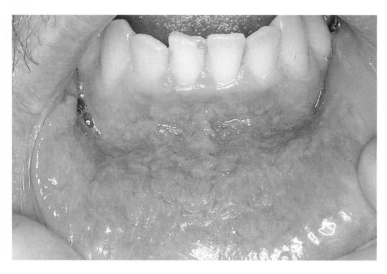

Fig. 26-27 The patient in Figs. 26-25 and 26-26 at examination. The lip mucosa shows hyperplastic folds with pointed extensions and inflamed fissures. The findings resemble bite wounds or irritation hyperplasia. As a consequence of chronic granulomatous cheilitis, the lips can be diffusely enlarged. In these cases, differential diagnosis with cheilitis granulomatosa of the Melkersson-Rosenthal syndrome must be considered. The two diseases may be interrelated.

Chapter 27

Inflammatory Changes of the Gingiva under the Influence of Sex Hormones

Gingivitis associated with puberty

Gingivitis associated with the menstrual cycle

Pregnancy gingivitis

The relation between the body and the oral mucosa is evident not only in systemic disease and correlated disease disturbances of the endocrine system; it also becomes evident in sex hormone-guided physiologic events and changes of the body. The gingiva shows a marked tendency for changes as a reaction to hormonal metabolism.

Clinical manifestations of hormonal influence generally occur in previously damaged gingiva by means of microbial plaque and/or other local irritative factors.

Gingival changes occur during puberty and can be observed both in boys and girls. In women, the oral mucosa is also affected by the menstrual cycle. Most noticeable are the effects of sex hormones on the hyperplastic inflammatory reactions of the gingiva during pregnancy. Estrogen and progesterone are assigned a major role in the as-yet incompletely explained cause of these findings. As a result of these hormones acting on the epithelium of the mucosa for a relatively long period (as during pregnancy), there is a decrease in the level of keratinization. There is increased vulnerability in relation to increased capillary permeability. The demonstrably increased sulcus fluid flow rate is possibly caused by increased permeability of the internal lining epithelium and terminal blood flow to the bordering vessels. The simultaneous increase of fluid and increased proliferation of the connective tissue facilitates the development of hyperplastic gingivitis.

Gingivitis associated with puberty (ICD-DA 523.11)

The dentist occasionally sees children and young patients with a noticeable marginal gingivitis that is considerably "thicker." It is mainly found in the inflamed and easily bleeding tissue of the vestibular anterior areas in the maxilla (Fig. 27-1) and more rarely in the mandible. The changes decrease in intensity toward the distal end on both sides (Fig. 27-2), so that there are normal gingival findings from the second premolar or first molar. The typical form of *juvenile hyperplastic gingivitis–gingival puberty hyperplasia* is found in children with anterior deep overbite whose teeth close together, in children who are mouth breathers, and also in girls and boys with normal anterior teeth and normal breathing through the nose. The extent of inflammatory infiltration and exudation determines the various clinical pictures.

Hyperplastic gingivitis can develop as early as puberty. Its greatest incidence is at the beginning of puberty. It then persists in the developmental years, and later there is a tendency toward spontaneous regression (Fig. 27-3).

Obviously, there is an endogenous reaction in certain children during growth. That is, the child is affected such that the gingiva reacts to slight stimuli (microbial) with increased tissue proliferation. Parents who are concerned with the unsightly oral conditions should be told that hyperplastic changes that start in puberty can regress.

Because puberty gingival hyperplasia as well as pregnancy gingival hyperplasia is primarily due to microbial plaque, therapy consists of removal of local irritative factors and instruction in oral hygiene. After conservative treatment in some cases, there can be surgical removal of the proliferative tissue by gingivectomy/gingivoplasty. By strictly following an intense oral hygiene regimen, recurrences should be eliminated.

Gingivitis associated with the menstrual cycle (ICD-DA 626.88)

The oral mucosa—particularly the gingiva—is affected by the menstrual cycle, and epithelial cell changes can be seen. These rhythmically changing keratinizations and desquamations are related to the cyclic changes in estrogen and progesterone. In some women, particularly young women shortly before the start of menstruation, there is usually an increase in gingival chronic inflammation, which is expressed clinically by painful swelling and reddening of the marginal gingiva and the interdental papillae (Figs. 27-4 and 27-5). These premenstrual-associated tissue reactions, and in rare instances reactions seen during other phases of the female reproductive cycle, usually decrease after menstruation so that only previously existing chronic inflammatory conditions remain. Their regular periodic return confirms the correlation with the menstrual cycle. The cyclic changes can also be observed by associated gingival changes.

Elimination of chronic gingivitis (by removal of all marginal irritations that encourage plaque retention and careful oral hygiene) will remove the cause of those cyclically conditioned inflammatory gingival reactions.

Pregnancy gingivitis (ICD-DA 646.80)

Pregnant women often show subacute oozing catarrhal inflammations, and less frequently ulcerative gingivitis. These conditions respond only partially to usual treatment procedures and often show an increase in intensity with increased exudation and bleeding tendency. In many cases this is only an exacerbation of a chronic gingivitis or marginal periodontitis that was present before pregnancy.

On average, every fifth to seventh pregnant woman—particularly younger ones—will have more or less characteristic inflammatory-hyperplastic gingival changes (so-called hyperplastic pregnancy gingivitis, gingival pregnancy hyperplasia). The massive, clinically impressive, usually soft tissue proliferation, which is red to dark red, is associated with overgrown granulation tissue rich in blood vessels. During the third month of pregnancy (sometimes also earlier) the lesion starts from the interdental papillae (Figs. 27-6 to 27-8) with rapid growth and reaches its largest size usually in the eighth month of pregnancy (Figs. 27-9, 27-10, and 27-12). The richness of blood vessels explains the increased tendency for bleeding with small traumatic irritations, which also increases because of the increased size of the tissue.

The inflamed gingival hyperplasia appears in generalized and sometimes localized form during the pregnancy. Preferential location is the maxillary anterior vestibule (Figs. 27-14 to 27-16). The interpapillary tissue sometimes enlarges to resemble a solitary epulis and is made up of soft tissue. Development usually occurs during the second trimester of pregnancy and then grows relatively rapidly. On the surface there are often small fibrin-covered ulcerations with a tendency to bleed.

The unfortunate terms "pregnancy tumor" and *"pregnancy granuloma"* (ICD-DA 646.81) have been given to these findings, which are similar in their clinical appearance to a granulomatous epulis (see chapter 14) or a telangiectatic granuloma (Fig. 27-11; see also chapter 22). It must be remembered that an epulis can also be present before pregnancy and can in increase in size during pregnancy. Endogenous and exogenous factors play a role with the development of inflammatory-hyperplastic gingival changes during pregnancy. Under endogenous determining causes fall flooding of the mother with steroid hormones produced by the placenta (estrogen, progesterone) and human chorionic gonadotropin (HCG; see diagram on page 585). Regarding the influence of female sex hormones and their metabolic products as cofactors, generalized as well as localized forms of gingival hyperplasia generally have a reversible course. Signs of reduced inflammation occur in the ninth month of pregnancy. Postpartum, there is further spontaneous reduction of the inflammatory hyperplasia (Fig. 27-13). If the remaining chronic gingivitis is untreated, recurrence is almost certain in a following pregnancy.

All pre-existing factors that facilitate the development of gingivitis are basically exogenous factors. The frequent appearance of pregnancy gingival hyperplasia in closed bite and in vertical overlap indicates that local chronic traumatic irritations also participate in the cause. Dental therapy must take the general conditions into consideration and must concentrate primarily on removal of local irritative factors. Other measures should eliminate the acute inflammatory component.

Because of the reduced salivary flow during pregnancy and the change in pH toward the acid, it is particularly important that pregnant women be instructed in intensive oral hygiene (especially plaque control). Surgical intervention is indicated only in exceptional cases and then only when chewing ability is affected because of the tissue growth or if there is major and frequent bleeding.

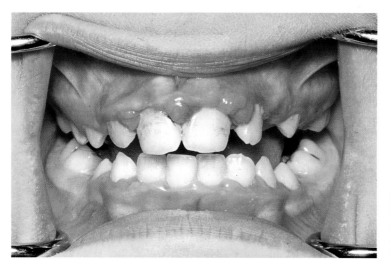

Fig. 27-1 Hyperplastic puberty gingivitis in a 10-year-old boy. The maxillary vestibular anterior area is preferentially affected.

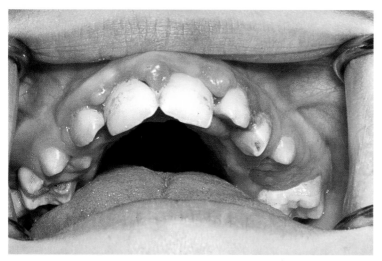

Fig. 27-2 The boy in Fig. 27-1 at same examination. With hyperplastic puberty gingivitis, the symptoms typically decrease bilaterally toward the posterior region.

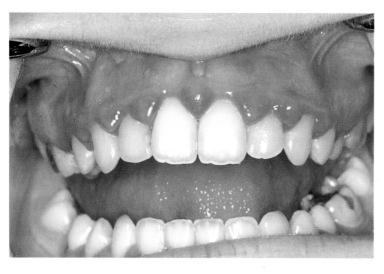

Fig. 27-3 Partially recurring hyperplastic gingivitis in a 20-year-old woman (appearance of gingival hyperplasia after puberty).

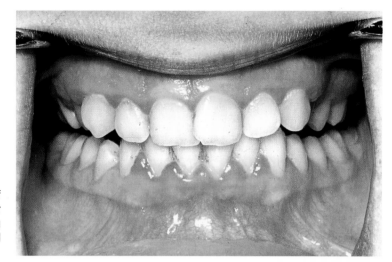

Fig. 27-4 Exacerbation of chronic gingivitis in the anterior area of the mandible recurring cyclically in the premenstrual phase in a 24-year-old woman.

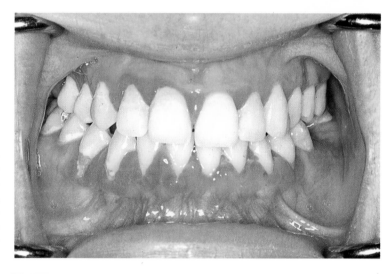

Fig. 27-5 Cyclic recurring exacerbation related to premenstrual phase of chronic gingivitis in a 32-year-old woman. Note the consequences of inadequate oral hygiene, particularly on the right side (right-handed patient).

Plasma concentration of estrogens during pregnancy. Östron = Estrone; Östradiol = Estradiol; Östriol = Estriol. (Adapted from: Gerhard I, Runnebaum B. Endokrinologie der Schwangerschaft. In: Runnebaum B, Rabe T (eds). Gynäkologische Endokrinologie. Berlin: Springer (after American sources), 1987:497.)

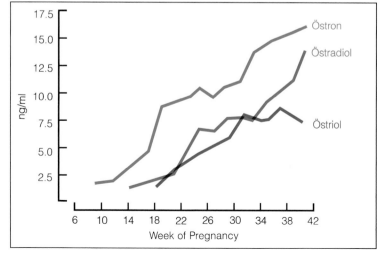

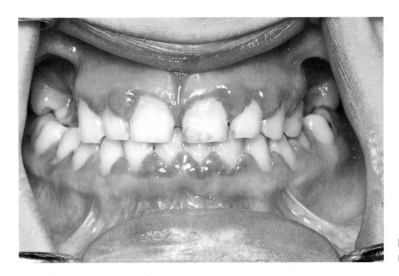

Fig. 27-6   Hyperplastic pregnancy gingivitis.

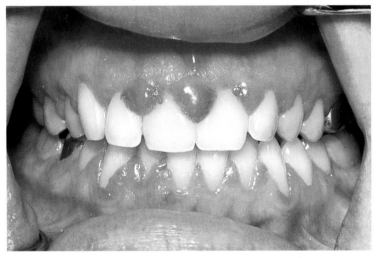

Fig. 27-7   Hyperplastic pregnancy gingivitis. Particularly in the area of the maxillary incisors, the interdental papillae are increasingly red and swollen and have a tendency to bleed.

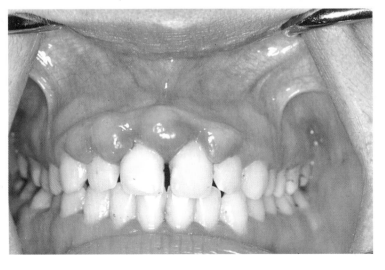

Fig. 27-8   Hyperplastic pregnancy gingivitis. Massive size increase of the interdental papillae in the anterior maxillary vestibule.

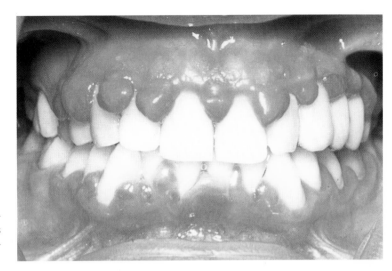

Fig. 27-9   Pronounced hyperplastic pregnancy gingivitis with marked inflamed interdental papillae.

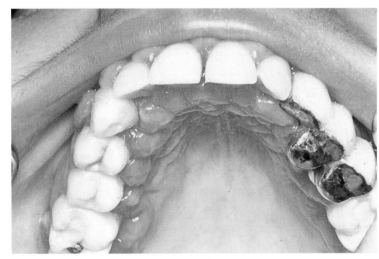

Fig. 27-10   The patient in Fig. 27-9 at the same examination. Note the pronounced gingival hyperplasia in the palatal area. Painful ulcerations and a considerable tendency to bleed led to impaired ingestion and caused the patient to neglect her oral hygiene.

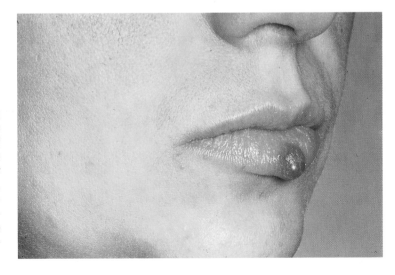

Fig. 27-11   The patient in Figs. 27-9 and 27-10 at same examination. At the bottom of an inflamed fissure was also the development (over a few weeks) of a slightly bleeding, superficially ulcerated soft formation on the lower lip. Histologic examination confirmed the clinical suspicion of telangiectatic granuloma.

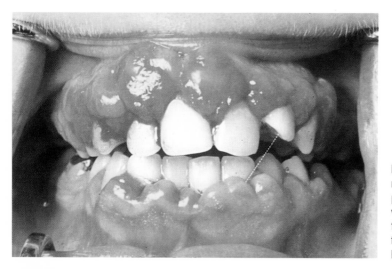

Fig. 27-12   Excessive pregnancy gingival hyperplasia, predominantly on the maxilla with extensive inflammatory infiltration and exudation. Note the tendency to spontaneous bleeding.

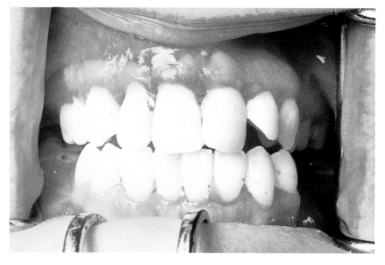

Fig. 27-13   The patient in Fig. 27-12, 3 months after delivery. The high level of inflammatory hyperplasia regressed spontaneously into a recurring chronic gingivitis that had been present before pregnancy.

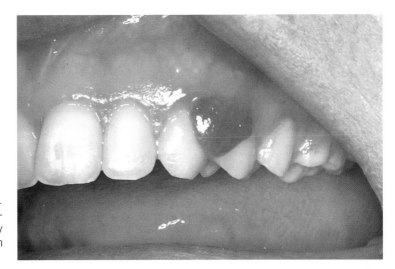

Fig. 27-14   Pregnancy epulis. The appearance of a granulomatous epulis was noticed by the patient only during the fifth month of pregnancy.

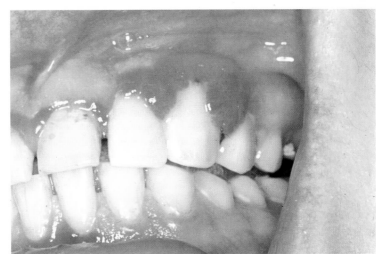

Fig. 27-15   Pregnancy epulis. The anterior maxillary region is the preferential zone for bleeding tendency of solitary soft tissue lesions.

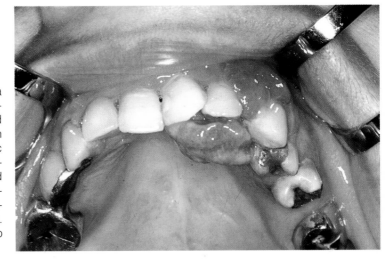

Fig. 27-16   Recurrence of a pregnancy epulis that was removed because of repeated bleeding–condition in the ninth month of gestation. Histologic examination of the dumbbell-shaped hyperplasia showed granulation tissue with extremely high vascularization resembling a capillary hemangioma. These findings correspond to telangiectatic granuloma.

Chapter 28

Oral and Perioral Manifestations of Some Dermatoses and Genodermatoses

---

Dermatoses
  Erythema multiforme
  Psoriasis

Genodermatoses
  Inherited keratoses
    Ichthyosis congenita
    Hyperkeratosis palmoplantaris, congenital type
  Epidermolysis bullous
    Epidermolysis bullosa hereditaria simplex
    Epidermolysis bullosa hereditaria dystrophica (Hallopeau-Siemens syndrome)

Dermatosis is the general term for skin diseases of any type. As has been described in other chapters, dermatoses are not limited to organs of the skin but can involve the mucous membranes. Even isolated involvement of the oral mucosa without simultaneous changes of the skin is possible.

The dentist must have certain basic knowledge about skin efflorescences to correctly interpret oral findings as partial manifestations of a dermatosis and thus be able to categorize it diagnostically. On the other hand, the dermatologist needs, as do other representatives of medical disciplines who value the oral cavity as a window to diagnosis, time and experience to understand the details of changes in the oral mucosa.

Because of its frequent appearance on the oral mucosa and its significance in the differential diagnosis of leukoplakias, lichen planus is described separately as an inflammatory dermatosis in chapter 16. In this chapter, with no claim to completeness, we differentiate from the group of (inflammatory) skin diseases an erythematous dermatosis (erythema multiforme) and a erythematous squamous dermatosis (psoriasis), which have very different frequencies of occurrence in the oral mucosa. Further, four genetically determined dermatoses (genodermatoses) will be presented that are of interest to dentists.

Dermatoses

The etiopathogenesis of most dermatoses is at present not completely clear. Knowledge of their causes could be considerably enlarged, which would help in simplifying of their nomenclature.

As medical empiricism proves, there are dermatoses with particular affinity for the oral mucosa (among others, lichen planus—see chapter 16; pemphigus vulgaris—see chapter 29; and erythema multiforme) and those in which oral manifestations are rare or appear only under exceptional circumstances (among others, dermatitis herpetiformis —see chapter 29; psoriasis).

Erythema multiforme, Stevens-Johnson syndrome (ICD-DA 695.1 and 695.10)

Erythema multiforme is at present unanimously considered an allergic reaction of polyetiologic basis. The acute initial dermatosis in its clinical appearance ("multiforme") and the severity of the disease course exhibit great variation, as do the different resultant disease forms. They are variant expressions of the same entity, from which one can easily differentiate *minor forms* from severe (major) ones. Predominantly affected are young people in their second or third decade of life, and men more frequently than women.

Pathogenetically, erythema multiforme consists of an allergic reaction that mostly takes place in the dermoepidermal and mucosal regions and corresponds to type III (immune complex reaction) according to the scheme of Coombs and Gell. In principle, however, with all allergic reactions it is difficult to apply the Coombs and Gell classification. Erythema multiforme is causally associated with infections and certain medications.

The infectious allergic forms are usually observed after previous infections from a virus of the herpes group—particularly herpes simplex *(postherpetic erythema multiforme*, Figs. 28-7 to 28-9). Within an interval of up to 2 weeks, there is the appearance of the dermatosis. Recurrences usually appear in spring and fall *(type annuus)*. The erythema multiforme that often develops at the conclusion of a bacterial infection, usually after a *Streptococcus* infection of the upper respiratory tract, frequently leads to the appearance of rheumatism *(type rheumaticus*, Fig. 28-11). Infection-related and drug-related forms were referred to earlier as Stevens-Johnson syndrome. They correspond to the major type of the disease. Sulfonamide, but also hydantoin pyrazolone derivatives, barbiturates, phenylbutazone, penicillin (Figs. 28-12 to 28-16), carbamazepine, and others should be considered as triggering medications.

The primary efflorescences of erythema multiforme are sharply circumscribed, light red, erythematous lesions ranging from the size of a lentil to that of a quarter. Because of the exudate, the lesion resembles an urticarial wheal (elevated erythema) from which the infection enlarges. This is followed by a cyanotic color change in the center. It is surrounded by a brown-red to dark-red intermediate zone, which blends peripherally into a light-red inflamed border. The efflorescence combination corresponds, at this point, to a mixed maculopapule in a concentric order. This targetlike form (Fig. 28-1) is typical of classic erythema multiforme of the skin. In addition, a centrally located blood-filled blister may develop.

In the case of the *minor form*, most often only a few foci are found scattered, grouped, or even confluent. The back and palm of the hand are the predominant locations of this manifestation. Lips and oral mucosa (most often the anterior part of the oral cavity) can also be affected. This disease, which runs an episodic course and often displays relapse, generally has a good prognosis with appropriate therapy. Healing follows most often in 2 or 3 weeks (Fig. 28-6).

The serious forms (major type) begin like the less serious forms. The more obvious exudative behavior appears in a rashlike spreading of skin efflorescences (Fig. 28-12) with rapid and extensive blistering similar to bullous dermatitis. Within 10 to 14 days, a sepsislike clinical picture appears with high fever, headache, and fatigue as well as possible bronchopulmonary and nephritic complications.

As the synonym *"ectodermous erosive pluriorificial"* implies, in all serious cases the mucous membrane of the orifices are also affected; the oral mucosa obligatorily, and the eyes and the nasal mucosa quite regularly, as well as the mucous membrane in the genitoanal region in half of all cases.

The major type of erythema multiforme has a special tendency to involve the oral mucosa, and the mucosal blisters—probably as a result of the marked exudative component—are prone to early bursting (Fig. 28-2) and subsequent bleeding. These blisters have only a short life (Fig. 28-3). They burst quickly and leave large, often confluent erosions or flat fibrin-covered ulcerations (Figs. 28-3 to 28-5, 28-7 to 28-16). In the lip seam region are hemorrhagic desquamative crusts of characteristic appearance (Figs. 28-4, 28-10, and 28-15). The stomatitis-like clinical picture (for this reason also the earlier term *"dermatostomatitis"*) is accompanied by unpleasant breath, increased saliva flow, and a lymphadenitis of the regional lymph nodes. Speaking and eating are often impaired because of the painful lesions.

The prognosis of the serious variant, which involves other organs for 5 to 6 weeks, is burdened by a mortality rate of approximately 10% even with modern therapy. For this reason, all serious cases require immediate hospitalization by a specialist.

Toxic epidermal necrolysis, which has flat blister formations and appears clinically as a large burn ("scalded skin"), is considered an extreme variation of erythema multiforme. Pathogenetically, the toxic epidermal necrolysis is considered to be a toxic-allergic combination of infection and an undesirable effect of medication. Further, there is the *Staphylococcus*-induced toxic epidermal necrolysis in newborns and children *(staphylococcal scaled skin syndrome)*.

In the case of involvement limited to the oral mucosa, the differential diagnosis of the erythema multiforme should include bullous dermatoses as well as bullous reaction to medication (see chapters 29 and 31). Even virally caused diseases must be ruled out. The secondary efflorescences in the form of fibrin-covered erosions or flat ulcerations must not be confused with a primary ulcerative stomatitits.

In minor forms, symptomatic therapy consists of the use of corticosteroid-containing ointments. In the case of severe symptoms, additional anesthetic preparations can be prescribed. Proper oral hygiene is especially important.

In the case of symptoms caused by suspected allergies to medications, all questionable substances must be strictly avoided. If antibiotic coverage is necessary, penicillin or ampicillin should not be used —only a broad-spectrum antibiotic—because the aforementioned pharmaceuticals are potential triggering factors. For all major forms, the advice of the dermatologist, who can also arrange for hospitalization, should be sought. Treatment consists of a large dose of systemic steroids and a precautionary covering against secondary bacterial infection using a broad-spectrum antibiotic, with compensatory electrolyte and water balance as well as support for the heart and circulatory systems.

Psoriasis (ICD-DA 696.1 and 696.10)

Aside from eczema, psoriasis is the most frequently occurring skin disease. It is characterized by inflamed redness and flaking *(erythematous squamous dermatosis)*. The morbidity rate is considered to be 1% to 2% of the population. Among dermatologists, 6% to 8% are specialists in psoriasis. The epidermal metabolic disturbances are based on a genetically determined predisposition to the disease in which the exogenous and endogenous factors are arranged in decreasing order. If a parent is affected, every fourth descendant will inherit psoriasis; if both parents are affected, 60% to 70% of the descendants will be affected.

Aside from the genetically based predisposition, the clinical manifestation of psoriasis is multifactorially triggered. Exogenous noxious agents (physical, chemical, contact allergies) and endogenous influences (infectious diseases, medications, hormonal changes, stress, and others) are blamed. The causes of the increased epidermal cell proliferation and the disturbance of the cell differentiation are still largely unexplained. The pathologic event within a lesion of psoriasis is clear; the volume of epidermis is increased from four to six times over the normal because the cell cycle (the time from one cell division to the next) is reduced from a normal 460 hours to 38 hours, which corresponds to a reduction of epidermal turnover from a normal 28 days to 3 to 4 days.

There are three stages of development in psoriasis: *(1)* latent psoriasis (genotypic), with a disposition for the disease but without clinical appearance; *(2)* subclinical psoriasis (genophenotypic), in which the diagnosis can be made with methods of experimental dermatology despite a lack of clinical findings; and *(3)* manifest psoriasis (phenotypical). The first manifestations of psoriasis are possible at any age but are most frequently noticed in the second or third decade of life.

The initial efflorescence of psoriasis is relatively uniform, but there are differences in size, configuration, and localization of the foci. Initially there is formation of a small, inflamed red spot with distinct borders, followed by a flat spot partly covered by a lidlike flake. The clinical diagnosis results from the so-called three psoriasis phenomena:

- "Candle spot" phenomenon (with careful scratching, the flake becomes whiter and clearer; because of the partial straightening of the hornified lamella, the light is more strongly reflected)
- "Last skin" phenomenon (after the relatively easy removal of flakes, the freed red papule is covered only by a damp, shiny layer of epithelium)
- "Bloody opening" phenomenon (after removal of the last layer of skin, a drop of blood protrudes from the open vessels of the dermal papillae)

Similar to that of lichen planus, production of the scaly lesion caused by *isomorphic sensitivity effect (Kobner phenomenon)* is possible. In patients with clinical manifestation of psoriasis, it is possible by local stimulation (in the easiest case by rubbing and scratching, experimentally by ripping off the horny layer with the help of tape) to produce a psoriatiform plaque in the irritated area. The typical efflorescence usually occurs after 10 to 14 days in the case of psoriasis, within a shorter period for lichen planus.

Psoriasis can take an acute or subacute course, with eruptive exanthematic clinical picture, or it can behave chronically. The spectrum of the clinical findings ranges from discrete changes to generalized skin involvement, possibly with the involvement of other organs.

Psoriasis can occur anywhere on the skin. Areas of predilection are physiologically and mechanically stimulated areas, such as the elbows and knee caps, but also the scalp, including the forehead and temples, which is observable by the dentist. Above all, the flaky papules can rest in bandlike layers along the hairline of the forehead (Fig. 28-17). Psoriatic changes of the vermilion of the lips are rare, and lesions of the oral mucosa (cheek, tongue, palate) are extremely rare and only to be expected in cases of generalized exudative extensive disease *(psoriasis pustulosa; Zumbuch type).* In these cases, foci can be observed, ranging in color from white to gray, that are well circumscribed with a central erosion (Fig. 28-18) as secondary efflorescences of short-lived pustules in the mouth.

Thirty percent to 50% of all patients with psoriasis show changes in the finger and toenails, which manifest themselves in the form of spotted nails or transparent subungual flaky papules ("oil spots"). Of special clinical significance is that the skin disease is associated in 5% to 7% of cases with serious changes of the joints *(psoriasis arthropathica)*, which can precede the skin symptoms and be extremely painful. The pathogenetic association of skin and joint changes is not adequately explained. Predominately affected are the small joints (fingers, toes). Involvement of the temporomandibular joint is also possible with serious osteolytic deformities, and in some cases, with periarticular soft tissue inflammation. Differentiation from primary chronic polyarthritis (PCP) can be difficult.

Therapy of psoriasis requires the control of the dermatologist. Local treatment is to be considered within the framework of systemic treatment. Lifelong control of psoriasis presents a difficult therapeutic problem, because even psychosomatic factors must be considered. An important point is avoidance of provoking factors of any type. Recurrence of psoriasis is unfortunately the rule; long-term healing cannot be achieved because of the inherited predisposition, which cannot be influenced. Prognosis is guarded only in the exudative more severe variants with tendency to generalization and in the special arthropathic forms.

Genodermatoses

It is proven that characteristics and predispositions can be inherited. It is also known that certain anomalies (e. g., true mandibular prognathism and complete vertical overlap), disposition to diseases (e. g., diabetes mellitus type I, atopy, and psoriasis), and diseases themselves (e. g., hemophilia) are gentically determined with regular occurrence in certain families and kinships. Clinical research on monozygotic and dizygotic twins has contributed significantly to the broadening of our knowledge.

Because of the achievements of modern genetics and molecular biology, not only is there a reliable explanation of hereditary diseases in humans, but also, in a steadily increasing number of monogenic diseases, information of the type and localization of the relevant gene defect on the corresponding chromosome is possible. On this basis, human genetics has developed into a recognized field of practical clinical medicine (genetic counseling of couples, prenatal diagnosis).

There are numerous and very different inherited diseases of the skin. Genodermatoses are designated inherited skin diseases with Mendelian inheritance, and keratoses and epidermolyses (bullous genodermatosis) are especially significant. This section provides interesting examples for the dentist from both groups.

Inherited keratoses

Among the inherited keratoses there are special forms, such as ichthyosis, the palmar-plantar keratosis including the Papillon-Lefèvre syndrome, and dyskeratosis follicularis (Darier morbus).

Ichthyosis congenita (ICD-DA 757.1 and 757.10)

Two types of ichthyosis (with further subordinate forms) are differentiated: ichthyosis vulgaris and ichthyosis congenita. In *ichthyosis vulgaris*, there is a generalized disturbance of keratinization through a *retention hyperkeratosis* (increased adhesion of the keratinized lamellae and therefore delayed shedding), which is inherited as an irregular autosomal-dominant condition.

In the course of the first years of life, firm, dry, flakelike deposits of varying degree of severity appear, which in extreme cases give the patient a reptilianlike appearance. The illness is progressive until puberty, after which it often shows a tendency toward regression.

The outward surfaces of the extremities are the preferred affected areas. The bend of the joints, the palms of the hands and soles of the feet, as well as the mucous membrane remain unaffected. Because of the decreased resistance of the keratin layer (altered by the disease), these patients frequently suffer from associated dermatitis.

A special form of the disease is X-chromosome dominant inherited ichthyosis. It originates in a genetic defect of the steroid sulfatase. A change in the surface lipids is the basis for the disturbance of keratinization of the skin.

The relatively infrequently occurring *ichthyosis congenita* with an autosomal-recessive pattern of inheritance is a *proliferation hyperkeratosis* (disturbed equilibrium between abnormal keratinization and exfoliation). The disease can occur clinically with varying degrees of intensity (ichthyosis congenita gravis, ichthyosis congenita mitis et tarda, ichthyosis congenita larvata). The most serious form, which involves prenatal formation of hornified armor, is not viable or barely viable (resulting in intrauterine death, prematurity). Milder courses are observed in all stages up to an almost normal skin type.

In contrast to ichthyosis vulgaris, the face (Fig. 28-19), joint bends, palms and soles, and mucous membrane are affected. Intraorally, cheeks and tongue are preferentially affected with leukoplakial deposits ranging from thick to discrete changes. In severely involved patients with dry, wrinkled skin and fishlike scales (Fig. 28-20), the oral cavity may show a considerable decrease in function, fragility of the epithelium, and formation of rhagades. The unavoidable complications for oral hygiene further predispose damage to the dentition. The genodermatoses can be associated with other symptoms (heart defects, defects of intelligence, epileptic seizures, dysgnathias, tooth aplasia).

Hyperkeratosis palmoplantaris, congenital type (ICD-DA 757.35)

Hyperkeratosis palmoplantaris (Papillon-Lefèvre type) belongs to the rare palmoplantar keratoses. These conditions form a group of inherited diseases that involve different degrees of hyperkeratosis on the inner surface of the hand and soles of the feet, and which differ from one another by mode of inheritance, clinical picture, and associated pathologic findings (see summary on page 612).

An independent disease is the autosomal-recessive inherited Papillon-Lefèvre syndrome in which simultaneous and obligatory serious damage to periodontal fibrous structures is the principal diagnostic sign. Further, the clinical picture is accompanied by excessive sweat secretion (hyperhidrosis), which can appear in combination with physical underdevelopment.

Palmoplantar hyperkeratosis usually appears between the first and third year of life. However, it does not always remain limited to palmoplantar areas but can spread to the dorsal surface (transgression; Figs. 28-21 and 28-22). Isolated lesions also occur in the joints (elbows, knees, ankles). Histologically, the findings correspond to hyperkeratosis and acanthosis.

Concurrent with the disrupted keratinization are serious inflammatory changes that develop in periodontal tissue shortly after eruption of the primary teeth. The clinical findings show an acute inflammation of the interdental papillae and marginal gingiva. Periodontal pockets then develop, from which pus leaks upon pressure. In a relatively short time, a *deep marginal periodontitis* develops that leads to premature tooth mobility, migration and tipping of the teeth, and finally to spontaneous tooth loss. Depending on the seriousness of the syndrome, the primary teeth exfoliate according to their order of eruption by the fourth or fifth year.

During the edentulous interval, between the loss of the primary teeth and the eruption of the first permanent teeth, the alveolar mucosa is unaffected. After eruption of the permanent teeth, there is a repetition of the destructive periodontal process (Fig. 28-23) so that the permanent teeth also exfoliate in order of eruption by the thirteenth to fifteenth year of life. The third molars are saved or can at least be maintained for a longer time. In accord with the clinical findings, radiographs show an advanced osteolysis of the alveolar and interdental bony structure (Fig. 28-24).

There is mutual dependence between the intensity of the keratosis and the acute inflammatory process of the gingiva and periodontal tissues. After loss of the last teeth, the hyperkeratosis on the palm and sole surfaces can regress somewhat.

The primary cause of this rapidly progressing juvenile deep marginal periodontitis presumably is the pre-existing inherited epithelial insufficiency of the gingivodental junction. Dental therapy (intensive local treatment, professional prophylaxis simultaneous with good plaque control on the part of the patient) can at best delay the course of periodontal destruction. According to present literature, hyperkeratosis and marginal periodontitis should respond to therapy with retinoid.

The group of hereditary keratoses includes *dyskeratosis follicularis (Darier's disease*; ICD-DA 757.32). This rare keratinization disturbance inherited as an irregular autosomal-dominant disease is not limited to hair follicles; it is also observed on follicle-free skin and the surface of the oral mucosa in a chronologically progressive course. It consists of itching keratotic papules that are usually symmetric. These papules can be as large as lentils and covered by a squamous crust ("thumbtack phenomenon"). Preferentially affected are the cutaneous areas of the head, which are rich in sebaceous glands (seborrheal location), the area next to the hair in the region of the forehead, nasolabial folds, and the retroauricular and temporal regions. The papules can easily degenerate into secondarily infected and intertriginous areas because of sweat secretion.

The impression of dirty, rough skin becomes evident with the increasing number and confluence of the single efflorescences. Clinical diagnosis is made through the demonstration of the interruption of the skin lines (papillary lines) on the inside of the hands and feet, which is typical of this disorder.

On the oral mucosa are sometimes lentil-sized hyperkeratoses appearing as a leukoplakia (see chapter 17).

Epidermolysis bullosa (ICD-DA 757.34)

Several diseases with varying inheritance patterns are included under epidermolysis bullosa, in which blisters develop on the skin and oral mucosa after insignificant mechanical stress. They can heal without a trace *(not dystrophic)* or with residual scarring *(dystrophic)*. This depends on the structures that are affected in the epidermis, basal membrane, or in the corium, and on the severity of lesions. In addition, there are dysplastic and bullous-keratotic forms, which will not be discussed here.

Epidermolysis bullosa hereditaria simplex

This relatively mild nondystrophic epidermolysis is the most frequently occurring disease (1 of every 50,000 viable births) of the genodermatosis bullosa. The dominant inherited disease shows lack of resistance to stress in the skin, which manifests with clefting above the basal layer with the formation of intraepithelial blisters. The blisters occur hours after mild trauma, show hemorrhagic changes, break, and then quickly heal. At the same time, intraepithelial blood blisters can be observed, even in the oral mucosa (Figs. 28-25 and 28-26), as can erosions that heal without leaving scars, just as occurs on the skin. The vulnerability of the mucosa almost regularly leads to secondary injury to the dentition (Figs. 28-25 and 28-26). Relapse can occur at any time; in many cases, improvement comes with aging.

Epidermolysis bullosa hereditaria dystrophica (Hallopeau-Siemens syndrome)

Epidermolysis bullosa hereditaria dystrophica runs a different, more severe course than the previously described clinical picture, always with atrophic-dystrophic sequelae. It is inherited as an autosomal-dominant disease and starts at an early age (the dystrophic *Herlitz* type is always fatal).

In all areas of the body exposed to pressure (fingers–Fig. 28-28 –toes, knees, elbows, buttocks) is the development of a subepidermal blister after minimal mechanical pressure. The blisters heal slowly. After repeated episodes at the same locations, long-term effects such as atrophy, sclerosis, pigment alteration, keloids, and contractures can develop (Fig. 28-28).

In approximately 20% of cases, the oral mucosa is affected, with the tongue (Fig. 28-27), cheeks (Fig. 28-29), and palate as favored locations. Forceful suction, or the use of a toothbrush, can trigger large blisters, which appear clinically a few hours after stimulus and often are hemorrhagic. They are–as are all blisters in the oral cavity–only of short duration and quickly change into erosions or ulcerations (Fig. 28-29). Slow healing is followed by atrophic-dystrophic changes in the oral mucosa. This leads to premature loss of papillary relief on the dorsum of the tongue (Fig. 28-27) and in the long run causes narrowing of the oral cavity (scarring, shallowing of the vestibule, decreased range of motion of the tongue, microstomia, jaw spasms secondary to scarring of the mucosa).

The genetically conditioned cause is a defect of anchoring fibrils (i. e., type VII collagen) in the area of the dermoepidermal interface of the skin, and particularly in the epithelial-connective interface of the mucous membrane.

The role of the dentist for severely impaired patients consists of giving advice about effective nutrition as well as providing motivation for nontraumatic but effective methods of oral hygiene, possibly by incorporation of chemical plaque inhibitors such as chlorhexidine-digluconate.

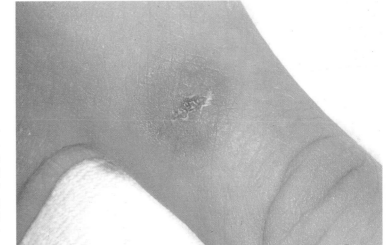

Fig. 28-1 Erythema multiforme. Typical targetlike efflorescence on the thumb. The layered concentric pattern of the individual maculopapular lesion arises from the differing intensity of the erythema that surrounds the central hemorrhage or blister.

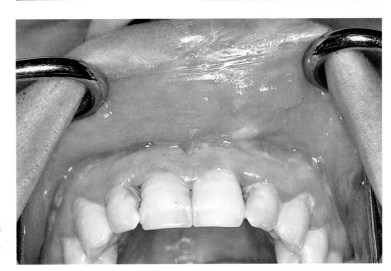

Fig. 28-2 Erythema multiforme. Stage of confluence of blisters on the mucous membrane of the upper lip.

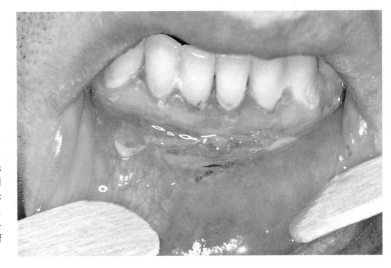

Fig. 28-3 The patient in Fig. 28-2 at the same examination. In the region of the mucous membrane of the lower lip and the vestibular fold, hemorrhagic blisters have already burst. Note the fresh erosion with remaining pieces from the top of the blister on the border.

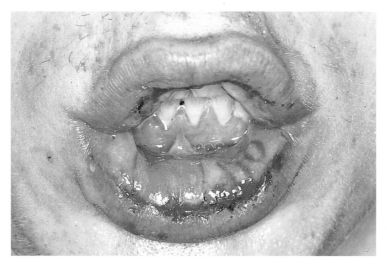

Fig. 28-4   Erythema multiforme. Targetlike mucous membrane efflorescences on the left
side of the lower lip. On the
right side there are more flat fibrin-covered erosions. In the
transition zone from the vermilion of the lips there are blood
crusts. The gingiva often remains unaffected by the changes.

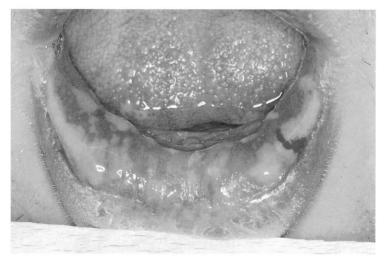

Fig. 28-5   Erythema multiforme. Extensive, painful erosions with fibrinous pseudomembranes on the entire
mucosal surface of the lower
lip.

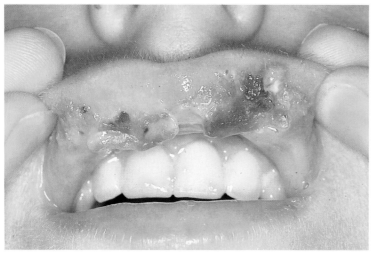

Fig. 28-6   Healing stage of
erythema multiforme on the
upper lip after an illness of
4 weeks.

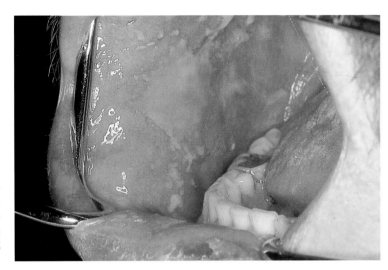

Fig. 28-7 Postherpetic ery-thema multiforme (Stevens-Johnson syndrome) with fibrin-covered erosions of varying sizes in the region of the cheek mucosa.

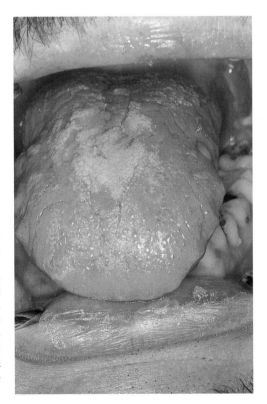

Fig. 28-8 The patient in Fig. 28-7 at the same examination. Peculiar appearance due to lo-cation of efflorescences on the dorsum of the tongue. More foci are identifiable on the bot-tom of the lip. The changes in the oral mucosa, which appear-ed 14 days earlier, developed 1 week after the eruption of a recurring herpes simplex infec-tion (allergic origin).

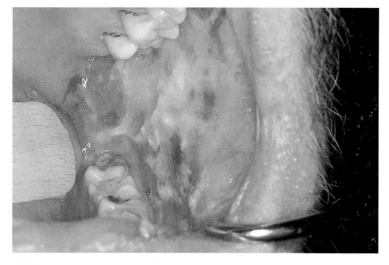

Fig. 28-9   The patient in Figs. 28-7 and 28-8 at the same examination. Bizarre, flat erosions with thick fibrin coat are also found on the mucosa of the left cheek. The dermatologic examination revealed further erosive foci on the genital mucous membrane.

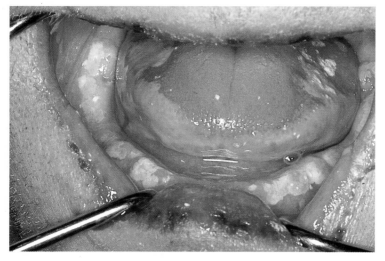

Fig. 28-10   Mucous membrane affected by erythema multiforme with diagnostically important blood crusts on the borders of the lips. The painfulness of the erosion, especially the flat ulcerations, results in decreased range of motion of the lips and tongue, hence speaking and eating are considerably impaired.

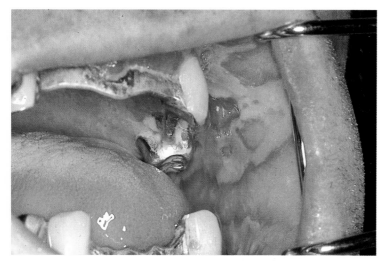

Fig. 28-11   Erythema multiforme appearing after acute streptococcal angina, with predominant involvement of the oral mucosa and systemic complaints of joint pain and fever.

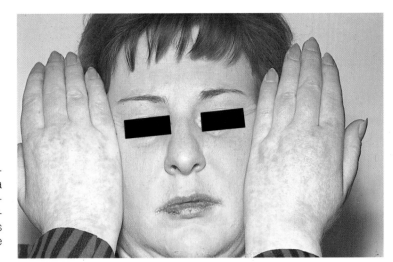

Fig. 28-12 Erythema multiforme as allergic reaction to a phenylbutazone-containing preparation. The symmetrically arranged exanthematous lesions were distributed over the entire trunk.

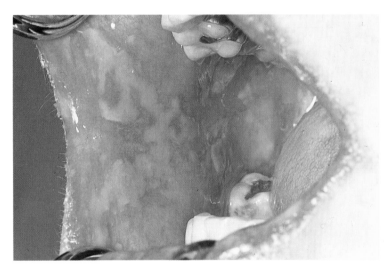

Fig. 28-13 The patient in Fig. 28-12 at the same examination. The extensive fibrin-covered erosions had been present on the right cheek mucosa for 14 days.

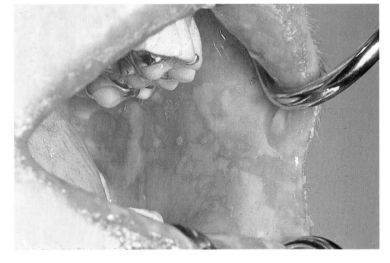

Fig. 28-14 The patient in Figs. 28-12 and 28-13 at the same examination. The painful, extensive fibrin-covered erosion, which is on the mucosa of the left cheek, underscores the stomatitis-like appearance, which was accompanied by halitosis, increased saliva flow, and lymphadenitis of the regional lymph nodes.

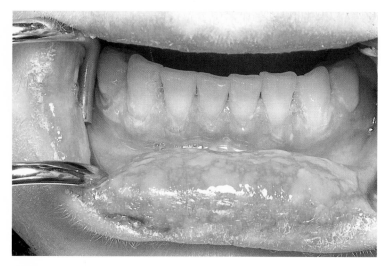

Fig. 28-15 The patient in Figs. 28-12 to 28-14 at the same examination. Similar changes are also found on the swollen inflamed lower lip. Note the bloody crusts on the lip border.

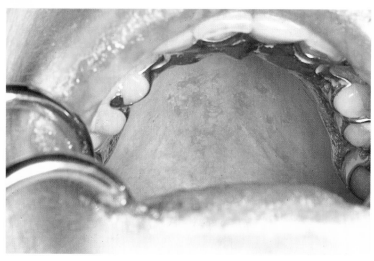

Fig. 28-16 The patient of Figs. 28-12 to 28-15 at the same examination. Erosive foci on the palate have been present for a long time but will not leave scars after healing.

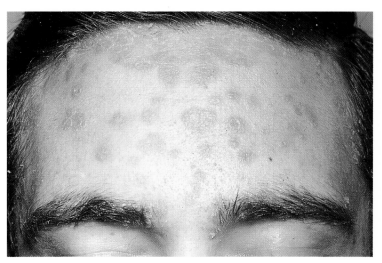

Fig. 28-17 Psoriasis vulgaris in classic location on the head. Aside from the hair-covered areas (including the eyebrows), which are always affected, there are band-shaped foci that hang together on the border of the forehead. Typical single lesions are recognizable in the middle of the forehead (round-to-oval flat papules with lidlike scales).

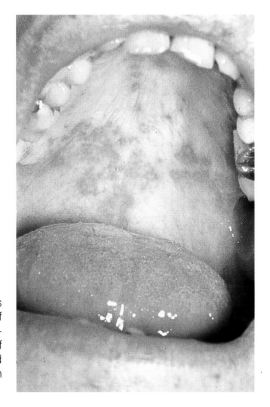

Fig. 28-18 Pustular psoriasis on the mucous membrane of the palate. Intraoral findings occur only in this major variant of psoriasis and are accompanied by a generalized eruption on the skin.

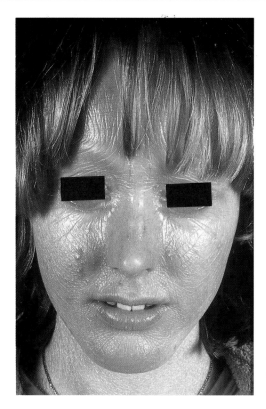

Fig. 28-19 Typical clinical picture of ichthyosis congenita. The face, hands, soles of the feet, and backs of joints are continuously affected.

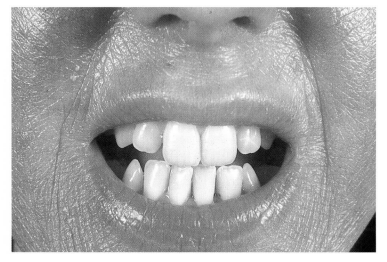

Fig. 28-20 The patient in Fig. 28-19 at the same examination. As a sign of genetically induced disturbed keratinization, an extensive scale formation exists on reddened, thickened dry skin (proliferation hyperkeratosis with abnormal keratinization). The intraoral changes vary from discrete leukoplakial findings to cobblestone-like keratotic scales.

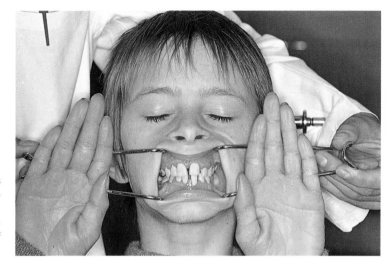

Fig. 28-21 Hyperkeratosis palmoplantaris of the Papillon-Lefèvre type in a 12-year-old boy. Frontal picture with discrete, shining hyperkeratosis of the palms of the hands.

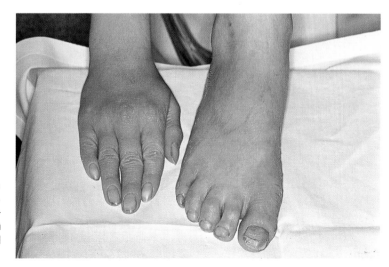

Fig. 28-22 The boy in Fig. 28-21 at the same examination. Clearly recognizable transgradience of the hyperkeratosis on the dorsal surfaces of hand and foot.

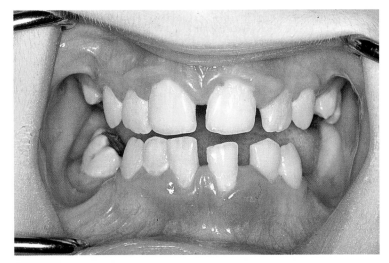

Fig. 28-23 The patient of Figs. 28-21 and 28-22 at the same examination. Advanced periodontitis marginalis profunda with loss of teeth 26 and 36 (19 and 14). The patient's history disclosed that the primary teeth were lost prematurely in a sequence corresponding to the eruption sequence.

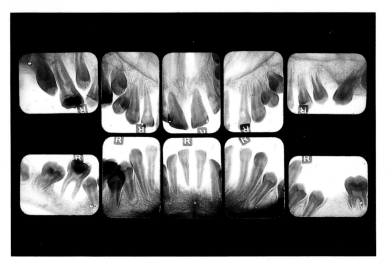

Fig. 28-24 Radiograph of the boy in Figs. 28-21 to 28-23 at the same examination. As in the clinical findings, the radiograph shows a severe destruction of the tooth-supporting bone with tooth movement and tipping. Loss of the other teeth is expected.

	Severity	Trans-gradience	Hyper-hidrosis	Tooth damage	Onset	Progr. Invol.	Handi-cap	Inheri-tance
Unna Thost disease	++	(+)	(+)	(+)	after 2 years	Progr. & inter-mittent	(+)	dominant
Mal de Meleda	+++	++	+++	Ø	post partum	Progr.	+++	recessive
Papillon Lefèvre syndrome	+	+	++	+++	1st year of life	Invol.	(+)	recessive
Greither disease	(+)	+++	+	Ø	1–8 years	Invol.	Ø	dominant

Clinical differential diagnosis of the flat palmoplantar keratosis. (From Schuerman H, Greither A, Hornstein O. Krankheiten der Mundschleimhaut und Lippen. München: Urban & Schwarzenberg, 1966:60.)

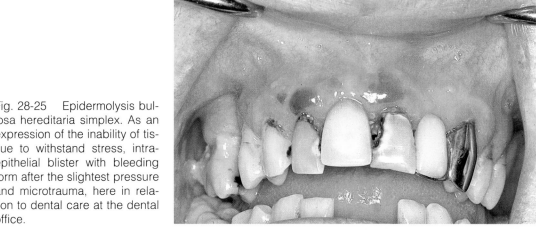

Fig. 28-25 Epidermolysis bullosa hereditaria simplex. As an expression of the inability of tissue to withstand stress, intraepithelial blister with bleeding form after the slightest pressure and microtrauma, here in relation to dental care at the dental office.

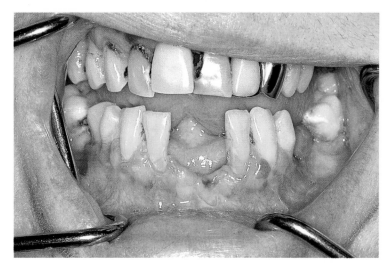

Fig. 28-26 The patient in Fig. 28-25 at the same examination. Appearance of the mandible. The blister formations heal without scars (nondystrophic form).

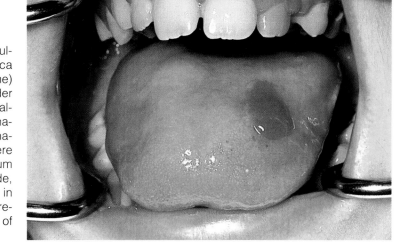

Fig. 28-27 Epidermolysis bullosa hereditaria dystrophica (Hallopeau-Siemens syndrome) in an 11-year-old girl. Under normal tongue function (swallowing, sucking) was the formation of large, usually hemorrhagic, subepithelial blisters. There is a fresh blister on the dorsum of the tongue on the left side, while on the right side is one in healing phase. The papillary relief of the tongue is in a stage of regression (dystrophic form).

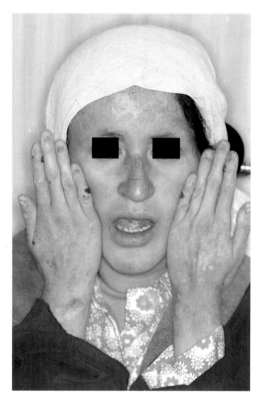

Fig. 28-28   Epidermolysis bullosa hereditaria dystrophica (Hallopeau-Siemens syndrome). Frontal picture of a woman also shows the hands. On mechanical exposure of body parts –represented here by the hands–the dystrophic repair leads to nail dystrophies with scarring and contractions resembling scleroderma. On the fingers are areas with fresh blisters. Alopecia is present in the area of the scarred scalp. The threshold of tissue susceptibility to microtrauma does not vary with aging. Patients are severely affected and therapy has no effect.

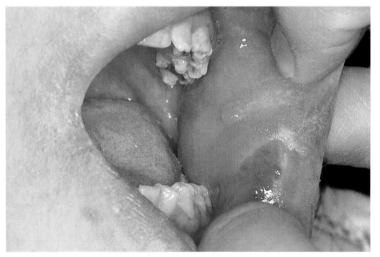

Fig. 28-29   The patient in Fig. 28-28 at the same examination. At the level of the occlusal surface, a fresh blister is developing. In the anterior mucosa region under this area is a large painful erosion as a secondary efflorescence delimited by a zone of epithelial repair. Note the scar at the corner of the mouth as a consequence of a repaired lesion. Scarring leads to microstomia, to flattening or disappearance of the vestibular region, and to mucosal jaw spasm.

Chapter 29

Bullous Diseases of the Oral Mucosa and Lips

Pemphigus group
   Pemphigus vulgaris

Pemphigoid group
   Bullous pemphigoid
   Benign mucosal pemphigoid

Desquamative gingivitis

Dermatitis herpetiformis

The classification used in this chapter is based on the morphologic criterion of the blister as a disease-specific efflorescence. It appears as a chronic disease with remissions and with scaly skin, which is presently thought to be largely dependent on autoimmune factors. Conditions to be considered in differential diagnosis and ruled out are mechanically conditioned (rubbing) blisters, thermically caused (burning) blisters (see chapters 32 and 33), blisters associated with an inflammatory dermatosis (such as oral lichen planus—see chapter 16—erythema exudativum multiforme—see chapter 28), blisters of bullous and medication reaction (see chapters 28 and 31), or those in relation to irradiation therapy.

   The apparently spontaneous blister formation is caused by a break of continuity inside the epidermis, at the dermoepidermal connecting layer or within the dermis (i. e., in the covering on the mucosa), within the epithelium, at the epithelium-connective tissue limit, or beneath it. These lesions are important for histomorphologic diagnostic differentiation of the interepidermal (intraepithelial), junctional, and subepidermal (subepithelial) blisters, which can be followed by immunologic confirmatory methods. Direct or indirect immunofluorescence methods using antibodies against immunoglobulin, complement component, basal membrane constituents, cell components, or collagen

Oral manifestation of blister-forming diseases*

Variable	Pemphigus vulgaris	Bullous pemphigoid	Benign mucosal pemphigoid	Desquamative gingivitis
Age (yr) at illness	30–60	>50	>60	40–60
Male: female	~1:1	1:1	1:2	1:3
Oral mucosa participation	Initial ~60%, later ~100%	20%–30%	in 90% only oral mucosal and/or conjunctiva	100%
Start; course; prognosis	Acute, first localized; progresses in leaps; generalized, if untreated, lethal	Acute to subacute; generalized; if not treated due to complications lethal in 50% of cases	Chronic course; local recurrences; local complications	Localized; chronic course; limited to gingiva; bordering areas of covering gingiva seldom affected
Mucosal findings	Loose; blisters of very short duration on unaltered mucosa; painful erosions, sometimes with vegetations	Plump distended blisters, often with hemorrhagic content; painful erosions on erythematous base	Plump blisters; hard erosions; shrinkage with scars	Short-lived; small blisters?; chronic erosions; scalelike desquamations
Histology	Acantholytic intraepithelial blister	Subepithelial blister	Subepithelial junctional blister	Only single subepithelial blister demonstrable; prominent desquamation
Immune status	Tzanck test positive; pemphigus antibodies	Tzanck test negative; pemphigoid antibodies	Tzanck test negative; pemphigoid antibodies	Tzanck test negative; no disease-specific antibodies demonstrable
Direct immunofluorescence antibodies in the area of disease	Positive (100%)	Positive (100%)	Positive (100%)	
Indirect immunofluorescence antibodies in serum	Usually positive	Usually positive (80%)	Usually positive	

* Modified from *Braun-Falco O, Plewig G, Wolff HH*. Dermatologie und Venerologie, ed 3. Berlin: Springer, 1984:445.

allow differentiation of the individual disease entities. Long-standing genodermatoses in the oral cavity are discussed in chapter 28.

In the chronic diseases discussed, oral mucosa involvement occurs quite often. Because the dentist cannot study the entire skin organ and mucosae outside the oral cavity, she or he is forced to make the diagnosis without this benefit. On the other hand, one must remember that the oral cavity can be (at the beginning of disease) the only manifestation point. Blister-forming diseases are easy to misdiagnose because the blisters on the oral mucosa are of short duration; this is because of unavoidable microtrauma and maceration effects of saliva. Blisters are seldom seen during intraoral examination. Mostly there are already secondary efflorescences in the form of erosions and ulcerations, although usually there are still (floating or rolled up) blister covers.

Pemphigus group

To the pemphigus diseases belong *pemphigus vulgaris, pemphigus vegetans*, and special forms *(pemphigus foliaceus, brazilian pemphigus, pemphigus erythematosus)* that will not be discussed here.

Common histomorphologic markers of this group are the *acantholytic intraepidermal (intraepithelial) blister-formation (positive Tzanck test)* and the corresponding immunologic criterion of the presence of antibodies, which act against certain parts of the intercellular substance of epithelial cells *(pemphigus antibodies)*.

Pemphigus vulgaris (ICD-DA 694.4 and 694.40)

Pemphigus is a relatively rare disease with no gender predilection that appears between the ages of 30 and 60 years. However, considerably younger persons can be affected. In almost every second patient, the disease starts in the oral cavity, and it can be limited to this site for many years. In 90% of patients with skin lesions, there is also participation of the oral mucosa.

The phenomenon of acantholysis (i. e., cohesion disturbance of epithelial cells) is clinically recognizable through two examination processes:

- On unaffected skin, lateral pressure will displace epithelium from the base *(Nikolsky's sign I)*.
- Pemphigus blisters are movable (because there is no definite separation, the blister remains slack) on light pressure within the tissue. The blister travels to a point in the tissue that seems normal *(Nikolsky's sign II)*. On the oral mucosa, the same effect can be obtained with the aid of an air jet *(air jet blister experiment)*.

  These phenomena are possible only during the active phase of the disease, not during remission periods!

The *Tzanck test* is a demonstration of acantholytic cells (pemphigus cells) that are released in the fluid of the blister by the dissolution of the intercellular bridges. The result of the Tzanck test is confirmed with histologic examination.

With the help of *direct immunofluorescence*, it is possible to find antibodies against immunoglobulins (primarily IgG type) as well as complement components on the blister cover and blister border area. There are also antibodies against intercellular components of layered epithelium in the serum of patients with pemphigus. The titer level of these pemphigus antibodies correlates with the activity of the disease. There is no longer any doubt of the autoimmunogenesis based on the specific pemphigus antibodies. Using these antibodies it is possible to obtain acantholytic blisters in animal experiments.

In pemphigus vulgaris, there is no specific oral predilection area. Obvious functional dependency preferentially affects the mucosa of the palate (prosthetically conditioned?), the cheeks, and lips (pressure in swallowing?) (Figs. 29-1 to 29-3). Characteristically, there are different large, slack blisters initially filled with clear contents that can be moved about within the tissue.

Because of their superficial location, the pemphigus blisters are easily ruptured. In the oral cavity, there can be rapid loss of the blister cover so that only secondary efflorescences in the form of extended and very painful erosions remain. These fibrin-coated or, in the absence of fibrin cover, very red erosions (Fig. 29-3) heal very slowly only to reappear in the same or new areas with renewed flare-ups. In the case of inflammatory complications caused by bacterial and mycotic superimpositions, there are recognizable remnants on the oral mucosa.

In *pemphigus vegetans* (ICD-DA 694.41) there is the development of erosions with secondary granulations and papillomatous growth (vegetations) that preferentially occur in the area of the maceration—corner of the mouth, nasolabial folds, and the larger skin folds—as well as in the genitoanal region. These special forms of pemphigus vulgaris appear because the autoimmune antibodies are directed against antigens other than the pemphigus vulgaris.

Pemphigus vulgaris must be differentiated from all other diseases discussed in this chapter (i. e., by Tzanck test, histology, immunology) as well as from erythema exudativum multiforme with its extension to the mucocutaneous borders, the bullous variants of medication exanthemas, fixed drug reactions, bullous erosive forms of lichen planus, and erosive lupus erythematoides. In the vegetative forms of pemphigus, there is the possibility of confusion with syphilitic papules as well as with acanthosis nigricans.

Obviously, there is a pathogenetic relation of pemphigus vulgaris with undesirable medication reactions (e. g., indomethacin, phenylbutazone, particularly penicillamine) and autoimmune diseases such as pernicious anemia, myasthenia gravis, and possibly even with malignant lymphogranuloma. Also, coexistence of pemphigus vulgaris and bullous pemphigoid seems possible.

Untreated, this dangerous progressive disease leads to death in up to 3 years. In spite of today's therapy advances, the prognosis is still serious even though mortality has been reduced to about half. Treatment consists of high doses of systemic steroids, use of immunosuppressive medication (preferentially azathioprin [Imurek]), as well as antibacterials and antimycotics for secondary infections. Newer immunosuppressive agents such as cyclosporine A must be studied to determine whether they are effective. There must also be sufficient liquid substitution and normalization of the nutritional state because the disease has a picture of a marked catabolic condition. In the case of suspected pemphigus, the dentist should refer the patient immediately to a dermatologist.

Pemphigoid group

As opposed to the pemphigus group, pemphigoid is characterized by a *subepidermal (subepithelial)* blister caused by disturbance of the cohesion between epidermis and dermis and/or between the mucosal epithelium and connective tissue. Therefore, there is a *negative Tzanck test result*, which means findings of a blister preparation without acantholytic cells but rather with blood cells in the lumen. Another differential sign is that in cases of pemphigoid blister there is generally a tightly filled *tension blister* in which Nikolsky's sign is not necessarily positive. With immunofluorescence, it is possible to demonstrate antibodies in the skin/mucosa, which are directed against parts of the basal membrane and can be distinctly differentiated from the antibodies of the pemphigus group *(pemphigoid antibodies)*. In 80% of patients, pemphigoid antibodies are also present in the serum.

The pemphigoid diseases of interest here are bullous pemphigoid and benign mucosal pemphigoid.

Bullous pemphigoid (ICD-DA 694.5 and 694.50)

Bullous pemphigoid is a chronic disease that progresses in stages and affects patients of both sexes over 50 years of age. Children are only rarely affected (juvenile pemphigoid). Even though the disease has a more favorable prognosis than pemphigus, and cases of spontaneous remission have been reported, weakening due to dysphagia, weight loss, and superinfection with fever (bronchopneumonia) can be debilitating to older persons and can reduce life expectancy.

Clinically, there is the development of filled, tightly distended, large blisters of the subepidermal type up to several centimeters in diameter on normal-appearing, but especially on inflamed reddish skin. A preferred region in the dental area is the lateral neck region. The oral mucosa is affected only in 20% to 30% of cases. Because the blister cover is made up of the whole epithelial layer, in comparison to the skin, the blisters of the mucosa are smaller, more resistant, and, therefore of somewhat longer duration than the pemphigus blisters (Figs. 29-4 to 29-8). Because of the split in the area of the papillary bodies, there is frequent bleeding in the blisters (Figs. 29-4 and 29-5). The secondary, roundish erosions that result from the blisters are sharply delimited and, because of the pain and their slow healing (Fig. 29-9), hamper the ability to eat.

Also in bullous pemphigoid are etiologic relations with drug reactions (e. g., penicillamine, laxatives). Associations with other autoimmune diseases (systemic lupus erythematosus, ulcerative colitis, chronic polyarthritis) are considered possible. Associations with malignant tumors in the sense of a paraneoplastic disease have also been described. There have been reports of patients with typical signs of bullous pemphigoid and dermatitis herpetiformis (so-called intermediary forms) simultaneously.

Regarding differential diagnosis and therapy, this disease belongs in the hands of the dermatologist. Treatment is the same as that of pemphigus (i. e., glucocorticoid, immunosuppressives).

A special form of pemphigoid is **Herpes gestationis** (ICD 646.8), which is explained by the peculiar immunologic conditions of pregnancy. They are rare gestational dermatoses (with an incidence of 1 in 5,000 to 10,000 pregnancies), in which polymorphic blisters develop during the second trimester of pregnancy (as opposed to the itchy skin changes of established pemphigus). In 20% of cases, the mucosa can be affected. The disease generally heals 2 to 3 weeks after delivery. It can also result from some contraceptive medications.

Benign mucosal pemphigoid (ICD-DA 694.6 and 694.60)

As the name indicates, this chronic blister-forming disease prefers the mucosa. In 90% of all cases, the main location, and often the only location over years, is the conjunctiva and/or the oral mucosa. Sometimes the mucosae of the nose, the pharynx and the larynx, and the genitoanal region can participate in the disease; participation of the skin is also possible but rare. Women are particularly affected (sex distribution 2:1) usually after age 60.

The attribute "benign" must be taken cautiously, because the scars and shrinkage resulting from the lesions in reality result in many serious problems as a consequence of this disease. Benign mucosal pemphigoid leads to blindness through increasing shrinkage and clouding of the cornea in 20% of patients.

Clinically it is not possible to differentiate a benign mucosal pemphigoid of the oral mucosa (Figs. 29-10 to 29-12) from oral pemphigus vulgaris. The blisters, which contrary to those in pemphigus vulgaris, are located subepithelially *(negative Tzanck test)*, last for 2 or 3 days before they burst, and then change into flat erosions or even deep ulcerations.

During healing of the scars, the mucosa shrinks. Depending on the location there can be scar tissue formation (Fig. 29-13) with a consequent slow reduction of tongue movements, impaired swallowing, a so-called mucosal jaw cramp, and microstomia in which eating ability can be affected.

According to current histopathologic and immunopathologic perceptions, benign mucosal pemphigoid is possibly a variation of bullous pemphigoid. The etiology is unclear, as are the causes for the prominent tendency to scarring, that is, scar atrophy of the mucosa.

The same points of view mentioned for bullous pemphigoid apply to differential diagnosis and therapy. Where there is threatening decrease of tongue mobility or ability to open the mouth, the mucosal scar can be removed, followed by plastic reconstruction.

Desquamative gingivitis (ICD-DA 523.13)

In the past, desquamative gingivitis was considered a special form of chronic gingivitis with a prominent desquamation. Later the terminology continued to be used to describe the clinical appearances of desquamative changes of the gingiva that, according to today's knowledge, are common manifestations of different nosologic entities. Improved immunologic examination methods have led to a considerable increase of knowledge and allow better classification in special cases. The lesions of desquamative gingivitis look histologically and immunopathologically like those of benign mucosal pemphigoides in about half of all patients. In other patients, the findings are identical to those of erosive lichen planus–or rarely–with those of pemphigus vulgaris or acquired bullous epidermolysis. Recently, *"chronic ulcerative stomatitis"* (CUS) has been described as a new disease, characterized by antiribonucleoprotein antibodies, therapeutic response to chloroquine, and that possibly appears with the same manifestations on the gingiva. The name "gingivitis desquamativa" should therefore be used today only for those cases that cannot be classified as another disease due to the lack of demonstrable specific antibodies.

Because most patients affected by desquamative gingivitis are women between the ages of 40 and 60, it is possible that disturbances in hormonal metabolism are at least cofactors. The clinical picture is variable. There is always the presence of a erythema in the region of the attached and/or marginal gingiva, usually on the vestibular side (Figs. 29-14 to 29-16). The epithelium that split from its base longitudinally through subepithelial separation can sometimes show clinically demonstrable blister formations with serous content; an air-blister experiment will then yield positive results. In other cases, no surface separation of the epithelium is noticeable.

When the epithelium has been previously damaged, and is therefore more vulnerable, there is the possibility of epithelial loss by wiping (for example, in the areas of dental treatment) or by slight mechanical irritation. There is the development of painful, even bleeding, erosions that have a poor healing tendency and only incomplete epithelial regeneration.

As opposed to other types of gingivitis, desquamative gingivitis can appear in plaque-free teeth. Not definitely explained is the question of changes persisting in the edentulous alveolar process. Finally, the etiology continues to be unclear. Autoimmune episodes against epithelium are possible.

A clinical diagnosis of desquamative gingivitis always requires pathohistologic and immunofluorescent microscopic examination by excision biopsy to distinguish similar clinical findings. Therapy should be planned in cooperation with the dermatologist.

In the forefront of dental treatment measures are first the removal of supragingival and subgingival plaque through professional prophylaxis and systematic periodontal treatment to remove bacterially induced inflammation. The patient is instructed to maintain careful oral hygiene, which is difficult because of the painful lesions. In this regard it must be remembered that many oral care preparations (i. e., toothpastes) as well as alcohol-containing mouthwashes induce desquamation. It is obvious that irritating materials cannot be used (Fig. 29-16). A positive effect can be obtained with a change of pH values by the use of alkaline toothpastes (also in form of periodontal packs with a deep sheet for carrying the pack). In some cases, cortico-steroid-containing ointments can also be of use, but they should only be used temporarily and should be discussed with the dermatologist. Finally, the therapy of desquamative gingivitis is only symptomatic, of long duration, and is usually unsatisfactory.

Dermatitis herpetiformis (ICD-DA 694.0 and 694.00)

Dermatitis herpetiformis is a rare, chronically recurring benign disease that appears on the trunk and the extremities with polymorphic skin changes. There are erythematous, urticarious, and papular efflores-cences of subepithelial-type herpetiform blisters appearing in groups. The disease is more common in men than women with a 2:1 ratio. There is a wide age distribution (between 20 and 70 years). Compared to the diseases of the pemphigus and pemphigoid groups, there is more severe itching and burning irritation. Participation of the oral mucosa is rare (Figs. 29-17 and 29-18). There is also formation of small, roundish, initially tight-filled, small blisters and fibrin-covered erosions, sometimes aphthous-like, that finally heal without scarring.

It is remarkable that in 70% of patients there are disturbances in the gastrointestinal tract (e. g., gluten-sensitive enteropathies), usually with demonstrable gliadin antibodies. Of dental interest is the sensitiv-ity of patients to a herpetiform dermatitis from iodine, that is, halogens, and nutrients. Iodine products trigger or increase the skin findings. The etiology is otherwise unknown. Autoimmunologic pathologic mechanisms are suspected.

The disease has a stagewise, usually chronic course over many years with intervals during which only rare, if any, lesions persist. Differential diagnosis, including immunopathologic examination, should be performed by the dermatologist. Therapeutically pre-scribed diaminodiphenylsulfone (Dapsone) has been the most suc-cessful treatment. The prognosis is good.

Finally, reference should be made to **IgA-linear dermatosis**, which also belongs to the group of chronic blister-forming diseases. Accord-ing to current knowledge, therapy-resistant, oral mucosal lesions develop in about 60% of cases. This dermatosis shows predominantly signs of dermatitis herpetiformis and also of bullous pemphigoids. It can be differentiated from dermatitis herpetiformis by a linear deposit of IgA on the basal membrane zone. There is also absence of a relation to gluten-sensitive enteropathy. Bullous pemphigoid can be distinguished from the IgA-linear dermatosis because the antibodies are not directed against the "pemphigoid antigen."

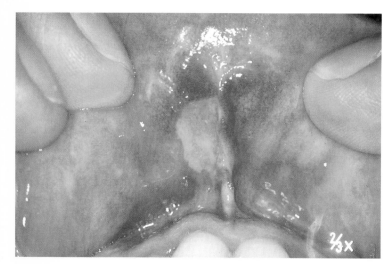

Fig. 29-1 Pemphigus vulgaris often starts in the oral cavity, which in some cases can be the sole area of manifestation. In primary skin changes, the oral cavity, in chronic and acute phases, almost always participates sooner or later. The pea- to grape-sized oral pemphigus blisters are fragile, hence erosions usually predominate in the clinical picture.

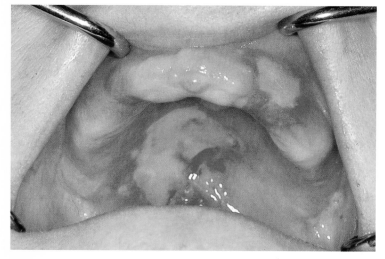

Fig. 29-2 Pemphigus vulgaris. Intraepithelial blisters caused by acantholysis (positive Tzanck test) in the mucosa are displaced laterally (Nikolsky's sign, air-blister experiment) by pressure. To confirm the diagnosis, histopathologic and immunologic examination by excision biopsy (unfixed specimen) is always recommended. The demonstration of pemphigus antibodies takes place in the diseased mucosa through direct immunofluorescence in serum through indirect immunofluorescence. When in doubt, refer to the dermatologist.

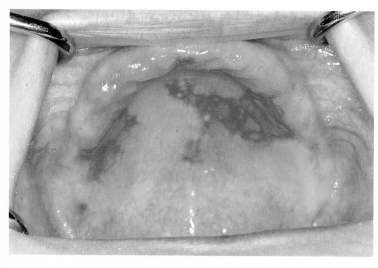

Fig. 29-3 Pemphigus vulgaris. The loose acantholytic pemphigus blisters are easily damaged and therefore of short duration in the oral mucosa. They change quickly into painful erosions covered with fibrinous material. When the fibrin cover is missing—as here—the erosions show their red surface. Often it is possible to see borders of floating parts of the blister cover. Untreated, pemphigus vulgaris leads to death within 3 years.

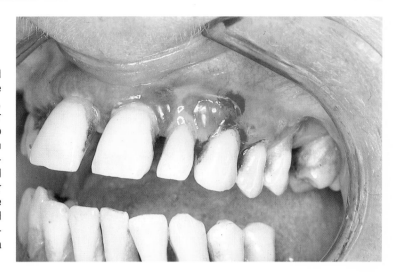

Fig. 29-4   Bullous pemphigoid in a 65-year-old woman. The chronic, usually generalized, bullous disease appearing after the fiftieth year of life leads to participation of the oral cavity in only 20% to 30% of cases. Because the blisters are located subepithelially and the blister cover is made up of the whole epithelial layer, the pemphigoid blisters are able to resist rupture longer in the oral mucosa than pemphigus blisters.

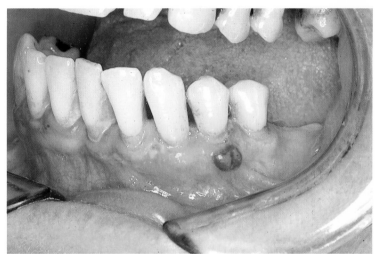

Fig. 29-5   The patient in Fig. 29-4 at the same examination. There is a well-delimited tight bullous efflorescence on the vestibular gingiva of tooth 34 (21). There are hemorrhagic blisters, usually caused by bleeding.

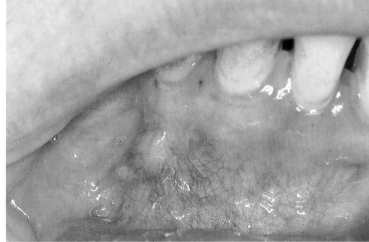
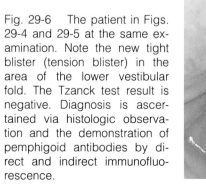

Fig. 29-6   The patient in Figs. 29-4 and 29-5 at the same examination. Note the new tight blister (tension blister) in the area of the lower vestibular fold. The Tzanck test result is negative. Diagnosis is ascertained via histologic observation and the demonstration of pemphigoid antibodies by direct and indirect immunofluorescence.

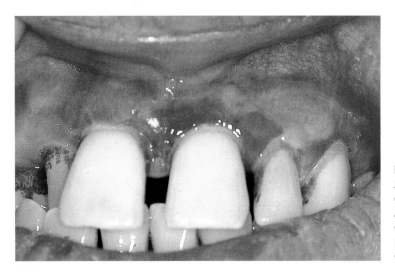

Fig. 29-7   The patient in Figs. 29-4 to 29-6 after 1 month. The disease progressed in stages. Advanced findings of vestibular gingiva with poorly healed, painful erosions are seen on an erythematous base.

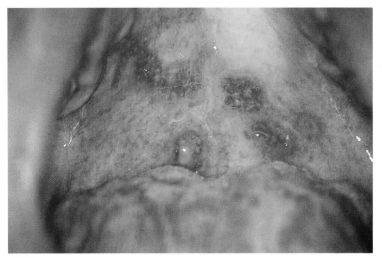

Fig. 29-8   The patient in Figs. 29-4 to 29-7 at same examination. As expression of a new stage, there are filled blisters on the palate and erosions as secondary efflorescences with borders containing partial blister covers. An older focus shows signs of an early epithelialization.

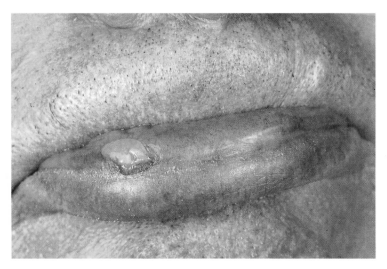

Fig. 29-9   Repair stage of bullous pemphigoid on the lower lip. Reepithelization of the fibrin-covered erosion takes 4 weeks. In the past there had been several previous blisters at the same spot.

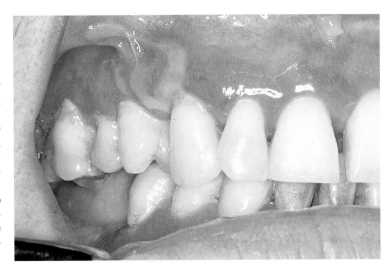

Fig. 29-10 Benign mucosal pemphigoid. Most frequently affected are the oral mucosa and the conjunctiva of the eye, primarily in women over 60 years. In the patient shown is a torn subepithelial distended blister. It extends from the gingiva in the region of teeth 15, 14, and 13 (4, 5, 6) to far into the vestibule. With the air-blister experiment, the rest of the epithelium lifted as a blister cover.

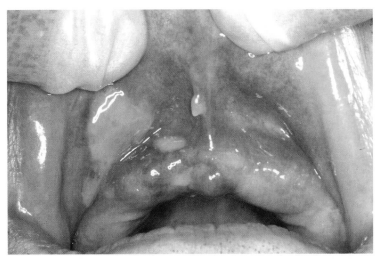

Fig. 29-11 Benign mucosal pemphigoid. Fibrin cover of erosive secondary efflorescences in mucosal area of the upper lip and maxillary alveolar process. The blister-forming disease progresses in stages, with the efflorescences often reappearing in the same spots. Immunologic findings correspond largely to those of bullous pemphigoid.

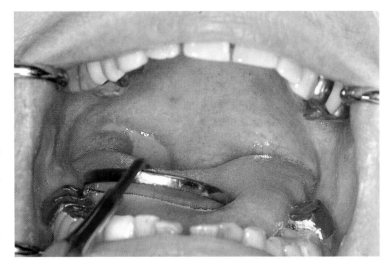

Fig. 29-12 Benign mucosal pemphigoid on the soft palate. Because the disease leads to scar shrinkage of the affected mucosal area, there are possible complications in the oral cavity (e.g., dysphagia, reduction of tongue mobility, mucosal-produced jaw clamping, microstomia).

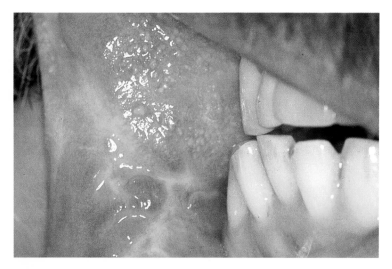

Fig. 29-13 Consequence of a benign mucosal pemphigoid. Extended scars in the area of the affected lip and cheek mucosa. These scar contractions can lead to microstomia.

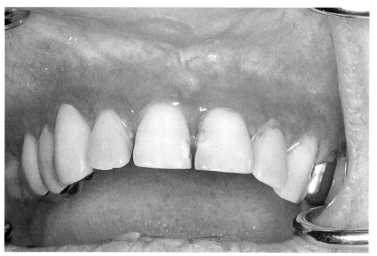

Fig. 29-14 Desquamative gingivitis. The slowly developing and then chronically progressing changes generally manifest in the area of the vestibular mucosa. There is reddening of fixed and free marginal gingiva with horizontal lifting of the epithelium. Because of the great possibility of tissue injury, there is easy epithelial loss with resulting erosions.

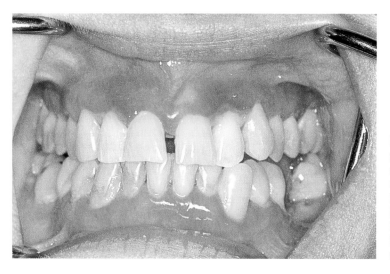

Fig. 29-15 Desquamative gingivitis. Independent of plaque accumulation is persistence of erythematous and desquamative gingival areas. In the air-blister experiment, the epithelium lifted as a sign of subepithelial split formation (Nikolsky's sign).

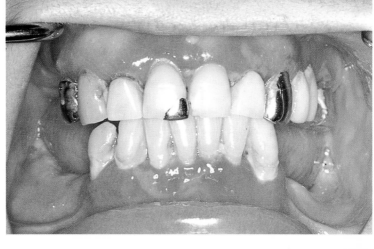

Fig. 29-16 Desquamative gingivitis often shows a superimposed inflammation caused by a pain-related lack of oral hygiene. An increase of desquamative gingival lesions due to inappropriately aggressive therapy methods (e. g., disinfecting with alcohol-containing mouth rinses) is also frequent, as shown here.

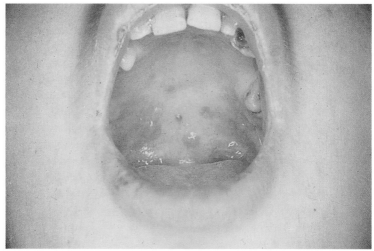

Fig. 29-17 Dermatitis herpetiformis. The very itchy dermatosis with acute or subacute onset offers a varied clinical picture. The polymorphic efflorescences that develop on the skin in groups of small blisters with herpetiform pattern give the disease its name. In rare cases there can also be pea-sized tightly filled vesicles (subepithelial) containing a clear fluid on the oral mucosa. Adjacent equal-sized erosions are seen with marginal vesicular remnants.

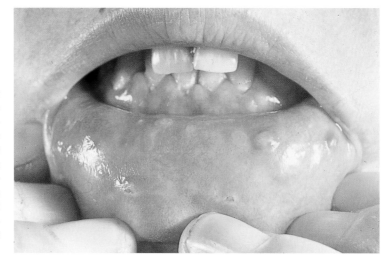

Fig. 29-18 The patient in Fig. 29-17 at same examination. The mucosa of the lower lip and the vestibular gingiva have primary and secondary efflorescences of dermatitis herpetiformis. The benign chronic recurring disease of unknown origin is associated with a gluten-sensitive enteropathy in 70% of cases. The frequent sensitivity to iodine and its relation to dermatitis herpetiformis is not explained at present.

Chapter 30

Oral and Perioral Manifestations of Other Autoimmune Diseases and Some Diseases of Unknown Origin

Autoimmune diseases
  Lupus erythematosus
  Discoid lupus erythematosus
  Systemic lupus erythematosus
  Sclerodermas
  Dermatomyositis
  Sjögren's syndrome
  Polyarteritis nodosa
    Giant cell arteritis
    Wegener's granulomatosis

Diseases without nosologic classification
  Lethal midline granuloma
  Langerhans' cell histiocytosis (e. g., eosinophilic granuloma)
  Melkersson-Rosenthal syndrome
  Hemifacial atrophy

When an etiopathology—whether because it is unknown or still unclear—is not available for nosologic classification of criteria, the initial clinical presentation is the next best organizational principle for diseases. The first part of this chapter describes diseases that, according to current knowledge, are based on autoimmune events. The term *autoaggressive diseases* (including the so-called collagen diseases) is also used. The second part of the chapter describes diseases without nosologic classification that affect the teeth, mouth, and jaw.

Autoimmune diseases

With an increasing number of diseases, it is currently possible to demonstrate autoimmune processes as well as reactions of the immune system against structures of the body that acquired the antigen character (autoantigen). The demonstration of autoantibodies cannot be equated automatically with a disease event in the clinical sense; for example, in more than 40% of clinically healthy persons over 60 years of age, there are antinuclear specific autoantibodies (ANA).

The immune system maintains the identity and integrity of the organism *(self-recognition)*. The aim of every immune reaction is elimination of extraneous antigens whereby cell-mediated and humoral events act together. This principle is known from the defense against infection (chapter 7), allergic reactions (chapter 31), immunohemolytic anemias (chapter 24), and blister-formation diseases (chapter 29). (Chapter 31 explains division of allergic basic reactions according to Coombs and Gell.)

The immune supervision of the body takes place through immunocompetent lymphocytes, which scan all anatomic extracellular structures, cell membranes, and cell parts or remnants of liberated intracellular parts. Between the recognition of *self* and *not-self* lies the *"altered self,"* to which the *"forbidden clones"* and damaged and altered body cell populations belong. Immune tolerance against self (cells, cell parts) and—with reservations—against "altered self" is the result of a complicated coordinated play of T and B lymphocytes, macrophages, antibodies, and immune complexes. Particularities of these only partially known reactions cannot be discussed here. Tolerance can be disturbed in different ways, which results in diseases. Body cells and cell parts can change so much from the tolerance state that they can no longer be protected. As altered self, they start to act as antigen and therefore cause the formation and persistence of specific antibodies. Similar phenomena occur at the level of the cellular arm of the immune defense with T-lymphocyte cytotoxic activity against body structures.

Aging-process neoplasms, viral infections, and medications play a causal role in changes in cells and in cell surfaces with consequent antigen-antibody reaction. According to current thought, autoimmune diseases depend first on an exaggerated and later on a pathologic reaction based on processes that, at a controlled level, are constantly taking place in the body. Regarding the disease, the clinical pictures vary from discrete to dramatic generalized pathologic events.

The following table includes dental diseases that may be associated with autoimmune events.

Diseases associated with autoimmune events

Autoantibodies against cells and tissue structures	Diseases
Erythrocytes	Hemolytic anemia
Leukocytes	Leukocytopenias (also as phenomenon in lupus erythematosus)
Platelets	Thrombocytopenias
Stomach mucosa	Pernicious anemia
−parietal cells	
Thyroid	Hashimoto's disease, immune thyroiditis
Pancreas	Insulin-dependent juvenile diabetes mellitus (type I)
−islet cells	
Intestinal mucosa	Regional enterocolitis (Crohn's disease)
Connective tissue localized-systemic	Lupus erythematosus, systemic scleroderma, dermatomyositis
Circulatory system	Polyarthritis nodosa, temporal arthritis, Wegener granulomatosis
Locomotion system	Rheumatoid arthritis (primary chronic polyarthritis), psoriasis arthropathica
Kidney	Glomerulonephritis
Heart	Endocarditis, myocarditis
Skin/mucosa	
−intercellular substance	Pemphigus vulgaris
−basal cell membrane component	Bullous pemphigoid
Mucosa (oral mucosa also affected)	Benign mucosal pemphigoid disease, Behçet's syndrome
Oral mucosa	Desquamative gingivitis (?)
	Chronic recurring aphthae (?)
Salivary glands	Sjögren's syndrome
Peripheral nerve system	Polyneuritis (?)
Central nervous system	Multiple sclerosis (?)

The autoimmune diseases that will be discussed have completely different histologic reactions in the area of the skin and mucosa with corresponding clinical findings. In lupus erythematosus on the dermal-epidermal junction, there is vacuolar degeneration and colliquation of the basal membrane, whereas in scleroderma the deep dermis is affected. In severe associated systemic forms with visceral organ involvement, for example in lupus erythematosus, there are often vessel changes with features of vasculitis, a finding not unusual in autoimmune diseases.

Differential diagnosis is difficult in the initial stages and demands interdisciplinary cooperation. Therapy of autoimmune diseases usually includes corticosteroids in high doses and immunosuppressive agents.

Lupus erythematosus

Lupus erythematosus encompasses several clinical pictures with different courses and prognoses. There are two main forms (with different subtypes not to be discussed here):

Discoid lupus erythematosus
Preferred location: Skin, seldom oral mucosa
Course: Usually chronic with remissions and
                                 flare ups
Prognosis: Good

Systemic lupus erythematosus
Preferred location: Systemic disease
Course: Subacute to acute
Prognosis: Serious to lethal

A transition from discoid to systemic form takes place in only 5% of cases during the progress of the disease, which lasts years to decades.

Discoid lupus erythematosus (ICD-DA 695.4 and 695.40)

This chronic progressive disease with remission and active stages is more frequent than the systemic form and is characterized by an inflammatory dermatosis, scaly erythemas, atrophic areas, and later scar formation. The autoimmune disease mostly affects young adults (20 to 40 years) and preferentially women. The requirement for manifestation of the disease is the combination of a genetic predisposition and exogenous factors. The main locations of the disease are the face exposed to light (cheek, forehead, nose, external ear, and less frequently the scalp) and the dorsum of the hand.

Skin lesions start as lentil-like to penny-size elevated erythemas that expand to disk forms and later become confluent. At the center one finds adherent scales, which correspond to a follicular keratosis and are characterized by the *"paper hanger nail phenomenon"* of discoid lupus erythematosus. In the continuing course, there is a central atrophic change and changes in pigmentation. At the border zone of the peripherally expanding process are telangiectases.

In typical cases, the foci on the skin of the midface show a butterfly pattern (Fig. 30-1). After many years of disease, there can be mutilations (particularly on the tip of the nose and external ear; therefore, the name, "lupus"). Lesions in the perioral region and on the lips are often noticed (Figs. 30-2 and 30-3). Reports of oral participation (cheeks, more rarely tongue, palate) vary considerably in the literature. "Stand-alone" intraoral findings are rare. The oral mucosal changes (Figs. 30-4 to 30-6) are discoid in one or more foci with an initial flat epithelial clouding of the dark-red edematous base. Later there is formation of hyperkeratosis milk-white stripes. The slightly raised border zone shows telangiectases with raised punctate or linear bleeding. In the depressed atrophic center are small, painful erosions or ulcerative lesions that continue for a long time.

Discoid lupus erythematosus on the oral mucosa may have varied clinical features, and there is a need for differential diagnosis from leukoplakia, lichen planus, other symptomatic leukoplakias, and the opaque plaques in syphilis II.

Laboratory findings vary from an increased but nonspecific erythrocyte sedimentation rate (ESR); sometimes it is possible to make a diagnosis with the use of indirect immunofluorescence testing to detect antinuclear antibodies in the serum. Histopathologic examination is decisive. In 70% to 90% of cases of discoid lupus erythematosus, direct immunofluorescence *(lupus band test)* from lesions of the skin show immunoglobulin and complement deposits in the basal membrane of the diseased region, while biopsy specimens of unaffected sun-exposed and non–sun-exposed skin show negative results. The lupus band test of non–sun-exposed skin has become less important since the development of new autoantibody techniques.

The prognosis of discoid lupus erythematosus is favorable; however, the disease leaves scars. Treatment is the task of the dermatologist.

Systemic lupus erythematosus (ICD-DA 710.0 and 710.00)

Even though discoid lupus erythematosus and systemic lupus erythematosus probably have the same pathogenesis, the course of the cellular and humoral immunoreaction in systemic lupus erythematosus leads to an acute and aggressive generalized condition (systemic disease). In Germany, every year there are five to 10 persons newly affected by systemic lupus erythematosus in every 100,000. Mostly young adult women are affected (women are affected eight times more frequently than men).

In addition to genetic predisposition, there are the suspected exogenous determining factors: sunlight, medications, and viral infections.

Presently there is thought to be an immunologic imbalance between B and T lymphocytes with marked increase of B-cell activity (polyclonal B-cell activation). There is an enhanced immune response with formation of antibodies that react with autoantibodies. Production of these antibodies may be induced by viral, bacterial, mycotic, chemical (pharmacologic), physical, and other factors. In the vessel walls and in the connective tissue, there is the deposit of immune complexes that activate the complement cascade and in the final stages lead to scarring of the tissue involved.

The central pathogenic finding is immune vasculitis, which is the key to understanding the many forms of clinical manifestations. The locomotion apparatus almost always takes part in the form of arthritis, which initially is often thought to be rheumatic disease. Later, almost all organ systems can be affected with a variable frequency (skin, kidneys, heart, lungs, central nervous system, gastrointestinal tract, and blood-forming organs).

In almost two thirds of cases, the skin changes previously described develop more acutely but with less tendency to disseminate. The often persisting erythema gives the patient a bloated appearance. There are also intraoral manifestations, which can be differentiated from discoid lupus erythematosus by the greater inflammatory symptoms and faster disease course.

In the preliminary diagnosis, the greatly increased erythrocyte sedimentation rate and blood changes (anemia, leukocytopenia, thrombocytopenia) are of significance. The diagnosis is based on the clinical picture, laboratory values, and the demonstration of antibodies. The many varied immunologic findings correspond to the variability of the clinical disease picture. Differential diagnosis and therapy of systemic lupus erythematosus is an interdisciplinary task in clinical medicine. The prognosis is essentially determined by kidney disease status.

Sclerodermas

Sclerodermas are chronic diseases that lead to fibrosis. The etiology is unknown. Two independent disease processes are clinically distinguished:

Circumscribed sclerodermas

Place of manifestation:	Skin, only seldom on mucosa
Course and prognosis:	Usually spontaneous arrest; spontaneous remission frequent

Systemic sclerodermas (progressive systemic sclerosis)

Place of manifestation:	Connective tissue structures and organ parenchyma
Course and prognosis:	Unpredictable; usually protracted, however also lethal

Circumscribed scleroderma (ICD-DA 701.0 and 701.00)

This disease, usually appearing in early adulthood and preferentially in women, starts with the formation of spotlike, reddish inflammations. After the erythema decreases, there is development of a yellow-white, discoid, firm lesion in the center of the inflammation. At the periphery of this ivory-colored irreversible change is a blue-violet ring ("lilac ring"). The oral mucosa is seldom involved. When it is involved, a circumscribed atrophic zone forms on the dorsum of the tongue.

There is a special form of circumscribed facial scleroderma, of interest to the dentist. It is perpendicular to the eyebrows, extending from the forehead to the hairline, and is usually a paramedially located groovelike depression of the connective tissue. This finding is known as *scleroderma en coup de sabre*. It can also appear more laterally or on the chin. Its relation to progressive hemifacial atrophy is discussed (Fig. 30-29).

Regarding differential diagnosis, there must initially be differentiation from chronic erythema migrans. The duration of the disease course, which is not influenced by therapy, is uncertain. Circumscribed scleroderma generally comes to a standstill after some years. Spontaneous regressions have also been observed. The prognosis in general is good.

Systemic sclerosis (ICD-DA 710.1 and 710.10)

This rare systemic disease of the connective tissue structures and blood vessels of the skin and parenchymal organs increases in frequency with age. Three to four times more women are affected than men. There are different forms of progressive systemic sclerosis with several variants. We will limit discussions to:

- Acrosclerosis
- Diffuse sclerosis
- Visceral sclerosis

Acrosclerosis is particularly important for the dentist. A characteristic early symptom and/or accompanying symptom of this disease is ischemia in the fingers due to cold *(Raynaud's phenomenon)*. The phenomenon appears in three phases with signs of painful ischemia, local cyanosis, and arterial hyperemia. Acrosclerosis is more frequent in the fingers. Vasomotor pain in relation to Raynaud's phenomenon follows development of a pasty swelling. Eventually, it is impossible to form a skin fold over the underlying tissue because the skin is tight, tense, waxy, and shiny. Sclerotic shrinkage causes clawlike hand contractures, which finally lead to a lack of function of the hand (Fig. 30-9). There is damage to the fingernails; in the area of the fingertips are small, persistent foci of necroses ("rat bite necrosis"). Later stump formation is possible.

Acrosclerosis manifests in the face with similar frequency. The fully developed disease picture shows characteristic masklike rigid facial features (Figs. 30-7 and 30-9), which are caused by tightly atrophic, shiny, pale skin distended over the bones. The nose becomes pointed, the skin of the cheeks appears wrinkled, the lips become thin, and the oral cavity decreases in size (i. e., *microstomia*–Fig. 30-8). Pigment disturbances (i. e., hyperpigmentation and telangiectasia) are the rule.

The oral mucosa may also be involved, with sometimes impressive pathologic changes. Initial bleeding disturbances with livid discoloration and edema are followed by tissue fibrosis, which finally develops into atrophic conditions and spontaneous amputation phenomena. The formerly movable mucosa is now white-yellowish and adherent to the lower layers. There is progressive sclerosis of the tongue and salivary glands and of the lymphatic throat ring, which leads to severe loss of function *(microglossia, xerostomia* with chewing, swallowing and speech disturbances). Disturbance in motility in the zone of the esophagus further increases the difficulty of eating.

In *diffuse scleroderma* and *visceral sclerosis*, the manifestions in the internal organs are the most important clinical findings. These forms show certain similarities with systemic lupus erythematosus. An early intraoral symptom of systemic scleroderma is the shortening and hardening of the tongue frenum (Fig. 30-10). The early participation of periodontal connective tissue manifests as a radiographically demonstrable enlargement of the desmodontal fissure. Other possible causes for this occurrence must be carefully ruled out by the dentist. There are also frequent reports of gingival recession.

The certainty of the diagnosis is obtained from the clinical picture, the demonstration of antinuclear antibodies, and the histologic findings. The course of systemic sclerosis cannot be predicted because the disease varies in severity and rate of progression. With the appearance of visceral changes (in the heart, lungs, and kidneys), the prognosis becomes poor.

Dermatomyositis (ICD-DA 710.3 and 710.30)

Dermatomyositis is a degenerative inflammatory systemic disease of the skin and musculature. Clinical course (usually with slow chronic progression but sometimes acute with remission phases) and disease symptoms can vary. The musculature may be affected without the skin being involved *(polymyositis)*. The autoimmunologic changes in the blood vessel connective tissue explain the involvement of the visceral organs (heart, lungs, digestive system, kidneys). Overlap with other autoimmune diseases can occur.

All age groups are affected, but primarily affected are children, women, and adults between 40 and 60 years. In about 20% of adults, there is coexistence with malignant tumors (carcinomas of the gastrointestinal tract, bronchi, breast, prostate; and lymphomas), hence dermatomyositis is considered a *"paraneoplastic syndrome."* The influence of the malignancies on the course of the systemic connective tissue disease is fairly obvious, and the dermatomyositis can regress after removal of the neoplasm and reappear when there are tumor recurrences.

Clinical signs include muscle and joint pain, weight loss, and often fever. Dermatomyositis leads to muscular weakness (primarily in the proximal area) with resulting limitation of movements. If the striated musculature of the pharynx or the upper part of the esophagus is involved, there is the possibility of dysphagia.

On the skin of the face (a typical place is the periorbital region), the neck, the nape of the neck, and the upper breast, there is development of spotty or more macular wine-red to violet edematous areas that later change into erythemas (Fig. 30-11). Occasionally the efflorescences of the face are in the form of butterflies, as in lupus erythematosus. The lilac-colored skin changes (therefore the name "lilac disease") later fade and leave atrophies, telangiectases, and abnormalities of skin pigmentation. Subacute calcium deposits (calcinosis) are possible. In every fourth patient the oral mucosa shows dark red, painful erythemas that may change into ulcerations.

The etiology of dermatomyositis is unknown. Results of new tests have given additional support for the existence of an autoimmune reaction that may also be related to the tumor. Participation of viruses in the pathogenesis is possible.

Diagnosis of the disease is based on clinical findings (weakness of proximal muscles, skin eruptions), histopathologic changes in the biopsy material, elevation of muscle enzyme levels in the serum, and abnormalites of the electromyogram. The prognosis of dermato-myositis/polymyositis is more favorable in children than in adults, but the disease is always serious.

Sjögren's syndrome; sicca syndrome (ICD-DA 710.2 and 710.20)

Sjögren's syndrome is a chronic disease progressing in stages. It is an inflammatory degenerative autoimmune disease characterized by autoimmune insufficiency of many exocrine glands as well as symptoms suggestive of rheumatoid arthritis (chronic polyarthritis). If the disease affects only eyes and mouth (dryness of the mucosa), it is called *sicca syndrome*. Every second patient with Sjögren's syndrome initially shows sicca symptomatology *(primary Sjögren's syndrome)*. In *secondary Sjögren's syndrome*, the sicca symptoms are associated with symptoms of other autoimmune diseases, such as rheumatic arthritis, systemic lupus erythematosus, systemic scleroderma, or other autoimmune diseases (in decreasing frequency). Every tenth patient with rheumatoid arthritis develops Sjögren's syndrome in the course of the disease. Patients with Sjögren's syndrome are at greater risk for lymphoma than is the general population.

Sjögren's syndrome appears most frequently in menopausal and postmenopausal women. It is presently thought that the disease is based on an exaggerated polyclonal activation of B lymphocytes. This leads to deposition of pathologic immunocomplexes in different tissues, resulting in inflammatory reactions and tissue destruction. In 60% to 100% of patients, one finds antinuclear antibodies. Further on, it is possible to find antibodies against the cytoplasm of the epithelium of the salivary gland ducts (30% to 60% of patients), against pancreas cells (20% to 40%), against smooth muscle (20% to 40%), against liver cell membranes (5% to 25%), against thyroid microsomes (10% to 20%), and against striated musculature (up to 10%), whereby the manifold possibilities of organ participation can be explained.

Initially the disease is insidious with progressive greater involvement of the glands of external secretion; the mucosa is dry and becomes atrophic. The expected damage due to inflammatory complications is initially slight, possibly because the B-cell hyperactivity results in increased synthesis of IgA.

Predominant features of the clinical picture in primary Sjögren's syndrome is dessication of the sclera and cornea due to decreased secretion of tears *(xerophthalmia* with *keratoconjunctivitis sicca)* and dryness of the oral mucosa because of diminishing saliva secretion *(xerostomia).* Lips and tongue (Fig. 30-12) are also dry and have an atrophic, shining surface that is covered with sticky, retained mucous rests and crusts. Erosions appear after removal of the deposits. There is development of rhagades but not only in the area of the corner of the mouth (Fig. 30-12).

In one-third of patients there is chronic enlargement of the parotid salivary glands with a tendency to develop stones in the duct system. Destruction of hard tooth substance due to the change in the oral environment occurs in time. Sjögren's syndrome can lead to loss of taste and smell.

With participation of the nasopharynx and larynx, there are problems of swallowing and speech as well as hoarseness. In advanced stages, the dryness of the oral cavity can be so severe that normal eating is severely limited, and finally pain makes it impossible. The mucosa of the bronchi, the vulva, and the vagina can also exhibit symptoms of sicca. As in other autoimmune diseases, the visceral manifestations determine the general course of the disease.

Sjögren's syndrome is clinically obvious when the classic symptoms (dryness of the mouth and eyes, rheumatic joint pain) exist. The qualitative determination of reduced saliva does not allow diagnostic conclusions for an early sicca syndrome. In this context, it must be considered that many general diseases, untoward drug reactions, and psychologic influences can lead to dry mouth or can give the patient the feeling of decreased saliva secretion (that is, ropy, gluey saliva). More relevant, but not diagnostic, is the decrease in flow of tears. Important signs are manifest by the great immunologic activity of the blood serum. The diagnosis is determined histologically by excision biopsy of the easy-to-find small salivary glands of the lips (atrophy of the glandular tissue with focal infiltrates of lymphocytes and plasma cells).

The dentist must use prophylactic measures against caries and periodontal disease to reduce the inevitable effects of mouth dryness; advise the patient regarding necessary, tooth-saving nutrition; and acquaint the patient with the use of artificial saliva.

Polyarteritis nodosa (ICD-DA 446.0)

Polyarteritis nodosa belongs to a larger group of allergic-hyperergic vasculites. Despite the fact that polyarteritis nodosa is a disease that does not have major importance in the dental field, its important signs must be discussed to better understand two other diseases of the same nosologic group.

It is a febrile systemic disease of middle-sized arteries that show segmental necrotizing inflammation of the vessel walls. It preferentially starts in the media of the bifurcation of the vessels and then extends to the intima and adventitia. There is a progressive swelling of the layers of the vessel walls and a proliferation of the intima. The resulting closure of the vessel lumen leads to decreased blood circulation, formation of thrombi, ischemic lesions, and tissue necrosis. Because each arterial region can have the disease, the clinical picture is determined by the location and seriousness of the vascular damage. Most frequently affected are kidneys, heart, central nervous system, and gastrointestinal tract, but any other organ can be affected. Because of the variety of organs that can be affected, the clinical signs are sometimes confusing. In about every fifth patient there are also skin changes (e. g., bleeding, signs of inflammation, and necrosis).

The cause of the disease, which starts at the age of 40 or 50 and is three times more frequent in men than in women, is not completely known. An immune reaction is assumed because there is accumulation of immunocomplexes and complement components in the altered vessels. Viral infections (particularly hepatitis B), foreign proteins, and medications have been considered as initiating antigens.

The course is acute, subacute, or chronic; the prognosis, despite today's therapeutic measures, is very serious. Untreated cases usually end in death within a short time.

Giant cell arteritis (temporal) and Wegener's granulomatosis are two disease pictures that currently belong to the group of polyarteritis nodosa diseases.

Giant cell arteritis (ICD-DA 446.5); temporal arteritis (ICD-DA 446.50)

Giant cell arteritis is considered a variation of polyarteritis nodosa. The disease is based on a giant cell granulomatous inflammation, which develops in the intima and media of the larger arteries. It starts with inflammatory thickening of the intima, leading to a decrease and finally displacement of the blood vessel lumen with the clinical consequence of partial or complete arterial closure. Giant cell arteritis is a typical disease of aging. It usually appears only after the sixth decade and increases in frequency with increased age. Women are four times more frequently affected than men. The incidence in Europe is 3 to 12 cases a year per 100,000 inhabitants. Every large artery can be affected. Favored are the small and middle-sized branches of the carotid arteries, and particularly the cranial vessels (most frequently the temporal and occipital arteries).

The disease starts insidiously or acutely with generalized prodromal symptoms such as migraine-type pain, subfebrile temperature, loss of appetite, and depression. Initial symptoms can give the picture of an influenza infection. The unilateral or bilateral drilling or throbbing headache (usually increased at bedtime) can be associated with dizziness, hemiparesis, and eye symptoms. Palpation discloses a hardened, pulsating cord in the area of the temporal artery (Fig. 30-13) in 40% of cases. The clinical diagnosis must be confirmed by biopsy (histology: giant cell arteritis). Depending on location, arterial closure can create different complications. There is possible development in the cranial vessels of a cerebral insult, blindness (usually both eyes), or even an infarct of the soft tissues. In the area of the masticatory musculature and the tongue, there can be ischemic necrosis (Fig. 30-14) under physiologic stress with the appearance of pain (claudication). Early initiation of therapy with corticosteroids is promising.

Wegener's granulomatosis (ICD-DA 446.4 and 446.40)

Wegener's granulomatosis is considered one of the diseases in the group of polyarteritides nodosa. It is a disease of unknown origin and may be found in young adults. The disease may have an insidious or acute course with localized granulomatous inflammation, particularly of the upper respiratory tract. Two of three patients complain of symptoms in the area of the nasal passages (chronic, therapy-resistant, crusty, slightly bleeding rhinitis, as well as sinusitis), which often are associated with a general feeling of malaise often with fever and weight loss.

After some weeks or months, the disease may enter a generalized phase. There is development of a disseminated necrotizing granulomatous vasculitis of the small arteries, capillaries, and veins. An initially focal glomerulitis quickly becomes a diffuse glomerulonephritis. The resulting progressing kidney insufficiency is the main point of the disease and determines the course progress. Lung manifestations are generally ill-defined infiltrates, inflammatory necrotizing skin changes are frequent, and other organ participation is possible. Oral mucosa syndromes are generally absent in the beginning and are usually associated symptoms of the generalized stage of the disease (Figs. 30-15 and 30-16). Destruction of cartilage and bone is only rarely observed.

The histologic picture is typical (epithelioid cells, Langerhans' cells, foreign body giant cells). Deposits of immunocomplexes are demonstrated in blood vessels and glomeruli. The diagnosis is made from the combination of patient history and clinical, radiographic, histopathologic and immunologic findings. Demonstration of antibodies against cytoplasmic parts of neutrophilic granulocytes (ANCA = anti neutrophil cytoplasmic antibodies) is important.

With modern therapeutic possibilities (immunosuppressive agents and corticosteroids), it is possible to improve the poor prognosis and in some cases even to obtain long-lasting remissions. In most cases the prognosis is unfavorable.

Diseases without nosologic classification

In the following section certain diseases without nosologic classification, whose etiopathology is totally unknown, will be discussed. Certain similarities exist among these conditions which, despite the predominating single clinical symptoms, can be considered systemic diseases. Further, the oral cavity and/or the perioral region show, in these cases, characteristic and predominant manifestations of diagnostic significance.

Lethal midline granuloma, malignant granuloma (ICD-DA 446.3 and 446.30)

In the past, malignant granuloma and Wegener's granulomatosis were considered the same disease. The separate listing of malignant granuloma today appears to be justified because there are the following differences with respect to Wegener's granulomatosis:

- The disease is not based on a disseminating (autoimmune) vasculitis
- Tissue necrosis begins in the connective tissue and leads to extensive soft tissue, cartilage, and bone destruction
- Kidney and lungs are not primarily involved in the disease
- According to new knowledge, some cases represent a highly malignant non-Hodgkin's lymphoma (T-cell type)

The rare, usually deadly, destructive lesion is observed mostly in middle-aged individuals, and in men twice as frequently as in women. The preferred location is in the nasal cavities and palate.

The months-long prodromic phase starts with intermittent, nonspecific nasal, oral, or facial complaints and is accompanied by noncharacteristic systemic changes such as tiredness, lack of appetite, fever, weight loss, and headaches. The patients often complain of a persistent cold with hampered nasal breathing and purulent discharge. Intraoral development consists of a painless or near-painless firm swelling that later ulcerates (Fig. 30-18), usually found on the mucosa of the hard palate (seldom on other parts of the maxilla or retromolar area).

The subsequent active disease phase consist of enlargement of the lesion, which undergoes necrosis and is associated with a penetrating, sweet-fetid smell. The mildly painful necrotizing process proceeds without stopping in the connective tissue and results in severe soft tissue and bone destruction (Figs. 30-17, 30-19, and 30-20). Depending on the primary location, the malignant granuloma destroys either the palate or nose and perinasal region over the palate starting at the base of the nose. In two of three patients, the palate is primarily or secondarily involved in the course of the disease and the changes are not always in the midline ("midline granuloma"). In advanced stages, the lesion develops into a noma-like destruction of the midface.

High doses of antibiotics as well as surgical interventions are usually useless. Radiation therapy is presently thought to be the most appropriate means of delaying or bringing the disease process to a standstill. Most patients die of cachexia or sepsis.

Regarding differential diagnosis, necrotizing ulcerative stomatitis (an intraoral initial finding) and the very rare noma must be considered together with Wegener's granulomatosis and the highly malignant non-Hodgkin's lymphomas and carcinomas (see chapter 19, Figs. 19-27 and 19-28).

Langerhans' cell histiocytosis (e. g., eosinophilic granuloma)

Within the concept of Langerhans' cell histiocytosis, there are three diseases characterized by the proliferation of histiocytes and belonging to the group of histiocytic diseases. These are Letterer-Siwe disease (acute disseminating histiocytosis), Hand-Schüller-Christian disease (chronic disseminating histiocytosis), and eosinophilic granuloma (local histiocytosis. Their most important signs are presented in summary form.

Letterer-Siwe disease (ICD-DA 202.5X or M 9722/3)

Age of presentation:	Newborns and small children
Histology:	Diffuse proliferation of lipid-rich histiocytes (neoplastic)
Course:	Acute, generalized, sepsislike; many organs participate (skin, mucosa, internal organs, bones); panmyelopathy due to bone marrow involvement
Prognosis:	Fatal

Hand-Schüller-Christian disease (ICD-DA 227.8)

Age of presentation:	Almost only children and growing youths
Histology:	Granuloma-type histiocytic lesion with eosinophilic granulocytes; later foam cells and fibrosis
Course:	Chronically progressing, disseminating; multiple osteolytic bone lesions throughout the skeleton possible; skull bones preferentially involved; the classical symptom triad: "geographic skull," exophthalmus (due to involvement of the orbit), diabetes insipidus (due to participation of the sella turcica), not infrequently involvement of the lymph nodes and internal organs (liver and spleen) Oral: from mucosal changes (bumpy or diffusely enlarged gingiva) up to destruction of the alveolar bone and lost teeth
Prognosis:	The younger the patient, the less favorable; death in about half of cases

Eosinophilic granuloma (ICD-DA 227.8)

Age of presentation:	After growth, particularly young men
Histology:	Polymorphocellular granulation tissue among other eosinophilic granulocytes; spontaneous healing with fibrosis possible

Course:	Local; mildest form among the diseases of the Langerhans' cell histiocytosis group. Chronic with solitary or multifocal osteolysis, particularly in flat bones such as top of the skull, mandible, ribs. Usually no evidence of systemic disease
Prognosis:	Good; local complications (pathologic fracture) possible

Only the eosinophilic granuloma of the jaws will be discussed in depth.

Eosinophilic granuloma of the jawbones; oral manifestations (ICD-DA 277.80)

Despite the similarity of name, there are no similarities with the *facial eosinophilic granuloma*, which appears in the form of a single or multiple focus of granulation tissue only on the face. Eosinophilic granuloma can affect either jaw, but it appears more frequently in the mandible. Frequently there are solitary osteolytic processes, which are located *centrally* or *peripherally*. Foci located in the central portion of the bone are usually discovered accidentally via radiography. They appear radiologically as sharply circumscribed round or oval cystlike areas or as more spotty transparencies with fuzzy border contours. The peripheral (alveolar) location (Figs. 30-21 to 30-23) appears as an expanded, irregular, horizontal, vertical, and circumapical bone destruction. Also, after loss of the involved tooth, these lesions remain in the radiographic picture as a half-round, light area not associated with the empty alveolus.

Expanding changes in the oral mucosa appear only in the alveolar forms of the eosinophilic granulomas. The diseases process that occurs in the alveolar process can appear as a progressive, deep, marginal periodontitis (Figs. 30-21 and 30-22). One can observe mucosal-bone defects (Fig. 30-23) or "cookie cutter" ulcerations on the periosteum of the fixed oral mucosa; the dental support apparatus is initially spared.

Eosinophilic granuloma does not stop progressing with tooth extraction—which is often done for lack of knowledge of the underlying bony defect—or after spontaneous exfoliation of the tooth, but often continues with progressive destruction in the jaw. In these cases, there is danger of a pathologic fracture.

To quickly confirm the clinical suspicion of eosinophilic granuloma, histologic examination of a biopsy specimen is necessary. Despite a few cases of spontaneous healing described in the literature, a waiting attitude is nondefensible. The most appropriate treatment decision can be made after evaluating the results of the general examination. In the case of single lesions, one can consider the enucleation of the solitary focus and eventually radiation therapy. When multiple bones are involved, cytostatic and corticosteroid medication may be used.

Melkersson-Rosenthal syndrome (ICD-DA 351.8X)

This disease, characterized by a classical clinical triad of recurring facial swelling, facial paresis (only in one-third of all cases), and a furrowed tongue (in less than half of the cases), is rarely observed. Incomplete (monosymptomatic and oligosymptomatic) forms are more the rule than the exception. They manifest primarily in the lip and oral mucosa. There is a large number of variable, accompanying symptoms, which emphasize the systemic character of this edema-associated, recurring granulomatosis. Melkersson-Rosenthal syndrome often appears only with single episodes but is able to generalize into chronically recurring courses. What was originally considered a separate condition and called *Miescher's cheilitis granulomatosa* is today incorporated into Melkersson-Rosenthal syndrome based on the consensus of clinicians and histologists.

The disease starts with recurring lip swellings and/or facial swellings (in decreasing frequency occurring on cheeks, eyelids, forehead, chin, in some cases, half of the face or all of the face) or it starts with a recurring, usually unilateral, peripheral facial paresis. In about every fourth patient are concurrent facial paralysis and swelling.

The changes on the lip and adjacent soft tissue areas (*cheilitis granulomatosa*, Figs. 30-24, 30-26, and 30-27) are characterized by a sudden and usually prodromataless, painless, circumscribed or relatively diffuse swelling of pillowlike soft, elastic consistency. The unilateral or bilateral swelling of the lips, often associated with a reddening of the adjacent skin, remains for several days and then regresses. After an interval of varied duration (weeks, months, or even years), there are recurrences, often in the same location. With each new episode the swelling loses some of its intermittent character and finally persists. However, it can be permanent from the beginning and enlarge over time. In severe cases, the *macrocheilia* can lead to trunk formation (tapir snout).

The oral mucosa can be involved. On the cheek mucosa are coarse humpback enlargements with formation of lobes and furrows and on the mucosa of the hard palate hard nodular elevations. With participation of the tongue *(granulomatous glossitis)*, there is *macroglossia* (Fig. 30-25). Associated edematous enlargement of the gingiva *(granulomatous gingivitis)* is not rare in the anterior region (Fig. 30-28).

The histologic substrate of the swelling is made up of a diffuse edema of the interstitial connective tissue with interspersed, nonconfluent, epithelioid cell granulomas as well as lymphocyte nodules. There are many neurologic, psychiatric, ophthalmologic, otorhinolaryngologic, or visceral symptoms associated with the already described disease picture. The diagnosis of Melkersson-Rosenthal syndrome is only possible clinically from evaluation of the course, and therefore, retrospectively.

The syndrome manifests itself primarily in young patients and affects both sexes equally. The etiopathology is, so far, unexplained, and there are many arguments for a polyetiologic disease. It is suspected that there is a basic congenital constitutional predisposition or local vasomotor dysfunction upon which microbial damage or allergic reactions can precipitate the disease. A possible association with Crohn's disease is being considered.

In the symptomatic treatment, corticosteroids are used systemically or injected into the foci. Some authors also suggest surgical repair of the foci. A persisting macrocheilia can be corrected surgically from the mucosal side. The prognosis of the syndrome is not serious regarding life expectancy; however, it is very guarded in relation to the cosmetic consequences.

The dentist's first responsibility is to include this disease in the differential diagnosis and when in doubt to search for further clarification and to initiate a referral. Knowledge of Melkersson-Rosenthal syndrome, the patient's history, and the clinical picture should protect against misdiagnoses because granulomatous cheilitis could be confused with secondary inflammation and edema of the lip due to dental disease (inflammatory infiltration or collateral inflamed edema–see chapter 6, Fig. 6-12). Regarding differential diagnosis, there are also: stasis edema as a consequence of a chronically recurring facial erysipelas (see chapter 7), with transitory appearance of a Quincke's edema (see chapter 31, Fig. 31-18), a pressure urticaria (see chapter 31, Fig. 31-44), and lymphangiomas.

Hemifacial atrophy (ICD-DA 744.80)

The etiology and nosologic position is still unknown for this very rare disease, which generally affects half of the face or a part thereof and is characterized by a slowly progressing noninflammatory atrophy. The forehead and eyes remain unaffected. It is thought that this is a nevoid defective development.

After frequent occurrence of neuralgiform, facial pain, there is development in the temple-cheekbone area of an initially spotty depigmented or hyperpigmented thinning of the skin. This slowly increases in size on the surface and becomes more depressed. In the nearly asymptomatic course, there can be paramedial development of a semilunar atrophy or scar such as can form in circumscribed scleroderma. Skin and underlying muscle and bone can be affected by this process. With participation of the jawbone is the possibility of a noticeable asymmetry of the facial skeleton (Fig. 30-29). The skin is often atrophic and distended and the sweat secretion locally decreased.

In most cases, the progressive facial hemiatrophy starts in the first or second year of life. With the early start of the disease, there is a delay of dental development and eruption in the affected side of the jaw. Later there is development of regressive-atrophic changes on the gingiva and marginal periodontium, which always have inflammatory changes and which lead to an increased caries incidence *("half side periodontal disease").* Hemiatrophy of the jawbone also occurs in the alveolar process (Fig. 30-30). There is frequently hemifacial reduction with or without regression of associated papillary relief (Fig. 30-31) on the tongue.

The disease can sometimes affect other body parts on the same side—particularly the neck, chest, and upper arm region. In exceptional cases, it can also spread to the other side.

Spontaneous arrest of the disease is possible at all times. The cause of the progressive facial hemiatrophy is associated with neurotrophic disturbances (of traumatic or inflammatory nature), particularly in the innervation area of the trigeminal nerve. A pathogenetic relationship with circumscribed scleroderma is suspected.

Patients who are concerned about the deformation in the facial area should be advised by competent specialists on the possibility and timing of esthetic plastic-reconstructive surgical intervention.

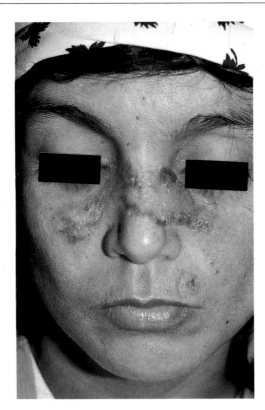

Fig. 30-1   Discoid lupus erythematosus. Typical location in
light-exposed   midface.   The
skin findings characteristically
include erythema, follicular keratosis, and atrophy.

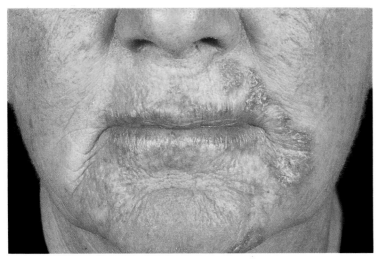

Fig. 30-2   Perioral manifestation of discoid lupus erythematosus. After a long time, there
are atrophic changes and abnormal pigmentation in the center of the foci, while in the border zone of the peripherally
progressing process there is
development of telangiectases.

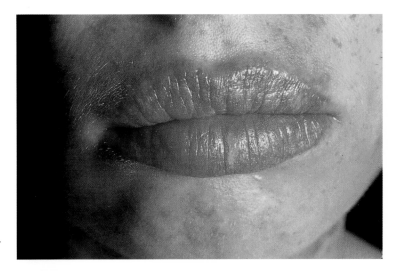

Fig. 30-3   Discoid lupus erythematosus in the lip area.

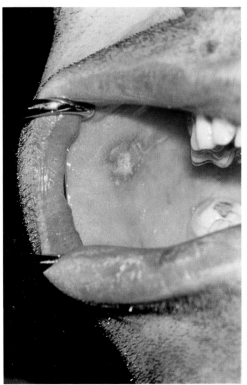

Fig. 30-4   Discoid lupus erythematosus on the right cheek mucosa.

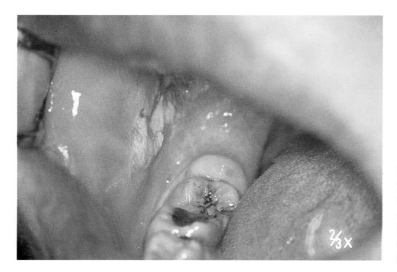

Fig. 30-5   Discoid lupus erythematosus in the area of the
right cheek mucosa. White lines
can be seen as a sign of hyperkeratosis. The border zone
shows   telangiectases   with
points of bleeding.

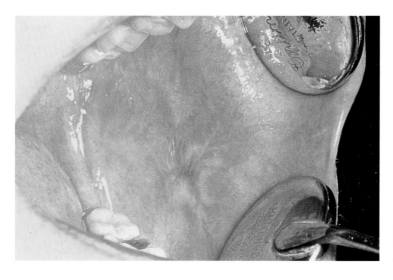

Fig. 30-6   Recurrent discoid
lupus erythematosus on the left
cheek mucosa.

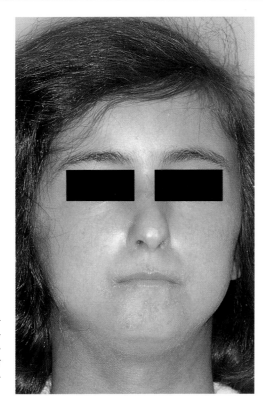

Fig. 30-7   Systemic scleroderma. The masklike facial expression is caused by tight distended atrophic shiny skin over
the facial bones. The nose becomes pointed.

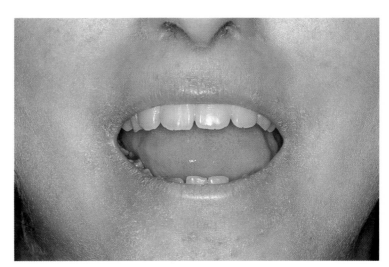

Fig. 30-8   The patient in Fig.
30-7 at the same examination.
The lips are small, and the
mouth opening is distinctly nar-
rowed   (microstomia).   The
tongue is in an advanced
sclerosing process.

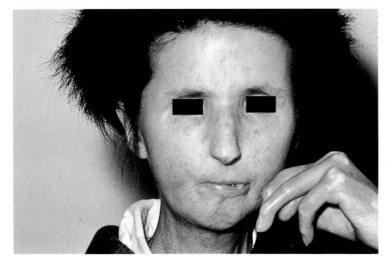

Fig. 30-9   Progressive syste-mic scleroderma in a 34-year-old woman. Condition after sev-eral years. Note the masklike expression of the small pointed face. The sclerosed shiny skin with pigmentary alterations is drawn tautly over the bones. The fingers have become flex-ed by contracture.

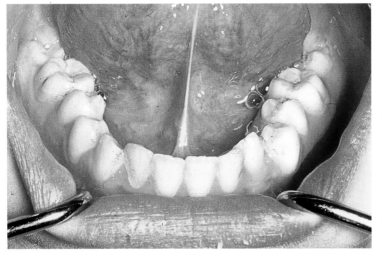

Fig. 30-10   Systemic sclero-derma. Stringy, white, shiny, sclerosing tongue frenum as an early intraoral symptom. The early participation of periodon-tal connective tissue will de-velop into a radiologically identifiable enlargement of the desmodontal fissure, which, however, is a nondiagnostic cri-terion. Laboratory findings im-portant for the diagnosis are the demonstration of antinu-clear antibodies and histologic examination of a biopsy speci-men.

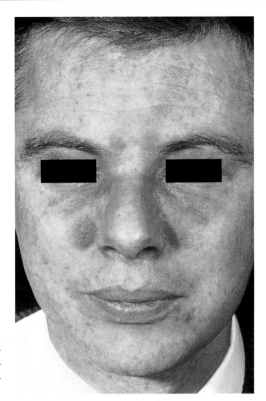

Fig. 30-11 Dermatomyositis. Partially spotty, partially macular wine-red edema that changed into erythema. The face appears slightly bloated.

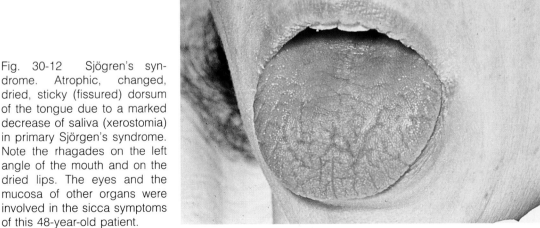

Fig. 30-12 Sjögren's syndrome. Atrophic, changed, dried, sticky (fissured) dorsum of the tongue due to a marked decrease of saliva (xerostomia) in primary Sjörgen's syndrome. Note the rhagades on the left angle of the mouth and on the dried lips. The eyes and the mucosa of other organs were involved in the sicca symptoms of this 48-year-old patient.

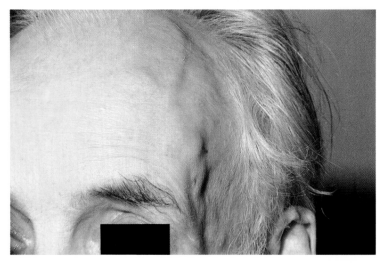

Fig. 30-13 Temporal arteritis. The patient complained of acute throbbing headache and dizziness. The leading diagnostic finding was a hardened, pulseless, temporal artery, a finding observed only in a few cases. The diagnosis must be confirmed histologically (giant cell arteritis) via biopsy. With early recognition and adequate therapy, the disease has a good prognosis.

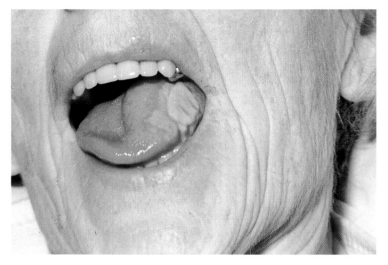

Fig. 30-14 Cranial arteritis with vessel closure and ischemic tissue necrosis in the left half of the tongue of a 74-year-old patient. The infarct was preceded by pain in the tongue, throat, and masticatory musculature of the affected side (claudication). The disease was associated with lack of appetite, weight loss, and depression. Feared complications of an arterial closure in the area of the cranial vessels are sight loss and cerebral damage.

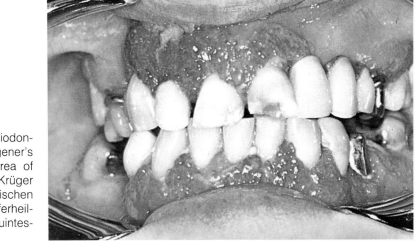

Fig. 30-15 Gingivoperiodontal manifestation of Wegener's granulomatosis in the area of the anterior teeth. (From Krüger E. Lehrbuch der chirurgischen Zahn- Mund- und Kieferheilkunde, vol. 2. Berlin: Quintessenz, 1988.)

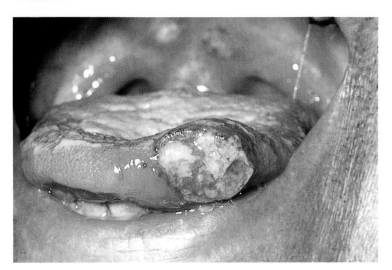

Fig. 30-16 Intraoral manifestation of Wegener's granulomatosis. The 61-year-old patient complained for 3 weeks of hampered nasal respiration and recurring nose bleeds, which were soon followed by a nodular infiltrate on the left border of the tongue as well as other slime-covered ulcerations and necrosis of the oral and throat mucosa. After hematologic disease was excluded, the patient was referred to an internist because of unexplained septic temperatures. The patient died in the clinic after 6 weeks as a consequence of a generalized vascular disease that the available therapy could not influence.

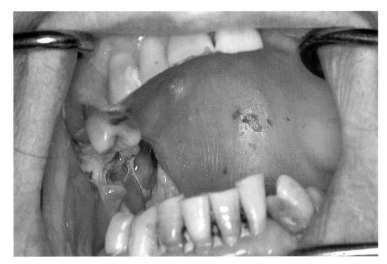

Fig. 30-17 Gangrenous granuloma. This case of necrotizing process in the retromolar region of the right side of the maxilla led to extended nomalike soft tissue and bone destruction.

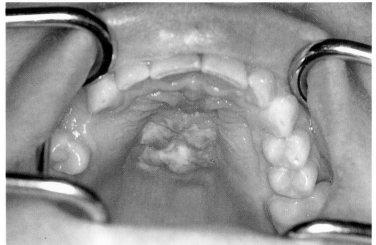

Fig. 30-18 Granuloma gangraenescens (lethal midline granuloma). The 47-year-old woman complained for 4 weeks of weight loss and diffuse pain in the anterior area of the maxilla. Soon after, she noticed the appearance of a slightly painful swelling in the middle of the hard palate from which blood and pus sometimes emptied. The change appears as a exophytic growing, ulcerated tumor. Histologic examination of the biopsy specimen showed necrotizing inflammation and no indication of malignancy.

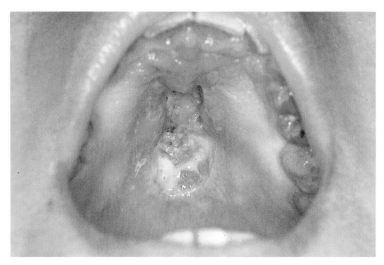

Fig. 30-19 The patient in Fig. 30-18 after 3 weeks. Despite high doses of antibiotics and surgical intervention, it was not possible to stop the progressing necrotizing perforation of the palate. After several biopsies (to exclude diseases such as Wegener's granulomatosis), radiation therapy (cobalt) was initiated and in this manner the lesion was finally halted.

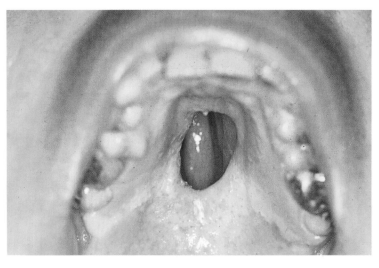

Fig. 30-20 Lethal midline granuloma with destruction of the hard palate in the midline with involvement of the nasal septum. For months, the 45-year-old patient had noticed a nonpainful, slowly enlarging palate perforation with a fetid smell. From the differential diagnostic viewpoint with such a finding and history, one must especially consider a late syphilis (gumma).

Fig. 30-21   Alveolar form of an eosinophilic granuloma in the mandible of a 20-year-old patient. The disease of the alveolar process leads to tooth movement, mobility, and spontaneous exfoliation. The clinical and radiologic changes should not be mistaken for a deep marginal periodontitis. The eosinophilic granuloma does not stop growing after tooth extraction or tooth loss but continues to grow. Note the nonhealing extraction wound 2 months after removal of teeth 41 and 42 (25 and 26).

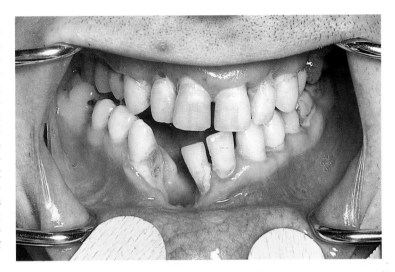

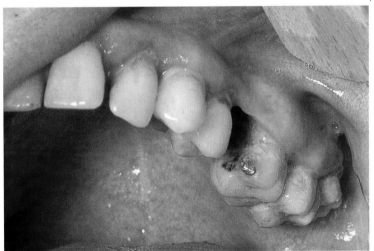

Fig. 30-22   The patient in Fig. 30-21 at the same examination. The radiographic findings show central bone lesions in both jaws. General examination revealed osteolytic processes in the area of the shoulder girdle.

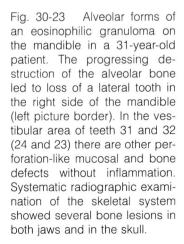

Fig. 30-23   Alveolar forms of an eosinophilic granuloma on the mandible in a 31-year-old patient. The progressing destruction of the alveolar bone led to loss of a lateral tooth in the right side of the mandible (left picture border). In the vestibular area of teeth 31 and 32 (24 and 23) there are other perforation-like mucosal and bone defects without inflammation. Systematic radiographic examination of the skeletal system showed several bone lesions in both jaws and in the skull.

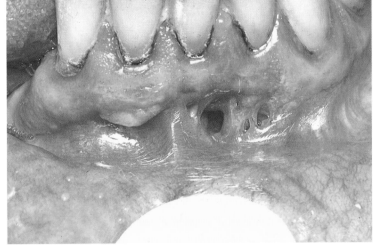

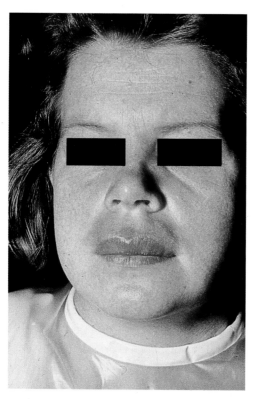

Fig. 30-24 Melkersson-Rosenthal syndrome. Trunklike thickening of the upper lip with reddening of the surrounding skin as well as swelling of the left side of the face. The sudden and unexplained swelling of the upper lip recurred several times and finally became permanent as demonstrated in here.

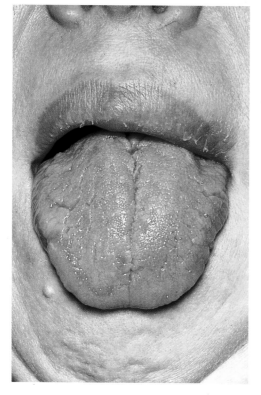

Fig. 30-25 Melkersson-Rosenthal syndrome. Furrowed tongue and early macroglossia caused by granulomatous glossitis with associated granulomatous cheilitis on the left side of the upper lip. The furrowed tongue, which is part of the classic triad of Melkersson-Rosenthal syndrome, is seen only in one-third of cases. The appearance of the tongue is similar to the furrowed tongue seen in constitutionally healthy patients (see chapter 2).

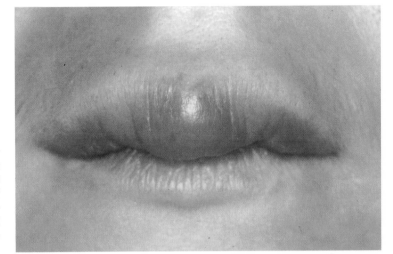

Fig. 30-26   Melkersson-Rosenthal syndrome. Lip swelling from granulomatous cheilitis as a monosymptomatic form of Melkersson-Rosenthal syndrome. (Furrowed tongue and recurring peripheral facial pareses were not present.)

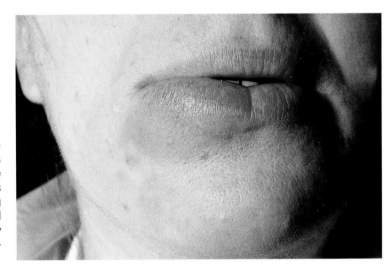

Fig. 30-27   Melkersson-Rosenthal syndrome. Edematous swelling of the right side of the lower lip from granulomatous cheilitis with distinct reddening of the adjacent skin (unrelated contact dermatitis?). After many recurrences, the now stable pillowlike swelling is soft.

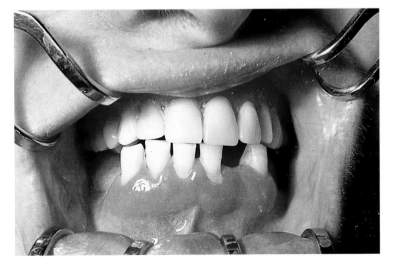

Fig. 30-28   The patient in Fig. 30-27 at the same examination. Concurrent edematous tissue thickening of the gingiva (granulomatous gingivitis) in the vestibular region of the mandibular anterior teeth. The edentulous areas of the mandible are also affected. The mucosa beneath the maxillary full denture is normal.

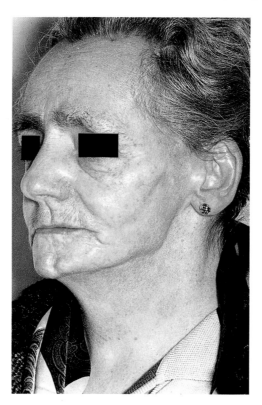

Fig. 30-29 Left-sided progressive facial hemiatrophy of the skull and its covering soft tissues with distinct asymmetry of the face in a 68-year-old woman. Eye and forehead are not affected. For differential diagnosis, circumscribed scleroderma must be considered.

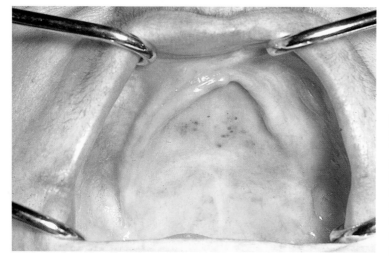

Fig. 30-30 The patient in Fig. 30-29 at the same examination. The appearance of the edentulous maxilla shows related involutive changes after tooth loss and a distinct hemiatrophy of the skeleton. The atrophy did not appear as clinically distinct on the mucosa as it did on the skin (and skin appendages).

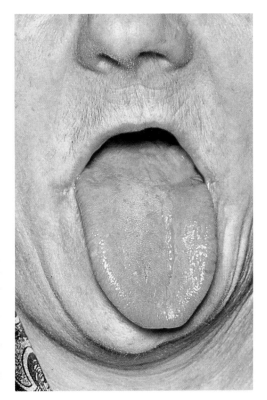

Fig. 30-31 The patient in Figs. 30-29 and 30-30 at the same examination. Based on the hemiatrophy of the musculature, the tongue is unilaterally thinned. In this patient, the perleche-like lesion at the mouth may be due to a too-low occlusion on the complete denture, which was responsible for continuous, nonphysiologic wetting of the corner of the mouth with saliva (see chapter 34).

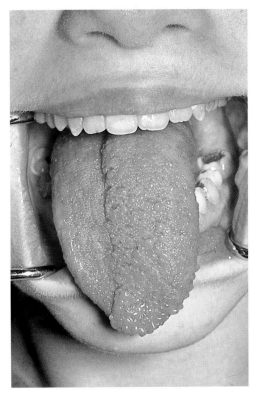

Fig. 30-32 Differential diagnosis of tongue findings in progressive facial hemiatrophy: left side hemihypertrophy of the tongue. The giant growth of half of the tongue associated with an enlargement of the tongue papillae of unknown origin makes the normal right side of the tongue seem atrophic (see chapter 3—phakomatosis).

Chapter 31

Undesirable Drug Reactions

Toxic damage and local tissue reaction to medication and consequences of dental treatment

Increased sensitivity due to dental medications and oral hygiene materials

Pseudoallergic reactions

Allergic reactions to drugs, dental medications, and materials

Other adverse effects of drugs typical for the oral cavity

Drug-induced xerostomia
Drug-induced fibrous gingival hyperplasia
Adverse effects of antibiotic therapy

Even when medications are used according to instructions, any effective medical therapy involves the risk of undesirable side effects. Medications that have no side effects are also of questionable therapeutic value. Some drugs' untoward reactions affect patients as well as the physician or dentist. Since antiquity, there has been a maxim that the risk of a disease must be evaluated carefully in each case against the risk of the drug effect. Today the concept is applied to symptomatic conditions as well as minor diseases to reduce drug treatment as much as possible.

Analgesics and antibiotics play a major role in medication prescription by dentists.

Today's knowledge of side effects and their frequency is known to both patients and dentists from the literature accompanying the medication. The importance of such information in the office, particularly when multiple drugs are used, is evident when prescriptions need to be changed at recall appointments.

The demand for safe medications has increased in the area of self-medications—primarily those drugs used for symptomatic therapy of vague disturbances of general conditions as well as for minor, generally self-healing conditions. In this connection, physicians and dentists must always consider nonprescription medications taken by the patient together with the effects of the medication prescribed. In relation to dental treatment, undesirable side effects have also been described. Dental medications are subject to the advantage-risk ratio and safety should be a high priority, which increasingly leads to a preference for single drug preparations and to the reduction of topical dental medications. The changes in therapy practice in endodontics and periodontics are a good example of this.

For dental materials, the pharmacologic concept of "effectiveness" can be only used conditionally. Because dental materials rest on physical properties, the term "appropriateness" may better apply. This disputable point does not exclude the rare possibility of the appearance of undesirable side effects that can be explained as a antigen-antibody reaction (allergy).

The discussions of toxic damage from dental materials are more speculative than scientific. Definitive restorative materials, which are placed in the oral cavity in plastic condition (amalgam, composite resin, cements) release trace amounts of compounds during hardening. In composite resins and cements, there is leaching of the reaction products. In amalgam, as in any metallic product, components are released by corrosion. The possibility of intoxication by traces of these materials has not yet been demonstrated. Compound damaging from multiple agents is only possible in relation to quantitative data, from scientifically sound precise analysis. However, the quantities discussed here may result in sensitization with ensuing allergic reactions in predisposed individuals. Diagnosis of such an event should be supported by objective symptoms that suggest allergy. Electrochemical side effects are also singled out and described.

Over-the-counter external medications, mouthwashes, and cosmetics can also cause undesirable reactions in the oral cavity and perioral tissues. Identification of the substance responsible requires a complete listing of the products used by patient.

The dentist must be aware of composition and effectiveness when recommending medications and oral hygiene preparations with prescription drugs and changes of prescriptions for the oral cavity.

Toxic damage and local tissue reactions to medication and consequences of dental treatment (ICD-DA 976.7)

There is local medication damage of the skin and mucosa that is *obligatory*—independent of individual reaction—and appears in every person. It is explained by the chemical (physical)-toxic properties of the materials. The effect is dependent on dose, concentration, time, and site of application. The irritation threshold for toxic substances is lower on the oral mucosa than on the skin. With allergic substances, the situation is inverse; the reaction limit of the oral mucosa in relation to skin is considerably higher. The difference between the skin and mucosal reactions results from structural differences of the epidermal and mucosal keratinization as well as from the physiologic differences of the skin and oral mucosal surfaces (lipid coating on the former; saliva covering and stretching during swallowing on the latter). Previous damage to the skin and oral mucosa play a major role in the phenomenon.

Of the many possible chemical-toxic noxious agents, only a few will be discussed. The *damaging effect of arsenic on vessels* causes a slow-onset, painless tissue necrosis that has been used for the devitalization of diseased pulp. Incomplete closure of the cavity, protracted use, or incorrect dosage may possibly create undesirable effects on the tissue by diffusion (Fig. 31-1). Similar damage is known after use of *formaldehyde-containing combination preparations* for devitalization. Through polymerization of the major component, there is a reduction of activity and uneven therapeutic effects after long storage. The use of formaldehyde in root canal treatment leads to overfilling and contact with nerve tissue, resulting in permanent damage.

Acids and other etching substances lead to a *coagulation necrosis* with sharply delimited areas of denaturation of the tissue proteins (Figs. 31-2 to 31-5). By not using vitamin C tablets (ascorbic acid) according to recommendation, a circumscribed erosion of the oral mucosa can result (Fig. 31-9). Bases can cause coalescence and uncontrollable progressive coagulation *necrosis* because of base-protein reaction followed by scar formation. This type of damage often takes place as a consequence of lack of knowledge of the mechanism of action or by a mix-up of concentrations. The use of etching protein precipitating substances and solutions in the treatment of marginal periodontal diseases is considered obsolete today. With repeated use, the inflammatory changes of the gingiva increase rather than improve because of the additional chemical trauma (Figs. 31-3 to 31-5). In addition, there is the danger of the acids acting on dental substances (Fig. 31-5). Self-treatment of gingivitis and marginal periodontitis using astringents has no demonstrable therapeutic effect on the disease course. Depending on concentration and viscosity, the same substances may act as astringent or as etching materials.

Mucosal damage by *phenol derivatives* is dependent on cytotoxic properties (Figs. 31-6 to 31-8). Pharmacologists consider phenol a relic of the Lister era. Its use as a disinfectant is variable in dentistry. In endodontics its selected concentration is based on the need to reach the nonaccessible root canal system with minimal but effective concentrations.

Lesions can be produced by *alcohol-type mouthwashes and alcohol-containing mouth disinfectants* if directions for use are not followed because the medications are prepared based on their hygroscopic properties and have discrete protein denaturing properties. Under certain conditions, serious tissue lesions can be produced (Figs. 31-10 and 31-11). In extreme cases, there are effects that resemble bullous diseases (Fig. 31-11).

Medical/dental prescribed medications can also lead to mucosal damage when incorrectly used by the patient, for example, *acetyl salicylate pain-killing tablets* placed on the cheek mucosa ("aspirin burn," Figs. 31-12 and 31-13). Findings, patient history, and the rapid healing tendency of the surface damage allow a secure differentiation from leukoplakial mucosal changes.

In the perioral region, there have been some cases of toxic skin damage when highly concentrated disinfecting solutions of organic mercury preparations were spilled on the skin during root canal irrigation (Fig. 31-14). These products have since been abandoned. Etching is also possible following an interaction between mercury preparations and halogen ions, metallic aluminium, as well as zinc and their combinations.

In the perioral region, the dentist can also occasionally see the consequences of a phototoxic reaction of the skin after contact with cologne and other bergamot-containing preparations. Furocumarin is the substance responsible for the *photodermatitis (berlogue-dermatitis)*, with an often permanent pigmentation.

Increased sensitivity due to dental medications and oral hygiene materials

It is occasionally difficult to differentiate local tissue reactions caused by increased reactivity of the tissues from obligatory changes. Such local tissue reactions depend on the biologically disturbed irritation threshold and should not be confused with allergy. A well-known example of biologic modifier of the irritation threshold reaction of the skin is sunburn. Also, externally and internally used medications can react differently depending on the individual. Within a population with average reactivity to the drug are smaller groups of persons who have a higher or lower threshold to the drug. In cases of a lower threshold, there can be development of local changes, which are considered "irritations."

It is currently thought that deviations from the standard reaction pattern are genetically determined and are caused by metabolic changes variant from the norm, for instance patients with the very rare glucose-6-phosphate-dehydrogenase deficiency. They develop hemolytic anemia after ingestion of certain medications (e. g., weak analgesics).

Among the externally used dental materials are the *essential oils*, which are irritating (Fig. 31-15) but also act as true allergens. The same is true for many coloring agents and conditioning additives in cosmetic products.

Another important finding for the dentist is *perioral acne*, which is observed after noncritical, protracted external use of corticosteroid-containing products. This is found almost exclusively in women. The change is caused by a complex of medication side effects (steroid acne) and the special condition of the skin in the perioral region.

Irritation of the oral mucosa in exceptional cases is also possible through electrochemical stimuli, which is the result of corroding metals (Figs. 33-12 to 33-14, 33-15 to 33-19). In patients with lichen planus of the oral mucosa, these electrochemical events sometimes are blamed as isomorphic irritation effects.

The frequency of the possibly genetically determined idiosyncrasy, including the individuals who are atopic, is considered to be 10% in the general population. *Atopic* persons are those with an increased allergy risk to drugs. This patient group also tends to have increased occupational skin diseases, which are also an important area of intervention for the dentist.

Pseudoallergic reactions

Pseudoallergic reactions are defined today as undesirable reactions to drugs without previous sensitization—that is, without antibody formation—and without generation of memory cells according to the rules of a true immunologic event. The mechanism is that of the allergic reaction. The clinical appearance cannot be differentiated from true allergy. There is a predominance of anaphylactoid type I-similar cases. Pseudoallergies are not rare. About 30% to 40% of the cases of urticaria are based on them. The underlying factor is probably a genetic predisposition.

Pseudoallergies are also referred to as analgesic intolerance, because all local-acting analgesics and nonsteroid antiphlogistics can create such reactions (for example, under the clinical appearance of an asthma attack—"salicylate asthma"—or an anaphylactoid complication). Preservative materials (PAB, PAB-ether, sorbitol acid, and sulfites) and coloring materials can result in pseudoallergic reactions, as can intravenous application of radiographic contrast media and narcotics.

Allergic reactions to drugs, dental medications, and materials (ICD-DA 995.1 to 995.3; 692)

It is a widely accepted practice to include under "allergy" any exceptional findings that are difficult to interpret without further proof. This unfortunate habit has led to a watering down of the allergic reaction concept and also creates confusion.

Allergy is based on the *antigen-antibody reaction or a reaction of the antigen with specific T-lymphocytes followed by illness.* The original, meaningful protective mechanism of immunization delivers an aberrant reaction to the body, which can vary from harmless itching to shock followed by death. The allergen is, in principle, independent of dosage, independent of the laws of pharmacodynamics, and is substance-specific (substance group specific). Broadening of the list of triggering substance caused by cross reaction or group allergies is possible and is clinically of great importance (paramaterial group allergies: allergy to compounds with benzene ring).

An allergic reaction can only be considered as such when antibodies against antigens exist and are specifically directed against medications or foreign proteins, and antigen-sensitized lymphocytes can be demonstrated in blood. These humoral and cellular phenomena are definitive proof of an antigen-specific immune response against foreign substances.

In dentistry, allergens of low molecular weight play a major role. To this belong, for example, reactive substances from the large group of materials used by the dentists, and metals, as well as a series of medications used in dental practice. To acquire true antigenic properties, these products of low molecular weight, referred to as *haptens*, require coupling with high molecular carrier substances. This includes soluble substances or membrane component glycoproteins, which can be specific for certain medication groups. Requirements for coupling ability with low molecular weight materials are labile and reaction-capable forms. The extent of the affinity depends on the sensitization index of the different substances.

The risk of development of medication-induced allergy depends on the predisposition of the individual, on the allergic potential of the substance, as well as on the form of application, application interval and condition, and also on quantity applied. Concerning the mode of delivery, the risk increases from perioral use to intravenous, intramuscular, subcutaneous, and topical use. Regarding the interval between applications, the risk of allergy in intermittent use is considered higher than in continuous use. Despite the dose-independency rule, there is increased risk with increased quantities because the amount delivered may surpass the threshold level.

In summary, local intermittent use of greater quantities of medication with allergizing potential–for example, antibiotics in external use, surface anesthetic of procaine type–have a very high sensitization risk.

If a drug-induced allergic reaction of systemic, local, or organ dependent type takes place, it is dependent, among other things, on where and in which form the antigen is presented to the immune-competent cells. The specificity of the antigen-antibody reaction has the extraordinary multifaceted clinical appearance of an allergic event. According to individual reactivity, each medication can cause almost any form of allergic reaction. Certain drugs seem to cause more frequent allergic reactions and prefer certain types of reactions. This finding in no way signifies that one can determine the causal agent from the type of allergic reaction. In other words: skin and mucosa allergic manifestations are not medication-specific.

Coombs and Gell in 1963 classified the basic allergic reactions with their corresponding clinical manifestations in four groups (see table on page 679). According to the reaction type, there is development of the effector phase, which as rule is the immunologically induced clinical picture that will be discussed below.

Type I allergic reaction

The immediate anaphylactic reaction (type I) is mediated through humoral antibodies (IgE); the antibodies are localized in mast cells and basophilic cells. Upon re-exposure to the allergen, there is liberation of mediators (H-substances such as histamine, serotonin, and others) that cause vasodilation, increased permeability, and contraction of smooth muscle. To this clinical picture belong: *allergic rhinitis and conjunctivitis, urticaria, Quincke's edema, bronchospasm, bronchial asthma gastrointestinal immediate reaction,* and finally *anaphylactic shock.* The appearance of these phenomena is to be expected within seconds. Causes are medications, food, food additives, foreign proteins (in vaccines, pollen) as well as insect poisons.

Basic allergic reactions*

Type		Participating factors	Location of reaction	Clinical picture
I	Anaphylactic (immediate reaction)	IgE, vasoactive amines	Mast cells and basophilic leukocytes	Urticaria, Quinckes edema, bronchial asthma, gastrointestinal immediate reaction, anaphylactic shock
II	Cytotoxic reaction	IgG, IgM, complement	Cell membranes of blood cells (i. e., platelets, leukocytes)	Granulocytopenia-agranulocytosis, thrombocytopenia/pathy, immunohemolytic anemia, autoimmune diseases
III	Immune complex reaction, Arthus reaction Serum sickness	IgG, IgM, complement, neutrophils	Complement activation in vessels	Allergic vasculitis, pulmonary alveolitis, nephritis, serum disease with fever, arthritis, lyphm node swelling
IV	Cell-mediated tuberculin reaction	T lymphocytes, lymphokines macrophages	T lymphocytes in dermis, in the tissue	Allergic exanthemas, microbial exanthemas, transplantation rejection, autoimmune disease
	Contact dermatitis	T lymphocytes, lymphokines, Langerhans' cells	Langerhans' cells and T lymphocytes	Acute allergic, contact dermatitis, chronic allergic contact eczema, hematogenous allergic contact dermatitis

* Modified from *Coombs RRA, Gell PGH*. Classification of allergic reactions responsible for clinical hypersensitivity and disease. In: *Gell PGH, Cooms RRA. Lachmann PJ* (eds). Clinical Aspects of Immunology, ed 3. Oxford: Blackwell, 1975: 761.

Additional information for the dentist

The best protection in daily dental practice against rare life-threatening events is to obtain a careful patient history ("allergic reactions?") and directed past medication history. Shock and allergic reactions—particularly urticarial reactions—sometimes also appear in association with the area of dental medication therapy (Figs. 31-16 to 31-18). Therapy for shock and allergic reactions can be found in medical and surgical textbooks in dentistry.

Type II allergic reaction

In cytotoxic reactions (type II), humoral IgG and IgM antibodies act with antigens on the cell surface of the blood cells or other cells and membranes (pemphigus and pemphigoid group), leading to complement activation during re-exposure. The result is cell membrane damage and cytolysis. Clinically, this is the picture of *allergic granulocytopenia-agranulocytosis* (see chapter 24), *allergic thrombocytopenia/pathy* (see chapter 25), and *acute immunohemolytic anemias* and of *autoimmune diseases*. The phenomena are almost completely related to medications and develop within a few hours.

In pemphigus vulgaris, there are antibodies against glycoproteins on the squamous cell surface, and in bullous pemphigoid there are antibodies against "pemphigoid-antigens" in the basal membrane, which are triggered by the same mechanism with the characteristic blister formation.

Additional information for the dentist

This type of immunologic complication can also be triggered by dental use of medications (primarily analgesics). With pyrazolone derivatives, the incidence of complications is approximately 1:1,000,000. If after prescribing antipain medication, there is development of undesirable general reactions, the dentist should consider the possibility of an allergic reaction to the medication and demand a careful medical explanation (i.e., blood picture).

Type III allergic reaction

The immune complex reaction (type III) is divided into two clinical forms, the *Arthus type* and the *serum sickness type.* IgG, IgA, and IgM antibodies form immune complexes (i.e., antigen, antibody, and complement components) with the corresponding antigen in proximity to the vessels. Through a complex mechanism of chemotaxis, phagocytosis, and leukocyte cell lysis, there is tissue damage from local enzyme release. The Arthus reaction appears clinically as *vasculitis, nephritis, pulmonary alveolitis, and possibly as Stevens-Johnson syndrome.* The symptoms generally develop within 6 hours (see diagram on page 705).

In serum sickness type, *fever, arthritis, lymph node swelling, and in undesirable cases anaphylactic symptoms* occur 1 to 14 days after the triggering event. Originally, foreign proteins, for example, in vaccines or antisera, protein-containing medications, and deposit of long-acting preparations are blamed. Microbial antigens are also frequent causes.

Additional information for the dentist

Diagnostic certainty of an allergic vasculitis is only possible in cooperation with other specialists. The disease can also appear in the facial skin and oral mucosa (Figs. 31-19 and 31-20).

Stevens-Johnson syndrome is considered a drug-induced allergic variant of erythema exudativum multiforme that is associated with this type of reaction (see chapter 28.)

Type IV allergic reaction

The cell-mediated reaction (type IV) is divided into two types, the *tuberculin type* and the *contact dermatitis type.* The cells involved are sensitized T lymphocytes. The allergic reaction is delayed (about 24 to 72 hours after re-exposure—see diagram on page 705—seldom after longer time).

In the tuberculin type, there is tissue damage caused by release of enzymes. The clinical manifestations include *microbial exanthemas, medication exanthemas, autoimmune diseases,* and *transplantation rejection.* Causes are drugs, microbial antigens, and autoantigens.

In the contact dermatitis type, the antigen is presented through the epidermal Langerhans' cells. This antigen presentation leads to interaction with sensitized T lymphocytes specific for this antigen. From this interaction, there is liberation of lymphokines, which cause a lymphohistiocytic infiltrate of the skin of varying degree of extension and intensity. The typical clinical pictures of this phenomenon are *acute allergic contact dermatitis* and, in case of persistence of the antigen, *chronic allergic contact dermatitis.*

Additional information for the dentist

The greatest number of allergic reactions to medications and dental therapeutic materials fall under type IV. This group, with its different clinical presentations, should therefore be discussed further. The many clinical and morphologic forms of acute *medication exanthemas* are based either on an antigen-antibody reaction of type I or III or an antigen T cell—mediated reaction of type IV. Some forms cannot be definitely assigned to one of the basic reactions described by Coombs and Gell. The exanthemas and enanthemas that resemble the rash of infectious diseases are of types I and III and only infrequently of type IV. Allergic reaction to medication that manifests as a disseminated symmetrically distributed skin eruption resembles scarlet fever, measles, and German measles (scarlatiform, morbiliform, rubeolaform medication exanthemas, see Figs. 31-21 to 31-26). In comparison to the skin reactions, the associated enanthemas on the oral mucosa are clinically much less distinct. The intraoral findings can be so discrete that they can barely be seen on the mucosa of the soft palate (Fig. 31-22).

In sensitized patients, there is such a type IV reaction 2 to 3 days after re-exposure. In rare cases, they can be confused with type I reactions. In nonsensitized individuals there may be development of medication exanthemas after 9 to 18 days' challenge with the drug. Sensitized memory cells remain for life.

In *acute allergic contact dermatitis* and *chronic allergic contact eczema* are inflammatory, noncontagious changes of the skin that are localized both in the vascularized papillary layer of the upper dermis and the vessel-free epidermis. The external antigen triggers the allergic reaction at the site of its penetration. In some cases of *allergic dermatitits,* the antigen is introduced parenterally or in other areas by contact with blood (e.g., endoprosthesis, metal-containing spirals as contraceptive devices, implants). After enough sensitization, there can be development of reactions of the skin, but they are rare.

In addition to the relatively monomorphic and symmetric disseminated findings of exanthemas, there are polymorphic efflorescences in very different combinations, and nonsymmetric distribution by the eczema.

Explanation of the allergic origin and identification of the culprit antigen are functions of the allergist/dermatologist. She or he decides which test is indicated, which allergy should be tested, and in which sequence and concentration. The examination results are recorded in the allergy report.

Typically, contact dermatitis of the skin is caused by disinfectants, adhesives (Fig. 31-38), rubber-containing materials (gloves), and substances in disposable mouthguards (Fig. 31-39).

Important in the dental field are metal ions (nickel, chrome, cobalt, mercury), composite resins, topical anesthetics, and essential oils (e.g., clove oil). The allergic predisposition of the patient as well as those of the dentist and his or her coworkers can be increased through previous damage of the skin, which facilitates percutaneous resorption of the potential antigens. Facilitating factors in such an event are soaps and cleaning materials (wash trauma). The current use of protective gloves has decreased the incidence of allergic contact eczemas on the fingers of dentists. But new problems must be taken into consideration due to the development of allergy to vulcanization products and rubber and latex gloves. Sometimes an allergic contact eczema in the lower lip/chin region can develop when there is leakage over the skin of saliva admixed with medications introduced in the oral cavity (Figs. 31-31 and 31-32).

Despite the larger resorptive capacity of the oral mucosa, under similar exposure, with some exceptions, allergic reactions of the mucosa are distinctly weaker than skin reactions, or may even be completely absent. Reddening or a slight, passing edema on the oral mucosa may be observed as a sign of allergic reaction and often is clinically limited to a small area that can barely be distinguished from the surroundings. When placed in the oral cavity, free antigens (e.g., in certain medications for wound repair—antibiotics, sulfonamides, surface anesthetics, iodoform), metallic portions of restorative materials and dental materials, and by-products of composite materials do not cause an actual reaction on the oral mucosa; however, these substances, when in contact with the skin in the perioral region or in other skin-covered areas, result in an impressive allergic contact dermatitis (Figs. 31-27 to 31-30, 31-33 to 31-35, 31-36 and 31-37).

Regarding the clinically detectable intensity of the allergic manifestations of the skin and oral mucosa, there is also no parallel, despite their identical etiopathogenesis. The response threshold of the oral mucosa is considered to be five to 12 times higher than that of the skin. Therefore, the conclusions obtained with intraoral test methods (epimucosal test) are unreliable.

Reactive products in composite resins (particularly polyester based) can result in local intolerance of allergic origin in patients and in the dentist (Figs. 31-40 to 31-42). Causes for allergy are sulfonic acid esters of different chemical structure. They act as catalysts in dental materials of epoxy resins for provisional crowns and fixed partial dentures as well as compound impression materials of polyether-rubber base. Cross allergies against different chemical structure catalysts are known. In general, allergic reactions to composite resins, restorations, and provisional restorations are rare. They take place far less frequently than patients and sometimes dentists assume. These reactions are even more uncommon in prostheses constructed of composite resins. There is, however, a higher incidence of allergy to the many materials that contain nickel. The reason for this is considered to be earlier sensitization by nickel-containing jewelry (e.g., ear studs).

Exceptions are the *fixed drug eruptions* of unknown pathogenesis, which are probably type IV and which appear on the oral mucosa. With renewed antigen supply is recurrence of a local reaction in the form of a distinctly circumscribed edematous spot always in the same area (Fig. 31-43), which later can become an area of hyperpigmentation. The cause of the limited reaction with lack of generalization continues to be unclear.

In dentistry, it is significant that a substance-specific antigen-antibody reaction can develop in a *substance group specific allergy.* It is also important that a known example is the paramaterial group allergy, that is, the allergy to medications the chemical substance of which is based on a benzene ring with para-positioned reactive (NO_2-, NH_2- or OH groups). This configuration appears in many medications (derivatives of p-amino benzoic acid as local anesthetic, sulfonamides, aniline derivatives, preservative materials).

There are also *cross allergy groups* to certain antibiotics as well as metals. There is also *polyvalent allergy* with sensitization to completely different chemical substances. The essence of allergies with their different reaction forms have been discussed to call attention to the possible dental side effects when planning and completing treatment procedures. There is also the possibility of substituting or omitting those medications and treatment materials that can endanger the patient. This demands knowledge of the composition as well as the interactions of medications and stresses the need for a careful use of medication in the attempt to avoid allergic complications and treatment risks.

If there is suspicion of an existing allergy from prior events (history of allergic conditions), the culprit substance must be avoided in the future.

Other adverse effects of drugs typical for the oral cavity

Drug-induced xerostomia (ICD-DA 527.71)

To objectively substantiate the symptoms of dry mouth is a difficult problem for the dentist. The amount of saliva normally secreted varies greatly. The complex events determined by the central nervous system show not only a distinct day-night rhythm but a great influence from outside conditions. The sight of something appetizing induces a "mouth-watering" sensation; with a scare, "spit" dries up and viscous saliva leaves us with the sensation of a gummy tongue. A foreign body in the oral cavity increases saliva secretion. These individual and situation-conditioned physiologic and psychological variations make more difficult the already difficult task of quantitative and qualitative evaluation of saliva secretion.

The values for normal saliva secretion are given as 700 to 1,500 mL/d, which gives an average quantity of 0.5 to 1 mL/min. With increased age, the quantity decreases to 0.3 mL/min. A reduction of saliva flow bewlow 0.2 mL/min is no longer enough for the physiologic protective functions within the oral cavity. This hypofunctional dryness is called xerostomia.

Among the general diseases that lead to insufficient secretion by the large and small salivary glands, and therefore to xerostomia, a classic example is Sjögren's syndrome (see chapter 30). As a consequence of reduced saliva secretion, the oral mucosa is covered by a sticky coating and becomes atrophic. Rhagades of the tongue, lips, and corners of the mouth appear. There is a high incidence of caries development (cervical caries—i.e., circular caries, smooth surface caries).

Quantity, composition, and flow properties of saliva can be influenced by many medications. With increased sympathicotonic medication, there is a reduction of saliva, and in the same manner the mucous saliva component increases in relation to the serous component. The corresponding active substance for the parasympathetic synapse is acetylcholine, and for the sympathetic synapse is noradrenaline. Therefore, medications that can be used legally can cause as side effects (temporary) hyposalivation and xerostomia. The following medications belong to this group: parasympatholytics, sympathomimetics, antidepressives, neuroleptics, anticonvulsives, muscle relaxants, anti-Parkinson drugs, antihistamines, appetite reducers, tranquilizers, and antihypertensives.

In everyday practice, the *tricyclic* and *tetracyclic antidepressive drugs* are the most frequent cause of dry mouth, and this again underlines the importance of obtaining a good patient history. In many cases it must be assumed, however, that in association with the depressive condition there was a psychological reduction of the saliva secretion before the use of medication so that the patient had been aware of the feeling of dry mouth. These patients complain of speech problems and difficulty in eating. Patients who had problem-free prostheses now have difficulties. Caries frequency also increases. There are also complaints of an unusual taste, a burning sensation, and frequently bad breath. The series of complaints that appear with medication-induced xerostomia is sometimes difficult to substantiate. Even so, consideration should be given to the possibility of reducing the dosage of the medication responsible for this side effect. Wetting of the oral cavity with fluids only leads to a short period of improvement, whereas a dry mouth caused by leg disturbed liquid balance (fever, dryness with systemic diseases) reacts well to increase of perioral and parenteral fluid.

Drug-induced fibrous gingival hyperplasia (ICD-DA 963.1, 966.1, and 972)

In anticonvulsant therapy of long duration with *hydantoin derivatives* such as *phenytoin (diphenylhydantoin),* there is characteristic gingival enlargement in almost every second case of epilepsy. The fibrous gingival growth usually appears in the area of the interdental papillae and later involves the other gingiva (Fig. 31-45). It can, in some cases, become a tumorlike enlargement so that finally the tooth crowns are partially or totally covered by the tissue mass and eating is severely restricted (Fig. 31-46). Pre-existing local irritation factors always play an aggravating role. The changes are more frequently seen in the anterior region and are more extensive in the side regions. The other areas of the oral cavity as well as the mucosa of the edentulous jaws show no clinical change.

There is development of pseudopockets by the fibrous gingival hyperplasia that are a hiding place for microbial plaque. In these pseudopockets, which are difficult to clean, there can be secondary inflammatory processes, which can alter the originally inflammation-free picture of the hyperplasia and take over (Fig. 31-46), particularly with deficient oral hygiene. The frequent side effect of phenytoin-induced gingival hyperplasia is without question. It must be considered, however, that in children with severe brain damage there can also be development of gingival enlargement independent of medication.

Regarding therapy of low-grade findings, it is possible to maintain a waiting attitude. The main task of the dentist is to eliminate systematically the local irritation points and to maintain regular and thorough oral hygiene for the patient. In advanced stages with excessive hyperplasia, gingivoplasty is the treatment of choice (Figs. 31-47 and 31-48). Postoperative, subtle oral hygiene with gingival massage is necessary but difficult to accomplish, in many cases because of lack of motivation of these patients. Treatment success is long-standing only if cooperation with the neurologist offers the possibility of a reduction of the hydantoin dosage or the change to another medication.

Fibrous gingival hyperplasia is also caused by medication with *cyclosporin* (immunosuppressive agent) as well as with the calcium antagonist *nifedipine,* and in coronary drugs (Figs. 31-49 and 31-50). Directions for use are included in the packaging.

Adverse effects of antibiotic therapy (ICD-DA 960)

In the oral cavity of the healthy person, there is, as in all other microbial-covered mucosa, a balanced relation between the saprophytic, facultative-pathogenic microorganism, and the host body (macroorganism). With antibiotic therapy, there can be oral mucosal changes of nonallergic nature because of the disturbed biologic equilibrium of the oral flora. The cause of a hairy tongue is discussed in chapter 2. The use of bacteriostatic or bactericidal antibiotics can also facilitate the appearance of *Candida* mycosis because it limits the development of bacterial microflora and therefore facilitates the development of saprophytic fungi. About 8 days after the administration of penicillin, an acute exacerbation of chronic marginal periodontitis is usually observed and leads to a shift of the resistance relationship. In typical cases, there is development of multiple pocket abscesses.

Antibiotics can influence the intestinal flora where the alteration of balance results in different types of symptoms. While all changes so far discussed are of passing type, changes caused by *tetracycline* lead to permanent dental changes if the medication is given during the mineralization phase of the enamel and dentin of primary or permanent teeth. Because of the high affinity of tetracycline for calcium ions, there is formation of tetracycline-calcium-orthophosphate in cartilage, bone, and tooth substances that are in the process of mineralization. The irreversible, dental deposits demonstrable by fluorescence microscopy take place according to the growth lines in enamel and dentin. They create gray-brown, brown, or yellowish changes of the affected dental areas (Figs. 31-51 to 31-53) and allow a back-dating to the antibiotic effect by their location.

Type, extent, and intensity of the discoloration depends on the time of tetracycline administration during dental development and on its intensity and duration as well as on the derivatives used. Continuous development of tetracycline preparations has resulted in preparations such as doxycycline having a weaker tendency to cause discoloration. Higher doses can—in combination with the underlying systemic disease—cause additional mineralization disturbances in the form of noticeable enamel hypoplasias because of a functional impairment of the ameloblasts (Figs. 31-51 and 31-52).

To reduce this type of iatrogenic dental damage, prescription of tetracycline should be avoided (as long as there is no compelling medical indication) during pregnancy and during the critical phase of crown development of the permanent incisors and canines between the first and fifth year of life.

Regarding differential diagnosis, one must consider dental discolorations due to rhesus factor incompatibility (fetal erythroblastosis, see chapter 24, Fig. 24-3) as well as to congenital erythropoietic porphyria. Above all, in cases of other mineralization disturbances, one must consider hereditary and acquired enamel and dentin defects of different origin (Figs. 31-54 and 31-55). During moderately protracted use of chlorhexidine gluconate, there is development of exogenous deposits of brown discoloration on the tongue and teeth; these, however, can be removed.

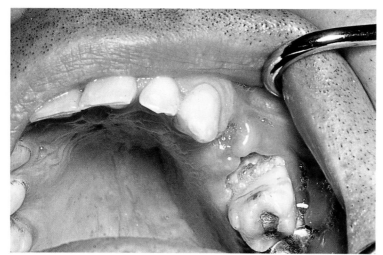

Fig. 31-1 Necrosis of bone and mucosa in the region of extracted tooth 25 (13) and the mesial root part of tooth 26 (14), which had been devitalized 2 weeks previously with a preparation containing arsenic. Cause: improperly sealed cavity with subsequent undesirable diffusion of arsenic oxide in the surrounding tissue. Indications for use of arsenic-containing preparations are extremely rare today. It is considered only as an adjuvant to pain reduction when the vital pulp cannot be extirpated. Safe closure of the cavity must be assured and the time of treatment monitored.

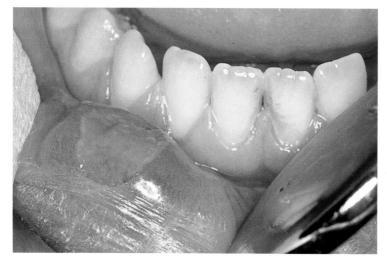

Fig. 31-2 Chronic recurring aphthae after etching with silver nitrate (Höllenstein). The earlier etching therapy practiced with different chemicals mitigates the pain in the short run through destruction of the sensitive nerve endings. However, it causes additional tissue damage, delays cure, and facilitates scar formation. Because of the unexplained etiology and, therefore, inadequate therapy capable of decreasing the incidence of recurrences, chronically recurring aphthae that spontaneously heal should not be treated with medication that has aggressive properties and/or undesirable side effects (see chapter 12).

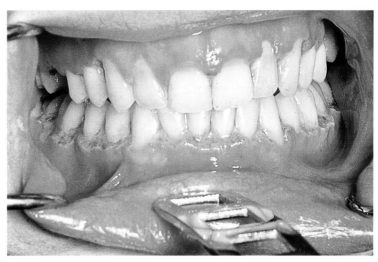

Fig. 31-3 Chromic-acid-induced gingival burn in the mandible with extensive damage of the gingival architecture. The periodontal damage in the maxilla is caused by inadequate oral hygiene and also by chromic acid.

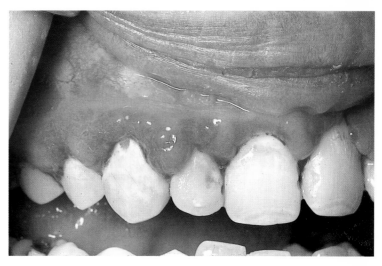

Fig. 31-4 Gingival condition after several months of unsuccessful treatment of hyperplastic gingivitis with chromic-acid solution. Note that the resulting inorganic acid injury did not damage only the periodontium but also the dental hard tissues (the surface is partially chalky because of the demineralization of the enamel).

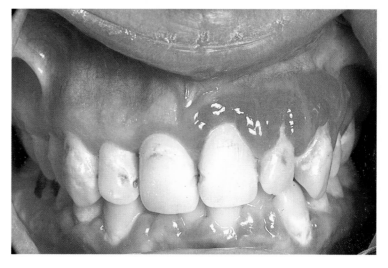

Fig. 31-5 The patient in Fig. 31-4 after periodontal surgery in the right maxillary region. On the still-untreated contralateral side, it is possible to recognize the marginal periodontitis caused by deficient oral hygiene and incorrect treatment. The inflammation has already extended to the free gingiva.

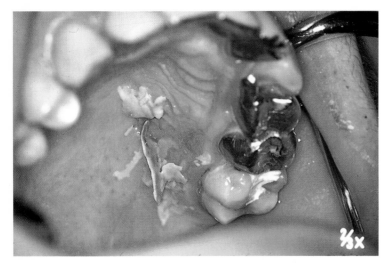

Fig. 31-6   Damage of the palatal mucosa with loss of epithelium due to contact with a camphorated chlorophenol-containing medication. Cause: during endodontic treatment of tooth 26 (14), a circumscribed area of the palatal mucosa was coated with the medication. Consequence: chlorophenol-containing solutions, the use of which is still accepted for endodontic treatment, will cause mucosal damage due to coagulative effect.

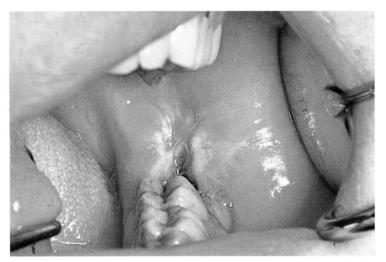

Fig. 31-7   Superficial irritation with chemical erosion of the oral mucosa, caused by application of a gauze strip soaked in a solution containing camphorated phenol. This was used because of disturbed healing of an extraction socket following removal of tooth 38 (17). The degree of damage of the mucosal surface decreases from the point of application toward the periphery. Cause: excessive soaking of the gauze strip in the medication.

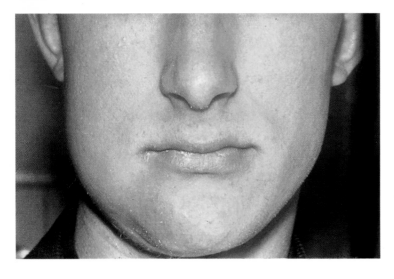

Fig. 31-8   Skin irritation of the lower lip and chin resulting from a solution of camphorated phenol. A gauze strip soaked in this solution accidentally touched the skin before it was introduced into the oral cavity.

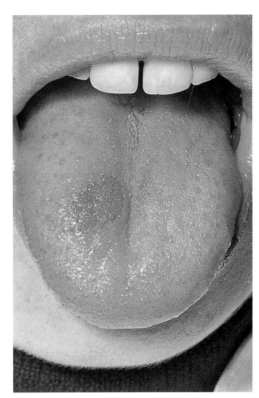

Fig. 31-9 Round lesion of specialized mucosa of the dorsum of the tongue in the area of action of an ascorbic acid tablet (vitamin C). Cause: The woman allowed the vitamin C tablet to slowly dissolve on the tongue and thereafter complained of a "burning feeling." Because of the pH (2.1 to 2.6) of the solution of ascorbic acid, a harmless erosion on the dorsum of the tongue was produced.

Fig. 31-10 Circumscribed mucosal damage of the upper vestibular fold from the use of an alcohol-containing mouthwash. Because of the hygroscopic and coagulative potential of the alcohol, a superficial

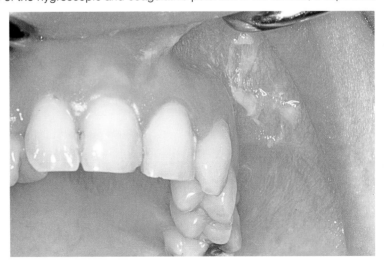

chemical trauma of the mucosa can occur even with prepared solutions if the fluid is retained in the mouth for too long a time. Directions for use of the mouth disinfectant must be followed exactly. In most cases, instructions for the use of the preparations are not adequately explained to the patient (exception: chlorhexidine gluconate). When mouthwashes—ut aliquid fiat—are prescribed, the possible untoward results should be remembered and solutions without risk of side effects should be recommended.

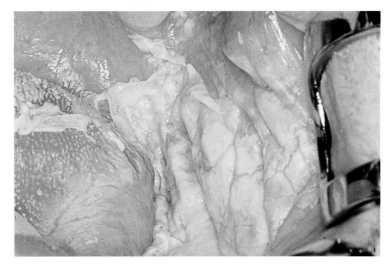

Fig. 31-11   Large superficial chemical burn of the oral mucosa following repeated applications of a nondiluted antiseptic mouthwash. Cause: misuse by the patient based on a "more is better" attitude. Alcohol content must be indicated today in ready-to-use preparations.

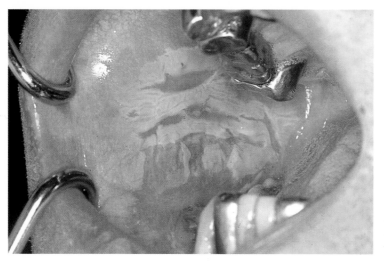

Fig. 31-12   Superficial etching of the cheek mucosa by acetylsalicylic acid in a pain-killing tablet (aspirin burn). Cause: the patient placed the tablet in the upper vestibular region and allowed it to dissolve slowly. The acetylsalicylic acid in solution with a pH value of 3.5 to 3.7 caused the noticeable mucosal lesion.

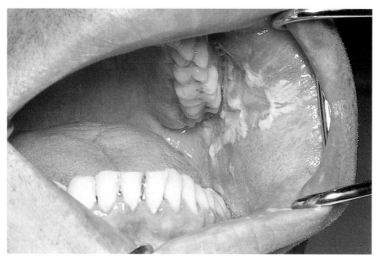

Fig. 31-13   Aspirin burn of the oral mucosa caused by a pain killer containing acetylsalicylic acid that was not used according to instructions. After ingestion of acetylsalicylic analgesics according to instructions, frequently there are gastric symptoms due to erosive changes of the gastric mucosa. This finding is associated with mild upper gastrointestinal bleeding.

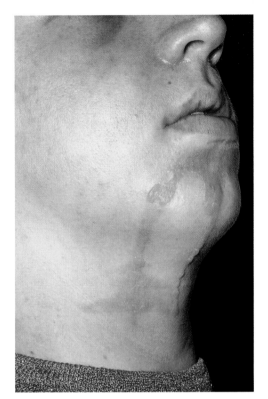

Fig. 31-14 Toxic-irritative contact dermatitis from an organic mercury compound. The disinfectant was used in high concentration to rinse a prepared root canal, and it trickled under the rubber dam onto the skin of the chin and neck. Etchings are also possible when, for example, a halogen-containing antiseptic is used and the affected tissue is then placed in contact with mercury-containing substances (interaction between mercury and halogen).

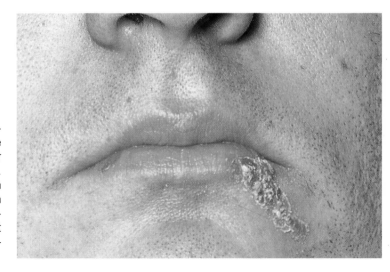

Fig. 31-15 Healing of a crust-covered acute dermatitis in the area of the left side of the lower lip (skin and vermilion border). Cause: irritation as expression of an increased reaction to an essential oil-containing impression material. This should not be confused with an allergic reaction.

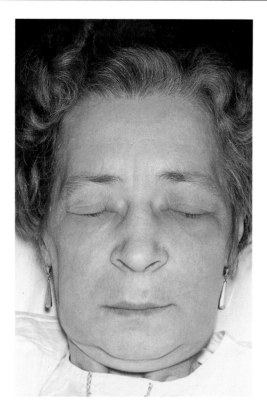

Fig. 31-16   Quincke's edema 3 hours after parenteral application of a penicillin-streptomycin compound. In addition to the facial edema illustrated, there was moderate glottis edema as a partial manifestation of allergic shock (anaphylactic type I allergic reaction).

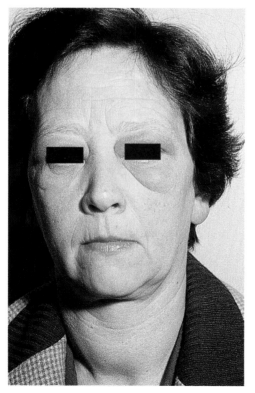

Fig. 31-17   Partial anaphylactic picture in the form of eyelid edema, thyroid swelling, shortness of breath, and tachycardia after local use of a sulfonamide preparation in the oral cavity (anaphylactic type I allergic reaction).

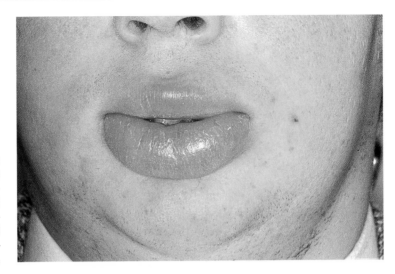

Fig. 31-18   Quincke's edema of the upper and lower lips as expression of an antigen-antibody reaction to the dental prescription of pyrazolone-containing analgesics. Food, food additives, and inhalation allergens can also cause this effect.

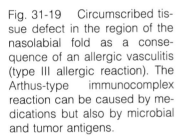

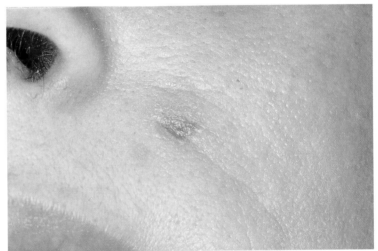

Fig. 31-19   Circumscribed tissue defect in the region of the nasolabial fold as a consequence of an allergic vasculitis (type III allergic reaction). The Arthus-type immunocomplex reaction can be caused by medications but also by microbial and tumor antigens.

Fig. 31-20   Intraoral finding of the patient in Fig. 31-9 at the same examination. In the vestibular mucosa-periosteum area of the alveolar process and in the area of teeth 23 to 25 (11 to 13) is an allergic vasculitis with superficial tissue necrosis. The relations of this immune complex vasculitis to other immunologic conditions with local clinical expression (e.g., certain hemorrhagic diatheses, see chapter 25) are many. Their diagnostic explanation requires interdisciplinary work in which the dentist is involved.

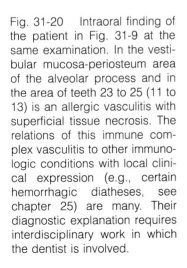

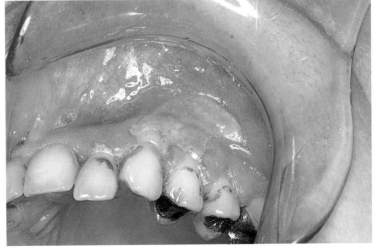

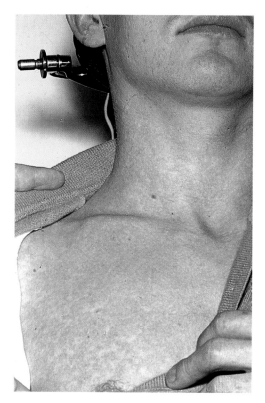

Fig. 31-21 Small spotted scarlatiniform drug exanthema following administration of a sulfonamide preparation. The exanthema, which resembles the skin efflorescences of certain infectious diseases, is usually itchy and maculous. Such exanthemas are frequently seen but are harmless. They affect either an antigen-antibody reaction of type I to III or an antigen T-cell–mediated reaction of type IV. Medication exanthemas appear in sensitized patients 2 or 3 days after a reexposure, in persons not previously sensitized after 9 to 18 days. Causal medications are analgesics, antibiotics, psychopharmacologics, or sulfonamides, among others.

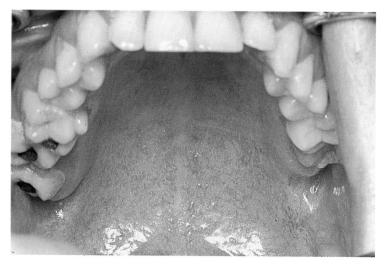

Fig. 31-22 Intraoral examination of the patient in Fig. 31-21 at the same examination. There is a small-spotted enanthema on the soft palatal mucosa that is synchronous with the exanthema. Note the obvious vascularity. This generalized allergic side effect of medication can involve other organs such as the myocardium, kidneys, liver, and the hematopoietic system. These occurrences are considered transitional forms to humoral immune reactions.

Fig. 31-23 Maculourticarial exanthema caused by a drug reaction 2 days after penicillin therapy. The clinical findings on the skin are caused by increased exudation with an urticarial-vesicular pattern. Transition to Stevens-Johnson syndrome has been discussed. The Lyell syndrome shows an acute course and an extremely variable drug exanthema. In rare cases, there is progressive formation of large blisters with loss of the epidermis after previous febrile infections and the prescription of drugs (toxic-allergic combination effect). The resulting skin lesion resembles burns (burned skin) and often leads to death.

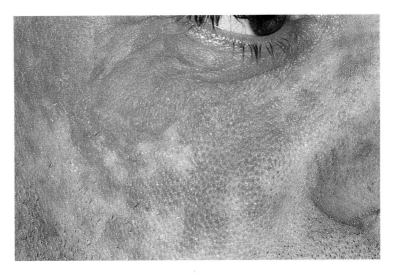

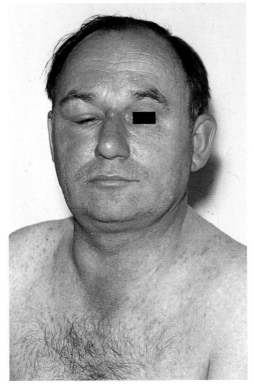

Fig. 31-24 Macular drug eruptions with small and large spots and unilateral eyelid edema 3 days after local intra-oral application of a sulfonamide tampon. This type of reaction can be caused by several drugs, among them antibiotics, sulfonamides, analgesics, hypnotics (barbiturates), and psychopharmacologic drugs.

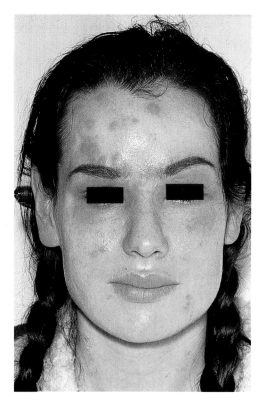

Fig. 31-25   Urticarial drug exanthem 10 days after parenteral application of a penicillin-streptomycin compound. The skin efflorescences are caused by perivascular inflammation mediated by sensitized T lymphocytes. The clinical picture varies depending on the level of the inflammation, vessel involvement, and permeability (macular, maculourticarial, vesicular, and bullous forms). These undesirable drug reactions should be cleared with the allergologist and recorded in the patient history. There is no indication today for the use of combined penicillin-streptomycin preparations in the dental clinic.

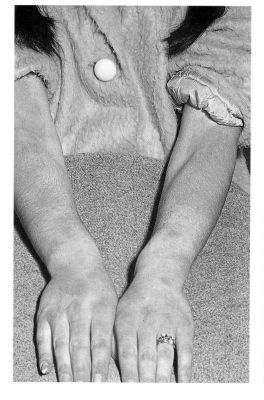

Fig. 31-26   The patient in Fig. 31-25 at the same examination. The usually itchy drug exanthemas are triggered by blood-borne antigens and are disseminated and systemically distributed. They manifest preferentially on the extension surface of the extremities (as here in the lower arms and hands). The skin reactions clinically associated with enanthemas on the oral mucosa are much less striking.

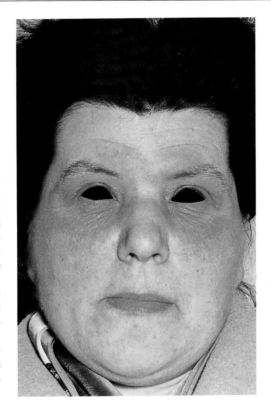

Fig. 31-27   Blood-borne allergic contact dermatitis of the facial skin in spectacle-shaped configuration. These changes are caused by type IV allergic reaction to mercury in silver-amalgam restorations that were in place for 5 or more years. The patient had a hypersensitivity to mercury, nickel, and hard rubber, which was demonstrated by skin patch tests. With the rigidly controlled elimination of the above antigens was regression of the blood-borne contact dermatitis.

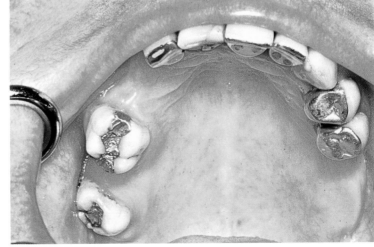

Fig. 31-28   Intraoral condition of the patient in Fig. 31-27 at the same examination. Despite the contact dermatitis of the systemically sensitized organism, the oral mucosa usually remains clinically free of clinical disease. The reason for this is discussed in the introduction of this chapter. However, the patient complained of metallic taste and burning tongue.

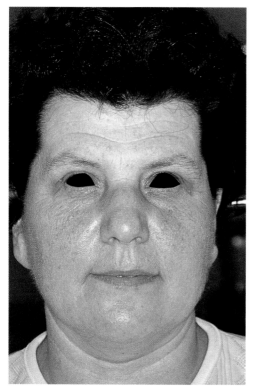

Fig. 31-29   The patient in Figs. 31-27 and 31-26. After a symptom-free interval of 1 year, a recurrence of the periorbital allergic contact dermatitis in weaker form occurred. The woman was a farmer, and the cause was accidental contact with seeds that had been treated with organic mercury. This demonstrates the high degree of sensitization to mercury, which was independent of the origin of the carrier material.

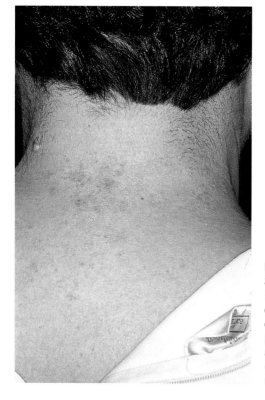

Fig. 31-30   The patient in Fig. 31-29 at the same examination. In the neck region are other foci of contact dermatitis. Because of the known nickel allergy, the patient had abandoned use of any nickel-containing articles (note the zipper in her blouse, made of composite materials).

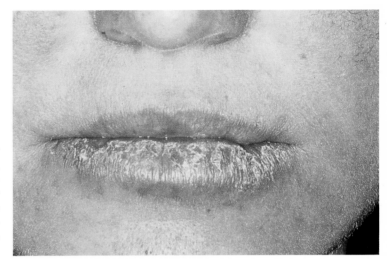

Fig. 31-31 Chronic allergic contact dermatitis of the lower lip (allergic contact cheilitis). A skin patch test confirmed mercury as the allergic cause. After elimination of all amalgam restorations, the reaction disappeared. Thus, the diagnosis was confirmed.

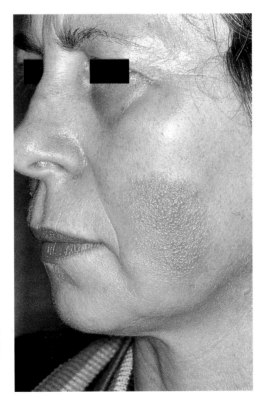

Fig. 31-32 Allergic contact dermatitis in the area of the left cheek. Cause: Essential oil in a product used on the skin to improve blood circulation.

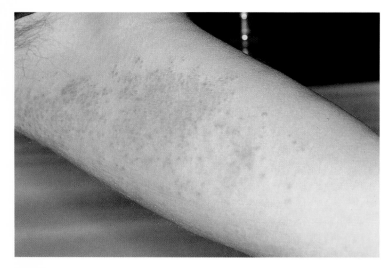

Fig. 31-33   Blood-borne allergic contact dermatitis (type IV reaction) on the inside of the upper arm with papulovesicular efflorescences. The woman had demonstrated (through allergy documentation) polyvalent allergy to nickel and cobalt as well as to wood, animals, rosin, and Peru balsam.

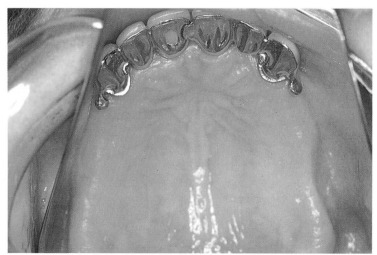

Fig. 31-34   Intraoral findings of the woman in Fig. 31-33 at the same examination. A combination fixed/removable maxillary prosthesis has been worn for years. The fixed part was made of a high-content gold alloy, the removable prosthesis—with exception of the connectors—was made of a chrome-cobalt-alloy with less than 1% nickel content. The mucosa is free of findings. The patient did not complain of any problems in the oral cavity.

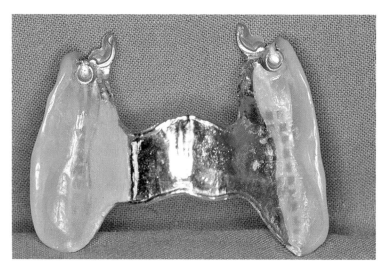

Fig. 31-35   Appearance of the prosthesis (palatal side) of the patient in Figs. 31-33 and 31-34. Because there were no current reasons for an allergic contact dermatitis, the chrome-cobalt alloy of the removable prosthesis against a high-gold alloy was replaced with a high-gold alloy (elimination test). The chronic allergic contact dermatitis regressed after this treatment.

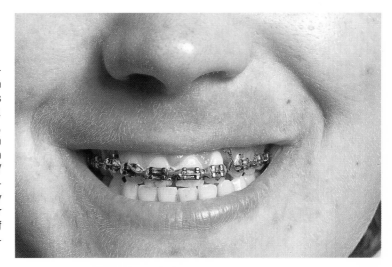

Fig. 31-36 Orthodontic therapy of an 11-year-old girl with fixed multibanded appliances with a nickel-containing alloy. Two months after treatment, there was the appearance of an itchy eczematous skin lesion that later proved to be a type IV allergic reaction to nickel. Development of the nickel allergy was facilitated by an earlier ear piercing for earrings and use of nickel-containing costume jewelry.

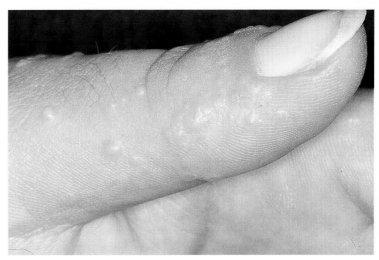

Fig. 31-37 The girl of Fig. 31-36 at the same examination. Blood-borne allergic contact dermatitis is visible on the thumb with prevalently papular efflorescences as partial manifestation of a type IV allergic reaction. Dyshidrotic eczema should be excluded. The skin changes regressed after elimination of the nickel-containing multibanded appliances.

Type and clinical course of immunoreactions. Drawing based on the diagram of Macher E, from Braun-Falco O, Plewig G, Wolff HH. Dermatologie und Veberologie, ed 3. Berlin: Springer, 1984: 240.

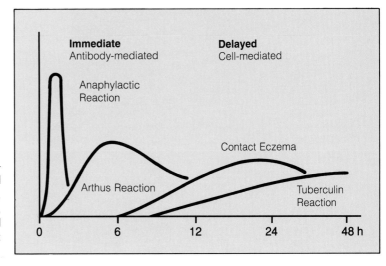

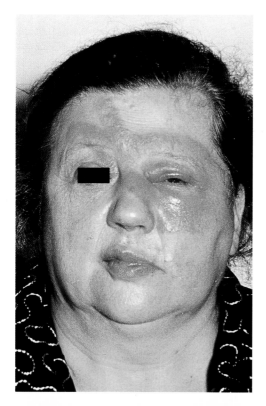

Fig. 31-38 Acute allergic contact dermatitis caused by an adhesive bandage. Because of a left side facial paresis, the patient used a so-called watch-glass bandage as eye protection, which was removed 24 hours later because of a skin reaction. Antigens are the resins in the glue. Special bandages are currently available for allergic patients. The acute type IV allergic contact dermatitis should be differentiated from a microbial skin infection under the bandage.

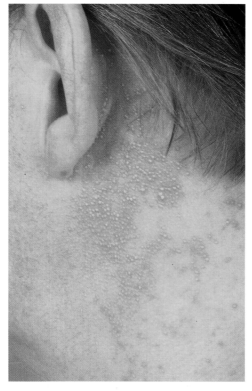

Fig. 31-39 Allergic contact dermatitis in the lateral neck region. Cause: cloth component of a disposable operation mask.

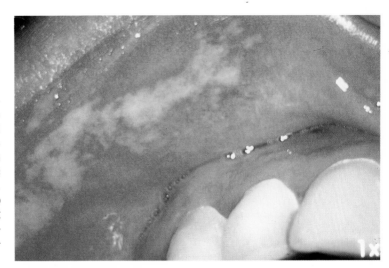

Fig. 31-40   Acute contact allergic reaction of the lip mucosa to material of a provisional crown of polyester base (epoxy-composite resin). The main findings of the contact allergic dermatitis are urticarial lesions. These do not remain limited to the oral cavity but can manifest on the larynx and cause swellings with concomitant breathing difficulties.

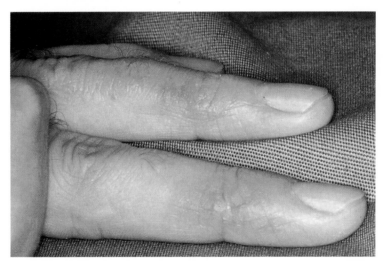

Fig. 31-41   Job-related chronic contact allergic dermatitis on the fingers of a dentist. Cause: sulfone acid-ester catalyst in dental materials. The sensitization is facilitated by cumulative toxic damage of the skin after mechanical use and washing trauma. In associated "wet jobs," sensitization to nickel, benzocaine, and other materials is common.

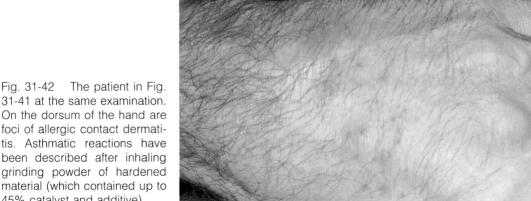

Fig. 31-42   The patient in Fig. 31-41 at the same examination. On the dorsum of the hand are foci of allergic contact dermatitis. Asthmatic reactions have been described after inhaling grinding powder of hardened material (which contained up to 45% catalyst and additive).

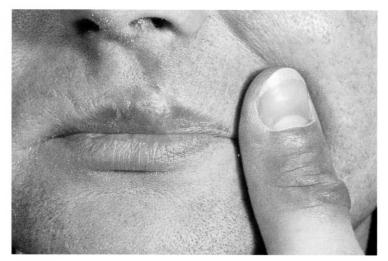

Fig. 31-43   Fixed drug eruption on the upper lip and thumb after injection of a pyrazolone derivative. After renewed antigen supply, there is always recurrence of the clinical manifestation in the same area. The causes of the local response in absence of generalization of the allergic reaction are unknown.

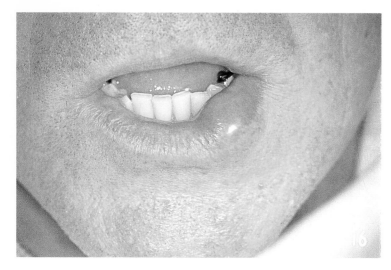

Fig. 31-44   Pressure urticaria on the upper lip appearing after dental treatment. Mechanical influence and temperature stress (cold urticaria, heat urticaria) can lead to liberation of vasoactive substances from mast cells. The consequent swelling imitates urticaria due to an allergic condition. Pressure urticaria can appear clinically as much as 6 hours after the determining condition.

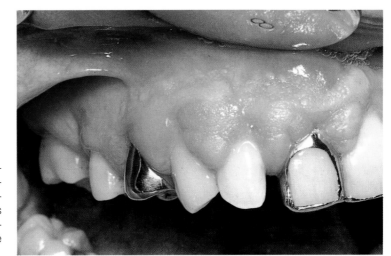

Fig. 31-45 Clinically inflammation-free hydantoin hyperplasia of the gingiva in a 30-year-old patient. The fibrous growth generally starts interdentally as hard swelling of the gingival connective tissue.

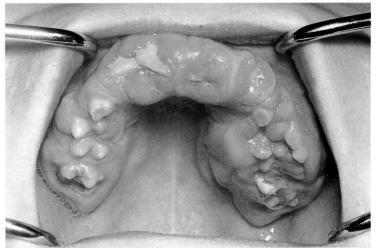

Fig. 31-46 Severe gingival hyperplasia in a 10-year-old boy after several years of anti-epileptic therapy with phenytoin (diphenylhydantoin). The palatal view shows the appearance of fibrous gingival enlargement with secondary inflammation. Differentiation from idiopathic fibrous gingival hyperplasia (gingival fibromatosis) may be achieved with the help of the patient's history. (See Fig. 15-9.)

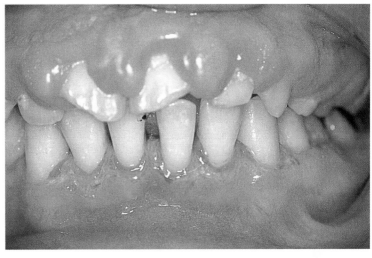

Fig. 31-47 Fibrous gingival hyperplasia caused by phenytoin in a 13-year-old boy. Condition 8 days after mandibular gingivoplasty. The enamel-dentin fracture of teeth 11 and 12 (8 and 9) is the consequence of a fall during an epileptic seizure.

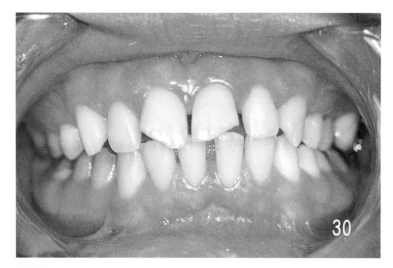

Fig. 31-48   The patient in Fig. 31-47. Condition of the maxilla 5 weeks after and in the mandible 7 weeks after gingivoplasty with re-establishment of the gingival architecture.

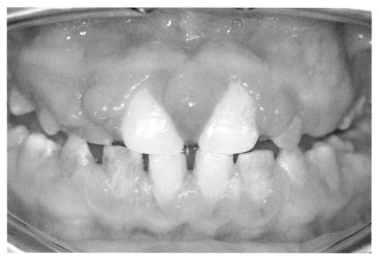

Fig. 31-49   Extensive inflammatory gingival hyperplasia in a 15-year-old patient undergoing immunosuppressive therapy with cyclosporine and concurrent treatment with the calcium antagonist nifedipine. Both drugs were used in a combination medication following kidney transplantation.

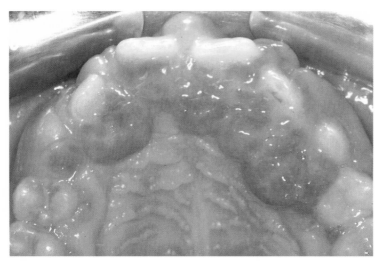

Fig. 31-50   The patient in Fig. 31-49 at the same examination. The palatal view shows severe inflammatory hyperplastic tissue reactions also present in the palatal gingiva. In agreement with the treating clinic, control of gingival hyperplasia is limited to oral hygiene measures.

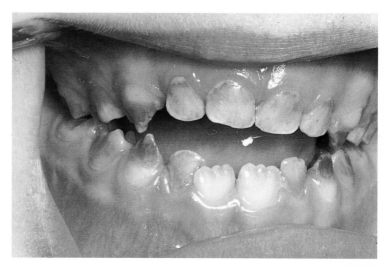

Fig. 31-51   Tetracycline discoloration of primary teeth. This 6-year-old girl was given tetracycline for 4 days after birth. This led to the yellow-brown discoloration of the teeth, which were in the process of mineralization. Also note the disturbances in the formation of hard substance in the discolored sections.

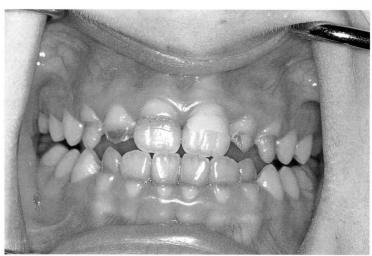

Fig. 31-52   Ringlike areas of discoloration and mineralization disturbance caused by tetracycline in the permanent anterior teeth in a 12-year-old girl. The enamel-dentin defect on tooth 21 (9) was corrected with a composite resin restoration. The antibiotic was prescribed for 3 weeks at the end of the second year. The color tone can vary from gray brown to brown or to a more yellow variation.

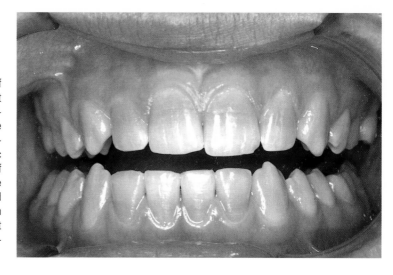

Fig. 31-53   Discoloration of the tooth crown of permanent incisors in a 16-year-old boy after many months of tetracycline administration during childhood. The long-term antibiotic therapy followed an episode of spastic bronchitis. Tetracycline derivatives should be avoided in the critical mineralization phase of dental development (i.e., during pregnancy, infancy, childhood).

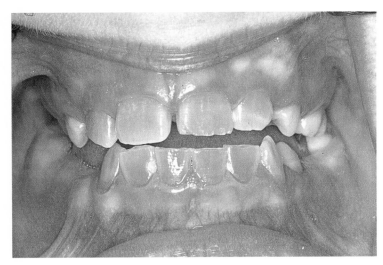

Fig. 31-54 Differential diagnosis of dental discoloration from tetracycline. Dentinogenesis imperfecta hereditaria is the most common form of hereditary dentin malformation. In this developmental disturbance of the dentin, the tooth crowns are gray-brown to gray-blue and amber and are translucent. Secondarily, there are multiple enamel ruptures with splinters in different sizes, leaving uncovered dentin surfaces (destruction of the support zone). The radiographic picture shows premature and extensive obliteration of pulp chambers. As in all enamel-dentin hereditary defects, the changes occur in both primary and permanent dentitions.

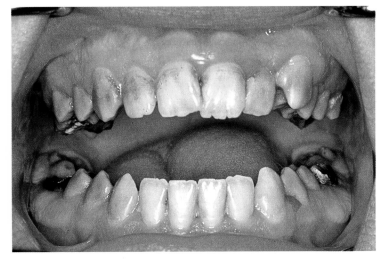

Fig. 31-55 Differential diagnosis of dental discoloration caused by tetracycline: hypomineralization as manifestation of hereditary enamel malformation (amelogenesis imperfecta hereditaria) in a 13-year-old girl. At the time of eruption, the teeth showed a normal crown configuration, but the surface had chalky or yellow-brown discolored enamel zones. The discoloration increases with age. There are enamel defects of various sizes, depending on the extension of the mineralization disturbance.

Chapter 32

Findings in the Oral Cavity and Perioral Region as a Result of Self-Inflicted Lesions and Other Undesirable Influences

Consequences of physical influences

Consequences of chemical influences

Consequences of habits and psychogenic disturbances

Consequences of seizures

This chapter covers changes in the oral cavity and perioral tissues that are either self-inflicted wounds because of unusual external associated conditions and influences or are effects of habits and psychological disturbances. All findings have a more or less similar mark in that they are unusual not in the morphology of the lesion but in the manner and background of the cause. Discovering the causal relationship is sometimes difficult and troublesome. The psychosomatic viewpoint is discussed in chapter 1.

Consequences of physical influences

There are many diseases, undesirable drug reactions, and independent events that adults encounter in the workplace or home and that also threaten children and young adults. Accidents involving children at home as well as self-inflicted wounds unfortunately have not decreased as much as similar events in the workplace, where there are accident-protection measures and programs. In the workplace, protective measures are accepted, while in the home and during hobby activities they are often neglected.

For typical accidental wounds of the jaw-face region, refer to traumatology books. Only a few, unusual, self-inflicted wounds from thermal, electrical, mechanical, and behavioral influences will be discussed here.

A large group of wounds consists of *thermal self-inflicted wounds*. Occurring most frequently are lip and oral mucosal burns from contact with hot food and drinks. The temperatures at which food may become harmful are as follows: with soups and hot drinks, the serving temperature should be from 75 to 85 °C. Ingestion temperature, for example in sipping, is about the same. At 60 °C, cooling drinks are still perceived to be hot because of the immediate initiation of counter reflexes and the rapid cooling of the mixture with saliva. Overly hot watery food and drinks usually lead only to minor lesions in the anterior part of the oral cavity, particularly on the tongue and palatal mucosa where their effect is limited to 1 or 2 days of burning sensation.

Oven- and pan-prepared foods containing fat have a higher temperature; the dilution effect of saliva is minimal. If these foods are placed in the mouth by mistake when too hot and remain there temporarily, there will be a consequent noticeable first- or second-degree burn (e. g., "pizza burns," Figs. 32-1 and 32-2).

Circumscribed burn damage is found on the lip, hard palate, and dorsum of the tongue when a lit cigarette or cigars is placed with its burning end in the oral cavity (Fig. 32-3). Particularly in India, the Caribbean, and in South America, "reverse smoking" is practiced. This habit leads to the development of oral precancerous lesions and carcinomas at a significantly high rate.

There are many sources (e. g., grills, fondue) for thermal self-injury. The possible causes range from exposure to direct flame and explosions (Figs. 32-4 to 32-6) to lesions caused by liquid metals (Figs. 32-7 to 32-9) and hot objects (ICD-DA 941 and 947.0X).

Electric burns (ICD-DA 941 and 947.0X) seldom occur today, thanks to prescribed safety rules in the electrical supply industry for household goods. To this group of injuries belongs severe burn necrosis with consequent development of tissue defects, which may occur when small children playing with electrical conductors and cables place the cords in their mouths (Fig. 32-10).

Self-inflicted wounds can occur during mastication. *Acute mechanical tissue traumas* are not infrequently caused by mouth and dental care procedures. Damage can be inflicted by inappropriate manipulation of toothpicks, needles, and other pointed objects. Inflammatory reactions may occur when the foreign material remains in the traumatized tissue. These findings may be caused by loose toothbrush bristles or fish bones (see also Fig. 6-20).

Particularly with children (who place everything in their mouths), piercing wounds are not infrequent in the period during which the child learns to walk (Fig. 32-11). These findings can be associated with tattoos (see Figs. 4-35 to 4-37).

Among job-related mechanical injuries, there are known anomalies of dental occlusion and forms that can be brought about through certain habits with machinery and material (e. g., nails, thread). The oral mucosa and lips can be affected in the form of rhagades, fissures, ulcerations, and hyper- and dyskeratoses.

Professional musicians have characteristic dental, jaw, and soft tissue changes from playing wind instruments with wood or metal mouthpieces for many years. With glass blowers, the extension of the cheek mucosa can frequently lead to typical mechanically conditioned epithelial changes in the area of "overblown cheek pockets."

Increased sun exposure can lead to different degrees of *sunburn* depending on skin type (Fig. 32-12). The influence on the skin of a tanning lamp is most intense in the lower lip, which is not protected by natural pigmentation, and sunburn in this area can lead to more severe acute or chronic light damage (*actinic cheilitis*, ICD-DA 892.70, Fig. 32-13).

Consequences of chemical influences

Self-inflicted chemical burns (ICD-DA 947.0X), because of their frequency, are of major importance. Oral tissue damage from typical chemicals such as acids and bases (Fig. 32-20) is not as frequent as in the past (because of improved work laws for accident prevention and their careful observation); however, the danger of self-inflicted wounds with the use of household cleaning materials has increased. Frequently affected are children who, in the oral phase, place unknown objects in their mouths. All such materials should have child-proof covers and a description of the chemical composition of the product.

An important, common problem for the dentist is the local chemical self-inflicted wound from alcohol solutions. They take place not only as described in chapter 31 but by not following directions for alcohol-containing mouthwashes and other topical alcohol products. In some cases, alcohol solutions for dermatologic use are incorrectly used on the mucosa.

Despite the extensive use of pain-relief tablets, even today some people relieve toothache pain with old-fashioned home remedies, in which a swab soaked with spirits, rum, schnapps, or Carmelite water is held in the vestibular mucosa for a long time. The result is superficial mucosal erosions to deep-reaching tissue necrosis, which finally lead the patient to the dentist (Figs. 32-14 to 32-19).

An unusual cause of chemical mucosal damage is from accidental application to the oral cavity of a chemical preparation in spray from for cold permanent waves application (Fig. 32-21). Unusual too is the hemorrhagic oral mucosal inflammation from a wasp sting (Figs. 32-22 and 32-23).

Consequences of habits and psychogenic disturbances

Contrary to the frequency of self-mutilation on the facial skin (Fig. 32-24), the soft covering of the oral cavity is seldom the location of deliberate self-mutilation. This may be explained by the fact that the oral mucosa is not a major eye-catcher, therefore the aim of creating an impression is lost. Also, demonstrable self-mutilations (artifacts) of the oral mucosa would generally cause pain and interfere with vital functions such as swallowing, eating, and talking. However, the literature does provide descriptions of oral mucosal manifestations of self-mutilations in psychopathic persons. Also, there are disturbed children who under local anesthesia, despite explanations, not accidentally (Figs. 33-43 to 33-45) but deliberately harm themselves and by self-mutilation develop lip defects from biting (Fig. 32-25).

In persons attempting suicide, severe lesions from firearms or chemically effective substances that greatly limit the physiologic function of the mouth are not uncommon. They will not be described here.

Differentiation should be made between these deliberate self-inflicted wounds and the oral mucosal mutilations caused by *parafunctional habits, tics,* and those caused during psychogenic disturbances. The background from which these findings originate often remains undiscovered in the diagnostic process. Especially in these cases, it should not be expected that the patient will be willing to provide information on his or her history. From experience, a repeated focused investigation is often needed.

Recognition of a fictitious mucosal injury creates special difficulties when there is a deliberate effort to hide the cause. Some patients remain silent about their history, because they are ashamed of it and will not admit to certain habits. Uncertainty about the cause also makes the process of obtaining the history more difficult. This can easily lead to a false diagnosis by the physician/dentist.

Behind self-inflicted wounds in children, there are frequently hidden, psychosocial conflict situations (home, school). These relationship disturbances can often be handled only by specially trained pediatricians or psychologists.

The question of why wounds are inflicted in the oral cavity can be explained by the fact that from birth the oral region is a highly sensitive recognition and exchange organ for air and nourishment and is also of particular significance for interpersonal contact. It is therefore not surprising that relationship disturbances are often manifested in the

718   Diseases of the Oral Mucosa

oral cavity and perioral region. Manifestations of *relationship distur-bances* include pleasure habits (sucking, licking) and acts of aggression (biting, tearing, pressing, crunching). In other cases, there is compulsive motor activity, as in chain smoking and constant pencil chewing. The severity of the problem ranges from mild to pathologic.

Typical examples are rubbing of the tongue tip against the expansion screw of an orthodontic appliance or a prosthesis clamp (Figs. 32-26 and 32-27), lip licking (Figs. 32-28 to 32-29), cheek chewing (Figs. 32-30 and 32-31), as well as lip biting (*cheilophagia*, Figs. 32-32 to 32-35). In cheek biting (ICD-DA 528.93), the clinical findings range from discrete leukoplakial changes to distinct erosions with floating epithelial rests and hyperkeratotic areas caused by a gnawing of the surface (Figs. 32-30, 32-31; see Figs. 34-14 to 34-16). In lip biting (ICD-DA 528.93), particularly on the lower lip, a chronic ulcer with inflamed infiltated border zone develops because of continuous tissue trauma, which requires a careful differential diagnosis from a carcinomatous ulcer. The location of the lesions relative to a particular group of teeth establishes an important diagnostic sign (Fig. 32-35).

Local dental therapy of these changes on the lip and oral mucosa is often achieved by the discovery of the cause as well as a discussion about stopping the behavior. Correct evaluation of the history and of the findings is complicated by a frequent shift of symptoms and may require cooperation with specialists from other disciplines.

One occasionally finds in the dental practice patients who have hallucinogenic ideas about abnormal enlargement of the tongue or about a disturbing foreign body in the oral cavity. Others may have a cleaning or control compulsion. Overly frightened people or people predisposed to hypochondria sometimes suffer from the presence of a harmless change, for example development of colored tongue coating, a furrowed tongue, or a slightly inflamed, irritated lateral tongue tonsil, with ideas of serious disease (*cancerophobia* ICD-DA 300.2). These patients (predominantly women) tend to perform exaggerated self-examinations. Their thoughts and actions are determined by fear and the firm belief that they have tongue cancer. Triggering factors for the imagined disease are often the death of a relative or close friend. In these cases, one must obtain help from sources competent to eliminate the possibility of the feared disease in order to guide the patient back to a normal everyday life. This task requires great experience—also in medical circles—and a high degree of sympathetic understanding.

Another important differential diagnostic problem in dental practice are complaints of *burning tongue (mucosal burning)* without demonstration of local diseases. Primarily affected are women between 40 and 60 years of age (perimenopausal or postmenopausal age), much more rarely men, and almost never young people and children. In most cases of burning tongue (*glossopyrosis*, ICD-DA 529.60), the cause is psychogenic. The suspicion of a psychiatric disturbance can, however, be made only when all possible local and systemic conditions have been excluded, including local tongue changes that can be misinterpreted by the patient. Also, there are hormonal-vegetative factors such as menopause or surgical interventions (e. g., hysterectomy) to be considered and clarified by referral to a gynecologist. Burning symptoms also appear in neuropathies, particularly in diabetes mellitus, in vitamin B_{12} deficiency, and in alcoholism, where the condition of an early phase of severe liver parenchymal damage plays a role. In regard to the possibility of other systemic causes, internal medicine and neurologic examinations usually are not very productive.

Tongue burning can be the somatic expression of depression (monosymptomatic, hypochondriac depression). The projection of misperception in the tongue area is explained by the association with the high central nervous system representation or the deep psychological significance of this organ. Symptoms of this type—as well as cases of so-called low prosthetic tolerance—border with the fields of psychosomatics and psychiatry.

The psychiatric patient offers tongue burning as a symptom and clings to this somatic sign. Through constant new attempts and through ignorance of local dental treatments (which inevitably are doomed to failure), the patient thinks his or her idea of serious—even if local—disease has been confirmed, and that no doctor can help.

Therapy belongs in the hands of a physician educated in psychosomatics or a psychiatrist. To avoid a problem for the dentist, the patient must be convinced that there is no need for dental treatment.

Consequences of seizures

Unintentional self-inflicted wounds of the oral mucosa, particularly of the tongue, can appear with seizures associated with epilepsy and the lack of consciousness. The best known are tongue bite wounds in epileptic patients (Figs. 32-36 and 32-37). Since the advent of improved therapeutic modalities, grand mal seizures and with them these findings are less frequently observed today.

The nosologic classification of endogenous and exogenous factors that lead to epilepsy (ICD-DA 345) is extensive, and the clinical symptoms vary in many aspects. We shall only note here that as a consequence of certain epileptic forms with seizures of focal nature, symptomatic rhythmic chewing and tongue and mucosal movements with intensified saliva production can occur at the time of lapse of consciousness.

In advanced stages of cerebral bleeding disturbances (e. g., after apopletic stroke), self-mutilations in the oral mucosa have been seen (Fig. 32-38). This is explained by the lethargy of the patient, psychomotor disturbances, and disorientation and is often associated with lack of oral care.

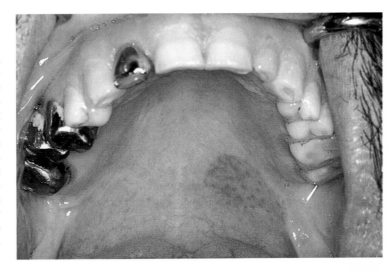

Fig. 32-1 "Pizza burn." A piece of oven-fresh pizza introduced into the mouth was too hot and remained attached to the palatal mucosa for a short time. Typically there is the development of a first-degree burn, which produces intense pain for several days. Burns from hot soups and drinks occur preferentially on the tongue tip, tongue border, and to minor extent on the palate. There are discrete mucosal changes (erythema, desquamation).

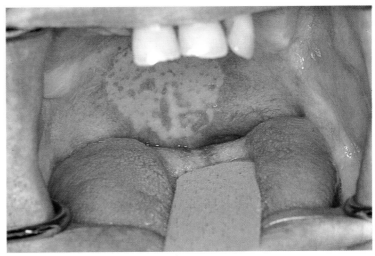

Fig. 32-2 "Pizza burn." First- to second-degree burn of the palatal mucosa from hot, fat-containing food with sticking tendency. The epithelium is lost and erosive areas can be seen. Second-degree burns, compared to first-degree burns, cause greater pain and require a longer healing time of the oral mucosa. The healing here and in Fig. 32-1 led to total repair.

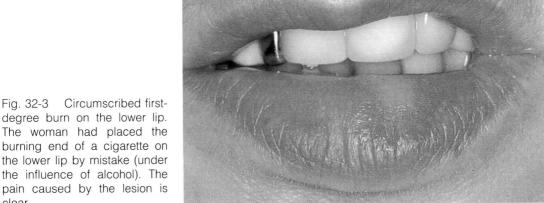

Fig. 32-3 Circumscribed first-degree burn on the lower lip. The woman had placed the burning end of a cigarette on the lower lip by mistake (under the influence of alcohol). The pain caused by the lesion is clear.

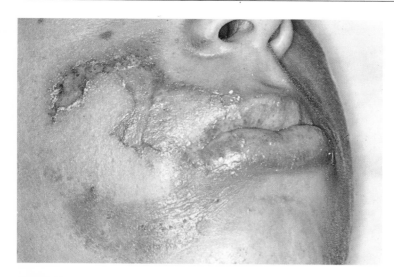

Fig. 32-4   Fresh burn (first and second degree) of the lips and perioral region in a 13-year-old boy who handled explosives carelessly and was burned.

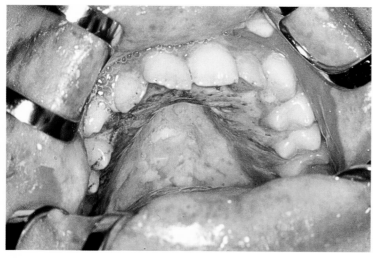

Fig. 32-5   Intraoral conditions of the patient in Fig. 32-1 at the same examination. The flame was inhaled into the open mouth at the time of the explosion. Second-degree burn lesions (burn blisters) can be seen over the entire heat-exposed mucosa and the pharynx. Swelling, blistering, and superficial necroses with impacted shrapnel fragments are especially noticeable on the palatal mucosa.

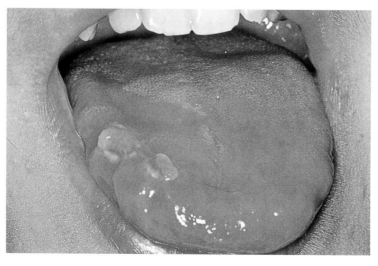

Fig. 32-6   The patient in Figs. 32-4 and 32-5 three weeks after the accident. Two ulcerations persist on the right side of the tongue. Impressions of the teeth at the margin of the tongue indicate persistent significant swelling. The anterior and lateral portions of the tongue have not yet recovered their papillary relief.

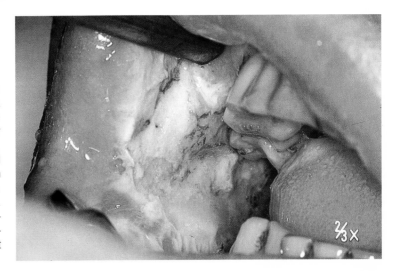

Fig. 32-7   Third-degree burn of the mucosa and submucosa in the cheek region. While handling an aluminum melter (melting temperature 660 °C), the 35-year-old man squirted aluminum into the oral cavity. In the area of the burned tissue, there is no blood circulation. Depth and extension of the tissue destruction depend on intensity and length of the heat influence.

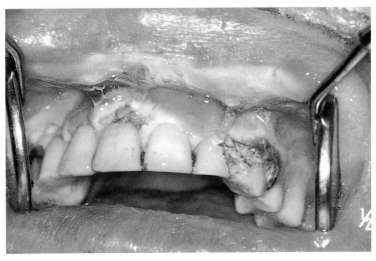

Fig. 32-8   The patient in Fig. 32-7 at the same examination. Third-degree burns on the upper lip and vestibular alveolar process. Note the white burn scales in the contact area of the liquid aluminum. The deep tissue necrosis extends to the alveolar bone. The interdental area of teeth 22 and 23 (9 and 10) is covered with hardened metal. Because nerve structures are also destroyed in a third-degree burn, there is initial analgesia.

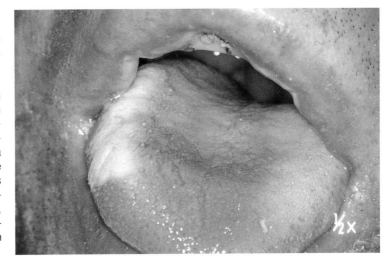

Fig. 32-9   The patient in Figs. 32-7 and 32-8 at the same time of examination: Third-degree burns on the tongue and lips. The slow healing process, which only takes place through secondary intention, is often disturbed by secondary infection and usually leads to atrophic scars on the oral mucosa with permanent loss of tongue papillae. Atrophic burn scars on the skin often tend to produce keloids. In this patient, there was scarring with microstomia and reduction of mouth opening.

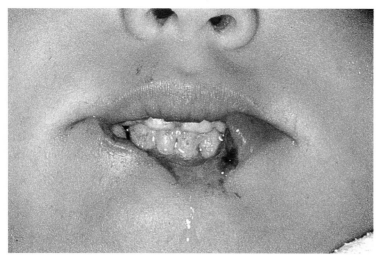

Fig. 32-10   Electric thermal lip injury. The 2-year-old child had put a live electrical plug into his mouth 2 weeks earlier. When current flowed, the heat released caused a marked tissue defect on the lower lip. This area was previously covered with necrotic tissue; other injuries were noted on the mandibular alveolar process and the tongue. The accident also caused short loss of consciousness and cardiac rhythm alterations.

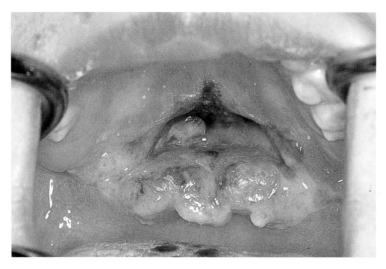

Fig. 32-11   Impaling wound of the soft palate in a 4-year-old child. Cause: the child fell while holding a sharp wooden toy in the mouth. In treating the wound, the intruded foreign body must be located. Any possible perforation reaching the nasal cavities should be carefully repaired.

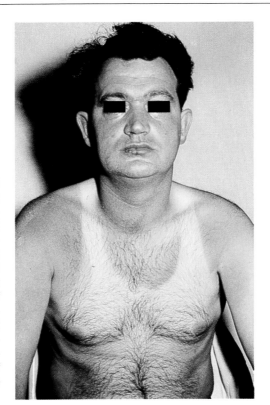

Fig. 32-12   Sunburn caused by long sunlight exposure. By overdosing with short-wave ultraviolet waves, after 12 to 24 hours there is a prostaglandin-mediated erythema, which is limited to the exposed skin; 48 to 72 hours later there is onset of pigmentation. Intensity of erythema and browning depends on skin type. The patient also shows a keratoconjunctivitis as well as recurrence of herpes labialis, an expression of the temporary weakening of the immune defenses of the skin.

Fig. 32-13   Chronic actinic cheilitis in a 63-year-old farmer. The lower lip is the area most exposed to sun rays and is not protected by pigment. Acute damage (e.g., glacier burn) is therefore more likely to leave residual chronic damage in this area. In the chronic form of actinic cheilitis, the lower lip shows partially crust-covered foci with rhagade formation and atrophic changes and scales at the boundary between skin and the vermilion. Development of carcinoma in these cases of chronic damage is possible. For this reason, these findings must be regularly supervised.

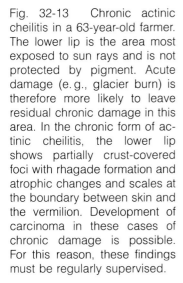

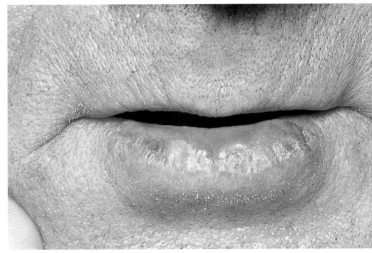

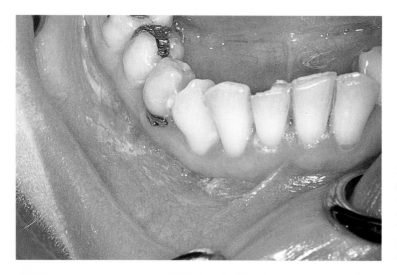

Fig. 32-14 Superficial mucosal damage in the area of the lower vestibular fold caused by chemicals. The patient's self-treatment for pain involved placing a swab soaked with an alcohol solution.

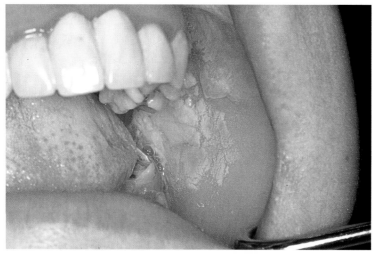

Fig. 32-15 Chemical self-inflicted wound of the cheek mucosa. A cotton wool pledget that had been soaked in a caraway seed–corn alcohol solution was placed in the upper cheek mucosal fold for relief of dental pain.

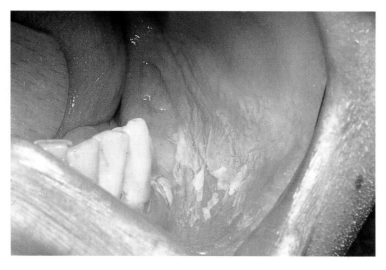

Fig. 32-16 Mucosal damage caused by the hygroscopic and fixed action of a high-proof rum-soaked cotton wool pledget applied to the mucobuccal fold. Using this home remedy, the 35-year-old man attempted to reduce pain in a poorly healing extraction site.

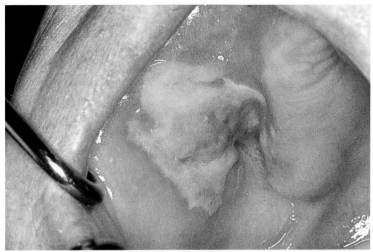

Fig. 32-17 Extensive fibrin-coated necrosis of the cheek mucosa with surrounding induration. Only persistent questioning explained the cause. It was a chemical tissue damage due to a cotton wool pledget soaked in Carmelite water and placed in the vestibular fold in an attempt to reduce pain.

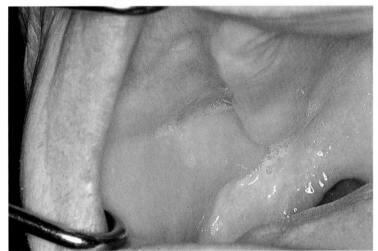

Fig. 32-18 The patient in Fig. 32-17 two weeks later. Rapid and almost complete healing of the mucosal lesion occurred after the damaging self-treatment was stopped.

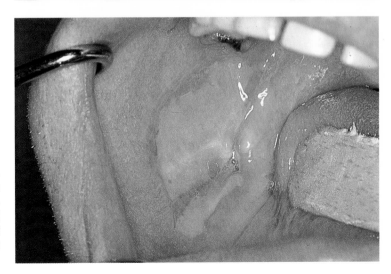

Fig. 32-19 Superficial mucosal necrosis caused by a cotton wool swab soaked with Carmelite spirit left in place for several hours. Without knowledge of patient history, such findings can lead to diagnostic errors.

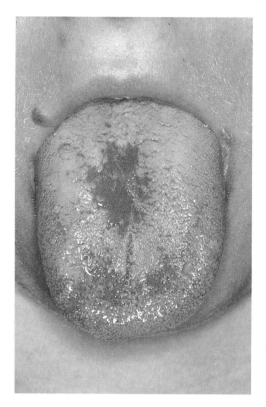

Fig. 32-20 Circumscribed self-inflicted wound of the tongue caused by lye, which reached the oral cavity while pipetting. Mouth pipetting is not allowed at present.

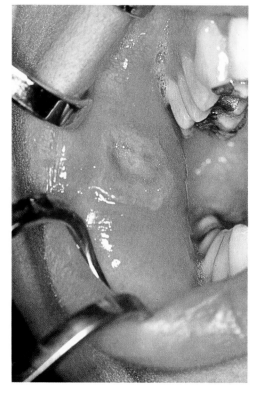

Fig. 32-21 Circumscribed coated ulceration on the retro-angular buccal mucosa in a 27-year-old woman. Cause: hair-spray (an alcoholic cold-wave spray solution) accidentally sprayed into the open mouth.

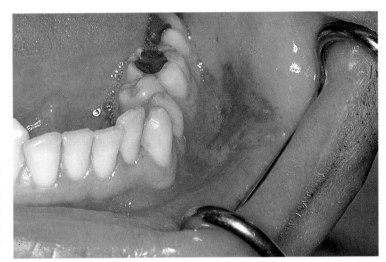

Fig. 32-22 Condition after a wasp sting on the lower vestibular mucosa of a 26-year-old patient with local edema and hemorrhagic inflammation. The wasp entered the mouth on top of a piece of fruit pie.

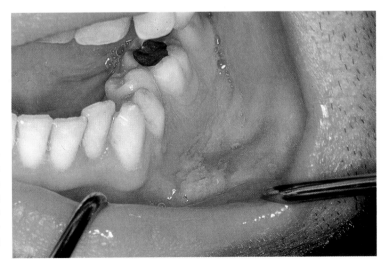

Fig. 32-23 The patient in Fig. 32-22 six days later. There are still signs of the regressing hemorrhagic inflammation. The risks associated with a wasp sting depend on the localization (pharynx, larynx with danger of asphyxiation due to severe swelling) and a possible allergic immediate reaction caused by the foreign proteins of the insect poison (anaphylactic shock) as well as the toxin effect (faster absorption through oral mucosa).

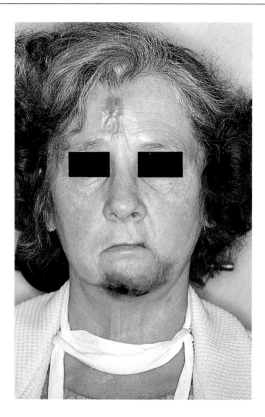

Fig. 32-24   Several old lesions (self-inflicted wounds) in the face of a psychotic patient.

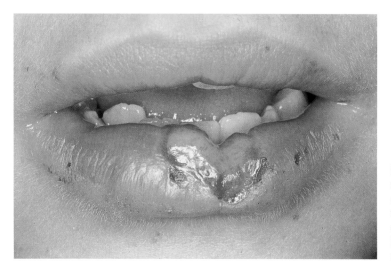

Fig. 32-25   Deep cleft-like tissue defect on the lower lip as a consequence of a self-inflicted wound produced by a disturbed 11-year old girl while under local anesthesia. Findings 10 days after the event.

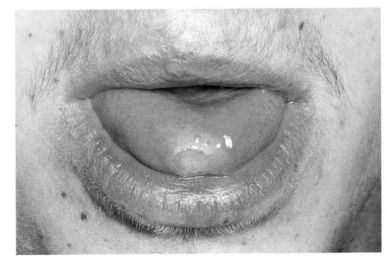

Fig. 32-26   Ulcer of the tip of the tongue with surrounding leukoplakia (stress hyperkeratosis) in a 13-year-old retarded boy. Cause: uncontrollable persistent friction on the expansion-screw of an orthodontic appliance.

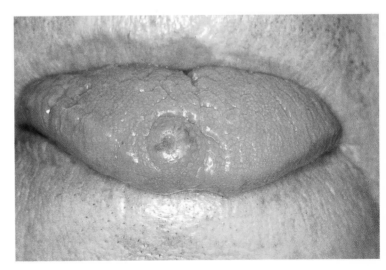

Fig. 32-27   Appearance of a chronic self-inflicted wound on the tip of the tongue of a 61-year-old woman. Cause: continuous friction with the tip of the tongue on a broken prosthesis clamp.

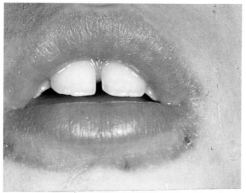

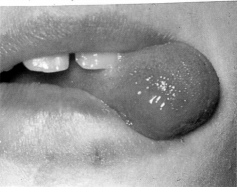

Fig. 32-28 Maceration of the skin with fissures near the lip margin in a 8-year-old boy. Cause: continuous licking with the tongue. After onset of maceration, the irritated skin provides another motivation for habit maintenance in addition to the psychogenic disturbance. A secondary mycotic infection may occur, as in perleche (see chapter 34) as long as the condition continues. The clearly defined arch-shaped lesion related to the movement of the tongue permits the exclusion of eczema (e. g., resulting from mouthwash solution).

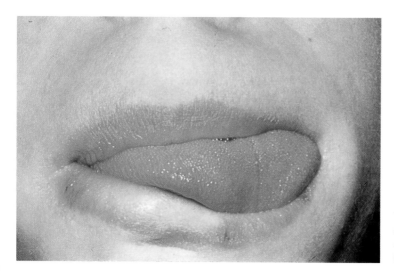

Fig. 32-29 Perioral dermatitis from lip licking. These findings are often combined with mouth angle fissures (also see Fig. 34-11).

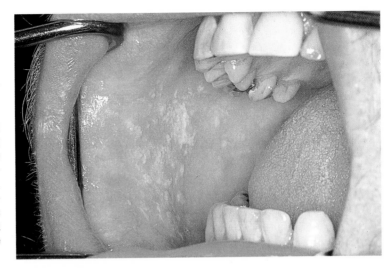

Fig. 32-30   Typical cheek mucosa finding in cheek biting. The squeezing of the mucosa, which leads to whitish epithelial thickening, follows the gnawing and tearing of epithelium, so that there are noticeable epithelial remnants and erosions. These habit-related, self-inflicted wounds are limited to areas of the cheek and lip mucosa that can be reached by the teeth.

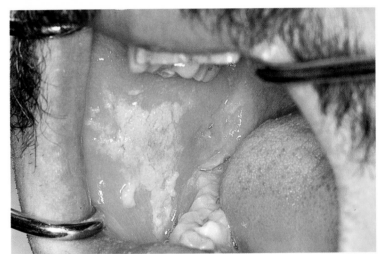

Fig. 32-31   Cheek mucosal findings after cheek biting with a leukoplakial appearance where there was no tearing of the epithelium.

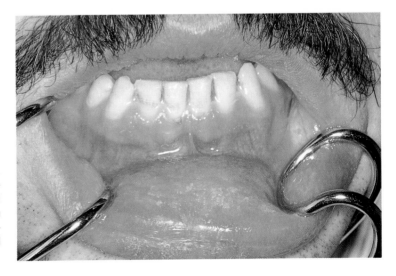

Fig. 32-32   The patient in Fig. 32-31 at the same examination. Typical discrete mucosal lesions on the lower lip caused by lip biting. Patients are often ashamed of their lack of self-control when they are informed of the cause these findings.

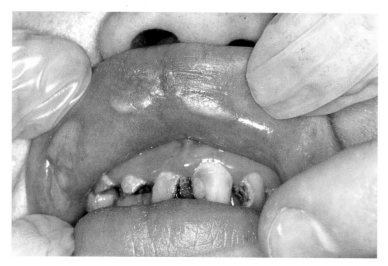

Fig. 32-33   Lesions on the upper lip of a 12-year-old girl caused by constant sucking of the mucosa and lip biting. This bad habit was facilitated by the sharp corners of the carious incisors.

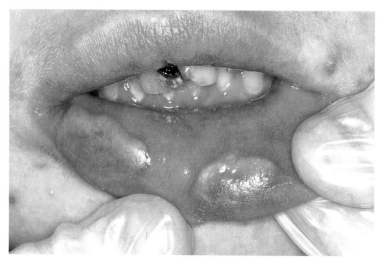

Fig. 32-34   The patient in Fig. 32-33 at the same examination. The flat pillowlike swelling of the lower lip can be attributed to the dental findings in the maxilla.

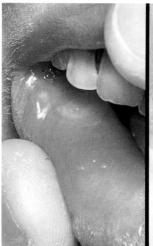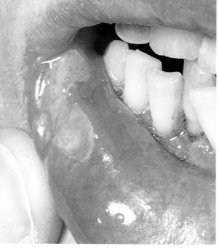

Fig. 32-35   Chronic ulceration on the lower lip in a 44-year-old woman. Cause: habitual, painful self-inflicted injury caused by lip biting (cheilophagia). The extension of the lesion corresponds to the impression of the protruding right maxillary anterior teeth from this habit.

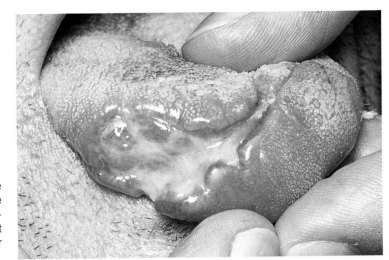

Fig. 32-36   Injury to tongue caused by a grand mal seizure in a 27-year-old epileptic patient. The smear-covered cleft injury remained untreated for 10 days.

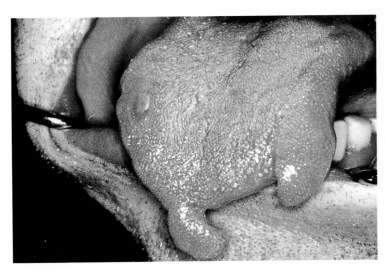

Fig. 32-37   Condition after repeated tongue biting injuries in a 53-year-old epileptic with generalized grand mal seizures. During a previous grand mal seizure, a part of the tongue was bitten off. The right side of the tongue shows consequences of earlier injuries.

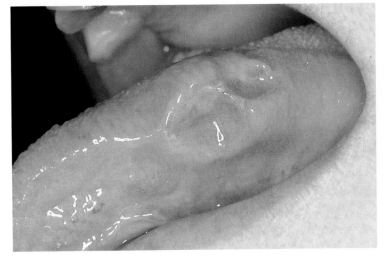

Fig. 32-38   Chronic craterlike bite injury in a patient needing care after a stroke. The finding was associated with the two remaining elongated molars in the left side of the maxilla. Differential diagnosis with a neoplasm is necessary.

Chapter 33

Findings Related to Therapeutic Measures

In the framework of conservative treatment

In the framework of orthodontic treatment

In the framework of prosthodontic treatment

In the framework of local anesthesia

In the framework of oral surgery

In the framework of other forms of therapy

In this chapter a series of lesions are presented that are directly or indirectly related to the following therapeutic measures: conservative treatment, orthodontics, prosthodontics, local anesthesia, oral surgery, and other therapies. It is not the aim of these illustrations to call attention to points of forensic importance. Instead, ways of avoiding incorrect therapies and errors are discussed. It remains to be decided on an individual case basis whether there has been an unexpected change or an avoidable complication as a result of inadequate examination or incorrect planning, carelessness, or inattention to detail, or whether there has been a definite violation of recognized rules of the healing arts. The alert observer will know how to differentiate without further explanation.

A patient's attitude toward hygiene may be a deciding factor in the development of pathologic changes, for example, under complete dentures. In other cases, especially with mucosal lesions in the region of the lips, various and sometimes complex etiologies must be considered.

Finally changes as a result of drastic therapeutic measures (irradiation, for example) deserve attention because such changes may lead to further complications. Some conditions are discussed that, because of technical progress in therapy with ionizing radiation, belong to the past.

All the symptoms that may be the result of dental treatment

measures—as well as undesirable drug effects—are important for differential diagnosis. Without expert knowledge of special problems in dentistry, misinterpretation is easy. Because treatment-associated problems may have a varied presentation, it is desirable to illustrate iatrogenic disease conditions extensively without coming to any conclusions as to the frequency of their occurrence.

Fig. 33-1 Cotton-roll stomatitis (ICD-DA 998.90) with fibrin coating and hyperemia in surrounding area on tooth 23 (11). The diagnosis resulted from the patient's history: the findings occurred 24 hours after use of a cotton roll to dry the field for treatment of tooth 23. Cause: tearing of the epithelium during removal of the dry roll, which stuck to the mucosa (mechanical factor). Chemicals (e. g., bleaching materials) can also have an effect. An allergic reaction was considered but appears unlikely.

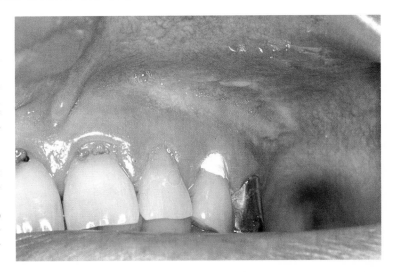

Fig. 33-2 Cotton-roll ulceration in the vestibule of the oral cavity in the region of tooth 44 (28) shown 24 hours after placement of a cervical amalgam restoration on tooth 44. The condition is found more frequently in the maxilla because the capillary suction effect of the cotton roll on the mucosa is smaller in the mandible as result of greater salivary flow. The painful erosion or ulceration sometimes accompanied by soft tissue swelling may be prevented by soaking the cotton roll with water before removing it.

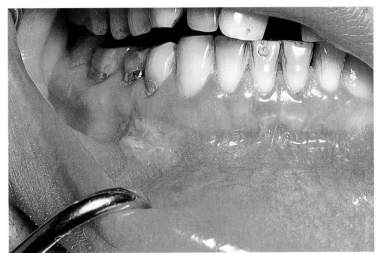

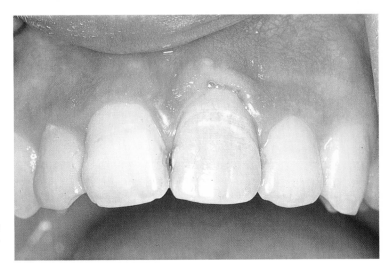

Fig. 33-3 Mechanical trauma of the gingiva of tooth 21 (9) after removal of the rubber dam.

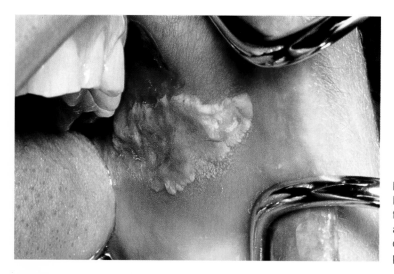

Fig. 33-4   Second-degree burn of the cheek 24 hours after cavity preparation with the aid of local anesthesia. Cause: overheated contra-angle handpiece.

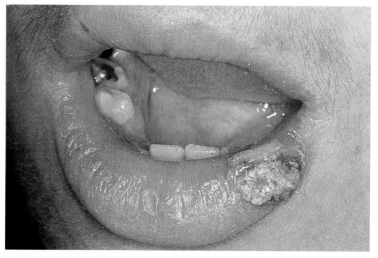

Fig. 33-5   First-degree burn of the upper lip. Situation 2 days after cavity preparation with the aid of local anesthesia. Cause: overheated handpiece. The finding should be differentiated from a self-inflicted wound under local anesthesia (see Fig. 33-43).

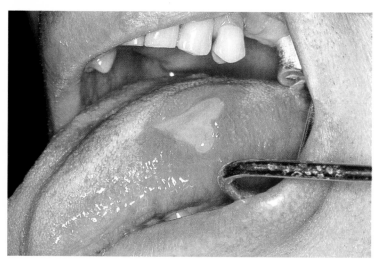

Fig. 33-6   Injury of the tongue caused by a rotating instrument during preparation of a canine for a crown under local anesthesia. Situation 4 days after event.

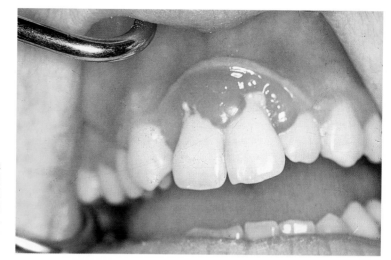

Fig. 33-7 Faulty closure of a medial diastema with nonfixed elastic band. The slow apical movement of the elastic band has already entrapped the circumscribed tissue and caused severe periodontal damage.

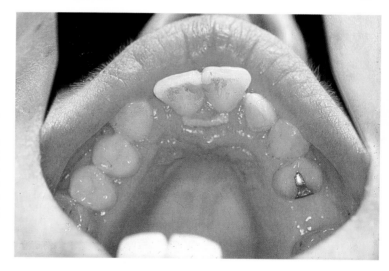

Fig. 33-8 The patient in Fig. 33-7 at the time of examination. On the palatal mucosa are parts of the elastic band that have moved deep into the tissue and tied up the teeth. Both maxillary central incisors are extruded and loose. In most cases, loss of the teeth becomes inevitable (principle of bloodless extraction).

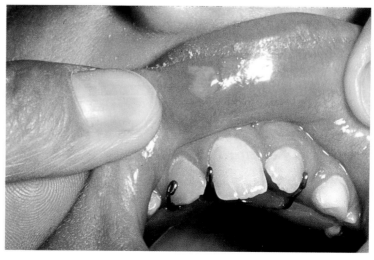

Fig. 33-9 An aphthae-like finding caused by a protruding wire element of an orthodontic appliance and mistaken for an erosion on the upper lip mucosa.

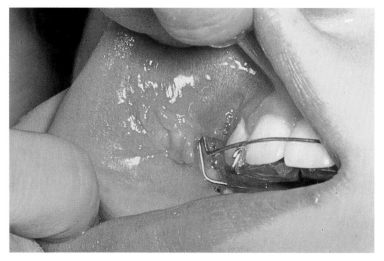

Fig. 33-10   Part erosive-ulcerative, part inflammatory-hyperplastic cheek mucosal change as a result of chronic traumatic irritation by wire elements of an orthodontic appliance.

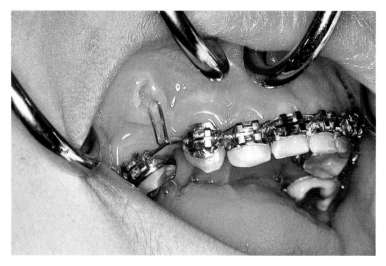

Fig. 33-11   Circumscribed pressure lesion of the vestibular mucosa from a tightly placed closing loop on a multibanded appliance.

Fig. 33-12 Upper lip mucosal erosion corresponding to a gold crown on tooth 12. This mucosal change had been present for 3 months and began to heal only after removal of the gold and palladium–based fixed partial denture. Cause: electrochemical effects between different metals in a patient with a low mucosal threshold. On the basis of the patient's history and assessment of the course, a single healing aphthous lesion and a mechanically induced erosion may be excluded in the differential diagnosis as can thermal damage from smoking.

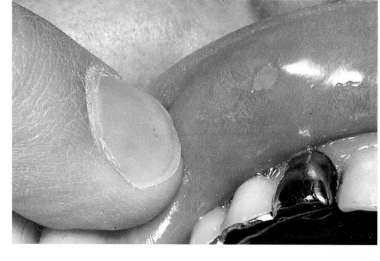

Fig. 33-13 Poorly healing ulcer corresponding to precious metal crown on tooth 22 (10) after local radiation therapy of the left side of the upper lip. Irradiation was ordered because of a mucosal change in the oral vestibule. This change was said to be carcinomatous on the basis of clinical findings alone; no histologic study was done. This type of procedure is considered obsolete today.

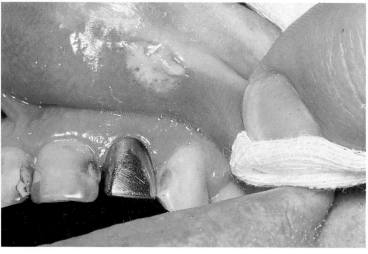

Fig. 33-14 The patient in Fig. 33-13. Appearance after surgery of a lip ulcer and change of the old crown for a provisional composite resin crown. Repair of the change within 2 months. Histologic examination provided no evidence to support the presence of a malignancy. Retrospectively it was thought that the mucosal change in the tissue adjoining the gold crown on tooth 22 was elicited by mechanical and electrochemical reactions on tissue weakened by radiation therapy.

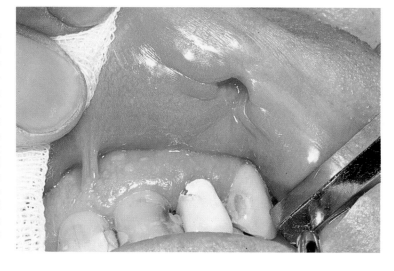

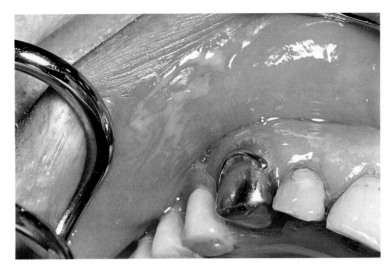

Fig. 33-15   Unusual mechanical-electrochemical reaction of the lip mucosa from metallic materials. The patient complained over a 4-week period of erosive changes of the lip mucosa associated with focal fibrin-coated swelling of the upper lip in the area of teeth 13 (6) and 23 (11). A bullous disease was excluded. The change illustrated is located in the area of the crown of tooth 13.

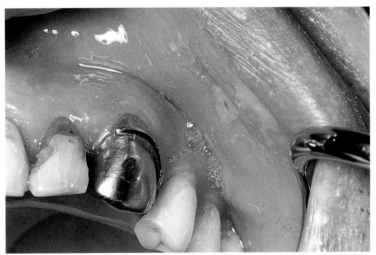

Fig. 33-16   The patient in Fig. 33-15 at the time of examination. Appearance of the left side of the maxilla. The erosion-ulceration on the upper lip mucosa corresponds to the metal surface of the crown on tooth 23 (11). The gingiva is not affected. The patient (a cigarette smoker) wore the prosthesis shown for 5 months: ring collar crown made of precious metal alloy on teeth 13 and 23 as well as mucosal-supported composite resin prosthesis with curved steel clamp. (Observation year is 1967.)

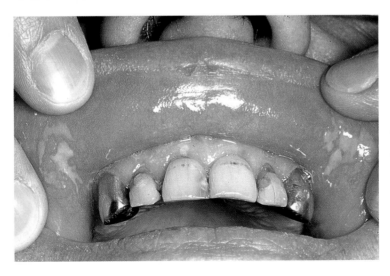

Fig. 33-17   Patient of Figs. 33-15 and 33-16. Situation 2 weeks later while retaining the maxillary partial prosthesis. The change in the area is decreasing, but the erosive efflorescence with partial fibrin cover is unchanged. A mechanical influence from the steel clamps is therefore considered to be secondary.

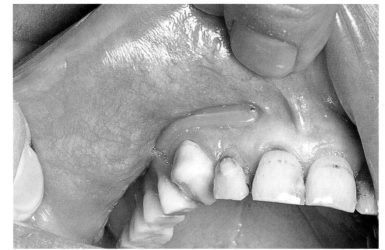

Fig. 33-18   The patient in Figs. 33-15 to 33-17. Situation 6 weeks later and 4 weeks after removal of the collar crowns with substitution of the change of the retention element with compositie resin. Again, there are no noticeable changes in the mucosa of the upper lip.

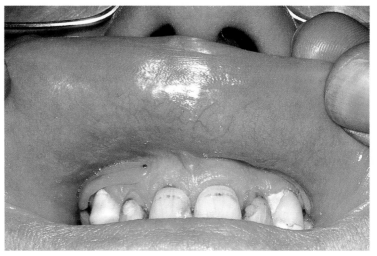

Fig. 33-19   The patient of Figs. 33-15 to 33-18. Situation 12 weeks after the patient was placed under temporary care. The mucosal lesions have now completely disappeared. Examination of the metal in both discolored collar crowns showed considerable corrosion and casting defects primarily in the area of the solder. In addition, superficial deposits of iron are demonstrable. Conclusion: unusual and rare mucosal reactions from electrochemical events on metal surfaces.

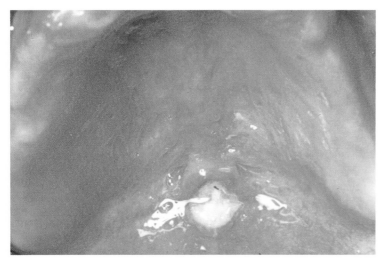

Fig. 33-20 Mechanically caused ulcer (pressure area, decubitus) in the area of the posterior border of the denture. The situation 24 hours after insertion of a relined complete prosthesis. If after elimination of the disturbing prosthesis border there is no rapid healing, ulcerations must be evaluated to exclude other causes.

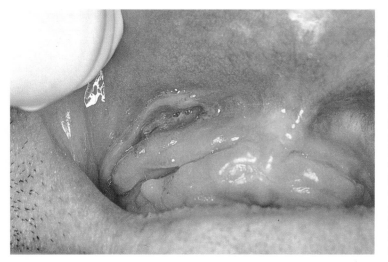

Fig. 33-21 Chronic, prosthesis-induced pressure area in the anterior region of the edentulous maxilla. An overextended or sharp prosthesis border led first to a traumatic ulceration. If the causative irritation is not eliminated, the body tries to heal the now chronic ulceration with development of abnormally inflamed hyperplastic tissue, which is known as a denture irritation hyperplasia, prosthesis irritation fibroma, or prosthesis border fibroma (ICD-DA 523.86).

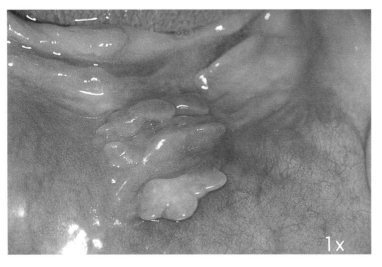

Fig. 33-22 Rimlike denture irritation hyperplasia ("flabby fibroma") in the area of a disturbing prosthesis border in the mandible. Most of these prosthesis-induced changes occur on the vestibular side directly localized on the jaw border. After correction of the prosthesis border and retention of the prosthesis, in many cases regrowth of the irritation hyperplasia occurs. This does not change the basic indication for surgical therapy, but it does reduce the extent of the intervention.

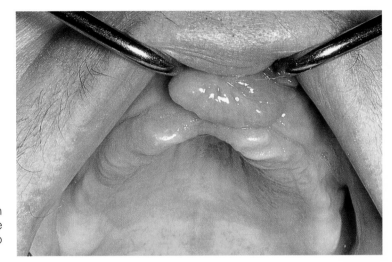

Fig. 33-23   Denture irritation hyperplasia in the fornix of the maxilla with extension to the lip mucosa.

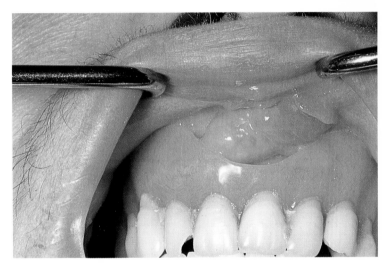

Fig. 33-24   The patient in Fig. 32-23 with a complete prosthesis in place. The extent of the inflammation of the connective tissue corresponds precisely to the damaging prosthesis border. Findings of this extent can be explained only by the patient's high pain and irritation threshold.

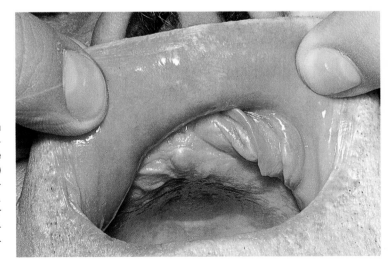

Fig. 33-25   Extended irritation hyperplasia (the so-called lobulated fibroma) in the area of the vestibule of tooth 21 (lack of 9) to 24 (lack of 12) involving transition zone of the lip mucosa. Cause: damaged vestibular prosthesis border of an otherwise functionally deficient maxillary prosthesis.

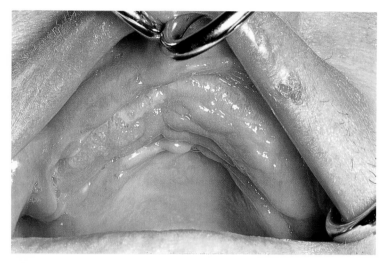

Fig. 33-26   Large rimlike irritation hyperplasia (so-called lobulated fibroma) in an edentulous maxilla with shallow ulcerated zones in the furrows. Cause: functionally insufficient maxillary prosthesis.

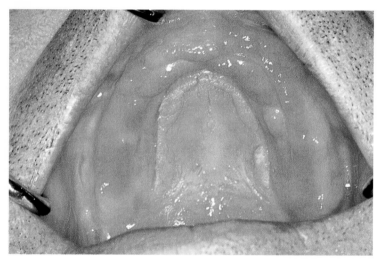

Fig. 33-27   Distinctive resorption of alveolar crest with flabby ridge a few months after placement of a useless palate-free prosthesis. Additional finding: smoker's leukokeratosis in the palatal region not covered by the prosthesis.

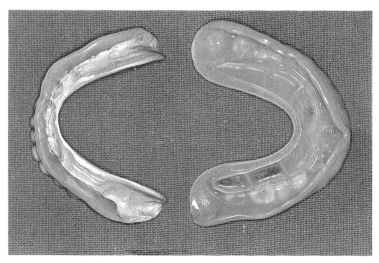

Fig. 33-28   Prosthesis of patient in Fig. 33-27. Appearance of the incorrectly made palate-free complete denture in which attempts at improvements were made by etching on the inside. This type of prosthesis construction made to please the patient can lead to a rapid resorption of the alveolar process and, as a consequence of the considerable pressure, stress to chronic inflammatory tissue hyperplasia as well as destruction of the prosthesis support.

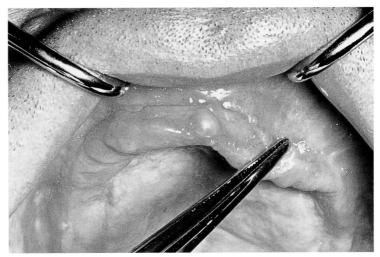

Fig. 33-29 Typical flabby ridge (ICD-DA 523.85) under a maxillary complete prosthesis. In the prosthetic-deficient mandible, there was a remnant dentition. A flabby ridge develops during resorption in the bony alveolar process because of traumatic occlusion and abnormal loading.

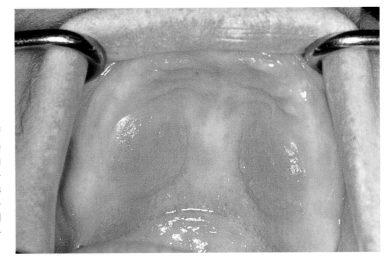

Fig. 33-30 Bilateral growth of the mucosa of the hard palate corresponding to the vacuum chamber of a complete prosthesis (see Fig. 33-31). This type of vacuum chamber stimulates proliferation of tissue and regularly leads to these changes.

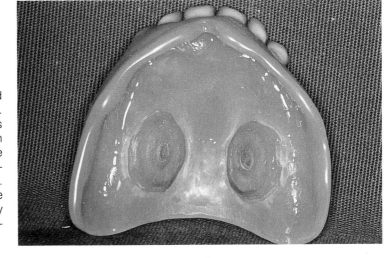

Fig. 33-31 Prosthesis related to the findings in Fig. 30-30. Preparation of the prosthesis for the use of a rubber suction cup is rejected today because of fundamental changes of impression making techniques. The small improvement of the prosthesis support as felt by the patient produced irreparable tissue damage.

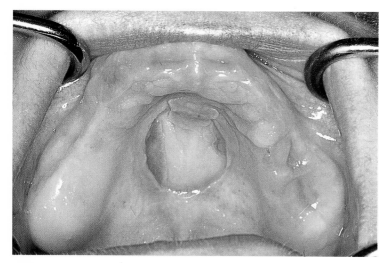

Fig. 33-32 Damage produced by rubber suction cup. The maxillary partial prosthesis was not replaced with a complete denture after loss of the last teeth; a suction device was used to obtain support. The damaging influence of the rubber disk led—particularly because it coalesces after long use—to impressions, ulcerations, and chronic proliferative inflammation processes with bone resorption. The perforation of the hard palate toward the nasal cavity is demonstrated.

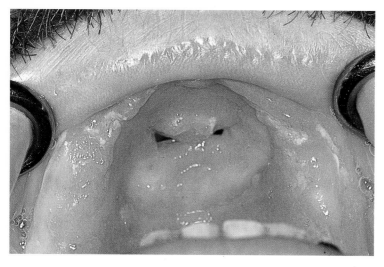

Fig. 33-33 Palatal perforation by a rubber suction cup. Destroyed palate roof with large fistula into the nasal cavity. Lack of attention and therefore conditioned, unavoidable rocking movement of the alveolar process leads to resorption events. There are indications in the literature of a causal relation between the extended use of a rubber suction cup and the development of carcinomas.

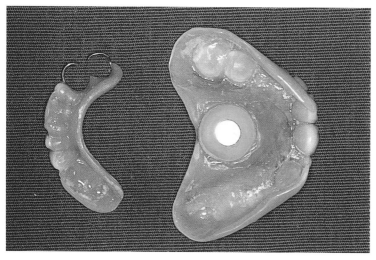

Fig. 33-34 Prosthesis of patient in Fig. 33-33. Completely inadequate construction of the base and function border of dentures in the maxilla and mandible. The rubber suction cup suggests negligence on the part of the practitioner.

Fig. 33-35   Denture stomatitis (ICD-DA 528.91) under a transverse connector. The continuous nonphysiologic covering of the mucosal area by the prosthesis led to findings that included reddening (erythema) and atrophy of the mucosa, which occurs more frequently in the maxilla than mandible. In the multifactorial etiology, mechanical and microbiologic influences play a major role. This emphasizes the importance of careful mouth and prosthetic hygiene. In some texts, the increased *Candida albicans* colonization under prostheses in patients with denture stomatitis

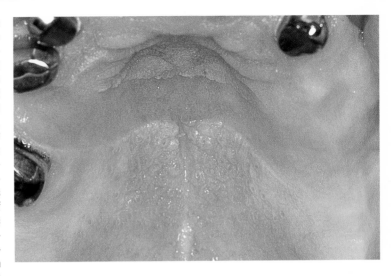

is given such a high causal value that these disease findings are also called *chronic atrophic candidiasis* (ICD-DA 112.03). The results of antimycotic therapy are, however, of little comfort. The original lesion probably requires another explanation. The covered mucosal region remains protected from the other changes, such as the smoker's leukokeratosis involving the remainder of the mucosa.

Fig. 33-36   Denture stomatitis under complete prosthesis. Inflammatory mucosal changes under complete prostheses are found in 30% to 40% of all prosthesis wearers. Focal reddened spots and diffuse inflammatory reactions over the whole prosthesis area are observed particularly in the palatal mucosa. There is also a hyperplastic-type of denture stomatitis (see Fig. 33-37). Many patients have no complaints despite obvious objective findings. A most important differential diagnosis is with allergy to prosthetic components and prosthetic cleaning materials. They occur, however, less frequently than is usually suspected in practice. As opposed to denture stomatitis, the allergic reactions caused by prosthetic intolerance inflammation always involve the support area of the prosthesis. They are always associated with symptoms.

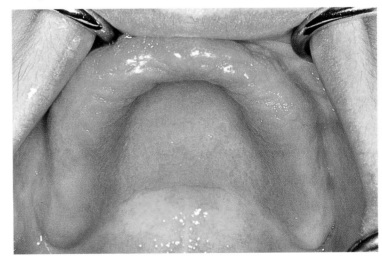

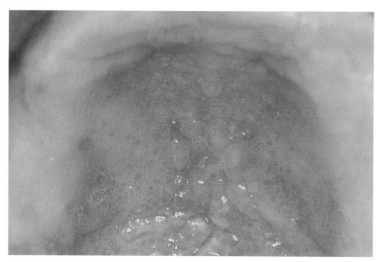

Fig. 33-37   Denture stomatitis of the hyperplastic type (papillary hyperplasia). The papillary hyperplasia of the palate (ICD-DA 528.92) under the complete maxillary denture—particularly in the area of the suction chamber and noncontact areas—is not uncommon (occurs in about 3% to 10% of cases). This hyperplastic variant of prosthesis stomatitis shows a nodular configuration, rough granulation, or small corny to mosslike surface structures. It is usually surrounded by inflamed mucosa and is not painful. This condition is most often seen in patients who use their prosthesis day and night. There is not always a lack of prosthetic hygiene. Fungi are almost always demonstrable. In some cases, these findings can also be observed in nighttime prosthesis users. Papillary hyperplasia is currently considered a benign change. In extensive findings, surgical intervention is recommended. Low-grade papillary hyperplasia will regress after removal of local irritative factors, repair, and disinfection of the prosthesis base in some cases complemented by an additional application of a *Candida*-specific antimycotic on the inside of the prosthesis.

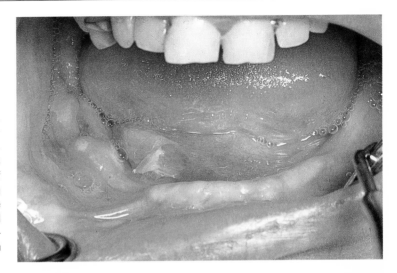

Fig. 33-38   Circumscribed lesion of the mucosa of the floor of the mouth close to the mandibular ridge of teeth 44 to 46 (28 to 30) as a consequence of improper use of a spray-form surface anesthetic. The nozzle of the spray can was placed too close to the mucosa, causing local tissue damage with superficial erosion.

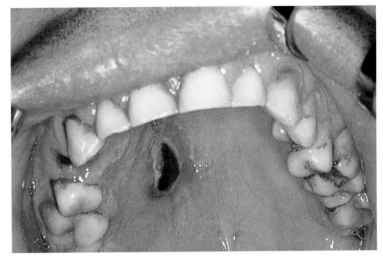

Fig. 33-39   Sharply delimited area of mucoperiosteal necrosis in the hard palate after local anesthesia for the removal of the maxillary right first premolar. Cause: excessive pressure during infiltration anesthesia in the region of the palatal mucosa tightly adhering to the bone.

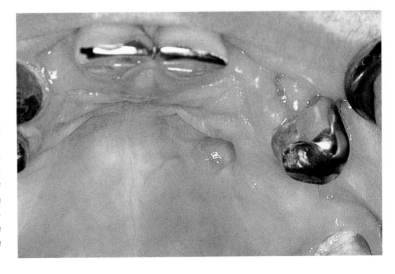

Fig. 33-40   Necrosis reaching the bone at the point of injection during infiltration anesthesia in the hard palate. Cause: excessive pressure caused by injection of too much fluid in the area of the tightly adhering palatal mucosa. With appropriate injection technique, this tissue damage can be avoided.

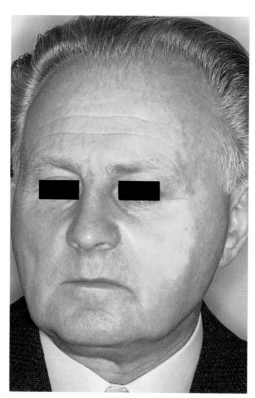

Fig. 33-41 Circumscribed anemic zone of the facial skin from angiospasm after infiltration anesthesia on the left infraorbital foramen. This temporary symptom can occur by direct irritation of the arterial wall or reflexively through contact with vessel nerves during injection.

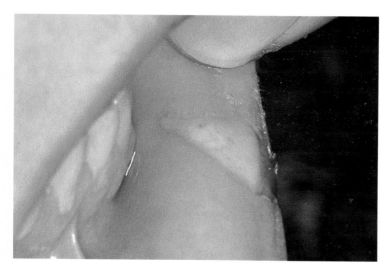

Fig. 33-42 Triangular necrosis on the upper lip of a 23-year-old woman with acute angle toward the vestibular fold. Situation 3 days after an infiltration anesthesia for removal of tooth 36 (19). There is no obvious bite wound. Form and extension of the mucosal change points to an ischemic tissue necrosis as expression of a pathergic response of the local vessel system to adrenalin. An organic tissue damage and infarct can also be excluded as possible factors.

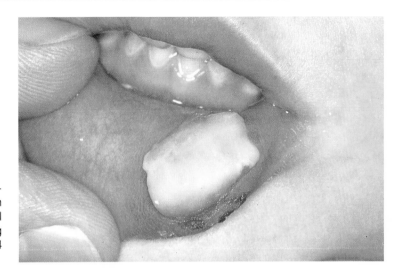

Fig. 33-43 Unintentional self-inflicted wound (bite wound) on the lower lip of a 7-year-old girl under local anesthesia. Finding of lip defect with fibrin cover 24 hours after the event.

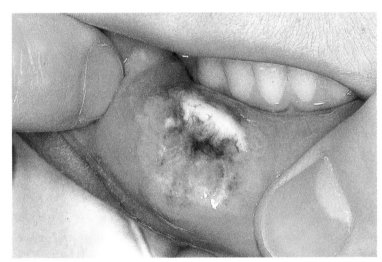

Fig. 33-44 Extensive ulceration of the lower lip with central necrosis in an 11-year-old boy 48 hours after unintentional self-inflicted wound (bite wound) under local anesthesia.

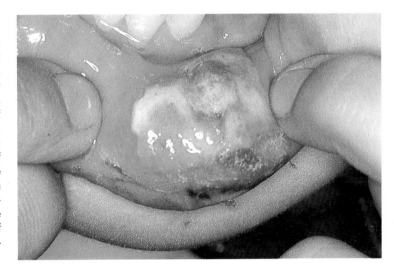

Fig. 33-45 Extensive fibrin-coated ulceration with central necrosis on the left side of the lower lip in a 10-year-old boy shown 3 days after infiltration anesthesia for the extraction of teeth 73, 74, and 75 (K, L, M). In children, bite injuries during the period of effectiveness of long-acting anesthetics are the most common cause of such lesions. Children and accompanying adults should therefore be warned of the possibility of self-inflicted injuries to the locally anesthetized lips.

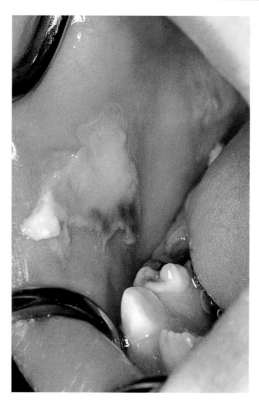

Fig. 33-46   Condition 2 days after self-inflicted wound (bite wound) under local anesthesia in the right cheek region in a 9-year-old girl. In habitual cheek biting, findings in adults are more discrete (see Figs. 32-30, 32-31 and 34-14, 34-16).

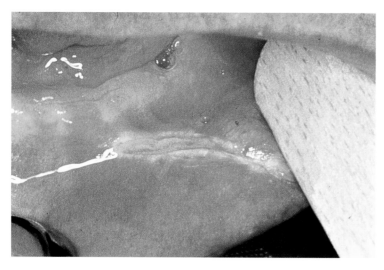

Fig. 33-47   Line-shaped ulceration extending from the left side of the lower lip to the alveolar ridge, with surrounding leukoplakia. Because of trigeminal neuralgia, this 64-year-old man underwent exeresis of the alveolar mandibular nerve. Cause of the present lesion: chronic bite injury in the permanently anesthetized region.

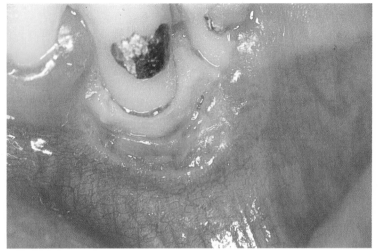

Fig. 33-48   Bone necrosis after incorrect use of electrosurgical equipment for gingivectomy. Bone and/or dental root contact with the working electrode must be avoided. The performance of the equipment must be adjusted to the work region.

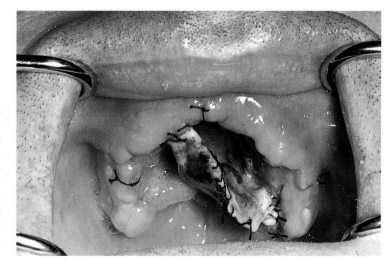

Fig. 33-49   Necrosis of the entire mucosa of the hard palate after a faulty incision for the removal of a palatally impacted canine with a follicular cyst. The palatine artery was cut bilaterally. The necrotic palatal flap remains attached on the left side by a few stitches while on the right side it has sloughed off.

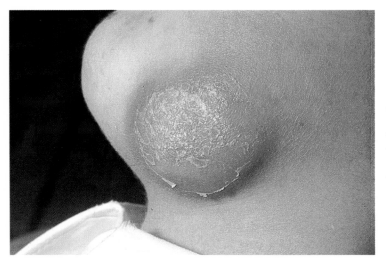

Fig. 33-50 Circumscribed necrosis of the skin covering a submandibular abscess that was not surgically treated in time. Instead of the needed incision, the abscess was treated with inadequate and irregular doses of antibiotics and by external warm applications for 14 days. As a rule such "conservative" treatment does not stop the progress of the disease.

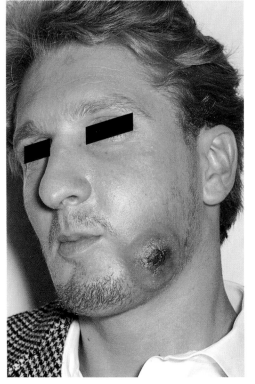

Fig. 33-51 Circumscribed necrosis of the skin covering an abscess of the cheek about to perforate spontaneously. The abscess arose from nonvital tooth 36 (19). The acute inflammatory condition was treated with inadequate and irregular doses of antibiotics, and the abscess was treated "conservatively" for 3 months with external warm applications.

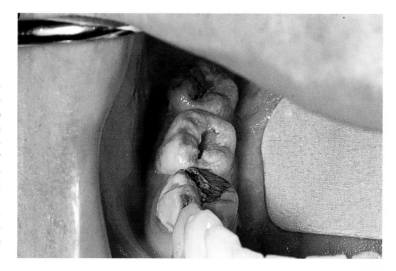

Fig. 33-52 Tooth damage after deep radiation therapy (tumor dose), which also led to cessation of salivary flow. In each area that has been treated by radiation, even a minor dental-surgical intervention carries a danger of severe wound repair damage (osteomyelitis, osteo-radiation necrosis). Therefore, antibiotic therapy is prescribed obligatorily in these cases.

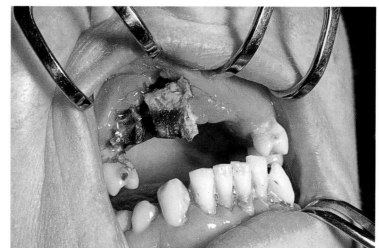

Fig. 33-53 Osteo-radiation necrosis of the right side of the maxilla after radiation therapy for lymphoma. Note the extensive exposed bone sequestrum bulging into the oral cavity. (Observation year is 1965.)

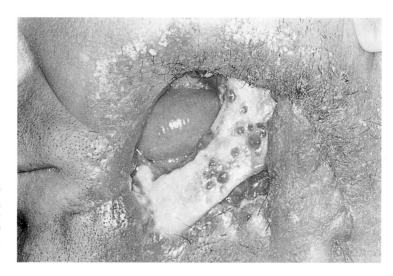

Fig. 33-54 Osteo-radiation necrosis of the left side of the mandible visible through a large cheek defect in a patient with advanced carcinoma of the cheek. (Observation year is 1963.)

Chapter 34

Problematic Angle of the Mouth

The angle of the mouth in children

The angle of the mouth in adolescents and young adults

The angle of the mouth with increased age

The angle of the mouth in systemic disease

Angle of the mouth and leukoplakias

The special anatomic and physiologic conditions of the angle of the mouth and the diseases that affect this problem zone require their own chapter. With this we consciously gave up a possible nosologic classification. For the many diseases affecting the region of the angle of the mouth, there are many synonyms: *angle of the mouth fissure, angle of the mouth rhagades, angle of the mouth cheilitis, angular cheilitis, perleche, infected angle,* and in some instances *interlabial mycosis.* In most cases, there is a polyetiologic disease picture, whose origin is recognized and, if need be, can be clarified in close interdisciplinary work.

Anatomy-physiology of the angle of the mouth

In regard to the epithelial covering there are three zones of the lip that can be recognized:

- Typical skin epithelium and skin appendages (hair, sweat, and sebaceous glands)

- A vermilion of the lip transitional zone, which is generally covered with a weakly cornified squamous epithelium and sometimes contains sebaceous glands without associated hair follicle unit; the sharply limited color of the vermilion of the lip is determined by the rich capillary network, which reaches almost to the surface of connective tissue papillae
- The area of the vermilion of the lip that blends with the oral region without a sharp demarcation but is associated with small seromucous glands under noncornified squamous cell epithelium (lip mucosa)

The corner of the mouth is the lateral border of the mouth slit and from a functional point of view is very important. In this region, the vermilion of the lip is the transition zone from the outer integument to the oral mucosa and is thinner than in any other zones of the lip (Figs. 34-1 and 34-2). This means that the skin of this area is influenced by the environment of the oral cavity. The lip orbicularis oris muscle tends to modulate with the other mimic musculature of the mouth opening with many extraordinary appearances. Form and movement of the lips are important for expression and body language. There is also an impressive change of the architecture of the mouth and perioral region during life. Besides natural changes in the skin and mucosa (loss of elasticity due to collagenization, decreased turgor), there are additional changes that influence the alveolar process of both jaws because of loss of teeth, opening of the mouth, the width of the vermilion of the lips, the position of the lips, and the mimic movements.

There is maximum extension of the angle of the mouth with extreme opening movement (Figs. 34-3 and 34-4), a condition that is damaging for fissure healing. There are other mechanical influences from the teeth, dental gaps, and prostheses to consider.

The mucosa at the angle of the mouth toward the retroangular region (Figs. 34-3 and 34-5) near the oral cavity corresponds embryonically to confluence regions of the maxillary and mandibular primordia. The cheek line derives ontogenetically from the epidermis, and the tendency to a so-called epidermization in nonphysiologic stress and in aging can be explained.

The skin of the angle of the mouth region is subjected to nonphysiologic wetting with saliva. This damage is an important determining factor for disease changes manifested on the skin of the area.

The angle of the mouth in children

First it is necessary to differentiate the most frequent paramedian pits in the angle of the mouth area (Figs. 34-6 to 34-8) from the rare *congenital lip pits* (ICD-DA 750.24). In this defect (remnants of the lateral lip sulci), there are blind-end tubes 0.5 to 2.5 cm long, from which there can be discharge of slimy secretion under pressure. Therapy consists of careful excision. In children, one must pay attention to *angular cheilitis* (ICD-DA 528.50), which is usually caused by streptococci (Figs. 34-9 and 34-10). Fungus colonization is rare at this age. These streptococcal infections of the skin of the angle of the mouth can develop into a contagious impetigo (see chapter 7).

A determining local factor is the continuous nonphysiologic wetting of the corner of the mouth with saliva, which brings with it a disturbance of the protective barrier of the skin and can result in maceration. This facilitates development of conditions for the colonization and entrance into the oral cavity of germs that are saprophytic but that develop facultative or obligatory pathogenic properties on the skin. In children, this compromised skin can originate from motor habits such as salivating, lip licking (Fig. 34-11), pacifier sucking, finger sucking, holding objects in the mouth (pencil, wood stick from sweets or popsicles) with resultant saliva flow. Without a change of behavior, any local therapy is of little value. Local treatment belongs in the hands of a pediatrician or dermatologist and should eliminate bacterial infection and return to normal the physiological environment of the skin.

In children and in adults, atopic eczemas are a predisposing factor to skin damage and angular cheilitis, based on predisposing genetic conditions.

The angle of the mouth in adolescents and young adults

From our experience with adolescents and young adults, *stress-related* parafunctional habits that involve the corner of the mouth are an important factor; for instance, the habit of continuously rubbing the skin with the tongue in this context, the habit of lip sucking, and the widely practiced habit of chronically nibbling on the lips and the cheek mucosa *(cheilophagia, cheek biting)*, to name a few (Figs. 34-14 to 34-16). Further discussion of the subject is found in chapter 32.

Self-inflicted wounds of the lips often lead to pain. The associated overloading of the angle of the mouth area sometimes leads to inflammatory changes in the region. Biting of foreign objects (pencils, paper clips, toothpicks, cigarette holders, pipes) can lead to additional erosive-fissural lesions in the area of the corner of the mouth. These habits also facilitate the flow of saliva (drooling) with resulting delayed healing.

Once lesions in the corner of the mouth have appeared, they have such a high irritative potential that even careful patients have a hard time stopping repeated touching with the tongue (Figs. 34-12 and 34-13) to check whether the painful lesion has regressed.

The angle of the mouth with increased age

With increased age, there are atrophic events on the skin and mucosa (decreased turgor, reduction of elasticity, deepening of the nasolabial fold) in addition to the reduction of the occlusal height related to tooth surface abrasion. This is especially the consequence of a lack of vertical support caused by partial or complete loss of dentition and sometimes as a consequence of an inadequate occlusion of a prosthesis. The phenomena are predisposing factors for the development of changes in the corner of the mouth. In this manner, the skeletal-dental support frame alters the mouth opening. In these cases, the lip can roll resulting in a narrow vermilion border, as seen in edentulous patients or when a denture is not properly cared for (Figs. 34-17 and 34-18).

The part of the corner of the mouth built by the skin is displaced intraorally. The altered skin tears because of constant wetting with saliva and because of stretching with increased mouth opening. The resulting fissures do not heal due to the nonphysiologic humidity (Figs. 34-17 to 34-19). These findings irritate the patient, making him or her instinctively place the tongue over the zone much of the time. This vicious cycle is the basis for infection.

The chronic angular cheilitis that occurs at this age usually is colonized by *Candida albicans* with development of chronic atrophic candidiasis (ICD-DA 112.03). This finding of a localized skin mycosis is frequently found in women at menopause (Fig. 34-20) and represents a noncontagious *interlabial mycosis*. Presumptive causes for the manifestation of the disease are the already-mentioned predisposing factors. Because *Candida albicans* is present in the oral cavity in 30% to 50% of people as a saprophyte, swabs from the oral mucosa are only a qualitative proof and offer no diagnostic certainty.

In the area of the corner of the mouth, one must differentiate an atrophy form (Fig. 34-20) from a chronic hyperplastic partially granulomatous form of this mycosis (Figs. 34-21 and 32-22). The interlabial mycosis can also be a partial manifestation of a more extensive candidiasis of the oral cavity.

The following therapeutic measures are based on the complex etiologic initial situation:

The first step in treatment should always be raising of the occlusion, that is, recreating the original occlusion to unfold the skin of the corner of the mouth and in this manner to eliminate maceration caused by saliva, improving the environment (making it dry). If there is then an improvement and there is no evidence of a systemic disease, the existence of a persisting interlabial mycosis should be considered.

This makes local treatment with a *Candida*-specific antimycotic agent desirable. However, antimycotic treatment without previous removal of local predisposing factors by adequate dental prosthetic measures leads to failure.

Regarding differential diagnosis, one must consider *cheilitis simplex*, which is preferentially located in the middle of the lower lip, from the changes of the corner of the mouth already described. Through lack of secretion and drying out *(desiccation cheilitis)*, there can be development of bleeding, wet cuts with crust formation ("opened lip") and also of deep persistent severely obstinate fissures (Figs. 34-23 and 34-24).

Cheilitis glandularis simplex must also be considered. It is based on a hyperplasia of the small mixed salivary glands in the contact surface of the lips, the lower lip in particular. The hyperplastic seromucous glands appear clinically as pinhead-sized reddish elevations. Under pressure there is spontaneous secretion discharge from their small openings (Fig. 34-25). In severe cases there can be development of macrocheilia, which facilitates the appearance of rhagades (Fig. 34-25). Conservative therapy of the disease offers little success. A limited surgical intervention is therefore indicated.

Herpes simplex labialis, which has a preferential location on the corner of the mouth (Fig. 34-26) with crust stage and possible secondary fissures, should be easily differentiated using the patient history and previous observations (Fig. 34-27). It is more difficult to differentiate damage to the corner of the mouth caused by mechanical conditions when the area is secondarily infected and history of previous intervention is not reported. For example, this is the case in *rhagade-forming pressure ulcerations,* which sometimes develop during dental treatment under local anesthesia because of a long, exaggerated push with a dental mirror or retractors (Fig. 34-28). As a rule, they heal rapidly and spontaneously.

The angle of the mouth in systemic disease

An important differential diagnostic problem is to distinguish the corner of the mouth fissures (not considering those already discussed) as a secondary symptom of a general disease. These findings are infrequent in *diabetes mellitus* (Fig. 34-29 and chapter 26). Perleche can also appear in *iron deficiency anemias* (Fig. 34-30 and chapter 24), in *vitamin deficiency,* and in *maldigestion and malabsorption syndromes* (see chapter 26). In these cases, there are usually also nonspecific oral concomitant symptoms such as mouth dryness and/ or burning tongue that, together with other findings, point to the endogenous cause and suggest the need for an internal medicine evaluation.

As an initial symptom of acute leukemia, there are often nonhealing ulcerations of the corner of the mouth region (Fig. 34-31). There are frequent concurrent and varied combinations of obvious oral mucosal changes (necrosis-ulcerations, tissue swelling processes as expression of leukemic proliferations in previously damaged gingivoperiodontal areas, bleeding) and general symptoms that lead the dentist to suspect a disease of the leukopoietic system (see chapter 24).

Obviously, with lesions linked to systemic disease any local treatment will be without effect as long as nothing is done about the main problem. This is true for *Candida albicans* interlabial mycosis during severe *consumptive disease* as well in *immunologic conditions* (see chapters 10 and 11). Also, certain diseases can show a deceptive perleche. A classic example of this phenomenon is the perleche appearance of highly infectious fissured papillae in secondary syphilis (see Fig. 8-6), which can be mistaken for polymorphic skin efflorescences in the perioral region as well as for modified changes in the oral cavity.

Many dermatologic diseases that facultatively or obligatorily are associated with lip and oral mucosa participation can also involve the corner of the mouth (Figs. 34-32 and 34-33). Systemic diseases in which atrophic skin and mucosal changes can develop also facilitate the formation of fissures in the corner of the mouth—among others, *Sjögren's syndrome* (Fig. 30-12), *systemic scleroderma* (Fig. 30-8), and *dermatomycosis*.

The same is true for the conditions after *irradiation therapy* in the jaw-face region. In *granulomatous cheilitis (Melkersson-Rosenthal syndrome)*, there are initially periodic, and later chronic lip swellings that are sometimes misdiagnosed as repeated episodes of angular cheilitis but that are actually part of the syndrome. In this manner, cause and effect can be confused.

The angle of the mouth and leukoplakias

Every pathologic cornification decreases the natural flexibility and loading capabilities of the mucosa of the corner of the mouth and the retroangular region. There can be simple (flat-homogeneous) leukoplakias (see chapter 17) as well as precancerous leukoplakias (see chapter 18), and they can develop on the basis of overstretching with rhagades and fissural epithelial damage. Through such secondary tears, homogeneous leukoplakia may assume the clinical picture of a suspicious precancerous lesion. Also to be considered is that epithelial defects of this type facilitate superimposed bacterial or mycotic infections. All of these conditions make more difficult the clinical evaluation of a leukoplakia in this region and complicate the diagnostic process for the dentist (Figs. 34-34 to 34-44).

A few cases are presented in which a growing carcinoma was falsely considered an angular cheilitis on the basis of a perfunctory examination (Figs. 34-45 to 34-49).

Figs. 34-1   Corner of the mouth at rest. Note the decrease in size of the lip zone toward the corner. There is more intense tissue turgor in adolescents. The mimic play of the musculature around the mouth gives an indication of personality.

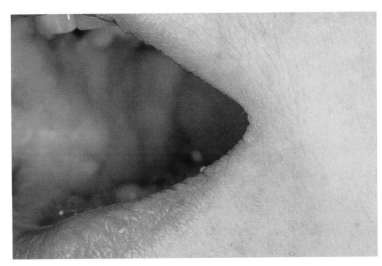

Fig. 34-2   Corner of the mouth slightly opened in the same adolescent. The corner of the mouth region is unfolded and allows recognition of the thinnest point of the vermilion of the lip.

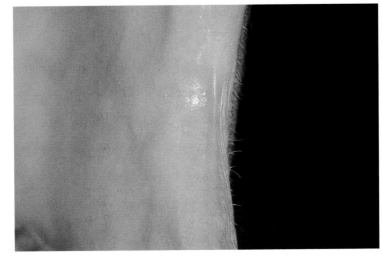

Fig. 34-3   Corner of the mouth of the same adolescent intraorally with wider opening of the mouth. The transition zone of the vermilion of the lip is maximally distended. Circumscribed keratinization in retroangular region.

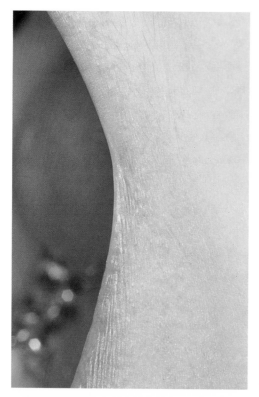

Fig. 34-4   Skin of the corner of the mouth with maximum distention.

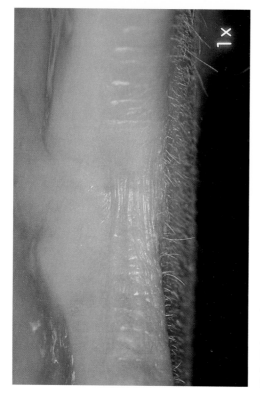

Fig. 34-5   Corner of the mouth in average mouth opening at higher magnification. Note the sharp limits of the hairy skin of the vermilion of the lip. Also note the relation of the upper and lower lips with the triangle in the retroangular mucosal segment center at the corner of the mouth.

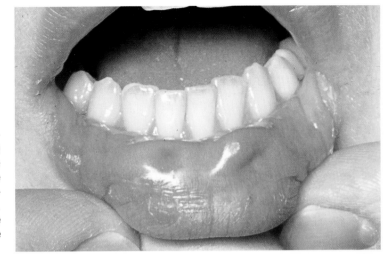

Fig. 34-6 Congenital paramedian mandibular lip fistulas. The funnel-shaped openings of the usually symmetric fistulas are easy to see within the circumscribed swelling of the lip. These congenital findings are associated with a cleft palate and reduced number of teeth.

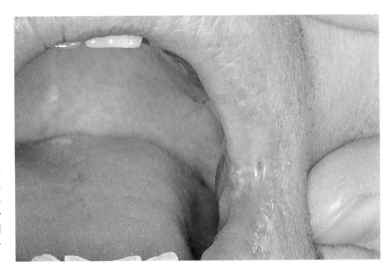

Fig. 34-7 Congenital lateral lower lip fistula with discrete retroangular leukoplakia. The fistulas are usually symmetrically placed. More often, the lateral findings are paramedian blunt-ending fistulas.

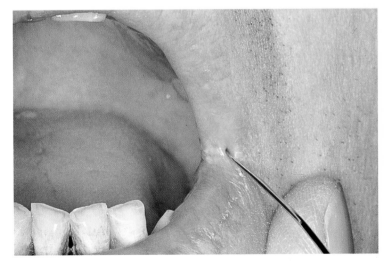

Fig. 34-8 Congenital lateral lower lip fistula with embedded blunt probe in the patient of Fig. 34-7. The fistula ends blindly after 0.7 cm. The discrete line-forming eczema of the skin in the border area of the upper lip vermilion is caused by chronic wetting.

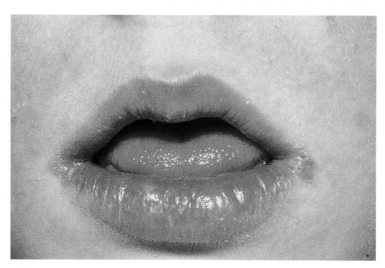

Fig. 34-9   Streptococcal angular infection in a school-age child.

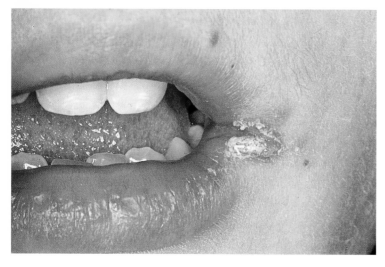

Fig. 34-10   Streptococcal angular infection with fissure formations in a 9-year-old child. These findings can progress to a contagious impetigo.

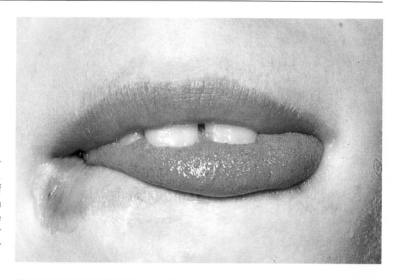

Fig. 34-11 So-called lip licking in an 8-year-old child. Sharply limited maceration of the skin with fissure formation from habitual rubbing of the tongue. Under the right corner of the mouth is an inflamed hair follicle unit.

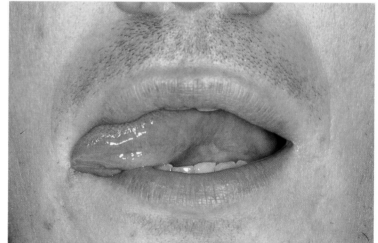

Fig. 34-12 Tongue licking produced perleche on the right corner of the mouth in a young adult. To confirm the diagnosis, it is desirable to allow a demonstration of movements of the tongue.

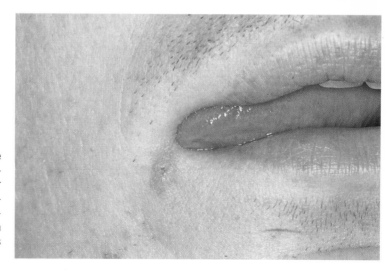

Fig. 34-13 Perleche in the patient of Fig. 34-13. The inflammatory change of the hair follicle (folliculitis) in the macerated area continues to give occasion to touch this area with the tongue creating a vicious circle.

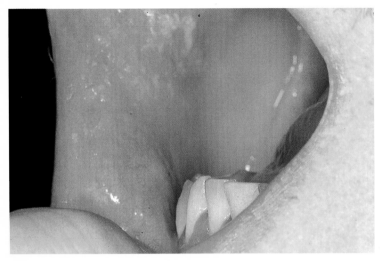

Fig. 34-14   Cheek biting. Only in the angle of the mouth is it possible to tear off epithelium. In the anterior third of the cheek, a focal whitish epithelial thickening is demonstrated by stretching the mucosa. These findings are frequently combined with bruxism.

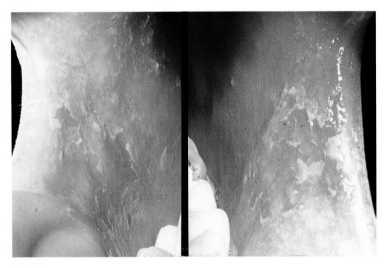

Fig. 34-15   Mucosal findings in the retroangular region of bilateral cheek biting. Cause: partially due to habit, partially due to shyness, constant gnawing and biting of the cheek mucosa. Note the gnawed oral mucosal parts with shallow erosions and floating epithelial remnants. Cheek-biting patients are usually not cooperative during the history taking; when in doubt, the suspected cause of the findings should be pointed out to them.

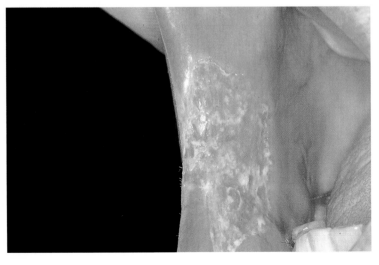

Fig. 34-16   The epithelial lesion from chronic cheek nibbling extends to the mucosa of the corner of the mouth. These findings of self-inflicted wounds are often mistakenly diagnosed as leukoplakia or candidiasis.

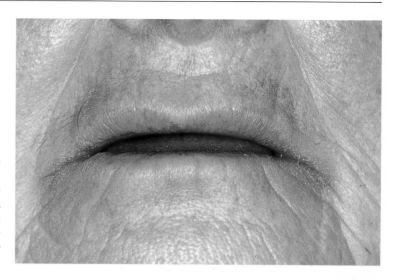

Fig. 34-17   Perleche in a 65-year-old woman caused by decreased occlusion. This situation leads to continuous saliva wetting, which after maceration of the skin area can lead to eczema. The first therapeutic step is to raise the occlusion.

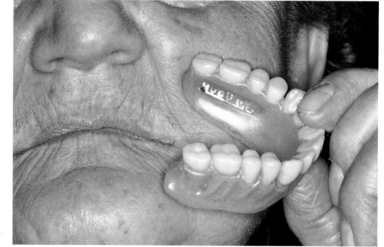

Fig. 34-18   Typical lip findings in a edentulous 69-year-old woman after removal of her prosthesis. Through the loss of vertical dimension of the jaws there is a narrowing of the vermilion border of the lips, wrinkling of the skin, and deepening of the nasolabial fold.

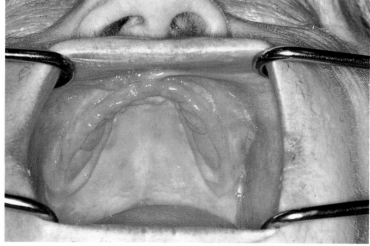

Fig. 34-19   Fissures at the corner of the mouth in the patient of Fig. 34-18. Stretching of the corner of the mouth can be recognized when the mouth is opened. The patient's nonfunctional palate-free complete prosthesis was rebased in an attempt to provide retention. As an expression of the mechanically conditioned inflammation caused by prosthesis malfunction, there is severe damage in the maxillary region of the prosthesis (flabby fibromatosis and flabby ridge associated with considerable bone loss).

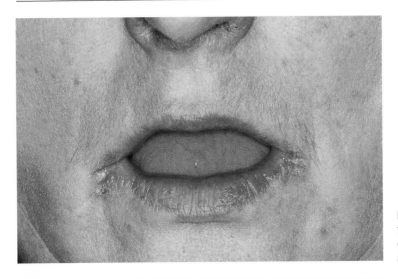

Fig. 34-20 Chronic-atrophic form of interlabial mycosis caused by *Candida albicans* in a 63-year-old woman.

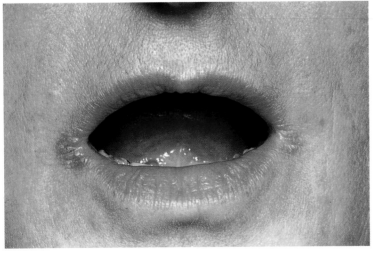

Fig. 34-21 Chronic-hyperplastic form of interlabial mycosis caused by *Candida albicans* in a 48-year-old patient. In these cases, there is usually an associated systemic problem.

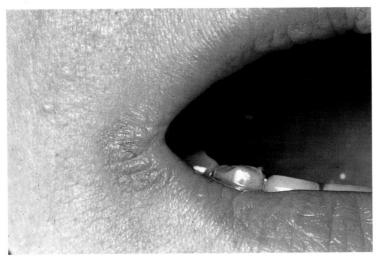

Fig. 34-22 Close-up view of the right corner of the mouth in the patient of Fig. 34-21. The well-demonstrated granulomatous tissue change has been present for 2 years. The local pathfinder in this case was the habit of constantly wetting the corner of the mouth with the tongue. As a facilitating systemic factor, it was possible to find a severe iron deficiency anemia. Diabetic metabolism disturbance as well as liver disease should be eliminated.

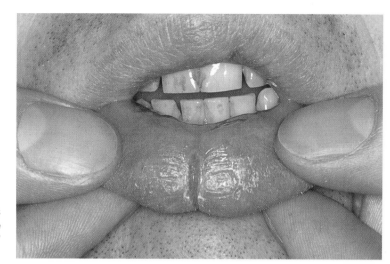

Fig. 34-23 Simple cheilitis with chronic deep fissure. The phenomenon of "opened lips" results from dryness.

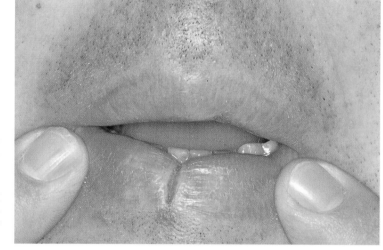

Fig. 34-24 Simple cheilitis with chronic, deep fissure in the patient of Fig. 34-23 at the same examination. The 2-month-old fissure extends to the skin-covered surface of the lower lip and has formed a circumscribed inflamed infiltration. These lesions often resist conservative local therapy so that excision may be necessary in difficult cases.

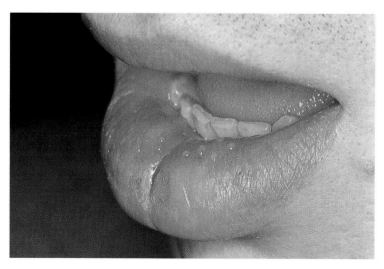

Fig. 34-25 Macrocheilia with median fissure in simple glandular cheilitis. A clear, viscous secretion empties spontaneously or under pressure from the dilated ducts of the small hyperplastic salivary glands.

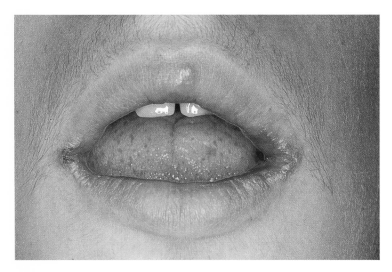

Fig. 34-26   Labial herpes with involvement of the corner of the mouth and the upper lip below the philtrum.

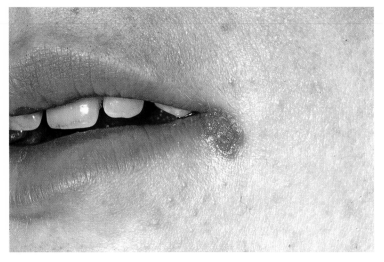

Fig. 34-27   Superimposed infection in a labial herpes of the angle of the mouth.

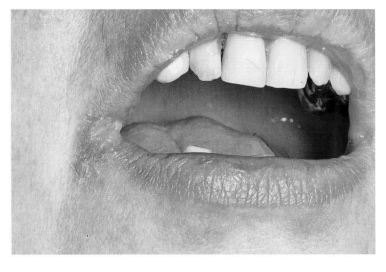

Fig. 34-28   Fissurelike pressure ulcerations in the area of the right angle of the mouth caused by extended pressure with a dental mirror during conservative dental treatment.

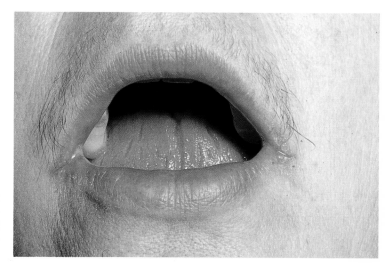

Fig. 34-29   Angular infection as a consequence of inadequately controlled mature-onset diabetes in a 52-year-old woman.

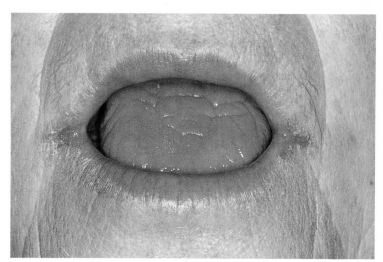

Fig. 34-30   Perleche in a 64-year-old woman. Cause: too-short occlusal distance in the prosthesis (local factor) and chronic iron deficiency (systemic factor). Note the atrophic, smooth tongue, a result of the systemic factor.

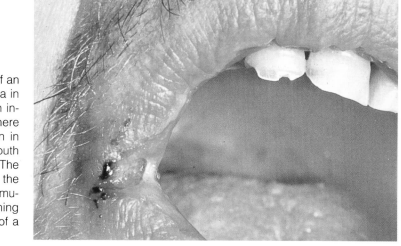

Fig. 34-31   Manifestation of an acute myelogenous leukemia in a 68-year-old woman. As an initial symptom, for 5 weeks there was a nonhealing ulceration in the right corner of the mouth with infiltrated borders. The spontaneous bleeding on the same side of the palatal mucosa associated with declining health led to the suspicion of a blood disease.

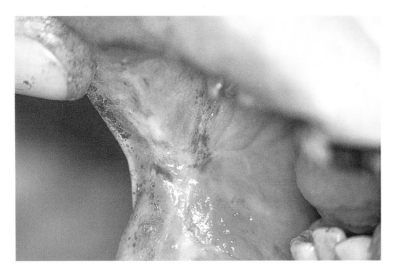

Fig. 34-32   Extensive scars in the right angular and retroangular regions as a consequence of a benign mucosal pemphigoid in a 51-year-old woman.

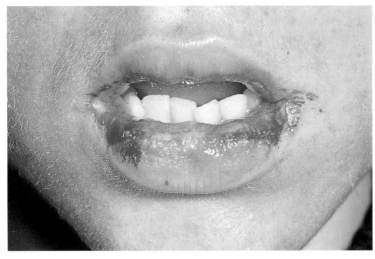

Fig. 34-33   Lip findings in a erythema exudativum multiforme. The oral mucosa and, in particular, the lips are always part of this severe form of erythematous dermatosis. In the corner of the mouth, there is often a delay in the healing of efflorescences.

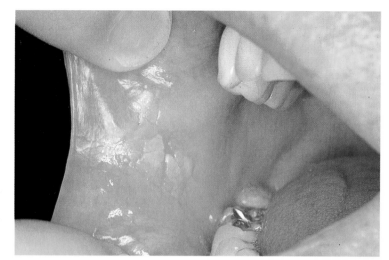

Fig. 34-34 Retroangular simple leukoplakia. The lesion in the distal area is a result of cheek scars associated with bruxism.

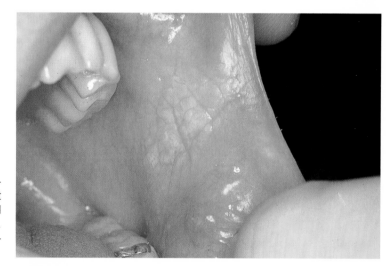

Fig. 34-35 Simple flat-homogeneous leukoplakia of the left retroangular region with typical fields in the patient of Fig. 34-34 at the time of examination.

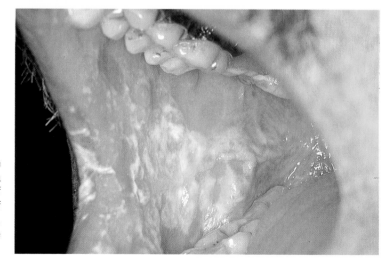

Fig. 34-36 Massive lichen planus of the cheek mucosa extending to the vermilion of the lip. In the posterior third of the cheek within the lesion, there is the impression of the occlusal surface of the teeth.

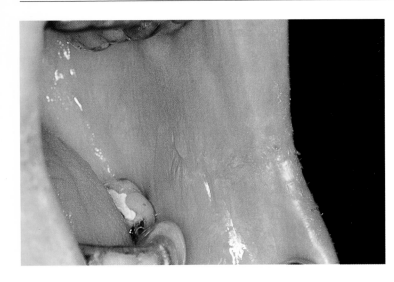

Fig. 34-37   The clinical appearance of a simple homogenous leukoplakia can be altered in the angular and retroangular region by secondary tears. The leukoplakial "rigid" mucosa is prone to formation of fissures during extension stress of the corner of the mouth.

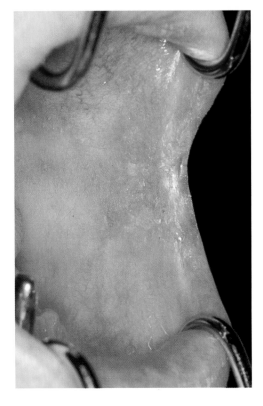

Fig. 34-38   Early clinical stage of a parakeratotic leukoplakia of the erosive type. These findings should not be confused with cheek biting.

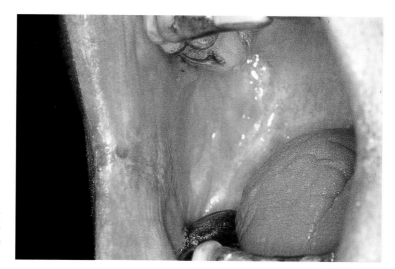

Fig. 34-39   Erosive-type pre-cancerous leukoplakia with participation of the corner of the mouth in a 56-year-old patient.

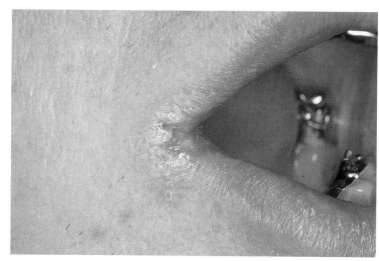

Fig. 34-40   Corner of the mouth fissures that had persisted for 2 years in a 46-year-old patient. They appeared during the process of obtaining a new maxillary prosthesis.

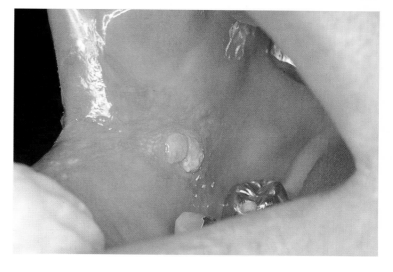

Fig. 34-41   Intraoral findings of the patient of Fig. 34-40 at the same examination. Precancerous leukoplakia reaching to the corner of the mouth with partially erosive, partially ulcerative lesions.

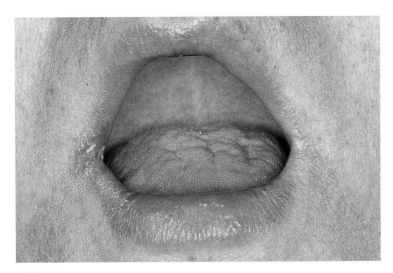

Fig. 34-42 Corner of the mouth changes on the base of a precancerous leukoplakia in a 52-year-old patient. There is an erosive change on the vermilion of the right side of the lip.

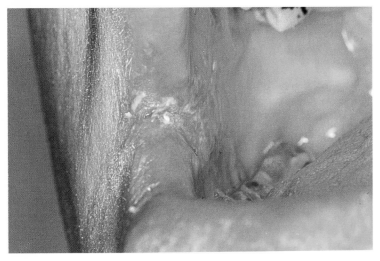

Fig. 34-43 The patient in Fig. 34-42 at the same examination. In the area of the corner of the mouth, there is an inflamed fissured area of precancerous leukoplakia partially covered by *Candida albicans*.

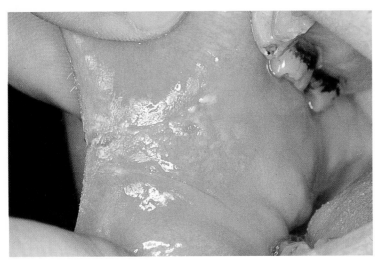

Fig. 34-44 Associated retroangular region of the patient in Figs. 34-42 and 34-43. Distinctly recognizable bumpy surface and interspersed erosive epithelial defects of precancerous leukoplakia. Histologically, there is no evidence of malignant transformation.

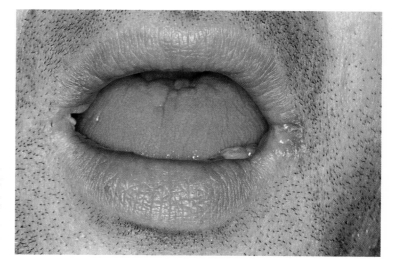

Fig. 34-45   Bilateral precancerous leukoplakia of the cheek mucosa in a 49-year-old patient. Frontal representation of the lip zone with defects of different depth in the area of the lip commissures.

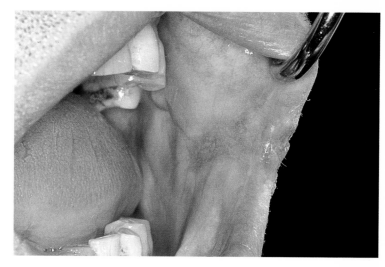

Fig. 34-46   Mucosal findings on the left side of the cheek in the patient in Fig. 34-45 at the same examination: precancerous leukoplakia of the papillary-endophytic type reaching to the corner of the mouth. Histologically there was no evidence of malignant transformation.

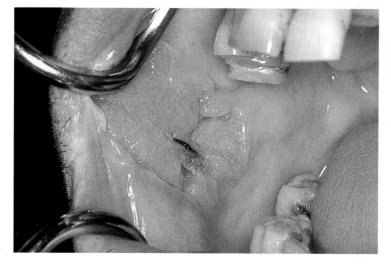

Fig. 34-47   Findings in the mucosa of the right cheek of the patient in Figs. 34-45 and 34-46. There are level tissue defects with a bumpy surface, reaching to the corner of the mouth. Tissue examination revealed an early squamous cell carcinoma arising from a papillary endophytic leukoplakia.

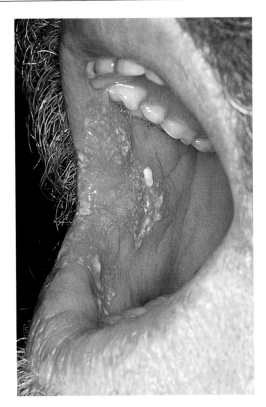

Fig. 34-48   Precancerous leukoplakia with histologically demonstrable carcinoma in situ in the mucosa of the corner of the mouth.

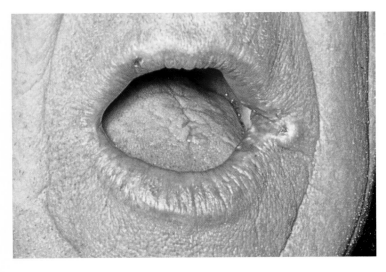

Fig. 34-49   Keratinizing squamous cell carcinoma of the mucosa of the cheek in the area of the left corner of the mouth to the external skin. With only a superficial examination, this finding could be confused with perleche.

Selected Bibliography

I.

Arnold, W. J., Laissue, J. A., Friedmann, I., Naumann, H. H. (Hrsg.): Diseases of the Head and Neck. Thieme, Stuttgart–New York 1987

Barrett, J. T.: Textbook of Immunology. 5. ed., Mosby, St. Louis 1988

Barthels, M., Poliwoda, H.: Gerinnungsanalysen. 3. ed., Thieme, Stuttgart–New York 1987

Becker, R., Morgenroth, K.: Pathologie der Mundhöhle. 2. ed., Thieme, Stuttgart–New York 1986

Begemann, H., Begemann, M.: Praktische Hämatologie. 9. ed., Thieme, Stuttgart–New York 1989

Begemann, H., Rastetter, J. (Hrsg.): Klinische Hämatologie. 3. ed., Thieme, Stuttgart–New York 1986

Bhaskar, S. N.: Synopsis of Oral Pathology. 7. ed., Mosby, St. Louis 1986

Bork, K., Hoede, N., Korting, G. W.: Symptome und Krankheiten der Mundschleimhaut und Perioralregion. Schattauer, Stuttgart–New York 1984

Brandis, H., Pulverer, G. (Hrsg.): Lehrbuch der Medizinischen Mikrobiologie. 6. ed., Fischer, Stuttgart–New York 1988

Braun-Falco, O., Plewig, G., Wolff, H. H.: Dermatologie und Venerologie. 3. ed., Springer, Berlin–Heidelberg–New York–Tokyo 1984

Braunwald, E. et al.: Harrison's Principles of Internal Medicine. 11. ed., McGraw-Hill, New York–Toronto–London 1987

Burkhardt, A., Maerker, R.: Vor- und Frühstadien des Mundhöhlenkarzinoms. Hanser, München 1981

Carl, W., Sako, K.: Cancer and the Oral Cavity. Quintessence Publ., Chicago 1986

Coombs, R. R. A., Gell, P. G. H.: Classification of Allergic Reactions responsible for Clinical Hypersensitivity and Disease. In: Gell, P. G. H., Coombs, R. R. A., Lachmann, P. J. (Hrsg.): Clinical Aspects of Immunology. 3. ed., Blackwell, Oxford–London–Edinburgh–Melbourne 1975

Dolby, A. E. (Hrsg.): Oral Mucosa in Health and Disease. Blackwell, Oxford–London–Edinburgh–Melbourne 1975

Dold, U., Sack, H.: Praktische Tumortherapie. 3. ed., Thieme, Stuttgart–New York 1985

Enzinger, F. M., Weiss, S. W.: Soft Tissue Tumors. 2. ed., Mosby, St. Louis 1988

Fleischer-Peters, S., Scholz, U.: Psychologie und Psychosomatik in der Kieferorthopädie. Hanser, München 1985

Fritsch, P.: Dermatologie. 2. ed., Springer, Berlin–Heidelberg–New York 1988

Gorlin, R. J., Pindborg, J. J.: Syndromes of the Head and Neck. McGraw-Hill, New York–Toronto–London 1964

Greenspan, D., Greenspan, J., Pindborg, J. J., Schiødt, M.: Aids and the Dental Team. Munksgaard, Copenhagen 1986

Haneke, E.: Zungen- und Mundschleimhautbrennen. Hanser, München–Wien 1980

Herrmann, D.: Allergien auf zahnärztliche Werkstoffe. In: Voß, R., Meiners, H. (Hrsg.): Fortschritte der Zahnärztlichen Prothetik und Werkstoffkunde, vol. 4. Hanser, München–Wien 1989

Hölzle, E., Kind, P., Plewig, G.: Pigmentierte Hautveränderungen. Klinik – Histopathologie – Differentialdiagnosen. Schattauer, Stuttgart–New York 1991

Hornstein, O. P. (ed.): Entzündliche und systemische Erkrankungen der Mundschleimhaut. Thieme, Stuttgart 1974

Kaufmann, R., Weber, L., Rodermund, O.-E.: Kutane Melanome. Editiones Roche, Basel 1989

Kayser, F. H., Bienz, K. A., Eckert, J., Lindemann, J.: Medizinische Mikrobiologie. 7. ed., Thieme, Stuttgart–New York 1989

Kirch, W.: Innere Medizin und Zahnheilkunde. Hanser, München–Wien 1986

Knolle, G. (Hrsg.): HLV III-Infektion – Problem für die zahnärztliche Praxis? Quintessenz, Berlin–Chicago–London–São Paulo–Tokio 1986

Krüger, E.: Lehrbuch der chirurgischen Zahn-, Mund- und Kieferheilkunde, vol. 1 und 2. 6. ed., Quintessenz, Berlin–Chicago–London–São Paulo–Tokio 1988

Laskaris, G.: Color Atlas of Oral Diseases. Thieme, Stuttgart–New York 1988

Lennert, K., Feller, A. C.: Histopathologie der Non-Hodgkin-Lymphome (nach der aktualisierten Kiel-Klassifikation). 2. ed., Springer, Berlin–Heidelberg–New York–London–Paris–Tokyo–Hong Kong 1990

Magnusson, B. O. (ed.): Pedodontics–A Systematic Approach. Munksgaard, Copenhagen 1981

Marxkors, R., Müller-Fahlbusch, H.: Psychogene Prothesenunverträglichkeit. Hanser, München–Wien 1976

Mittermayer, Ch.: Oralpathologie. 2. ed., Schattauer, Stuttgart–New York 1984

Mittermayer, Ch., Riede, U. N., Härle, F.: Präkanzerose der Mundhöhle. Hoechst AG, Frankfurt/M. 1980

Mueller-Eckhardt, C. (ed.): Transfusionsmedizin. Springer, Berlin–Heidelberg–New York–Paris–Tokyo–Hong Kong 1988

Müller-Fahlbusch, H., Marxkors, R.: Zahnärztliche Psychagogik. Vom Umgang mit dem Patienten. Hanser, München–Wien 1981

Pape, H. D.: Die Früherkennung der malignen Mundhöhlentumoren unter besonderer Berücksichtigung der exfoliativen Cytologie. Hanser, München 1972

Pindborg, J. J.: Cancer and Precancer. Wright & Sons, Bristol 1980

Pindborg, J. J.: Krebs und Vorkrebs der Mundhöhle. Quintessenz, Berlin–Chicago–Rio de Janeiro–Tokio 1982

Pindborg, J. J.: Atlas of Diseases of the Oral Mucosa. 4. ed., Munksgaard, Copenhagen 1986

Pindborg, J. J.: Atlas der Mundschleimhauterkrankungen. Dtsch Ärzte-Verlag, Köln 1987

Platz, H., Fries, R., Hudec, M.: Prognoses of Oral Cavity Carcinomas. Hanser, München–Wien 1986

Rappaport, H.: Tumors of the Hematopoietic System. In: Atlas of Tumor Pathology III/8. Armed Force Institute of Pathology, Washington D. C. 1966

Rateitschak, K. H., Rateitschak, E. M., Wolf, H. F.: Parodontologie. In: Rateitschak, K. H. (ed.): Farbatlanten der Zahnmedizin, ed., 1. 2. ed., Thieme, Stuttgart–New York 1989

Riede, U. N., Schaefer, H. E., Wehner, H. (ed.): Allgemeine und spezielle Pathologie. 2. ed., Thieme, Stuttgart–New York 1989

Schneider, G. (ed.): Klinische Syndrome der Kiefer-Gesichtsregion. VEB Verlag Volk und Gesundheit, Berlin 1975

Schroeder, H. E.: Orale Strukturbiologie. 3. ed., Thieme, Stuttgart–New York 1987

Schuermann, H., Greither, A., Hornstein, O. P.: Krankheiten der Mundschleimhaut und Lippen. 3. ed., Urban &Schwarzenberg, München–Berlin 1966

Schulze, Ch.: Anomalien und Mißbildungen der menschlichen Zähne. Quintessenz, Berlin–Chicago–London–São Paulo–Tokyo 1987

Schwenzer, N., Grimm, G. (Hrsg.): Zahn-Mund-Kieferheilkunde. ed. 2: Spezielle Chirurgie. 2. ed., Thieme, Stuttgart–New York 1990

Schwenzer, N., Pfeifer, G. (ed.): Fortschritte der Kiefer- und Gesichts-Chirurgie, vol. XXXIII: Mesenchymale Weichteiltumoren und Melanome. Thieme, Stuttgart–New York 1988.

Seifert, G., Burkhardt, A.: Orale Krebsvorstadien. In: Dohm, G. (ed.): Praenoplasien. Fischer, Stuttgart–New York 1980

Seifert, G., Miehlke, A., Haubrich, J., Chilla, R.: Speicheldrüsenkrankheiten. Thieme, Stuttgart–New York 1984

Siegenthaler, W. (ed.): Klinische Pathophysiologie. 6. ed., Thieme, Stuttgart–New York 1987

Thomas, L. (Hrsg.): Labor und Diagnose. 3. ed., Medizinische Verlagsgesellschaft, Marburg 1988

UICC: TNM-Klassifikation maligner Tumoren. Deutsche Übersetzung durch Hermanek, P., Scheibe, O., Spiessl, B., Wagner, G. 4. ed., Springer, Berlin–Heidelberg–New York–London–Paris–Tokyo 1987

van der Waal, I., van der Kwast, W. A. M.: Oralpathologie für Zahnärzte. Quintessenz, Berlin–Chaicago–London–São Paulo–Tokyo 1987

van der Waal, I., Pindborg, J. J.: Diseases of the Tongue. Quintessence Publ., Chicago 1986

Veltmann, G.: Dermatologie für Zahnmediziner. 2. ed., Thieme, Stuttgart–New York 1984

Weiss, L. (ed.): Cell and Tissue Biology. 6. ed., Urban & Schwarzenberg, Baltimore–Munich 1988

World Health Organization: International Classification of Diseases. 9. Revision, WHO, Genf 1977

World Health Organization: Application of the International Classification of Diseases to Dentistry and Stomatology. 2. ed., WHO, Genf 1978

II.

Aul, C., Schneider, W.: Neuere Gesichtspunkte in Pathogenese und Therapie chronischer Leukämien. Kampf dem Krebs, 24, 9 (1988)

Aul, C., Schneider, W.: Aktuelle Therapie: Leukämien und maligne Lymphome. Intern Prax 30, 783 (1990)

Bánóczy, J., Sugár, L.: Longitudinal studies in oral leukoplakias. J Oral Pathol 1, 265 (1972)

Bäurle, G.: Allergie im Arbeitsfeld des Zahnarztes. In: Akademie Praxis und Wissenschaft in der DGZMK (ed.): Umwelt, Arbeitswelt, Gesundheit. Hanser, München–Wien 1988

Beck, L.: Gynäkologische und perinatologische Fragen im Zusammenhang mit der Zahn-, Mund- und Kieferheilkunde. Dtsch Zahnärztl Z 32, 660 (1977)

Beutner, E. H., Jaremko, W. M., Kumar, V. et al.: Stratified epithelium specific antinuclear antibodies (SESANA) in chronic ulcerative stomatitis (Cus): is SESassociated Cus a new clinical entity? J Invest Dermatol 92, 403 (1989)

Bonorden, St. W., Machtens, E.: Maligne Speicheldrüsentumoren. Dtsch Z Mund Kiefer Gesichtschir 11, 361 (1987)

Brüster, H.: Trends, Arbeitshilfen und Automation in der hämatologischen Routinediagnostik. In: Reimerdes, E., Depner, W. (Hrsg.): Analysensysteme und Methoden. 3. ed., Giebeler, Darmstadt 1984

Clark, W. H.: A classification of malignant melanoma in man correlated with histogenesis and biologic behavior. In: Montagna, W., Hu, F. (ed.): Advances in the biology of skin. The pigmentary system. Pergamon Press, Oxford 1967

Clark, W. H., Elder, D. E., van Horn, M.: The biologic forms of malignant melanoma. Hum Pathol 17, 443 (1986)

Erpenstein, H.: Periodontal and prosthetic treatment in patients with oral lichen planus. J Clin Periodontol 12, 104 (1985)

Goerz, G., Lehmann, P., Schuppe, H. C., Lakomek, H. J., Kind, P.: Lupus erythematodes. Z Hautkr 65, 226 (1990)

zur Hausen, H.: The role of viruses in human tumors Adv Cancer Res 33, 77 (1980)

zur Hausen, H.: Viruses as tumor initiators and tumor promotors. Haematol Blood Transfusion 29, 306 (1985)

zur Hausen, H.: Concepts of Carcinogenesis. Interdisciplin Sci Rev 14, 203 (1989)

Heese, A., Peters, K. P., Koch, H. U., Hahn, H., Riedl, B., Hornstein, O. P.: Allergien und Intoleranzreaktionen gegen Latex-Handschuhe im medizinischen Fachbereich. Dtsch Ärztebl 86, 56 (1989)

Helm, E. B.: Das klinische Bild der HIV-Infektion. In: Klietmann, W. (ed.): Aids: Forschung, Klinik, Praxis, soziokulturelle Aspekte. Schattauer, Stuttgart−New York 1990

Herforth, A., Knolle, G., Straßburg, M.: Juvenile Parodontopathien und Hauterkrankungen. Dtsch Zahnärztl Z 28, 242 (1973)

Hornstein, O. P.: Orale Aphthen − örtliche und allgemeinmedizinische Aspekte. Dtsch Zahnärztl Z 34, 808 (1979)

Jablonska, S.: Typisierung von humanen Papillomviren und ihre Bedeutung. In: Macher, E., Knop, J., Bröcker, E. E.: Jahrbuch der Dermatologie, Regensberg & Biermann, Münster 1986

Jaremko, W. M., Beutner, E. H., Kumar, V., Kipping, H., Condry, P., Zeid, M. Y., Kauffman, C. L., Tatakis, D. N., Chorzelski, T. P.: Chronic ulcerative stomatitis associated with a specific immunologic marker. J Am Acad Dermatol 22, 215 (1990)

Kerl, H., Soyer, H. P., Hödl, S., Smolle, J.: Diagnostik dysplastischer Naevi. Dtsch Med Wschr 115, 1104 (1990)

Kind, P., Goerz, G., Straßburg, M.: Naevus spongiosus albus mucosae (Weißer Schwammnaevus). Dtsch Zahnärztl Z 45, 87 (1990)

Knolle, G., Schübel, F., Straßburg, M.: Infarkt an der fixierten Mundschleimhaut. Dtsch Zahnärztebl 23, 57 (1969)

Knolle, G., Schübel, F., Straßburg, M.: Selbstverletzungen an der Mundschleimhaut und ihre differentialdiagnostische Bedeutung. Österr Z Stomatol 68, 303 (1971)

Koch, H.: Blaue Nävi der Mundschleimhaut. Dtsch Zahnärztl Z 25, 1022 (1970)

Kövesi, G., Bánóczy, J.: Follow-up studies in oral lichen planus. Int J Oral Surg 2, 13 (1973)

Kuntz, F., Fehrenbach, J., Reichart, P.: Nekrotisierendulzeröse Gingivitis und progressive Parodontitis bei HIV-Infektion. Dtsch Z Mund Kiefer Gesichtschir 11, 157 (1987)

Löe, H.: Periodontal changes in pregnancy. J Periodontol 36, 209 (1965)

Maerker, R., Burkhardt, A.: Klinik oraler Leukoplakien und Präkanzerosen. Retrospektive Studie an 200 Patienten. Dtsch Z Mund Kiefer Gesichtschir 2, 206 (1978)

Meyle, J., Jenss, H., Scherwitz, C.: Funktionsstörungen neutrophiler Granulozyten bei oralem und intestinalem Morbus Crohn. Dtsch Zahnärztl Z 42, 751 (1987)

Nazzaro, V., Blanchet-Bardon, C., Mimoz, C., Revuz, J., Puissant, A.: Papillon-Lefèvre Syndrome. Arch Dermatol 124, 533 (1988)

Neuhauser, W.: Psychosomatik aus der Sicht des Zahnarztes. In: Ketterl, W. (ed.): Deutscher Zahnärztekalender, Hanser, München−Wien 1990

Orban, B., Sicher, H.: The Oral Mucosa. J Dent Educ 10, 94 (1945) and 10, 163 (1946)

Otto, H. F., Born, I. A., Schwechheimer, K.: Maligne mesenchymale Tumoren der Mundhöhle. In: Schwenzer, N., Pfeifer, G. (ed.): Fortschritte der Kiefer- und Gesichts-Chirurgie, vol. XXXIII: Mesenchymale Weichteiltumoren und Melanome. Thieme, Stuttgart−New York 1988

Radtke, J., Machtens, E.: Lymphome mit oromaxillofazialer Manifestation. Dtsch Z Mund Kiefer Gesichtschir 14, 111 (1990)

Raue, F., Komposch, G., Ziegler, R.: Schleimhautneurome an Lippen und Zunge. Dtsch Zahnärztl Z 41, 1000 (1986)

Rechmann, P., Florack, M.: Fokale epitheliale Hyperplasie (Morbus Heck) der Mundschleimhaut bei einem dreijährigen deutschen Mädchen. Dtsch Zahnärztl Z 43, 379 (1988)

Rechmann, P., Kind, P.: Ein großer Nävuszellnävus der Mundschleimhaut. Dtsch Zahnärztl Z 41, 1136 (1986)

Reinauer, H.: Erhöhte Blutzuckerkonzentration (Hyperglykämie). Internist 31, W 13 (1990)

Scharffetter, K., Kind, P., Wollny-Protzel, D., Schuppe, H. C., Lakomek, H. J., Goerz, G.: Die Sklerodermien. Z Hautkr 65, 237 (1990)

Schettler, D., Koberg, W.: Zur malignen Entartung des LIchen ruber planus (Bericht über 5 eigene Fälle). Dtsch Zahnärztl Z 25, 991 (1970)

Scheunemann, H.: Zur Früherkennung und Therapie des Mundhöhlenkarzinoms. In: *Ketterl, W.* (ed.): Deutscher Zahnärztekalender, Hanser, München–Wien 1991

Schirner, E., Hornstein, O. P., Simon, M.: Ätiologie und Prognose des Lichen planus oralis–Vorläufige Ergebnisse einer kontrollierten prospektiven Studie. Dtsch Zahnärztl Z 36, 130 (1981)

Schröder, H.: Diagnostische und therapeutische Probleme der generalisierten akuten eitrigen Parodontitis marginalis profunda. Dtsch Zahnärztl Z 34, 506 (1979)

Seifert, G., Burkhardt, A.: Vor- und Frühstadien des Mundhöhlenkrebses. Dtsch Ärztebl 78, 327 (1981)

Seifert, G., Rieb, H., Donath, K.: Klassifikation der Tubmoren der kleinen Speicheldrüsen. Pathohistologische Analyse von 160 Tumoren. Laryngol Rhinol Otol 59, 379 (1980)

Straßburg, M.: Zur oralen Manifestation allgemeiner Erkrankungen aus zahnärztlicher Sicht. Dtsch Zahnärztl Z 32, 648 (1977)

Straßburg, M., Knolle, G.: Symptom: Mond-Winkelveränderungen. Münch Med Wochenschr 120, 1653 (1978)

Straßburg, M., Knolle, G.: Welchen Aussagewert haben Mundhöhlensymptome für die Diagnose von Allgemeinerkrankungen? In: *Ketterl, W.* (ed.): Deutscher Zahnärztekalender, Hanser, München–Wien 1981

Topoll, H. H.: Therapie der desquamativen Gingivitis. Zahnärztl Mitt 78, 1621 (1988)

Wessels, M.: Beitrag zur Diagnose und Therapie des Granuloma gangraenescens. Med. Diss. Univ. Mainz 1980

Williams, R. C.: Periodontal Disease, N Engl J Med 322, 373 (1990)

World Health Organization: Cancer Unit: Definition of leukoplakia and related lesions: an aid to studies on oral precancer. Oral Surg 46, 518 (1978)

Picture Sources

Besides the colleagues of our clinic already mentioned in the Introduction (Prof. Dr. Armin Herforth, Prof. Dr. Franz Schübel, and Prof. Dr. Walter Weise), the following ladies and gentlemen (in alphabetical order) offered slides and, in this manner, participated in the completion of the picture materials, for which we thank them:

Priv.-Doz. Dr. Gabriele Bäurle, Erlangen (Figs. 31.36, 31.37),

Professor Dr. Dr. Rüdiger Becker, Münster (Figs. 8.3, 30.20, 31.11),

Dr. Dr. Ummo Francksen, Oldenburg (Figs. 25.16),

Professor Dr. Dr. Gerhard Frenkel, Frankfurt/Main (Figs. 11.54, 11.59 to 11.61, 11.63 to 11.69, 11.71),

Professor Dr. Dr. Claus-Udo Fritzemeier, Düsseldorf (Figs. 31.39),

Professor Dr. Günter Goerz, Düsseldorf (Figs. 30.1 to 30.3, 30.5, 30.11),

Professor Dr. Gustav-Adolf von Harnack, Düsseldorf (Figs. 7.7, 7.8, 11.42, 11.43),

Professor Dr. Jo Hartung, Hannover (Figs. 4.10, 4.14),

Professor Dr. Dr. Wolfgang Hoppe, Lübeck (Figs. 4.21),

Professor Dr. Otto Hornstein, Erlangen (Figs. 7.4, 22.64, 30.4),

Professor Dr. Helmut Ippen, Göttingen, at that time Düsseldorf, with Dr. Richter, Düsseldorf (Figs. 11.1 to 11.4)

Priv.-Doz. Dr. Roland Kaufmann, Ulm (Figs. 16.1, 19.60 to 19.62, 21.13),

Professor Dr. Jürgen Knolle, Flensburg (Figs. 26.20, 26.22, 30.13, 30.14),

Professor Dr. Gerda Komposch, Heidelberg (Figs. 5.5, 5.6, 33.7, 33.8, 33.11),

Professor Dr. Dr. Eberhard Krüger, Bonn (Figs. 3.12, 23.12),

Professor Dr. E. Landes, Darmstadt (Figs. 8.2),

Dr. Jan Laturnus, Düsseldorf (Figs. 4.38 to 4.40),

Professor Dr. Gerd Plewig, Düsseldorf (Figs. 12.15, 26.19, 29.1, 29.6 to 29.9, 29.13),

Professor Dr. Friedhelm Raue, Heidelberg (Figs. 3.26 to 3.28),

Professor Dr. Dr. Horst Scheunemann, Mainz (Figs. 23.10, 23.11, 23.17, 23.18, 30.18, 30.19),

Professor Dr. Albert Schimpf, Homburg/Saar (Figs. 8.6, 10.16, 12.16, 12.17, 29.17, 29.18),

Dr. Ulf Utech, Frankfurt/Main (Figs. 31.40).

Some no-longer identifiable slides come from the collection of Prof. Dr. Dr. Ulrich Rheinwald, Stuttgart, as well as the collection of Prof. Dr. Dr. Aloys Greither (deceased) and Dr. Dr. Alfred Rehrmann, both from Düsseldorf.

Kind permission from Carl Hanser Verlag allowed reproduction of published color photographs of a collection (Straßburg) from the *Dtsch Zahnärztl Z* (1977; 32: 650, 651 and 1990; 45: 87). For Fig. 4.22, permission for reproduction was secured from the Institute for Labor and Social Medicine of the University of Erlangen–Nurenberg.

We used some of the color pictures from the *Lehrbuch der chirurgischen Zahn-, Mund- und Kieferheilkunde* from Prof. Dr. Dr. Eberhard Krüger, Bonn, published by Quintessenz Verlag with kind permission from author and publisher. The same is true for the pictures of the contribution of Prof. Dr. Dr. Gerhard Frenkel, "Klinischer Verlauf der HTLV III-Infektion (Lymphadenopathie-Syndrom und AIDS)–Manifestation in der Mundhöhle und Mundumgebung" in the book by G. Knolle (ed) *HTLV III-Infektion–Problem für die zahnärztliche Praxis?*, which appeared by the same publisher. In these cases, the source is indicated in the legends.

Index